Geriatric Trauma and Critical Care

Jay A. Yelon • Fred A. Luchette
Editors

Geriatric Trauma and Critical Care

Springer

Editors
Jay A. Yelon
Department of Surgery
Lincoln Medical Center
Bronx, NY
USA

Fred A. Luchette
Department of Surgery
Stritch School of Medicine
Loyola University Medical Center
Maywood, IL
USA

Vice-Chair VA Affairs
Chief of Surgical Services
Hines, VA
USA

ISBN 978-1-4614-8500-1 ISBN 978-1-4614-8501-8 (eBook)
DOI 10.1007/978-1-4614-8501-8
Springer New York Heidelberg Dordrecht London

Library of Congress Control Number: 2013956123

Printed on acid-free paper

Springer is part of Springer Science+Business Media (www.springer.com)

Foreword

The new and well-written textbook, *Geriatric Trauma and Critical Care* (edited by Jay Yelon and Fred Luchette), is a timely and necessary addition to our current body of knowledge on this topic. The existing medical landscape in the United States includes a population of 315 million people, 793,648 physicians, and over 6,000 hospitals for acute care and elective management. With the overall population expanding by 25 million each decade, along with a projected steady increase of Americans over 65 years of age, a crisis is developing with respect to optimal healthcare for this very vulnerable and special population – the elderly.

Considering increased comorbidities and distinctly different physiologic responses/reserves, the geriatric patients will continue to present an array of challenges for all aspects of healthcare management. The highly accomplished specialists who have contributed to this excellent textbook are to be commended for providing the reader with the physiological basis for assessment and principles of management for this cohort of patients. The section and chapter formats are well presented, with each organ-based topic being complete and comprehensive. I, particularly, applaud the editors for including a separate section on the Impact of Aging on Health.

Undoubtedly, this textbook will be recognized as a definitive work in the field for years to come.

Norfolk, VA, USA L.D. Britt, MD, MPH, FACS

Contents

Contributors

Charles A. Adams Jr., MD, FACS, FCCM Department of Surgery, Alpert Medical School of Brown University, Rhode Island Hospital, Providence, RI, USA

Sasha D. Adams, MD, FACS Division of Acute Care Surgery, Department of Surgery, University of North Carolina, Chapel Hill, NC, USA

Aman Banerjee, MD Department of Surgery, MetroHealth Medical Center, Cleveland, OH, USA

Robert D. Barraco, MD, MPH, FACS, FCCP Department of Surgery, Lehigh Valley Health Network, Allentown, PA, USA

Matthew V. Benns, MD Department of Surgery, University of Louisville, Louisville, KY, USA

Karen J. Brasel, MD, MPH Department of Surgery, Medical College of Wisconsin, Milwaukee, WI, USA

L.D. Britt, MD, MPH, FACS Department of Surgery, Eastern Virginia Medical School, Norfolk, VA, USA

Marko Bukur, MD, FACS Department of Surgery, Cedars-Sinai Medical Center, Los Angeles, CA, USA

Eileen M. Bulger, MD Department of Surgery, Harborview Medical Center, University of Washington, Seattle, WA, USA

Charles Cassidy, MD Department of Orthopaedic Surgery, Tufts Medical Center, Boston, MA, USA

Michael C. Chang, MD Department of General Surgery, Wake Forest University Baptist Medical Center, Winston-Salem, NC, USA

William G. Cioffi, MD Department of Surgery, Rhode Island Hospital, Providence, RI, USA

Jeffrey A. Claridge, MD, MS, FACS Division of Trauma, Department of Surgery, Critical Care, Burns, and Acute Care Surgery, MetroHealth Medical Center, Cleveland, OH, USA

Northern Ohio Trauma System, Cleveland, OH, USA

Department of Surgery, Case Western Reserve University School of Medicine, Cleveland, OH, USA

Department of Surgery, MetroHealth Medical Center, Cleveland, OH, USA

Raul Coimbra, MD, PhD, FACS Division of Trauma, Surgical Critical Care, and Burns, Department of Surgery, University of California, San Diego Health Sciences, San Diego, CA, USA

Zara R. Cooper, MD, FACS, MSc Department of Surgery, Brigham and Women's Hospital, Boston, MA, USA

Trauma, Burn, & Surgical Critical Care, Brigham and Women's Hospital, Boston, MA, USA

Edward E. Cornwell III, MD, FACS, FCCM Department of Surgery, Howard University Hospital, Howard University College of Medicine, Washington, DC, USA

Todd W. Costantini, MD Division of Trauma, Surgical Critical Care, and Burns, Department of Surgery, University of California, San Diego Health Sciences, San Diego, CA, USA

Chasen A. Croft, MD Department of Surgery, Shands at the University of Florida, Gainesville, FL, USA

Kimberly A. Davis, MD, MBA Department of Surgery, Section of Trauma, Surgical Critical Care and Surgical Emergencies, Yale School of Medicine, New Haven, CT, USA

Marissa De Freese (Delgado), MD Department of Surgery, Stamford Hospital, Stamford, CT, USA

Thomas G. DeLoughery, MD Department of Medicine, Oregon Health and Science University, Portland, OR, USA

Demetrios Demetriades, MD, PhD Department of Surgery, Los Angeles County & University of Southern California Medical Center, Los Angeles, CA, USA

Michael F. Ditillo, DO Department of Surgery, Section of Trauma, Surgical Critical Care and Surgical Emergencies, Yale School of Medicine, New Haven, CT, USA

Samir M. Fakhry, MD, FACS Department of Surgery, Medical University of South Carolina, Charleston, SC, USA

William F. Fallon Jr., MD, MBA, FACS Department of Surgery, VA New Jersey Healthcare System, East Orange, NJ, USA

Jason P. Farrah, MD Department of General Surgery, Wake Forest School of Medicine, Winston-Salem, NC, USA

Peter E. Fischer, MD, MS Department of Surgery, Carolinas Medical Center, Charlotte, NC, USA

Joshua Gish, MD Department of Surgery, Lehigh Valley Health Network, Allentown, PA, USA

Stephanie R. Goldberg, MD Department of Surgery, Virginia Commonwealth University, Richmond, VA, USA

Stephanie Gordy, MD, FACS Department of Surgery, Trauma, Emergency General Surgery and Surgical Critical Care, Oregon Health and Science University, Portland, OR, USA

Vincente H. Gracias, MD Department of Surgery, Rutgers-Robert Wood Johnson Medical School, New Brunswick, NJ, USA

Wendy R. Greene, MD, FACS Department of Surgery, Howard University Hospital, Howard University College of Medicine, Washington, DC, USA

David G. Greenhalgh, MD, FACS Department of Surgery, University of California, Davis Medical Center, Shriners Hospital for Children Northern California, Sacramento, CA, USA

David T. Harrington, MD, FACS Department of Surgery, Rhode Island Hospital, Providence, RI, USA

Sharon M. Henry, MD Department of Surgery, Program in Trauma, R. Adams Cowley Shock Trauma Center, University of Maryland School of Medicine, Baltimore, MD, USA

Kenji Inaba, MD, FACS, FRCSC Division of Trauma and Critical Care, University of Southern California Medical Center, Los Angeles, CA, USA

Sudha P. Jayaraman, MD, MSc Department of Surgery, Brigham and Women's Hospital, Boston, MA, USA

Diana J. Jho Department of Neurosurgery, Allegheny General Hospital, Pittsburgh, PA, USA

Dirk C. Johnson, MD Department of Surgery, Yale New Haven Hospital, Yale University School of Medicine, New Haven, CT, USA

Ronald M. Jou, MD Department of Surgery, Stanford Hospital and Clinic, Stanford, CA, USA

Lewis J. Kaplan, MD, FACS, FCCM, FCCP Department of Surgery, Section of Trauma, Surgical Critical Care and Surgical Emergencies, Yale University School of Medicine, New Haven, CT, USA

Olivia Kates, MD Department of Orthopaedic Surgery, Tufts Medical Center, Boston, MA, USA

Leslie M. Kobayashi, MD Division of Trauma, Surgical Critical Care, and Burns, Department of Surgery, University of California, San Diego Health Sciences, San Diego, CA, USA

Nicole J. Krumrei, MD Division of Traumatology, Surgical Critical Care and Emergency Surgery, Department of Surgery, Perelman School of Medicine, University of Pennsylvania, Philadelphia, PA, USA

Department of Surgery, University of Pennsylvania Medical Center, Philadelphia, PA, USA

Anastasia Kunac, MD Division of Trauma, Department of Surgery, Rutgers – New Jersey Medical School, Newark, NJ, USA

Ryan A. Lawless, MD Department of General Surgery, Lehigh Valley Health Network, Allentown, PA, USA

Fred A. Luchette, MD, MSc Department of Surgery, Stritch School of Medicine, Loyola University Medical Center, Maywood, IL, USA

Vice-Chair VA Affairs, Chief of Surgical Services, Hines, VA, USA

Ajai K. Malholtra, MDDNB, FRCS, FACS Department of Surgery, VCU Medical Center, Richmond, VA, USA

Gary T. Marshall, MD Department of Surgery, University of Pittsburgh Medical Center, Pittsburgh, PA, USA

Department of Surgery, New York University, New York, NY, USA

R. Shayn Martin, MD Department of Surgery, Wake Forest School of Medicine, Winston-Salem, NC, USA

Cathy A. Maxwell, RN, PhD Vanderbilt University School of Nursing, Nashville, TN, USA

Nicolas Melo, MD, MS Department of Surgery, Cedars-Sinai Hospital, Los Angeles, CA, USA

Jay Menaker, MD, FACEP Division of Trauma/Surgical Critical Care, Department of Surgery, University of Maryland School of Medicine, R Adams Cowley Shock Trauma Center, Baltimore, MD, USA

James T. Miller, PharmD Department of Pharmacy Science, University of Michigan Health System, Ann Arbor, MI, USA

Frederick Moore, MD, FACS Department of Surgery, University of Florida, Gainesville, FL, USA

Anne C. Mosenthal, MD, FACS Department of Surgery, Rutgers – New Jersey Medical School, Newark, NJ, USA

Lena M. Napolitano, MD, FACS, FCCP, FCCM Department of Surgery, University of Michigan Health System, Ann Arbor, MI, USA

Robert K. Parker, MD Department of Surgery, Rhode Island Hospital, Providence, RI, USA

Michael D. Pasquale, MD Department of Surgery, Lehigh Valley Health Network, Allentown, PA, USA

Andrew B. Peitzman, MD Department of Surgery, University of Pittsburgh Medical Center, Pittsburgh, PA, USA

Erin L. Rader, RN, MSN, BSN Department of Geriatrics, MetroHealth Medical Center, Cleveland, OH, USA

Patrick M. Reilly, MD, FACS Division of Traumatology, Surgical Critical Care and Emergency Surgery, Department of Surgery, Perelman School of Medicine, University of Pennsylvania, Philadelphia, PA, USA

Department of Surgery, Hospital of the University of Pennsylvania, Philadelphia, PA, USA

Preston B. Rich, MD, MBA, FACS Division of Acute Care Surgery, Department of Surgery, University of North Carolina at Chapel Hill, Chapel Hill, NC, USA

J. David Richardson, MD Department of Surgery, University of Louisville, Louisville, KY, USA

Scott P. Ryan, MD Department of Orthopaedic Surgery, Tufts Medical Center, Boston, MA, USA

Ali Salim, MD, FACS Department of Surgery, Cedars-Sinai Medical Center, Los Angeles, CA, USA

Thomas M. Scalea, MD, FACS Department of Surgery, Division of Trauma/Surgical Critical Care, University of Maryland School of Medicine, R Adams Cowley Shock Trauma Center, Baltimore, MD, USA

Martin A. Schreiber, MD, FACS Department of Surgery, Oregon Health and Science University, Portland, OR, USA

Michael J. Sise, MD, FACS Trauma Service, Scripps Mercy Hospital, San Diego, CA, USA

David Spain, MD Department of Surgery, Stanford University Medical Center, Stanford, CA, USA

Andrew H. Stephen, MD Division of Trauma and Surgical Critical Care, Warren Alpert Medical School at Brown University, Rhode Island Hospital, Providence, RI, USA

Samantha L. Tarras, MD Department of Surgery, Wayne State University/Detroit Medical Center, Detroit, MI, USA

Donald Trunkey, MD, FACS Department of Surgery, Oregon Health Sciences University, Portland, OR, USA

Nancey Trevanian Tsai, MD Department of Neurosurgery, Medical University of South Carolina, Charleston, SC, USA

George Velmahos, MD, PhD Division of Trauma, Emergency Surgery, and Surgical Critical Care, Massachusetts General Hospital, Boston, MA, USA

Wendy L. Wahl, MD Department of Surgery, Saint Joseph Mercy Ann Arbor, Ann Arbor, MI, USA

Travis P. Webb, MD, MHPE Trauma & Critical Care Surgery, Froedtert Memorial Lutheran Hospital, Medical College of Wisconsin, Milwaukee, WI, USA

Jack Wilberger, MD, FAANS, FACS Department of Neurosurgery, Allegheny General Hospital, Pittsburgh, PA, USA

Anne M. Yawman, MD Department of Geriatric Medicine, Lehigh Valley Hospital Network, Allentown, PA, USA

D. Dante Yeh, MD Department of Surgery, Massachusetts General Hospital, Boston, MA, USA

Jay A. Yelon, DO, FACS, FCCM Department of Surgery, Lincoln Medical Center, Bronx, NY, USA

Syed Nabeel Zafar, MD, MPH Department of Surgery, Howard University Hospital, Howard University College of Medicine, Washington, DC, USA

Part I

Impact of Aging on Health

Changing Demographics of the American Population

1

Stephanie Gordy and Donald Trunkey

Introduction

Geriatric citizens in the United States are the most rapidly growing segment due to the aging baby boomer generation. This generation will live longer than the preceding and will have access to improved health care. Because these physically active elderly will remain living independently and longer, traumatic injuries can be expected to increase. In addition, there are numerous physiologic alterations that occur with aging, and special consideration should be given to the elderly patient from a medical and surgical standpoint. Multiple comorbidities may also be present in this population lending to higher complications, longer hospital stays, and a higher case fatality rate. Moreover, disposition barriers often exist and include the need for short- and long-term rehabilitation. Finally, traumatic injuries have the ability to change the patient's independent living status and increase the need for admission to skilled nursing facilities. Complex end-of-life decisions and discussions are often also required in this population. Trauma and acute care surgeons should be knowledgeable about the specific needs of the geriatric critically ill patient.

The Aging Population

The definition of elderly has not been definitively established in the trauma literature, but the consensus is that it lies somewhere between the ages of 45 and 75 years [1]. In 2010, the population over 65 years of age was 40.4 million. This represented 13.1 % of the American population at that time. As the "baby boomer" generation reaches the golden years, this demographic is expected to show continued growth. The 15.3 % increase from 2000 to 2010 in the over 65 portion of the population was nearly double the increase (8.7 %) for all ages younger than 65. It is projected that by 2020 this number will increase by 36 % to 55 million. In 2010, the 65–74 age category was ten times larger than in 1900 at 20.8 million. In contrast, the 75–84 demographic was 17 times larger at 13.1 million. Moreover, the >85 group was 45 times larger at 5.5 million. This reveals that the elderly population itself is getting increasingly older even within itself. By 2020, the >85 population is projected to increase from 5.5 million in 2010 to 6.6 million. Furthermore, the centenarian (greater than 100) population is steadily increasing. In 2010, 53,364 persons were 100 years old or greater which is greater than a 50 % increase from the 1990 values [2].

Since 1900, improvements and accessibility to healthcare services in addition to improved life expectancy have allowed the number of individuals over 65 years to more than triple. This is not only due to the post-World War II baby boom but to an increased life expectancy as well. A child born in 2009 can expect to live 78.2 years which is 30 years longer than the life expectancy of a child born in 1900. The older population will continue to increase due to maturation of the baby boomer generation (Fig. 1.1). While the population growth slowed in the Great Depression era, it will continue on the upswing as those born between 1946 and 1964 get older. The elderly population will have reached its peak by the year 2030 as the >65 population is expected to be 19.3 % of the entire population. As this population increases, the number of injured elderly is also likely to grow [1].

The Cost of Caring for the Elderly

As the elderly population increases, the need for healthcare services and the cost of health care are expected to grow. The elderly represented 40 % of all hospitalized adults in 2008 [3].

S. Gordy, MD, FACS
Department of Surgery, Trauma, Emergency General Surgery and Surgical Critical Care, Oregon Health and Science University, 3181 SW Sam Jackson Park Road, Mail Code L611, Portland, OR 97239, USA
e-mail: gordys@ohsu.edu

D. Trunkey, MD, FACS (✉)
Department of Surgery, Oregon Health Sciences University, 3181 SW Sam Jackson Park Road, L223, Portland, OR 97239, USA
e-mail: trunkeyd@ohsu.edu

J.A. Yelon, F.A. Luchette (eds.), *Geriatric Trauma and Critical Care*,
DOI 10.1007/978-1-4614-8501-8_1,

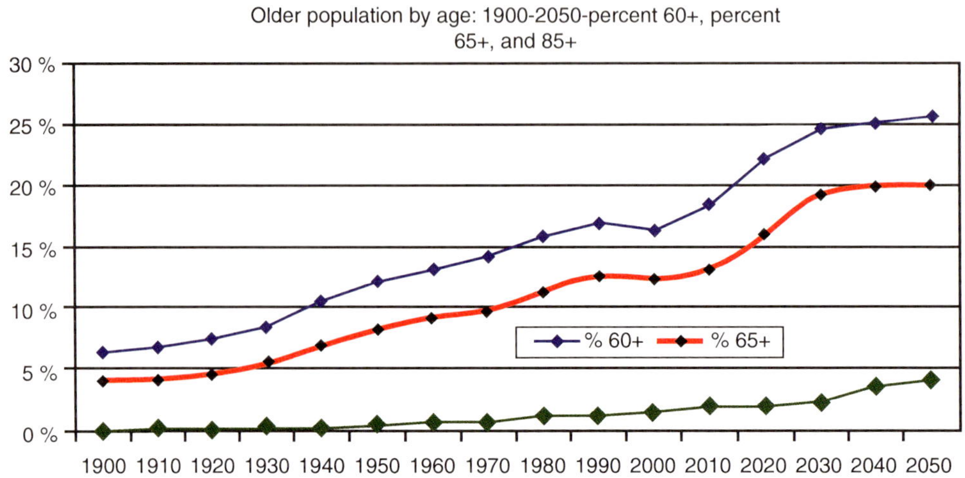

Fig. 1.1 The administration on aging

Similarly, even though this population comprises only 13 % of the population of the United States, nearly half of all healthcare dollars spent are on the elderly. Additionally, the population over 85 years of age represents only 1.8 % of the total population but accounts for 8 % of all hospital discharges. Hospitalizations and healthcare spending for older adults are expected to rise as the geriatric population grows [4].

More healthcare resources will be necessary to care for the aging population which will pose an additional burden on an already-strained system. This cost will not only be reflected in dollars but in resource utilization including acute and long-term care. In 2002, the elderly made up 13 % of the US population, but they consumed 36 % of the total US personal healthcare expenses. The average healthcare expense in 2002 was $11,089/year for elderly people but only $3,352/year for those younger than 65 years [5]. Furthermore, older Americans spend 13.2 % of their total expenditures on health, more than twice the proportion spent by the younger citizens (6.6 %) [2]. The five most expensive illnesses include heart disease, cancer, trauma, mental disorders, and pulmonary conditions. Heart disease and trauma ranked first and second as the two costliest diseases in terms of total healthcare spending [6].

Thirty percent of total Medicare payments each year are for 6 % of the beneficiaries who died that year. Payments for the last 60 days of life constitute 52 % of the total dollars spent annually by Medicare. Inpatient services consume 70.3 % of the Medicare budget of which the majority of the funds are spent on critical care [7]. In summary, the sickest, eldest patients with a high incidence of morbidity and mortality consume the majority of the Medicare budget [8].

Effects of Aging on Organ Function

Understanding the medical physiology pertinent to this population is particularly important, because it affects the physiologic reserve and compensatory mechanisms required to respond to a traumatic injury, an acute illness, and major operations. The elderly population has a high incidence of comorbidities which can confound the physicians' ability to assess for injury. In injured geriatric patients, the incidence of preexisting medical conditions is 66 %. Moreover, 81 % of nonagenarians have medical comorbidities [9]. Nearly every organ system is affected by changes due to aging. A detailed discussion of this is beyond the scope of this chapter, but a brief synopsis follows.

Traumatic brain injury (TBI) has a bimodal age distribution, with the first peak at 15–19 years and the second appearing in those over 65 years of age. The most common cause of TBI in older patients is falling from standing. Despite this low-energy mechanism, the brain is more susceptible to injury due to the progressive volume loss and atrophy that results in space for shear injury [10]. Elderly patients with traumatic brain injuries have worse outcomes when compared to similar injuries in the young [11]. Cardiovascular changes that occur in this population include arterial atherosclerosis which can lead to an elevation in baseline SVR. Disruption in coronary autoregulation from scarring can result in ischemia. The typical tachycardia in response to hypovolemia may also be blunted in these patients due to medications. The increase in SVR may produce a falsely elevated blood pressure. If these patients are chronically hypertensive, a normal SBP may be relatively hypotensive for an individual patient and may result in end-organ ischemia [12]. The effect of age on the pulmonary system is impaired gas exchange due to a reduced alveolar surface area [13]. Chest wall compliance is decreased and may result in a blunted cough reflex leading to increased risk for aspiration [14]. There is also a risk for renal failure following trauma. The renal tubular function declines with increasing age as indicated by a decrease in the glomerular filtration rate (GFR). Chronic diuretic use may predispose to electrolyte abnormalities and a contracted plasma volume. The collecting tubules may not concentrate or retain

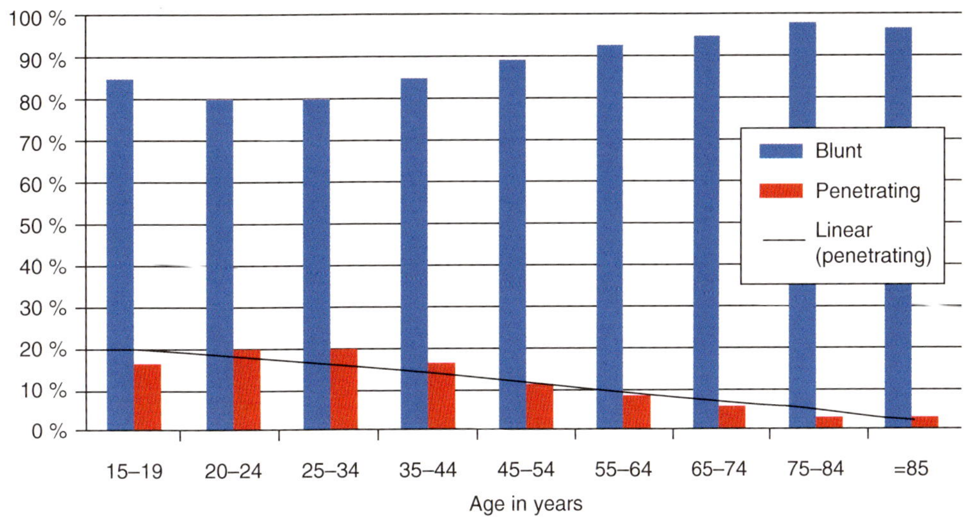

Fig. 1.2 Mechanism of injury (Adams et al. [1])

appropriate electrolytes and is at risk for acute kidney injury/failure due to medications and/or ischemia [15]. Changes in the gastrointestinal system result in increased reflux disease and dysphagia resulting in a higher risk for aspiration in the elderly. Aging causes a slower transit time and colonic disturbances ranging from constipation to diarrhea. The musculoskeletal system is also affected. Lean body mass decreases at a rate of 10 % per decade after the age of 50. The reduction in the number and size of myocytes results in progressive weakness with increasing age. This loss of muscle mass combined with osteoporosis leads to an increase risk of fall-related fractures. Hip fractures are a common injury in the elderly and result in an eightfold increase in all-cause mortality within 3 months after the fall [16]. The endocrine and immune systems are also affected by aging. Extensive hormonal changes occur and thermoregulation may be impaired. Elderly patients are also more susceptible to infections and concomitantly are less able to mount a normal immune response. Moreover, malnutrition is common in the elderly requiring nutritional supplementation to prevent profound catabolism [17]. In summary, every organ system is affected by aging and predisposed to injury, infection, and disability. Medications for preexisting illnesses may also complicate the physiologic response to injury and resuscitation. It is paramount to take these changes into consideration when caring for a geriatric trauma patient.

The functional decline that occurs with aging can lead to an increase in traumatic injuries due to changes in the ability to do activities of daily living (ADLs). ADLs include bathing, dressing, eating, and mobilization. They are important in assessing an individual's ability to function independently. In noninstitutionalized Medicare recipients, 27 % had difficulty in performing one or more ADLs. The ability to conduct ADLs is worse for institutionalized recipients, and 95 % reported difficulties with one or more activity. Additionally, 74 % of those surveyed had difficulty with three or more activities. Limitations in ADLs related to chronic conditions increase with age and can predispose to traumatic injuries [2]. An increase in the frequency of ground level falls in this group can reflect a decline in the ability to perform daily activities. This decline in their ability to perform ADLs suggests that the elderly may become more prone to injuries with advancing age.

Trauma in the Elderly

Trauma is the fifth most common cause of death in the elderly. The mechanism of injury in this demographic is primarily blunt forces, and falls are the most common mechanism of injury in this group (Figs 1.2 and 1.3) [1]. The increase in life expectancy and independent living will lead to an increase in elderly drivers. It is estimated that between 20 and 30 million licensed drivers are currently older than 65 [18]. This number is projected to increase to 50 million by 2030. This explosion in geriatric drivers will be associated with an increase in motor vehicle collisions and/or pedestrians struck and result in an increase in the mortality rate.

The geriatric trauma population poses a special challenge to the trauma team. The mechanism of injury is different than those seen in younger patients. Several studies have reported an age-related increase in mortality rates for all injury mechanisms and ISS scores (see Fig. 1.4) [19–21].

Multiple mechanisms that result in trauma exist in the elderly population. Of those patients that fall, it is usually a repeated occurrence and 71 % of falls result in an injury requiring medical care [22]. Additional mechanisms of blunt trauma include motor vehicle collisions, pedestrians struck, and burn injuries. According to the NTDB, <5 % of deaths are due to penetrating injuries in this age group [23]. Elderly patients who sustain blunt chest trauma with rib fractures

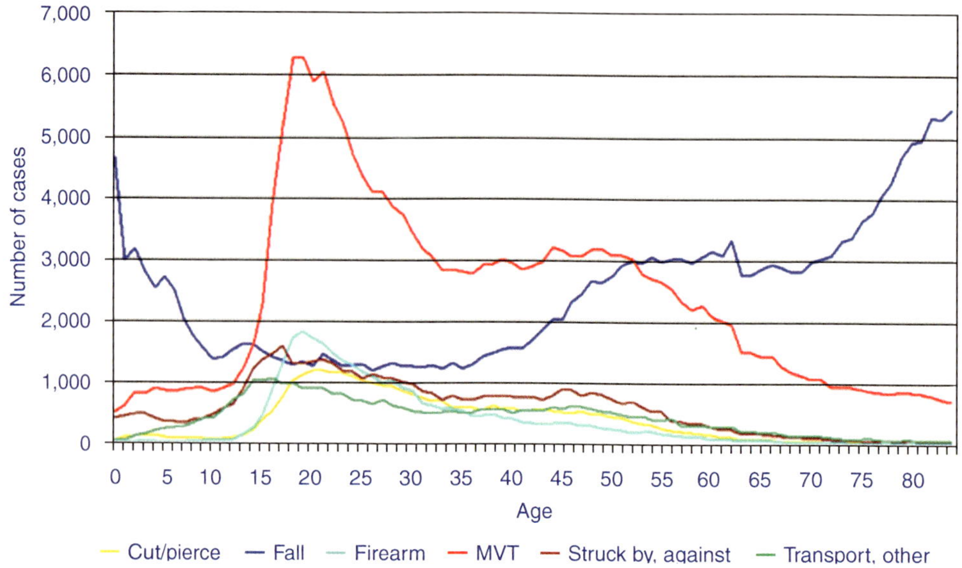

Fig. 1.3 Selected mechanisms of injury by age (NTDB® Annual Report 2010)

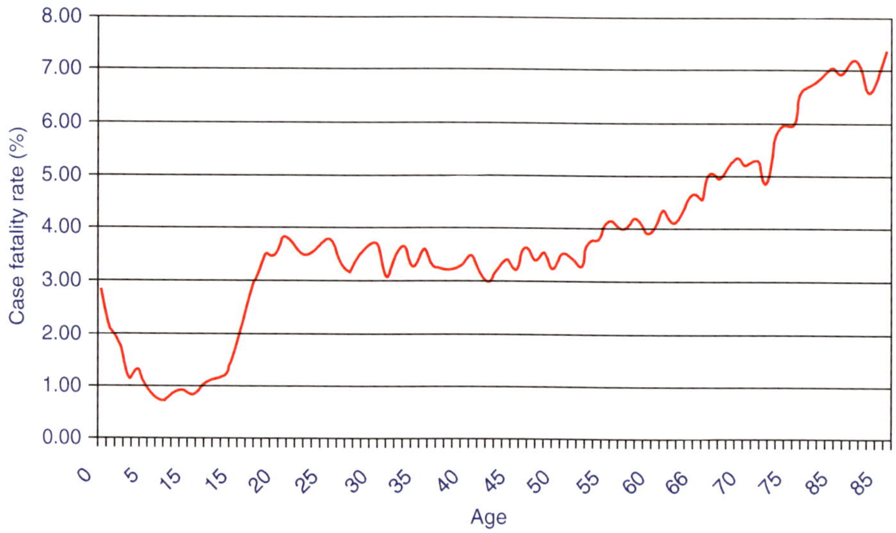

Fig. 1.4 Case fatality rate by age (NTDB® Annual Report 2010)

have a morbidity and mortality rate twice that compared to those younger than 65. For each additional rib fracture in the elderly, mortality increases by 19 % and the risk of pneumonia by 27 % [24]. Moreover, when considering rib fracture injuries, "elderly" has been shown to be as young as 45 and older [25]. Clinical pathways that aggressively treat the pain and attempt to prevent the respiratory complications have shown to be successful [21].

Once an elderly person is injured, the trauma system is not reliable in identifying those that are severely injured. This is primarily a difficulty in triage of these patients. Demetriades et al. found that 63 % of elderly patients that were severely injured (ISS >15) and 25 % of those critically injured did not meet the trauma center's standard trauma activation criteria. They concluded that patients older than 70 years should be considered for trauma team activation based on age alone [26, 27]. The EAST guidelines recommend that geriatric patients should be triaged to a trauma center, but do not use age as an impetus to activate the trauma team [28]. The state of Ohio has implemented a specific geriatric triage based on age [29]. Furthermore, once the elderly are in the emergency department, they may not be easily identified as in shock. Physiologic changes that occur in the elderly may alter the typical physiologic signs and manifestations of shock. Scalea et al. studied patients older than 65 involved in motor vehicle collisions and found their physiology allowed them to present with a higher than expected systolic blood pressure (SBP) due to an elevated systemic vascular resistance (SVR). Of those initially deemed stable with a normal SBP at presentation, 43%were found to actually be in cardiogenic shock and 54 % of these patients died [30]. Accordingly, base deficit may correlate better with mortality in the elderly trauma population. In those older than 55 years, a base deficit greater than ten was associated with an 80 % mortality rate. In contrast, a base deficit between three and five is equivalent to 23 % mortality [31]. Geriatric blunt trauma patients warrant increased vigilance despite normal vital signs on presentation. It has been suggested that criteria for the elderly include a heart rate greater than 90 or a systolic blood pressure less than110 mm [32].

Additionally, medications taken prior to admission can confound the diagnosis of significant injury as well as the resuscitation of these patients. Over 80 % of patients that fall are on a drug that could have contributed to the fall including antidepressants, antihypertensives, and sedatives [33]. Beta blockers prescribed for hypertension can blunt the normal tachycardic response to hemorrhage resulting in a false sense of security that the patient is stable. Anticoagulants, including warfarin, Plavix, and aspirin, can result in increased bleeding. This can be especially detrimental when traumatic brain injuries are present and expeditious reversal should occur. Those that do present on these anticoagulation medications have a higher risk of death [34].

Furthermore, delirium may also add to the difficulty in assessing this demographic of injured patients in the emergency department. Delirium affects up to 10 % of elderly patients in the emergency department and can confound assessment of these patients. Delirium is often the first presentation of sepsis in the elderly and is unrecognized which may lead to an increase in mortality [14]. As early sepsis can result in falls and therefore traumatic injuries, sepsis screening in the emergency department should be implemented early in these patients [35].

Once admitted to the hospital, geriatric patients pose a unique challenge to the trauma service due to their abnormal response to shock and injury. Bradburn et al. established a geriatric protocol that significantly reduced mortality in their patient population. The protocol included a geriatric consultation, a lactate level, arterial blood gas, and echocardiogram [36]. An additional study by Lenartowicz et al. showed that a proactive geriatric consultation resulted in decreased delirium and discharges to long-term care facilities [37].

In a large series of elderly patients, mortality was demonstrated to correlate closely with ISS. It was also influenced by blood and fluid requirements as well as the GCS score. Regression analysis revealed that ISS predicted adult respiratory distress syndrome, pneumonia, sepsis, and gastrointestinal complications; fluid transfusion predicted myocardial infarction; and need for surgery and transfusion requirements predicted sepsis. These complications, in turn, were significant risk factors for mortality [20].

Early Inpatient Rehabilitation

Weakness associated with impaired function is commonplace in the injured elderly. Admission to the intensive care unit (ICU) often results in increased muscle weakness, and the need for short- and long-term rehabilitation is frequent. Implementing early physical therapy in the ICU can result in increased strength as well as decreased length of ICU and hospital stay. More importantly, preventing core muscle wasting and preserving strength can reduce mortality [38].

Multiple hospitalizations increase in the last few months of life, as does the use of intensive care services, suggesting an increase in intensity of care. Other studies have also found an increase in the aggressiveness of care at the end of life. On the other hand, the sustained growth in hospice payments indicates that palliative and supportive care services are becoming utilized more as well. Some patients receive both types of care, undergoing aggressive treatment for some time and then entering a hospice program a short time before death. The relationship between hospice utilization and other services is unclear. Whereas hospice may substitute for more aggressive care in some cases, it may be used in addition to conventional care services in others [39].

Geriatric trauma patients have an overall higher mortality rate from equivalent injuries when compared to younger patients. Additionally, their likelihood of dying within 5 years after an injury increases significantly. Despite this elevated mortality rate, a portion are able to go home and resume a good quality of life. Of those that are discharged from the hospital, 52 % are to home, 25 % are to skilled nursing facilities, and 20 % are to rehabilitation facilities. The discharge process can be complex from a financial and emotional standpoint as a traumatic event often results in additional care and loss of independence.

End-of-Life Issues

Advanced care directives and honoring a patient's end-of-life wishes are salient in the geriatric population. Laws regarding these medical decisions arose to preserve a patient's autonomy in a critical care scenario. Patients often fear prolonged suffering, emotional and financial burdens on their families, and concerns about lack of control of their end-of-life care [40]. Of 3,746 older adults (>60 years old), 42.5 % required end-of-life decision making. Of these patients, 70.3 % lacked capacity. Patients with an advance directive were significantly more likely to want limited or comfort care and have their wishes honored [41]. Additionally, the elderly are more likely to have a do not resuscitate (DNR) status at time of death. Increased rate of DNR could be either a reflection of increased injury or poor physiology and inability to tolerate resuscitation [28].

As the elderly portion of the population has increased, the prehospital presence of advanced directive decisions has also increased. In 1994, the SUPPORT study showed that only 21 % of seriously ill patients had an advanced directive, while a 2010 study revealed that 67 % had an advanced directive [42]. A retrospective study by Trunkey et al. evaluated the decision-making process for those geriatric patients that were at risk for death. This study revealed that the elderly frequently have more concerns about long-term disability rather than death. Notably, the families were initially reluctant to discuss the topic of end-of-life care, but ultimately the majority of end-of-life discussions centered on withdrawal of therapies and establishing comfort care measures. Moreover, surgeon input regarding the projected quality and quantity of life was also instrumental when family members were establishing goals of care [43].

The legal aspects of end-of-life care vary from state to state. The POLST form was implemented in Oregon in 1991. This advanced directive addresses four treatment options: code status, transportation wishes, desire for antibiotic administration, and tube feeding. This form is an easily identifiable bright pink form, and the data collected is entered into a central database that can be easily accessed by EMTs and emergency physicians in case of injury. Multiple studies have evaluated this program's effectiveness in preventing unwanted treatments, hospitalization, and resuscitations. In a review of nursing home patients, 91 % had DNR orders, which were ultimately honored. Additionally in a survey of EMTs, 93 % of them regarded the POLST form favorably, and greater than half reported using the POLST to change a patient's treatment plan [44]. While this plan is more applicable to those in nursing home facilities, it can aid in decision making when the elderly are injured. Advanced care planning should be addressed upon admission as soon as the patient or their surrogate is present. It belies the trauma team to be proactive in addressing these issues early, so the patient's autonomy is protected, and specific interventions are not performed.

As the post-World War II generation continues to age and the geriatric population expands, our medical system must likewise mature to provide optimal care for them. The cost of health care will continue to increase and will place new strains on an already-stressed system. As trauma is a major cause of morbidity and mortality in the elderly, efforts to improve all aspects of acute care should increase to match the growing demands. A high index of suspicion is needed when caring for these patients as they may not follow the standard physiologic response when injured. Furthermore, end-of-life discussions are paramount when caring for the elderly, and if a prehospital advanced directive is not present, the discussion should occur early with the patient or their representative to discuss the goals of care. Expansion of geriatric-centered strategies to improve trauma prevention, triage, resuscitation, critical care, and rehabilitation in the elderly is necessary to meet the needs of this rapidly expanding, complex population.

References

1. Adams SD, Cotton BA, McGuire MF, et al. Unique pattern of complications in elderly trauma patients at a Level I trauma center. J Trauma Acute Care Surg. 2012;72(1):112–8.
2. Profile of older Americans. 2012. Available at: http://www.aoa.gov/aoaroot/aging_statistics/Profile/index.aspx. Accessed 17 Nov 2012.
3. Wier LM, Levit K, Stranges E, et al. HCUP Facts and Figures: Statistics on Hospital-based Care in the United States, 2008. Rockville, MD: Agency for Healthcare Research and Quality, 2010. Available at: http://www.hcup-us.ahrq.gov/reports.jsp.
4. Squires DA. Healthcare Cost and Utilization Project (HCUP) statistical briefs. Rockville: Agency for Health Care Policy and Research (US); 2006.
5. Projections of future growth of the older population. 2010. Available at: http://www.aoa.gov/aoaroot/aging_statistics/future_growth/future_growth.aspx#age. Accessed 17 Nov 2012.
6. The high concentration of U.S. health care expenditures. 2006. Available at: http://www.ahrq.gov/research/ria19/expriach4.htm. Accessed 17 Nov 2012.
7. Kane RL, Kane RL. Essentials of clinical geriatrics. New York: McGraw-Hill Medical; 2009.
8. Lubitz JD, Riley GF. Trends in Medicare payments in the last year of life. N Engl J Med. 1993;328(15):1092–6.
9. Bergeron E, Lavoie A, Clas D, et al. Elderly trauma patients with rib fractures are at greater risk of death and pneumonia. J Trauma. 2003;54(3):478–85.
10. Thompson HJ, McCormick WC, Kagan SH. Traumatic brain injury in older adults: epidemiology, outcomes, and future implications. J Am Geriatr Soc. 2006;54(10):1590–5.
11. Mosenthal AC, Livingston DH, Lavery RF, et al. The effect of age on functional outcome in mild traumatic brain injury: 6-month report of a prospective multicenter trial. J Trauma. 2004;56(5):1042–8.
12. Menon V, Greene T, Wang X, et al. C-reactive protein and albumin as predictors of all-cause and cardiovascular mortality in chronic kidney disease. Kidney Int. 2005;68(2):766–72.
13. Kulik AM, Kondrat'eva LN. Combined effects of hypoxia and hypercapnia on the functional state of the respiratory center. Biull Eksp Biol Med. 1975;79(4):39–43.
14. Han JH, Shintani A, Eden S, et al. Delirium in the emergency department: an independent predictor of death within 6 months. Ann Emerg Med. 2010;56(3):244–52.e1.
15. Marik PE. Management of the critically ill geriatric patient. Crit Care Med. 2006;34(9 Suppl):S176–82.
16. Haentjens P, Magaziner J, Colón-Emeric CS, et al. Meta-analysis: excess mortality after hip fracture among older women and men. Ann Intern Med. 2010;152(6):380–90.
17. Cahill NE, Dhaliwal R, Day AG, Jiang X, Heyland DK. Nutrition therapy in the critical care setting: what is "best achievable" practice? An international multicenter observational study. Crit Care Med. 2010;38(2):395–401.
18. Hakamies-Blomqvist L, Wiklund M, Henriksson P. Predicting older drivers' accident involvement – Smeed's law revisited. Accid Anal Prev. 2005;37(4):675–80.
19. Richmond TS, Kauder D, Strumpf N, Meredith T. Characteristics and outcomes of serious traumatic injury in older adults. J Am Geriatr Soc. 2002;50(2):215–22.
20. Tornetta 3rd P, Mostafavi H, Riina J, et al. Morbidity and mortality in elderly trauma patients. J Trauma. 1999;46(4):702–6.

21. Holcomb JB, McMullin NR, Kozar RA, Lygas MH, Moore FA. Morbidity from rib fractures increases after age 45. J Am Coll Surg. 2003;196(4):549–55.
22. Aschkenasy MT, Rothenhaus TC. Trauma and falls in the elderly. Emerg Med Clin North Am. 2006;24(2):413–32, vii.
23. American College of Surgeons: Trauma Programs: NTDB: NTDB® Data Points. 2012. Available at: http://www.facs.org/trauma/ntdb/datapoints.html. Accessed 17 Nov 2012.
24. Bulger EM, Arneson MA, Mock CN, Jurkovich GJ. Rib fractures in the elderly. J Trauma. 2000;48(6):1040–6; discussion 1046–7.
25. Testerman GM. Adverse outcomes in younger rib fracture patients. South Med J. 2006;99(4):335–9.
26. Demetriades D, Sava J, Alo K, et al. Old age as a criterion for trauma team activation. J Trauma. 2001;51(4):754–6; discussion 756–7.
27. Goodmanson NW, Rosengart MR, Barnato AE, Sperry JL, Peitzman AB, Marshall GT. Defining geriatric trauma: when does age make a difference? Surgery. 2012;152(4):668–75.
28. Jacobs DG. Special considerations in geriatric injury. Curr Opin Crit Care. 2003;9(6):535–9.
29. Werman HA, Erskine T, Caterino J, Riebe JF, Valasek T. Development of statewide geriatric patients trauma triage criteria. Prehosp Disaster Med. 2011;26(3):170–9.
30. Scalea TM, Simon HM, Duncan AO, et al. Geriatric blunt multiple trauma: improved survival with early invasive monitoring. J Trauma. 1990;30(2):129–34; discussion 134–6.
31. Martin JT, Alkhoury F, O'Connor JA, Kyriakides TC, Bonadies JA. "Normal" vital signs belie occult hypoperfusion in geriatric trauma patients. Am Surg. 2010;76(1):65–9.
32. Heffernan DS, Thakkar RK, Monaghan SF, et al. Normal presenting vital signs are unreliable in geriatric blunt trauma victims. J Trauma. 2010;69(4):813–20.
33. Nordell E, Jarnlo GB, Jetsén C, Nordström L, Thorngren KG. Accidental falls and related fractures in 65–74 year olds: a retrospective study of 332 patients. Acta Orthop Scand. 2000;71(2):175–9.
34. Ohm C, Mina A, Howells G, Bair H, Bendick P. Effects of antiplatelet agents on outcomes for elderly patients with traumatic intracranial hemorrhage. J Trauma. 2005;58(3):518–22.
35. Moore LJ, Turner KL, Todd SR, McKinley B, Moore FA. Computerized clinical decision support improves mortality in intra abdominal surgical sepsis. Am J Surg. 2010;200(6):839–43; discussion 843–4.
36. Bradburn E, Rogers FB, Krasne M, et al. High-risk geriatric protocol: improving mortality in the elderly. J Trauma Acute Care Surg. 2012;73(2):435–40.
37. Lenartowicz M, Parkovnick M, McFarlan A, et al. An evaluation of a proactive geriatric trauma consultation service. Ann Surg. 2012;256(6):1098–101.
38. Morris PE, Goad A, Thompson C, et al. Early intensive care unit mobility therapy in the treatment of acute respiratory failure. Crit Care Med. 2008;36(8):2238–43.
39. Riley GF, Lubitz JD. Long-term trends in Medicare payments in the last year of life. Health Serv Res. 2010;45(2):565–76.
40. Bok S. Personal directions for care at the end of life. N Engl J Med. 1976;295(7):367–9.
41. Silveira MJ, Kim SYH, Langa KM. Advance directives and outcomes of surrogate decision making before death. N Engl J Med. 2010;362(13):1211–8.
42. Gordy S, Klein E. Advance directives in the trauma intensive care unit: do they really matter? Int J Crit Illn Inj Sci. 2011;1(2):132–7.
43. Trunkey DD, Cahn RM, Lenfesty B, Mullins R. Management of the geriatric trauma patient at risk of death: therapy withdrawal decision making. Arch Surg. 2000;135(1):34–8.
44. Schmidt TA, Hickman SE, Tolle SW, Brooks HS. The Physician Orders for Life-Sustaining Treatment program: Oregon emergency medical technicians' practical experiences and attitudes. J Am Geriatr Soc. 2004;52(9):1430–4.

Cardiovascular Physiology

2

Jason P. Farrah, R. Shayn Martin, and Michael C. Chang

Introduction

Once thought to be predominately a disease of younger individuals, injury is now increasingly common in the geriatric population. There are thus a larger proportion of patients with a complicated array of medical comorbidities presenting to hospitals following acute trauma. Cardiovascular disease is the most prevalent and substantial comorbidity affecting posttraumatic outcomes in the elderly [1]. Recent epidemiological studies demonstrate that although persons aged 75 and older only account for roughly 6 % of the population, these individuals account for 30 % of all myocardial infarctions and 60 % of all deaths related to myocardial infarction [2]. The discussion that follows highlights the differences in anatomy and physiology demonstrated by the aging heart and the importance of these changes during the "stress" of exercise and illness. Common cardiovascular disease states are addressed as well as their impact in the setting of trauma and emergency care.

Left Ventricular Changes in Aging

Aging confers changes in cardiac function directly related to incremental increases in the workload on the heart [1, 3, 4]. Left ventricular changes result from increased afterload as aging blood vessels stiffen and lead to increased systolic blood pressure. Sustained increases in systolic pressure result in increasingly larger degrees of stroke work (stroke volume × blood pressure). This increased stroke work has been implicated as the etiology of left ventricular (LV) wall thickening in elderly patients [4]. Left ventricular hypertrophic remodeling is an accepted by-product to the aging process [4], but it is not known if this is adaptive or not.

Studies utilizing M-mode echocardiography and gated blood pool scans demonstrate that resting early diastolic filling rates decline with age [5]. However, this decrease in early ventricular filling rate does not correlate with overall end-diastolic volume reduction suggesting that atrial contraction ("atrial kick") likely makes a greater contribution to ventricular filling in the elderly patient [6]. In addition, early studies from the 1960s and 1970s demonstrate decreases in cardiac output in the elderly at rest. Unfortunately, these studies did not differentiate between patients with or without preexisting cardiac disease. Indeed, more recent studies proved that resting cardiac output is preserved in the elderly patient free of cardiac disease. These latter studies also demonstrate that, in the absence of preexisting cardiac disease, other indices of pump function (such as ejection fraction and ejection velocity) are also preserved. It was therefore concluded that modest hypertrophic changes in the left ventricular wall are adaptive in preserving cardiac function secondary to increased workload due to systolic hypertension. Furthermore, the aging left ventricle maintains cardiac output through prolonged contraction, atrial enlargement, and increased contribution to LV filling [5].

Recently, our understanding of elderly left ventricular function has been challenged by studies utilizing cardiac MRI technology. Cardiac MRI with tagging is the new standard for assessing LV structural abnormalities and can assess function in greater detail than echocardiography [7]. Recent work with cardiac MRI has investigated LV structure and function in large cohorts of ethnically diverse elderly individuals free of baseline cardiac disease. The largest of these studies demonstrated age-related decreases in absolute and indexed LV

J.P. Farrah, MD (✉)
Fellow in Acute Care Surgery, Department of General Surgery, Wake Forest School of Medicine, Medical Center Blvd., Winston-Salem, NC 27157, USA
e-mail: jfarrah@wakehealth.edu, jpfarrah1@gmail.com

R.S. Martin, MD
Department of Surgery, Wake Forest School of Medicine, Medical Center Blvd., Winston-Salem, NC 27157, USA
e-mail: romartin@wakehealth.edu

M.C. Chang, MD
Department of General Surgery, Wake Forest University Baptist Medical Center, 1 Medical Center Boulevard, Winston-Salem, NC 27157, USA
e-mail: mchang@wfubmc.edu, mchang@wakehealth.edu

J.A. Yelon, F.A. Luchette (eds.), *Geriatric Trauma and Critical Care*,
DOI 10.1007/978-1-4614-8501-8_2, © Springer Science+Business Media New York 2014

mass in both genders. In addition, there were increased mass to volume ratios in the presence of decreases in left ventricular end-diastolic volumes (LVEDV). End-systolic volumes (LVESV) also decreased slightly, generating a net decrease in stroke volumes that correlated with increased age. Ejection fractions were maintained or modestly elevated owing to reductions in LVESV that were substantially less than the decreases in LVEDV. Strain analyses demonstrated age-related impairment of both systolic and diastolic strain which was observed as decreased circumferential shortening during systole (age-related impaired contractility) and decreased circumferential lengthening in diastole (age-related impaired and relaxation). Finally, these data demonstrated that increases in the mass to volume ratio of the left ventricle were associated with a significantly increased risk of cardiovascular events independent of age [7].

Right Ventricular Changes in Aging

The heart is a single pump consisting of discrete cardiac chambers in series; therefore, an understanding of both ventricles is paramount to understanding global cardiovascular function. Under normal circumstances, the right ventricle is connected in series to the left ventricle and is therefore obligated to pump the same effective stroke volume. In the young, otherwise healthy, trauma patient, right ventricular flow is presumably equivalent to left ventricular flow. However, some authors have pointed out that in aged patients the right heart function may not always parallel or reflect left heart function. Estimates of left heart function from right heart measured flow variables may be unreliable in persons with right heart or pulmonary vasculature abnormalities. Recent studies utilizing modern echocardiographic techniques demonstrate that both systolic and diastolic right ventricular function may be impaired with normal aging. The tricuspid annular plane systolic excursion (TAPSE) is often used as an estimate of the longitudinal contractile properties of the right ventricle. Recent studies using M-mode echocardiography in combination with Doppler technology in healthy elderly volunteers have been able to elucidate explanations for impaired systolic function in the right ventricle. Using Doppler echocardiography and pulse tissue Doppler technology, there is a significant age-related reduction in TAPSE in otherwise healthy subjects. This is confirmed by pulsed tissue-derived measurements of the right ventricular systolic function and agrees with similar findings of older studies demonstrating reduced systolic function by echocardiographic criteria. Reduced right ventricular systolic function is secondary to a gradual age-related increase in pulmonary arterial vascular resistance, clinically evident by increased pulmonary artery systolic pressures in otherwise healthy aged adults [3, 8, 9]. These pressures exert a deleterious effect on the longitudinal systolic function of the heart. With less ability for longitudinal systolic contraction, the aged right heart invests more contractile effort into inefficient rotational motions as evidenced by recent studies utilizing cine magnetic resonance imaging [10]. Inefficient rotational motions and non-longitudinal muscular movement of the right ventricle contribute to the observed age-related decrease in systolic function of the right heart.

Age-related changes in the diastolic function of the right heart have also been reported. Tissue Doppler-derived measurements of flow velocities and time intervals are capable of characterizing diastolic functional properties of the right heart [11, 12]. Commonly used variables include right atrial pressure (RAP), tricuspid inflow velocity (E), myocardial early diastolic velocity (Ea), and atrial peak velocity (Aa) [13]. In healthy volunteers, age is significantly correlated with increases in Aa and decreases in Ea over time. Additionally, there is a negative relationship between the Ea/Aa ratio and increasing age, indicating less filling velocities in the ventricle despite higher atrial velocities. These findings have been reproduced in other studies utilizing pulsed tissue Doppler to evaluate right-sided heart function [14]. This study is the first of its kind to report increases in RAP with advancing age by demonstrating increases in the E/Ea ratio (an index of RAP). Just as systolic functional decline is attributed to increasing stiffness of the pulmonary vasculature with aging, diastolic functional changes are attributed to increased afterload [13].

Analysis of cardiac mass and function with cardiac MRI has demonstrated age-related changes in the right ventricle that parallel data from echocardiography and angiography. For example, Sandstede and colleagues found age-associated decreases in end-systolic volumes, end-diastolic volumes, and preserved right ventricular mass using cine cardiac MRI [10].

Vascular System Changes in Aging

A predominant feature of the aging cardiovascular system is increasing arterial stiffness with age. Patients with known cardiovascular disease demonstrate proportionally higher degrees of arterial stiffness and blood pressure increases; likewise, healthy elderly adults also demonstrate an age-associated increase in the relative stiffness of the central arterial tree. In the young, oxygen and nutrient-rich blood is transported through large, elastic vessels that, through cushioning effect intrinsic to their structural compliances, transform the pulsatile flow from the end aortic root to a steady stream of blood flow in the peripheral system [15]. The potential energy thus released during the cardiac cycle stretches the elastin fibers in the arteries and accordingly transmits this energy smoothly downstream to the muscular arterioles and capillary beds [15]. With aging, this elastin becomes depleted and replaced with increased amounts of non-distensible collagen and calcium [16]. This remodeling process causes age-associated dilation and stiffening of the arterial tree so that the once distensible, compliant vessels of youth are now replaced by thick-walled and stiff vessels affectionately compared to a "garden hose" [17, 18].

This pathophysiologic process is most clinically evident in the so-called systolic hypertension syndrome seen in the elderly patient. This syndrome is characterized by an age-associated increase in systolic pressures with a lowering or maintenance of the diastolic pressure level so that a widened pulse pressure is readily observed [19]. Additionally, changes in the vessel wall predispose to changes in blood flow, promoting non-laminar and turbulent flow and thus increasing tensile and shear forces on the vessel that further promotes progressive arterial disease. Cardiac chamber performance is altered in older patients to compensate for this arterial stiffening, and as a result, blood velocity increases as a function of increased age to overcome the increased afterload of the stiffened central arterial tree [20–22].

The decrease in central arterial elasticity that occurs with age is paralleled by increased pulse wave velocity. This occurs in the forward and backward (reflected) direction. Young patients, based on the intrinsic compliance of their vessels, have pulse wave reflections that occur with diastole that augment coronary perfusion and ameliorate tensile shear forces of pulsatile blood flow [22]. Blood flow in aged, less compliant vessels has enhanced shear due to turbulent flow and does not augment diastolic filling of coronary vessels that are already at risk due to atherosclerosis. A widened pulse pressure is the clinical hallmark of stiffened aging central arteries due to a cardiac impulse transmitted outward or downstream with greater force, which thus makes reflected waves return at end or peak systole [22]. This isolated systolic hypertension so often observed in the clinical setting is not benign, and it further stands to reason that compromised diastolic filling of aged coronary vessels (already at risk given occult or overt coronary artery disease) will compromise the ability of elderly patients to both generate and withstand the stress of injury.

Increased age is associated with a decreased ejection fraction (EF) reserve (i.e., ability to increase EF during exercise) [23, 24]. However, a recent study by Najjar and colleagues has examined the impact of age on the relationship between the heart and the vasculature (ventricular-arterial coupling) by comparing the ratio of arterial elastance (EaI) to left ventricular systolic elastance (ElvI) at rest and during exercise in 239 subjects ranging in age from 21 to 87 years of age. The study subjects were comprised of 136 men and 103 women, which were healthy, community-dwelling participants from the Baltimore Longitudinal Study of Aging. This study revealed that EaI/ElvI decreases less in older versus younger persons during exercise. Interestingly, men and women demonstrate different mechanistic reasons for a decreased coupling ratio. Compared to older men, women were able to attain a higher ElvI. However, in women the EaI is directly proportional to age, while there is no difference between younger versus older men. The authors thus concluded that normal aging is associated with less ability to attain and maintain maximal cardiac efficacy due to reductions in the reserve capacity as manifested by a lesser reduction in the coupling index [25]. In women, this is likely due to an increase in arterial elastance without an appropriate rise in ventricular elastance, whereas in men left ventricular elastance declines over time [25].

Age-Related Changes in Function and Physiology (See Table 2.1)

Cardiac Output

It had previously been held that in elderly adults free of coronary disease, there was no change in cardiac output or pump function despite age-related increases in systolic blood pressure and arterial stiffness [26]. This was thought to be due to adaptations including moderate increase in LV thickness, prolonged contraction times, atrial enlargement, and increased atrial contributions to LV filling [26]. It was further postulated that prolonged contraction during systole maintained the load-bearing capacity of the heart in the face of increased afterload that came with age-related increase in arterial stiffness. Most of these data, however, came from older technology such as M-mode echocardiography and gated blood pool scans. More recently newer technology such as cardiac MRI, 2-D ECHO, 3-D ECHO, and pulsed tissue Doppler echocardiography demonstrates that these previously held theories may not be as accurate as once thought. Indeed contemporary authors have shown that echocardiography is not as efficient as cardiac MRI in distinguishing between concentric remodeling and concentric hypertrophy [27–29].

Newer studies utilizing cardiac MRI demonstrate that left ventricular hypertrophy, once thought to be adaptive, may be suboptimal. Although older myocytes do increase in size, there is overall myocyte depletion (dropout) that is associated with increased collagen deposition and nonenzymatic cross-linking [30–33]. The older ventricle, while increasing in overall mass, does not increase in overall functional mass, as demonstrated by cardiac MRI findings that reveal increasing left ventricular mass to volume ratios and associated declines in LVEDV in relation to left ventricular mass. Additionally, although the EF is preserved, absolute stroke volume is not [7]. Although LVEDV and LVESV both decrease in age, the decrease in LVEDV is

Table 2.1 Age-related changes in function and physiology

Physiologic consequence of aging	Clinical importance	Impact on treatment and care
Decreased intrinsic heart rate, maximal heart rate, and response to beta-adrenergic stimuli	Reliance on stroke volume increase and ventricular filling to augment cardiac output during stress	Utilize early aggressive fluid resuscitation for optimization of ventricular filling-
Decreased baroreceptor sensitivity	Blunted stress response to injury	Beta-adrenergic inotropes likely more useful than vasoconstrictors; afterload augmentation may be necessary
	Poor tolerance of hypovolemia	Tachycardia an unpredictable response to hypovolemia
Left ventricular hypertrophy	High rates of occult diastolic/lusitropic dysfunction	Maintenance of sinus rhythm and volume repletion within a narrow range of utmost importance.
Left atrial dilatation	Increased reliance on atrial contribution to overall slowed ventricular filling	Dysrhythmias must be rapidly diagnosed and effectively treated
Right ventricular dilation	Poor tolerance of sustained tachycardia and dysrhythmias	Preserved EF poorly predictive of preserved overall cardiac function
Increased left ventricular mass to volume ratio	Predisposition for atrial fibrillation	
	Hypersensitivity to overaggressive fluid administration	
	Preserved or increased ejection fraction with overall decreased ventricular volumes and contractility	
Stiffening of the central arterial tree	Systolic hypertension syndrome with increased pulse pressure, pulse wave velocity, augmentation index	Increased sensitivity of coronary perfusion to low diastolic pressures
Increased prevalence of occult or overt cardiac disease and/or cardiomyopathies	May reduce cardiac function during stress of acute injury and illness	Maintain a high index of suspicion and employ liberal use of diagnostic modalities such as ECG, ECHO, and serial troponin measurements – especially during unexplained occurrence of sudden vital sign derangement
Atypical presentation of MI	Increased sensitivity to myocardial ischemia and acute coronary syndrome during periods of increased demand	
	Higher rates of "silent" MI	

proportionally greater than the decrease in LVESV, which leads to an overall age-related decline in stroke volume [7]. The phenomenon of ventricular adaptation and decreased function over time is not unique to the left ventricle. Echocardiography with pulsed tissue Doppler technology demonstrates that right ventricular systolic and diastolic function is similarly affected by an age-related decline [13]. It was previously held that elderly patients could respond to injury nearly as well as their younger counterparts based on lack of change in overall cardiac function at rest [26]. Recent findings of cardiac MRI and newer echocardiographic modalities show this to be false; however, the degree to which this affects the injured elderly patient has yet to be determined.

Baroreflex Function in Aging

Gribben and colleagues were among the first to investigate the effect of aging on baroreflex function in a study relating pulse interval to change in systolic blood pressure after phenylephrine injection. There is a linear relationship between pulse interval and change in systolic blood pressure and a distinct decrease in the baroreceptor reflex sensitivity in the elderly. Shimada and colleagues found that an age-related decline in baroreflex sensitivity is independent of systolic blood pressure and systemic noradrenaline levels [34]. Similar findings of decreased baroreceptor reflex sensitivity are found in a study of healthy volunteers examining cardiac response to angiotensin II (ANG II) infusions. The elderly, unlike their younger counterparts, do not exhibit decreases in heart rate when blood pressure is increased via ANG II infusion [35].

Beta-Adrenergic Response

Another inevitable consequence of normal aging is a decreased responsiveness to beta-adrenergic stimuli. Age-related decreases in maximal heart rate (HR max) are responsible for decreases in aerobic work capacity [7, 36, 37]. This decline is independent of gender, regular exercise, and other factors [7, 36, 37]. This decrease in chronotropic responsiveness to exercise contributes largely to age-related reduction in maximal cardiac output and is key in determining aerobic exercise capacity [37].

Although otherwise healthy, older adults exhibit decreased chronotropic responsiveness (HRmax) to exercise, the exact mechanism responsible has not been fully elucidated [37]. The elderly have decreased chronotropic and inotropic response to beta-adrenergic stimulation, and this decreased responsiveness to sympathoadrenal stimulation may explain the observed decrease in HRmax [37]. However, historical studies of B-adrenergic responsiveness consist of poorly matched heterogeneous groups and have inconsistent results. Additionally, differences in vagal tone do not seem to contribute at all to differences in HRmax in normoxic conditions. In fact, the elderly exhibit decreasing vagal tone when compared to younger counterparts [38], and incremental decreases in vagal tone accompany increased workloads during exercise. The net sum of these observations would theoretically increase the elderly patient's HRmax, not reduce it.

Insight into B-adrenergic responsiveness and resultant decreases in HRmax can be drawn from recent work from Christou and Seals. A 2008 study of a cohort of young and elderly men examined the role of reduced intrinsic heart rate (HRint) and decreased B-adrenergic responsiveness in age-associated decreases in HRmax. Maximal heart rate was tested during treadmill exercise to exhaustion. HRint was measured at rest after complete ganglionic blockade, and B-adrenergic responsiveness was likewise tested at rest via exogenously administered isoproterenol after ganglionic blockade. This study reveals that elder men are significantly more likely to have higher serum levels of norepinephrine at rest, lower HRmax, lower HRint, and decreased chronotropic responsiveness. Both decreased HRint and decreased B-adrenergic responsiveness are strongly related to decreased HRmax; however, HRint shows a higher degree of correlation ($r=0.87$ vs. $r=0.61$). These authors conclude that decreased maximal heart rate observed with aging correlates with reduced B-adrenergic responsiveness but is largely explained by a lower intrinsic heart rate in healthy elderly adults [37].

Decreases in HRint are thought to be clinical manifestations of occult sinoatrial node (SA node) dysfunction, possibly related to age-related myocardial fibrosis and collagen deposition at the SA node [39]. However, SA node dysfunction does not always accompany remodeling and may in fact indicate a molecular change in the pacemaker cells [39, 40]. Recent studies have shown reductions in calcium channel proteins which may lead to decreased sinus node depolarization reserve and thus suppression of action potential formation and propagation [41]. Additionally, connexin [42], a primary gap junction protein, is reduced in aged cells [42]. This reduction is hypothesized to restrict conduction of SA node action potentials within the myocardium.

Effects of Aging on Cardiovascular Performance After Injury

Although there is very little information regarding the impact of aging on the cardiovascular response to injurious stress, much is known of the cardiovascular response to exercise. Much of our understanding of the cardiovascular response to injury is extrapolated from these data.

The cardiac output response in the elderly during exercise is significantly reduced. However, subsequent studies excluding patients with coronary artery and cardiac disease show no significant age-related change in cardiac output during exercise. Cardiac output modulation is affected by age. Older patients cannot increase cardiac output with increases in heart rate due to decreases in HRint and B-adrenergic responsiveness. The elderly utilize the Frank-Starling mechanism and increase their end-diastolic volume and stroke volume during exercise, thereby increasing cardiac output without substantially increasing heart rate. The elderly do augment their stroke volume during exercise; however, the increase in ejection fraction is less than that observed in younger counterparts secondary to a decreased ability to reduce end-systolic volume. This is similar to what is seen in young patients given exogenous beta-blockade and then stressed with increasing exercise loads. In this scenario, the young similarly increase cardiac output by increasing stroke volume without appreciably increasing heart rate. Interestingly, the elderly have increased plasma levels of epinephrine and norepinephrine during exercise loading. This finding further underscores the elderly patient's lack of beta-adrenergic responsiveness.

Severe injury often leads to profound states of hypovolemia through blood loss and capillary leak. Critically ill elderly patients are also susceptible to further intravascular depletion from fever (free water loss), poor intake, pharmacologic vasodilation (home medications), and decreased plasma oncotic pressure (poor nutrition). Given the elderly dependence on the Frank-Starling modulation of cardiac output rather than chronotropy, the elderly patient is particularly sensitive to preload reductions secondary to hypovolemia. This is evident in work done by Shannon and colleagues in which elderly patients mount a blood pressure increase and slight HR increase similar to younger patients in tilt test. However, when the same test is performed subsequent to preload reduction with diuretics, elderly patients sustain a symptomatic fall in blood pressure due to an inability to mount a tachycardic response, whereas younger patients exhibit a profound increase in both heart rate and blood pressure [43].

Therefore, based on exercise data, elderly patients are capable of maintaining cardiac output in response to the stress of injury. This is not by heart rate augmentation but rather by effecting stroke volume by increasing end-diastolic volumes and contractility. Research from the early 1980s suggests that elderly patients were unable to mount a cardiac output response to stress. However, subsequent studies of carefully screened healthy elderly patients demonstrate an absence of significant changes in age-related cardiac output variables during exercise in the elderly [6, 62]. Newer technology including cardiac MRI pulsed tissue Doppler echocardiography in 2D and 3D demonstrates that while elderly patients can mount a cardiac output response to stress, this may be much less in magnitude than their younger counterparts due to decreased cardiac reserve [13, 25, 44, 45].

In a study of critically ill trauma patients, Belzberg and colleagues document age-related differences in cardiovascular response to injury [46]. In their 2007 study, they utilized noninvasive primarily transcutaneous devices to collect hemodynamic and oxygen transport variables on 625 consecutive trauma patients at the time of emergency department (ED) admission. Of these, 259 were deemed "high risk" and had pulmonary artery catheters placed for invasive hemodynamic monitoring. Hemodynamic patterns for elderly (>65) and non-elderly (<65) patients were analyzed. Data were stratified by survivors and non-survivors and then further divided by age (elderly vs. non-elderly survivors). Elderly trauma patients had significantly lower CI, HR, arterial oxyhemoglobin saturations (SpO_2), hematocrit (Hct), and oxygen delivery. Interestingly, while elderly survivors have significantly lower values of these parameters than young survivors, elderly and young non-survivors exhibit very similar hemodynamic and oxygen transport values. This study concludes that aggressive resuscitation titrated to hemodynamic and oxygen transport variables may improve outcomes and that the cardiac response to injury seen in elderly patients is much less robust than that of their younger counterparts [46]. It is obvious that elderly patients generate increased cardiac performance in the face of the stress such as surgery and injury; however, the magnitude of this response is attenuated and less robust than that of younger counterparts. It is unknown whether this is due to normal age-related decline in cardiovascular function or to an increased prevalence of cardiovascular disease. Extrapolation from exercise data suggests that it is a combination of both.

Post-injury Myocardial Depression

Real-time assessment of global cardiovascular function using dense data capture technology and bedside assessment of ventricular-arterial coupling demonstrates the occurrence of myocardial depression in the critically injured and post-traumatic septic shock patient [47]. Prior work by Tacchino and Siegel describes similar phenomena in multiply injured patients [5]. The authors reported a 32 % incidence of myocardial depression, as evidenced by a reduction in cardiac index (CI) and ejection fraction (EF), in patients 65 years and older, and a 21 % incidence in those 13–30 years of age. Furthermore, mortality rate rises to 60 % in the elderly group when myocardial depression occurs.

Cardiac Performance in Aging and Disease: Effect of Comorbidities on the Cardiovascular Response to Injury

Atrial Fibrillation

In critically injured elderly patients, atrial fibrillation (AF) is particularly troublesome because age-related changes in pump function and cardiac output rely heavily on prolonged contraction times and increased atrial contribution ("atrial kick") for adequate left ventricular filling. Age-related increases in left (and right) atrial size in healthy older patients are a risk factor for the development of atrial fibrillation [48]. Additional age-related risk factors include inflammatory cytokines, local and systemic stress, altered calcium handling, and electrical remodeling [49]. In the acute setting, pulsatile mechanical atrial stretch and inflammatory cytokines (from injury, sepsis, or ischemia) contribute to arrhythmogenesis [49]. Numerous cytokines may contribute to the development of AF. Postoperatively, elevated interleukin 6, interleukin 8, and hsCRP levels are highly correlated with AF [49]. Interestingly, these same cytokines are present in high levels in the serum of injured patients and can be used to predict progression to multiple organ dysfunction and failure in the multiply injured patient [50, 51]. In addition to inflammatory cytokines, injured patients are exposed to other risk factors that predispose to atrial fibrillation: large volume resuscitation causing increased atrial stretch, increased endogenous catecholamine release, rapid fluid and electrolyte shifts, hypoxia, hypercarbia, pulmonary artery catheter placement, as well as specific injury patterns [52, 53]. Another risk factor is withdrawal from chronic beta-blockade in the elderly [54].

Although this dysrhythmia is common in critically ill and injured patients, its exact pathophysiology in injured patients is unknown. Although the occurrence of AF after blunt thoracic injury with cardiac contusion is well described [55, 56], until recently there has been sparse data regarding atrial fibrillation in the injured patient. A 2011 study has given some insight into AF in trauma patients. In a retrospective review of trauma patients admitted to a large level one trauma center, AF occurred in 6 % of patients and was an independent risk factor for mortality. The sole risk factor for AF development in these patients was age greater than 55. Interestingly, there is a mortality benefit if these patients were "exposed" to beta-blockers sometime during their hospital stay. Unfortunately, the exact dosages and duration have yet to be defined. There is currently not a superior algorithm for treatment of AF in the elderly. AF should be treated according to current ACLS protocols with preference of beta-blockade for treatment if efficacious. AF should be diagnosed and managed expeditiously in the elderly due to greater expected reductions in cardiac output secondary to loss of atrial kick and need for longer diastolic filling times.

Ischemic Heart Disease

Injured patients are uniquely at risk for acute myocardial ischemia given that trauma and critical illness are associated with endogenous catecholamine release, systemic inflammation, and increased myocardial oxygen demand. Additionally, hyperdynamic blood flow during acute resuscitation and its resultant turbulent and non-laminar blood flow increase shear forces. This increased shear may theoretically confer instability on coronary and arterial atherosclerotic plaques and predispose to myocardial infarction (MI) [57]. This is further compounded in the elderly in whom arterial pulse wave indices do not favor diastolic filling of coronary vessels and in whom arterial stiffening only exacerbates conditions of turbulent arterial blood flow. Elderly patients are additionally at risk from age-related coronary artery disease and preexisting cardiac disease. MI represents an important disease entity to address as it is associated with poorer outcomes especially in the aged [58–60].

Currently, the elderly are the most at-risk group for MI occurrence, most likely to suffer poor outcomes should MI occur, and subsequently the most likely to benefit from intervention. MI is difficult to diagnose in critically injured patients and is even more difficult in the elderly secondary to atypical symptomatology and presentation. The physician treating these patients should maintain a high index of suspicion for MI and liberally use diagnostic modalities such as ECG and serial troponin measurements. This is particularly important in the face of unexplained vital sign decompensation after hemorrhage and hypovolemia are excluded. Diagnostic echocardiogram should be considered to diagnose wall motion abnormalities in the face of nondiagnostic troponin elevation [61]. Cardiology consultation should be obtained liberally in the setting of acute coronary syndrome as the patient may be a candidate for intervention.

Heart Failure with Preserved EF

Heart failure (HF) with preserved ejection fraction is defined by heart failure with an ejection fraction equal to or greater than 50 % and represents up to 40 % of patients with heart failure [62]. HF with preserved EF is more common in the elderly, females, and in persons with isolated systolic hypertension [63]. It is mentioned here for two reasons: (1) patients with HF with preserved EF at rest appear normal and (2) EF at rest is often erroneously used in these patients as a surrogate for achievable cardiac performance under stress. In several exercise studies of patients with HF and preserved EF, these patients are unable to adequately increase ElvI, lower peripheral resistance, increase heart rate, and ultimately demonstrate reductions in EaI/ElvI necessary to tolerate submaximal and maximal exercise workloads [64–67]. These patients express nonadaptive inotropic, lusitropic, chronotropic, and vasodilatory responses to the physical stress of exercise and likely have similar inadequate responses during physical stress of injury and severe illness as well [44].

Summary

Care of the elderly trauma patient is complicated by both intrinsic age-related changes in anatomy and physiology and a high prevalence of preexisting conditions. Derangements of the cardiovascular system are common after severe injury and result in an inability to adequately perfuse the organs of the body. Improving the function of the cardiovascular system after injury is of great importance, and the physician caring for these patients must be aware of the effects of aging on the cardiovascular system and the common cardiovascular issues encountered in the setting of traumatic injury.

The elderly exhibit a blunted response to adrenergic stimulation secondary to reductions in intrinsic heart rate and beta-adrenergic responsiveness. Their capability to augment cardiac output during exercise and increased demand is regulated more by Starling mechanisms with greater reliance on an increase in EDV and SV than an increase in chronotropy and EF. This is further complicated by age-related decreases in baroreceptor reflexes that render them more sensitive to hypovolemia and hemorrhage. The elderly exhibit predisposed sensitivity to myocardial ischemia due to increased prevalence of cardiovascular disease, and the clinician must be vigilant in the diagnosis of acute coronary syndrome in this patient population due to atypical presentation and unreliable clinical exam. Dysrhythmia is a common occurrence in the aged and usually heralds underlying physiologic derangement from infection, ischemia, or shock. Deleterious cardiac rhythms must be rapidly diagnosed and treated due to reliance on atrial contributions for adequate ventricular filling and cardiac output in the elderly. In treating these complicated patients, physicians must carefully adhere to the principles of resuscitation within a narrow therapeutic window. Every effort must be made to minimize the increased metabolic demands of hypovolemia, hypothermia, acidosis, pain, and the need for ventilatory support due to decreased ability to compensate for physiologic stress.

References

1. McGwin Jr G, MacLennan PA, Fife JB, Davis GG, Rue III LW. Preexisting conditions and mortality in older trauma patients. J Trauma. 2004;56(6):1291–6.
2. Crispell KA. Common cardiovascular issues encountered in geriatric critical care. Crit Care Clin. 2003;19(4):677–91.
3. Haddad F, Hunt SA, Rosenthal DN, Murphy DJ. Right ventricular function in cardiovascular disease, part I: anatomy, physiology, aging, and functional assessment of the right ventricle. Circulation. 2008;117(11):1436–48.
4. Lakatta EG. Do hypertension and aging have a similar effect on the myocardium? Circulation. 1987;75(1 Pt 2):I69–77.
5. Duggan J. Cardiovascular control. In: Horan MA, Little RA, editors. Injury in the aging. Cambridge: Cambridge University Press; 1998.
6. Rodeheffer RJ, Gerstenblith G, Becker LC, Fleg JL, Weisfeldt ML, Lakatta EG. Exercise cardiac output is maintained with advancing age in healthy human subjects: cardiac dilatation and increased stroke volume compensate for a diminished heart rate. Circulation. 1984;69(2):203–13.
7. Cheng S, Fernandes VR, Bluemke DA, McClelland RL, Kronmal RA, Lima JA. Age-related left ventricular remodeling and associated risk for cardiovascular outcomes: the Multi-Ethnic Study of Atherosclerosis. Circ Cardiovasc Imaging. 2009;2(3):191–8.
8. Davidson Jr WR, Fee EC. Influence of aging on pulmonary hemodynamics in a population free of coronary artery disease. Am J Cardiol. 1990;65(22):1454–8.
9. Dib JC, Abergel E, Rovani C, Raffoul H, Diebold B. The age of the patient should be taken into account when interpreting Doppler assessed pulmonary artery pressures. J Am Soc Echocardiogr. 1997;10(1):72–3.
10. Sandstede J, Lipke C, Beer M, et al. Age- and gender-specific differences in left and right ventricular cardiac function and mass determined by cine magnetic resonance imaging. Eur Radiol. 2000;10(3):438–42.
11. Hori Y, Kano T, Hoshi F, Higuchi S. Relationship between tissue Doppler-derived RV systolic function and invasive hemodynamic measurements. Am J Physiol Heart Circ Physiol. 2007; 293(1):H120–5.
12. Meluzin J, Spinarova L, Bakala J, et al. Pulsed Doppler tissue imaging of the velocity of tricuspid annular systolic motion; a new, rapid, and non-invasive method of evaluating right ventricular systolic function. Eur Heart J. 2001;22(4):340–8.
13. Innelli P, Esposito R, Olibet M, Nistri S, Galderisi M. The impact of ageing on right ventricular longitudinal function in healthy subjects: a pulsed tissue Doppler study. Eur J Echocardiogr. 2009; 10(4):491–8.
14. Lindqvist P, Waldenstrom A, Henein M, Morner S, Kazzam E. Regional and global right ventricular function in healthy individuals aged 20–90 years: a pulsed Doppler tissue imaging study: Umea General Population Heart Study. Echocardiography. 2005;22(4): 305–14.
15. O'Rourke M. Mechanical principles in arterial disease. Hypertension. 1995;26(1):2–9.
16. Greenwald SE. Ageing of the conduit arteries. J Pathol. 2007; 211(2):157–72.
17. London GM, Marchais SJ, Guerin AP, Pannier B. Arterial stiffness: pathophysiology and clinical impact. Clin Exp Hypertens. 2004;26(7–8):689–99.
18. Dao HH, Essalihi R, Bouvet C, Moreau P. Evolution and modulation of age-related medial elastocalcinosis: impact on large artery stiffness and isolated systolic hypertension. Cardiovasc Res. 2005;66(2):307–17.
19. Izzo Jr JL. Arterial stiffness and the systolic hypertension syndrome. Curr Opin Cardiol. 2004;19(4):341–52.
20. O'Rourke MF, Blazek JV, Morreels Jr CL, Krovetz LJ. Pressure wave transmission along the human aorta. Changes with age and in arterial degenerative disease. Circ Res. 1968;23(4):567–79.
21. Nichols WW, O'Rourke MF, Avolio AP, et al. Effects of age on ventricular-vascular coupling. Am J Cardiol. 1985;55(9):1179–84.
22. Nichols WW, Edwards DG. Arterial elastance and wave reflection augmentation of systolic blood pressure: deleterious effects and implications for therapy. J Cardiovasc Pharmacol Ther. 2001; 6(1):5–21.
23. Fleg JL, O'Connor F, Gerstenblith G, et al. Impact of age on the cardiovascular response to dynamic upright exercise in healthy men and women. J Appl Physiol. 1995;78(3):890–900.
24. Lakatta EG. Cardiovascular regulatory mechanisms in advanced age. Physiol Rev. 1993;73(2):413–67.
25. Najjar SS, Schulman SP, Gerstenblith G, et al. Age and gender affect ventricular-vascular coupling during aerobic exercise. J Am Coll Cardiol. 2004;44(3):611–7.
26. Duggan J, Kilfeather S, O'Brien E, O'Malley K, Nussberger J. Effects of aging and hypertension on plasma angiotensin II and platelet angiotensin II receptor density. Am J Hypertens. 1992;5(10):687–93.
27. Redfield MM, Jacobsen SJ, Borlaug BA, Rodeheffer RJ, Kass DA. Age- and gender-related ventricular-vascular stiffening: a community-based study. Circulation. 2005;112(15):2254–62.
28. Lang RM, Bierig M, Devereux RB, et al. Recommendations for chamber quantification: a report from the American Society of Echocardiography's Guidelines and Standards Committee and the Chamber Quantification Writing Group, developed in conjunction with the European Association of Echocardiography, a branch of the European Society of Cardiology. J Am Soc Echocardiogr. 2005;18(12):1440–63.
29. Alfakih K, Bloomer T, Bainbridge S, et al. A comparison of left ventricular mass between two-dimensional echocardiography, using fundamental and tissue harmonic imaging, and cardiac MRI in patients with hypertension. Eur J Radiol. 2004;52(2): 103–9.
30. Olivetti G, Giordano G, Corradi D, et al. Gender differences and aging: effects on the human heart. J Am Coll Cardiol. 1995;26(4):1068–79.
31. Olivetti G, Melissari M, Capasso JM, Anversa P. Cardiomyopathy of the aging human heart. Myocyte loss and reactive cellular hypertrophy. Circ Res. 1991;68(6):1560–8.
32. Anversa P, Hiler B, Ricci R, Guideri G, Olivetti G. Myocyte cell loss and myocyte hypertrophy in the aging rat heart. J Am Coll Cardiol. 1986;8(6):1441–8.
33. Anversa P, Palackal T, Sonnenblick EH, Olivetti G, Meggs LG, Capasso JM. Myocyte cell loss and myocyte cellular hyperplasia in the hypertrophied aging rat heart. Circ Res. 1990;67(4):871–85.
34. Shimada K, Kitazumi T, Sadakane N, Ogura H, Ozawa T. Age-related changes of baroreflex function, plasma norepinephrine, and blood pressure. Hypertension. 1985;7(1):113–7.
35. Duggan J, Nussberger J, Kilfeather S, O'Malley K. Aging and human hormonal and pressor responsiveness to angiotensin II infusion with simultaneous measurement of exogenous and endogenous angiotensin II. Am J Hypertens. 1993;6(8):641–7.
36. Higginbotham MB, Morris KG, Williams RS, Coleman RE, Cobb FR. Physiologic basis for the age-related decline in aerobic work capacity. Am J Cardiol. 1986;57(15):1374–9.
37. Christou DD, Seals DR. Decreased maximal heart rate with aging is related to reduced {beta}-adrenergic responsiveness but is largely explained by a reduction in intrinsic heart rate. J Appl Physiol. 2008;105(1):24–9.
38. Ford GA, James OF. Effect of 'autonomic blockade' on cardiac beta-adrenergic chronotropic responsiveness in healthy young, healthy elderly and endurance-trained elderly subjects. Clin Sci (Lond). 1994;87(3):297–302.

39. Kistler PM, Sanders P, Fynn SP, et al. Electrophysiologic and electroanatomic changes in the human atrium associated with age. J Am Coll Cardiol. 2004;44(1):109–16.
40. Haqqani HM, Kalman JM. Aging and sinoatrial node dysfunction: musings on the not-so-funny side. Circulation. 2007;115(10):1178–9.
41. Jones SA, Boyett MR, Lancaster MK. Declining into failure: the age-dependent loss of the L-type calcium channel within the sinoatrial node. Circulation. 2007;115(10):1183–90.
42. Jones SA, Lancaster MK, Boyett MR. Ageing-related changes of connexins and conduction within the sinoatrial node. J Physiol. 2004;560(Pt 2):429–37.
43. Shannon RP, Wei JY, Rosa RM, Epstein FH, Rowe JW. The effect of age and sodium depletion on cardiovascular response to orthostasis. Hypertension. 1986;8(5):438–43.
44. Chantler PD, Lakatta EG. Arterial-ventricular coupling with aging and disease. Front Physiol. 2012;3:90.
45. Innelli P, Sanchez R, Marra F, Esposito R, Galderisi M. The impact of aging on left ventricular longitudinal function in healthy subjects: a pulsed tissue Doppler study. Eur J Echocardiogr. 2008;9(2):241–9.
46. Belzberg H, Wo CC, Demetriades D, Shoemaker WC. Effects of age and obesity on hemodynamics, tissue oxygenation, and outcome after trauma. J Trauma. 2007;62(5):1192–200.
47. Martin RS, Norris PR, Kilgo PD, et al. Validation of stroke work and ventricular arterial coupling as markers of cardiovascular performance during resuscitation. J Trauma. 2006;60(5):930–4.
48. Lakatta EG, Levy D. Arterial and cardiac aging: major shareholders in cardiovascular disease enterprises: part II: the aging heart in health: links to heart disease. Circulation. 2003;107(2):346–54.
49. Hadi HA, Alsheikh-Ali AA, Mahmeed WA, Suwaidi JM. Inflammatory cytokines and atrial fibrillation: current and prospective views. J Inflamm Res. 2010;3:75–97.
50. Frink M, van Griensven M, Kobbe P, et al. IL-6 predicts organ dysfunction and mortality in patients with multiple injuries. Scand J Trauma Resusc Emerg Med. 2009;17:49.
51. Miller PR, Meredith JW, Chang MC. Optimal threshold for diagnosis of ventilator-associated pneumonia using bronchoalveolar lavage. J Trauma. 2003;55(2):263–7.
52. Solti F, Vecsey T, Kekesi V. Effect of atrial dilatation on the tendency of atrial arrhythmias. Acta Physiol Hung. 1989;74(1):49–55.
53. Amar D, Zhang H, Leung DH, Roistacher N, Kadish AH. Older age is the strongest predictor of postoperative atrial fibrillation. Anesthesiology. 2002;96(2):352–6.
54. Hadjizacharia P, O'Keeffe T, Brown CV, et al. Incidence, risk factors, and outcomes for atrial arrhythmias in trauma patients. Am Surg. 2011;77(5):634–9.
55. Elie MC. Blunt cardiac injury. Mt Sinai J Med. 2006;73(2):542–52.
56. Ismailov RM, Ness RB, Redmond CK, Talbott EO, Weiss HB. Trauma associated with cardiac dysrhythmias: results from a large matched case–control study. J Trauma. 2007;62(5):1186–91.
57. Moosikasuwan JB, Thomas JM, Buchman TG. Myocardial infarction as a complication of injury. J Am Coll Surg. 2000;190(6):665–70.
58. DeMaria EJ, Kenney PR, Merriam MA, Casanova LA, Gann DS. Aggressive trauma care benefits the elderly. J Trauma. 1987;27(11):1200 6.
59. DeMaria EJ, Kenney PR, Merriam MA, Casanova LA, Gann DS. Survival after trauma in geriatric patients. Ann Surg. 1987;206(6):738–43.
60. Perdue PW, Watts DD, Kaufmann CR, Trask AL. Differences in mortality between elderly and younger adult trauma patients: geriatric status increases risk of delayed death. J Trauma. 1998;45(4):805–10.
61. Alcalai R, Planer D, Culhaoglu A, Osman A, Pollak A, Lotan C. Acute coronary syndrome vs nonspecific troponin elevation: clinical predictors and survival analysis. Arch Intern Med. 2007;167(3):276–81.
62. Owan TE, Hodge DO, Herges RM, Jacobsen SJ, Roger VL, Redfield MM. Trends in prevalence and outcome of heart failure with preserved ejection fraction. N Engl J Med. 2006;355(3):251–9.
63. Klapholz M, Maurer M, Lowe AM, et al. Hospitalization for heart failure in the presence of a normal left ventricular ejection fraction: results of the New York Heart Failure Registry. J Am Coll Cardiol. 2004;43(8):1432–8.
64. Borlaug BA, Olson TP, Lam CS, et al. Global cardiovascular reserve dysfunction in heart failure with preserved ejection fraction. J Am Coll Cardiol. 2010;56(11):845–54.
65. Borlaug BA, Nishimura RA, Sorajja P, Lam CS, Redfield MM. Exercise hemodynamics enhance diagnosis of early heart failure with preserved ejection fraction. Circ Heart Fail. 2010;3(5):588–95.
66. Borlaug BA, Melenovsky V, Russell SD, et al. Impaired chronotropic and vasodilator reserves limit exercise capacity in patients with heart failure and a preserved ejection fraction. Circulation. 2006;114(20):2138–47.
67. Kawaguchi M, Hay I, Fetics B, Kass DA. Combined ventricular systolic and arterial stiffening in patients with heart failure and preserved ejection fraction: implications for systolic and diastolic reserve limitations. Circulation. 2003;107(5):714–20.

Pulmonary Anatomy

3

Vicente H. Gracias and Marissa De Freese (Delgado)

The respiratory system provides the body with oxygen to sustain aerobic metabolic function. Components of the respiratory system include diaphragm, chest wall and abdominal muscles, the nose and mouth, the pharynx and trachea, the bronchial tree, and the lungs. Specifically, the thorax includes the sternum, ribs, chest wall, thoracic vertebrae, two pleural cavities containing the lungs, and the mediastinum. The mediastinum consists of the pericardium, heart, esophagus, trachea, great vessels, thoracic duct, and thymus [1]. Defects in the muscles of respiration or chest wall structure cause derangements in respiratory function.

Comorbidities

Normal aging creates structural changes in the respiratory system that alter the pulmonary physiology. Aging leads to a progressive decrease in the compliance of the chest wall, in static elastic recoil of the lung, and in strength of respiratory muscles. Pulmonary comorbidities in the elderly also affect the basic anatomic landscape of the respiratory system. Medical conditions can influence the respiratory system directly or via influence on a different organ system.

V.H. Gracias, MD (✉)
Department of Surgery, Rutgers-Robert Wood Johnson Medical School, 89 French Street, 3rd Floor, Room 3274, New Brunswick, NJ 08901, USA
e-mail: graciavh@umdnj.edu

M. De Freese (Delgado), MD
Department of Surgery, Stamford Hospital, 30 Shelburne Road, Stamford, CT 06902, USA
e-mail: mdefreese@shipmds.org, defreema@hotmail.com

Chest Wall

The bony thorax and muscles of respiration comprise the chest wall. The ventral aspect of the chest wall includes the manubrium, sternum, and xiphoid process. The first seven pairs of ribs articulate directly with the sternum, the next three pairs connect to the lower border of the preceding rib, and the last two terminate in the flank and back. The ribs originate from the 12 thoracic vertebrae. The ribs are joined by three distinct muscles and a neurovascular bundle. The intercostal muscles begin superficially with the external intercostal muscle, then the internal intercostal muscle, and the innermost intercostal muscle, which is adjacent to the parietal pleura. The intercostal artery, vein, and nerve course along the inferior edge of each rib. Another important source of blood supply is the internal thoracic artery located just lateral to the sternum, which anastomose with the intercostal arteries along the lateral aspect of the chest wall [1].

Lung Anatomy

The lungs are paired organs located in the thoracic cavity. Each lung is conical in shape with a rounded apex and a broad base that rests on the diaphragm. The left lung is divided into two lobes by an interlobular fissure, which extends from the costal to the mediastinal surface of the lung both above and below the hilus. The right lung contains three lobes, superior, middle, and inferior, which are separated by two interlobular fissures [1].

Diaphragm

The diaphragm is a thin, dome-shaped fibromuscular organ that serves a number of anatomic and physiologic purposes. Foremost is its function in the respiratory system where it

J.A. Yelon, F.A. Luchette (eds.), *Geriatric Trauma and Critical Care*,
DOI 10.1007/978-1-4614-8501-8_3, © Springer Science+Business Media New York 2014

serves as the driving muscle to create a pressure gradient for air exchange. The diaphragm also separates the thoracic cavity from the peritoneal cavity. The phrenic nerves, originating from cervical vertebrae 3, 4, and 5, innervate the diaphragm [2].

Pulmonary Physiology

The bony thorax provides protection to the thoracic viscera from injury and provides fixation points for the associated musculature. Respiration occurs with contraction of the muscles (inspiration) and with muscle relaxation (expiration). This provides a bellows effect which entrains oxygen-rich air through the airways into the alveoli during inspiration and then elimination of carbon dioxide-rich air during expiration.

Airflow follows a pressure gradient from a region of higher pressure to an area of lower pressure. A pressure difference between the atmosphere and alveoli is established by the respiratory muscles and chest wall. The diaphragm functions as a piston. During inspiration, it contracts moving caudally in the thoracic cavity creating a negative intrathoracic pressure. As soon as the pressure gradient is sufficient to overcome the resistance in the airways, air flows into the lungs. With exhalation, the diaphragm relaxes and the elasticity of the lungs causes the contained volume to reduce. Intercostal muscles, scalenes, and other accessory muscles of respiration assist with increasing the thoracic volume when vigorous respirations are required such as during exercise or with conditions of increased metabolic demand (i.e., sepsis) [1].

Effects of Aging

The chest wall undergoes several physiologic changes as the patient ages. Bone loss in the thoracic cage and calcification in the costal cartilage change the mechanics of the chest wall. Kyphotic changes of the thoracic spine result in an increase in the anterior to posterior diameter of the thorax. Respiratory muscle strength decreases with age. The decrease in muscle strength results from a reduction in cross-sectional muscle fiber area, a decrease in the number of muscle fibers (especially type II fast-twitch fibers and motor units), alterations in neuromuscular junctions, and loss of peripheral motor neurons with selective denervation of type II muscle fibers. There is also a notable decrease in compliance of the chest wall and static elastic recoil of the lung [3].

Aging also has an effect on the airway. Older patients develop decreased sensitivity of respiratory sensory nerves. This reduction causes an increased risk of aspiration. Patients have less sensation of debris in the pharynx and have difficulty clearing secretions. Bronchiolar diameter decreases with age creating an increased resistance for airflow [3].

Pulmonary parenchyma also demonstrates changes with aging. There is an enlargement in the alveolar airspace diameter similar to that observed in emphysema. There are no inflammatory cell infiltrates identified in healthy older lungs unlike emphysematous lungs. "Senile emphysema" is the term applied to this pathologic change. Because elastic recoil of the lung decreases with normal aging, patients demonstrate an increase in residual volume similar to obstructive airway disease.

Pulmonary Function Testing

Utilization of pulmonary function tests provides practitioners with objective data about lung function. The data determined by these tests help health-care providers diagnose and monitor obstructive airway disease. The major types of pulmonary function tests include spirometry, measurement of lung volumes, and diffusion capacity. Airflow into and out of the lungs is measured during different breathing maneuvers to gauge expiratory flow rates and volumes.

Spirometry creates a tracing of the relationship between maximal expiratory airflow and time, termed a *spirogram*. It is the most common measure of ventilatory lung function. Good-quality test results are based on accurate equipment, good test procedures, an ongoing program of quality control, appropriate reference values, and good algorithms for the interpretation of results. Variability in spirometry is often based on patient cooperation and ability. The interpretation of lung-function tests usually involves comparing values measured in patients with reference ranges obtained from populations of healthy nonsmokers [4].

Diffusing capacity for carbon dioxide evaluates the alveolar membrane. DLCO measures the ability of the lungs to transfer gas from inhaled air to the red blood cells in pulmonary capillaries. This test is useful for the differential diagnosis of restrictive and obstructive lung volumes. Patients are instructed to rapidly inhale gas that is a combination of carbon monoxide (usually 0.3 %) and a tracer gas. The test gas is held for 10 s then the subject exhales. During the breath-holding period, the carbon monoxide continuously moves across the alveoli into the blood. A low DLCO correlates with a low mean lung tissue density. This is often found in emphysema. Conversely, a normal or high DLCO is seen in airway obstructive disease such as bronchitis or asthma.

Lung disease is typically classified as being either obstructive or restrictive. Obstructive lung disease carries a primary criterion of a reduced percent of FEV_1/VC. In a restrictive pattern, the lungs are small. The primary criterion for this diagnosis is a decreased total lung capacity (TLC). The presence of restriction is inferred from vital capacity since the TLC is calculated indirectly.

Pulmonary function tests are often performed at baseline and then with the administration of medications, frequently a bronchodilator. In airflow obstruction, the pulmonary function measurements may improve. This helps guide the medication prescription and monitoring of disease progression.

As patients age, utilization of pulmonary function tests becomes more complicated. Patients may be unable to cooperate with the test secondary to physical frailty or cognitive decline. Decreased physiologic reserve in older patients reduces the airflow measurements that is not necessarily indicative of underlying pulmonary parenchymal disease. Data for healthy older patients is unavailable for a reference to determine what an expected change in airflow measurements should be [4].

Airway Diseases

COPD

Chronic obstructive pulmonary disease is the fourth leading cause of death among Americans. The Global Initiative for Chronic Obstructive Lung Disease (GOLD)—a report produced by the National Heart, Lung, and Blood Institute (NHLBI)—and the World Health Organization (WHO) define COPD as a preventable and treatable disease with some significant extrapulmonary effects that may contribute to the severity of disease in individual patients. The airflow limitation is usually progressive and associated with an abnormal inflammatory response to noxious particles or gas. Risk factors for development of COPD are directly associated with exposures to fumes, gas, cigarette smoke, or cooking fire. There are several different types of COPD that include emphysema, asthma, and bronchitis. There is significant overlap between the disease processes, but there are hallmark features that classify them as COPD.

Clinical features that identify COPD are respiratory symptoms; coughing, sputum production, wheezing, and exertional dyspnea. The manifestations of disease are variable in each patient based on disease progression, risk factors, and comorbidities. Spirometry is essential for diagnosis once symptoms raise suspicion of COPD. When the FEV1/FVC ratio is less than 0.70, it generally indicates airway obstruction. Decreased inspiratory capacity and vital capacity, accompanied by increased total lung capacity, functional residual capacity, and residual volume, are indicative of hyperinflation. This can also be demonstrated on diagnostic imaging such as plain radiographs and computed tomography [5].

Alveoli

Emphysema is defined as abnormal and permanent enlargement of the alveoli that are distal to the terminal bronchioles. Most commonly, emphysema is the result of long-term cigarette smoking. It typically develops in the sixth and seventh decades. A key component of emphysema is destruction of airspace walls associated with inflammatory cells. This creates loss of elastic recoil and persistent dilation of the alveoli.

Bronchioles

Bronchitis is a persistent inflammation of the bronchial tubes. It can be divided into acute and chronic subtypes. Chronic bronchitis is defined as a productive cough that is persistent for at least 3 months in two consecutive years. The cough is due a loss of normal mucociliary function of the mucosa and reduced ability for expectoration of mucus. Cigarette smoking is a common cause of both emphysema and chronic bronchitis. Management of COPD is based on limiting exposure to exacerbating factors and monitoring progression of disease.

Asthma is a chronic inflammatory disease of the airways. It is one of the most common chronic diseases of childhood, affecting more than six million children. Key components of asthma include airway edema, bronchoconstriction, airway hyperresponsiveness, and airway remodeling. Airway inflammation contributes to airway hyperresponsiveness, airflow limitation, respiratory symptoms, and disease chronicity. Acute and chronic inflammation can affect not only the airway caliber and airflow but also underlying bronchial hyperresponsiveness, which enhances susceptibility to bronchospasm. Clinical manifestations and symptoms are variable, as are responses to treatment [6].

Adults aged 65 or greater have a prevalence of asthma of 4–8 %. Diagnosis of asthma in this population is more difficult than in younger adults secondary to comorbidities and other etiologies of dyspnea. Doctors may attribute symptoms to other diseases that are more common in old age such as emphysema, chronic bronchitis, and congestive heart failure. Differentiation of asthma versus COPD is important because the management is different. Older adults have two categories of asthma: one form of asthma preexists from childhood, whereas the second form is adult-onset asthma. Often there is no identifiable cause for adult-onset asthma. However, cigarette smoking is a known risk factor for developing asthma in adulthood [7, 8].

Restrictive Lung Disease

Restrictive lung diseases are a category of parenchymal or extrapulmonary diseases that limit the lung expansion resulting in decreased lung volumes. Clinical presentation is consistent with shortness of breath and cough. Diagnostic testing includes spirometry. FEV_1 and FVC are both decreased from normal. Primary pulmonary diseases that manifest as restrictive lung disease include pulmonary fibrosis, interstitial lung disease, acute respiratory distress syndrome, sarcoidosis, radiation fibrosis, and asbestosis. Restriction to lung expansion can also be secondary to extrapulmonary diseases. Pleural abnormalities and chest wall dysfunction, including neuromuscular diseases like myasthenia gravis, can create this pathophysiology. Treatment choices and prognosis differ based on the etiology.

Pulmonary Embolism

Pulmonary embolus (PE) can be a life-threatening complication. It is defined as blockage of the vasculature of the lung by a venous embolism. Pulmonary embolus is most commonly thrombotic in nature, but fat, air, medications, and amniotic fluid can cause the same result. Management of pulmonary embolus is based on prophylaxis, rapid diagnosis, and restoration of blood flow to the involved portion of the lung. Clinical symptoms include dyspnea, shortness of breath, chest pain, tachypnea, and cough or hemoptysis. In severe cases, hemodynamic instability and right heart strain may be evident [9].

Deep venous thrombus initiate at sites of venous stasis or injury. Continued growth of the thrombus is perpetuated by limitation of venous flow adjacent to the thrombus. If the clot becomes unstable, it can break off and migrate to the lungs. Prophylaxis is recommended for patients that have prolonged immobility or hypercoagulable processes. Incidence rates of VTE increase dramatically beginning at about age 55 and by age 80 are nearly 1 in 100 per year, approximately 1,000-fold higher than for those aged 45 or younger. Pulmonary embolus in this patient population may have deleterious effects given the compromise to physiologic reserve already observed with normal aging. Risk factors for developing VTE are the same as for younger patients: decreased mobility, trauma, cancer, indwelling venous catheters, and hypercoagulability states [10].

Diagnosis of pulmonary embolus is based on clinical findings, laboratory findings, and radiologic imaging. D-dimer is highly sensitive but not very specific. A negative elevation in D-Dimer will exclude pulmonary embolus as a diagnosis. Computed tomographic angiography (CTA) of the chest is utilized to visualize the vasculature of the lungs. CTA is the gold standard test for the diagnosis of PE with a sensitivity of 83 % and specificity of 96 %. Ventilation/perfusion (V/Q) scans are utilized when there is a contraindication to CTA. This imaging study evaluates pulmonary blood and airflow. A defect in perfusion requires a mismatched ventilation defect. A VQ mismatch is highly specific (97 %) for a pulmonary embolus.

Treatment for VTE is with anticoagulation unless there is a contraindication. Unfractionated heparin or low molecular weight heparin is administered in therapeutic doses. If patients have proven or suspected heparin-induced thrombocytopenia, direct thrombin inhibitors should be used. Oral anticoagulation with warfarin is started once a patient is therapeutic on parenteral anticoagulation. Warfarin is titrated to a therapeutic INR (2.5–4). The most serious complication of anticoagulation is bleeding. The risk of hemorrhage must be carefully weighed against the pulmonary effects of a pulmonary embolus in all patients. Elderly patients are at an increased risk for falls which can make them more susceptible to bleeding while anticoagulated. The most common fracture in the elderly trauma patient is a rib fracture. Traumatic injuries on anticoagulation can be lethal.

Infections

Pulmonary infections are common in the elderly secondary to normal physiologic alterations to the respiratory and immune systems. Older patient demonstrates predisposition to aspiration and impaired mucociliary clearance. Up to one third of elderly patients with a community-acquired pneumonia will not manifest leukocytosis.

Pneumonia is an infection of the alveolar portion of the lung. It is the fifth leading cause of death in older patients. It can be community acquired or health care associated. Several different pathogens can be the source for pneumonia including bacteria, virus, and fungus. Clinical symptoms include cough, fever, shortness of breath, and sputum production. Diagnosis of pneumonia is based on symptoms, physical examination, and radiographic findings. Community-acquired pneumonia can be treated with antibiotics as an outpatient. Patients that have suspected health-care-acquired pneumonia are at risk for resistant organisms [11].

Empyema is a pleural space infection. Parapneumonic effusions occur when the region of parenchyma involved with the pneumonitis abuts the pleural surface and alters the pleural membranes. In the majority of cases, pneumonia is treated with antibiotics and the parapneumonic effusion resolves. However, 5–10 % of patients hospitalized for pneumonia will develop a persistent parapneumonic effusion that progresses to an empyema. Empyema matures via three distinct phases: exudative, fibrinopurulent, and organization. All pathogens that cause pneumonia can also cause a parapneumonic effusion and empyema. Patients with traumatic injury to the chest are susceptible to pneumonia due to parenchymal damage such as contusion. Placement of a chest tube is also associated with a higher risk of empyema. Diagnosis of empyema is based on clinical history and chest x-ray or CT scan of the chest. Treatment is drainage of the empyema and antibiotic therapy guided by organism sensitivities. There is a high failure rate for chest tube clearance of the empyema, particularly when drainage is initiated during the organization phase [12].

Tuberculosis (TB) is an infectious disease caused by the atypical bacteria, mycobacterium tuberculosis. Chronic lung disease and cigarette smoking are significant risk factors for TB. Older patients are at a higher risk for tuberculosis because of abnormal lung function and immunocompromise. Tuberculosis may have two different conditions: latent or active disease. Latent tuberculosis is characterized by infection with mycobacterium but no symptoms. Approximately 5–10 % of patients with latent TB will transition to active disease during their lifetime. Persons with latent TB will have a positive skin tuberculin test or TB blood test. Active disease in the lungs manifests symptoms such as cough, fever, weight loss, night sweats, and hemoptysis. TB can also have extrapulmonary symptoms based on spread of the bacteria. Diagnosis of tuberculosis is based on clinical history, high index of suspicion, radiographic findings, AFB microscopy, and culture data. First-line agents for treatment of TB are isoniazid, rifampin, pyrazinamide, and ethambutol. Patients need to be followed closely for treatment response and failure [1].

Aspiration Pneumonitis

Risk factors for aspiration include altered mental status, dysphagia, and disorders of the upper gastrointestinal tract. Older patients are at an increased risk for aspiration events. Pulmonary aspiration of gastric content will produce a chemical pneumonitis. Most pneumonia arises following the aspiration of microorganisms from the oral cavity or nasopharynx. Diagnosis is based on history and chest x-ray or bronchoscopy findings. Treatment is supportive for aspiration (chemical) pneumonitis. Bacterial infection or pneumonia following an aspiration event should be treated with antibiotics for 7–10 days [13].

Cancer

The peak incidence of lung cancer is in the elderly. The likelihood of developing lung cancer is 1 in 2,500 in men younger than 39 years of age and 1 in 15 in men between the ages of 60 and 79 years. There is a high mortality rate associated with lung cancer secondary to the inability to diagnose the disease at an early stage, when it may be potentially curable [14]. Lung cancer patients can expect a high symptom burden, particularly from fatigue and breathlessness. The aging patient with a primary lung malignancy has challenging management issues secondary to the high rates of comorbidities found among the aging patient including cardiovascular disease (23 %), COPD (22 %), and other malignancies (15 %) [15].

Risk factors for lung cancer include environmental and lifestyle exposures. Lung cancer is strongly associated with smoking, radiation exposure, and occupational exposure to arsenic, asbestos, nickel, uranium, chromium, silica, beryllium, and diesel exhaust. Cigarette smoking is estimated to account for approximately 90 % of all lung cancers. Diagnosis of malignancy is via radiologic and invasive testing. Patients may manifest common signs and symptoms of lung cancer such as cough, hemoptysis, wheeze, stridor, or dyspnea. Chest x-ray is the initial screening tool based on clinical findings. When an abnormality is identified with initial chest x-ray, a CT scan will help precise anatomic localization. Histologic diagnosis is important prior to staging workup. Depending on the location of the tumor, histology can be achieved with sputum cytology, bronchoscopic biopsy, CT-guided transthoracic biopsy, or operative biopsy [1].

Lung cancer is primarily divided into two categories: small cell lung cancer (SCLC) and non-small cell lung cancer (NSCLC). Approximately 5 % of malignancies arise from other cell types in the lung. Small cell histology tends to be more aggressive but also more responsive to treatment. NSCLCs include squamous cell carcinoma, adenocarcinoma, and large cell carcinoma. Staging of lung cancer allows for accurate prognosis and treatment options. The staging system for NSCLC is TNM staging. SCLCs are classified as limited disease or extensive disease based on the high likelihood of early metastasis. Positron emission tomogram (PET) scanning is utilized for metabolic staging and can identify occult metastases.

Treatment management for NSCLC is based on staging (Table 3.1). Staging is based on anatomic extent of disease during clinical-diagnostic stage, surgical-pathologic stage, retreatment stage, or autopsy stage. T1 tumors are ≤3 cm in greatest dimension, do not invade the visceral pleura, and are without bronchoscopic evidence of invasion more proximal than a lobar bronchus. T2 tumors are >3 cm but ≤7 cm in greatest dimension, invade a mainstem bronchus with its proximal extent at least 2 cm from the carina, invade the visceral pleura, or are associated with either atelectasis or obstructive pneumonitis that extends to the hilar region without involving the entire lung. T3 lesions are larger than 7 cm in greatest dimension; invade the chest wall (including superior sulcus tumors), diaphragm, phrenic nerve, mediastinal pleura, parietal pericardium, or a mainstem bronchus less than 2 cm from the carina without invasion of the carina; are associated with either atelectasis or obstructive pneumonitis of the entire lung; or are a separate tumor nodule located in the same lung as the primary nodule. T4 lesions are any size

Table 3.1 Treatment of NSCLC

Stage	Operative intervention	Radiation	Chemotherapy
Stage I	Surgical resection for cure	Primary radiotherapy in patients not fit for operation with intent to cure	
Stage II	Surgical resection for cure	Radiation with intent to cure in patients with inoperable disease	Cisplatin-based adjuvant improves survival
Stage II	Surgical resection for cure	Radiation with intent to cure in patients with inoperable disease	Cisplatin-based adjuvant improves survival
Stage IIIA (incidental, potentially resectable, unresectable)	Thoracotomy and potential resection	Adjuvant radiation unclear outcomes	Adjuvant chemotherapy
Stage IIIB	Not surgical candidates	Radiation appropriate	Primary treatment or palliation
Stage IV	Not surgical candidate	Not radiotherapy candidate	Survival improvement with supportive care

tumor with invasion to surrounding or distant structures. Nodal involvement ranges from N0 to N3. N0 has negative pathology in the lymph nodes. N1 involves ipsilateral intrapulmonary, peribronchial, or hilar lymph nodes. N2 status indicates involvement of ipsilateral mediastinal or subcarinal lymph nodes. N3 involves contralateral mediastinal or hilar lymph nodes or involvement of either ipsilateral or contralateral scalene or supraclavicular lymph nodes. M status describes metastatic extent. M0 has no distant metastasis. M1 is divided into a and b. M1a includes malignant pleural effusion, pleural nodes, pericardial effusion, or contralateral lung nodules. M1b classifies distant metastasis [16].

The seventh edition of the TNM staging system (Table 3.2) is the most recent version. It was developed by the International Association for the Study of Lung Cancer and approved by the American Joint Committee on Cancer and the International Union Against Cancer.

SCLC is often metastatic at the time of diagnosis. Patients with limited disease are typically treated with chemoradiotherapy. Cisplatin, etoposide, and thoracic radiation are used to improve survival. Surgical resection is not a mainstay of treatment for SCLC. Patients with extensive disease are treated with several cycles of etoposide and a platinum-based chemotherapeutic agent.

Elderly patients with associated comorbidities and physiologic decline in other organ systems are less tolerant of aggressive treatment options. However, recent studies have shown improved survival outcomes for aging patients when all appropriate treatment options are considered. Chronologic age alone should not be a determinant of the therapeutic decision in patients with lung cancer.

Table 3.2 TNM staging of NSCLC

T/M	Subgroup	N0	N1	N2	N3
T1	T1a	Ia	IIa	IIIa	IIIb
	T1b	Ia	IIa	IIIa	IIIb
T2	T2a	Ib	IIa	IIIa	IIIb
	T2b	IIa	IIb	IIIa	IIIb
T3	$T3_{>7}$	IIb	IIIa	IIIa	IIIb
	$T3_{Inv}$	IIb	IIIa	IIIa	IIIb
	$T3_{Satell}$	IIb	IIIa	IIIa	IIIb
T4	$T4_{Inv}$	IIIa	IIIa	IIIb	IIIb
	$T4_{Ipsi\ Nod}$	IIIa	IIIa	IIIb	IIIb
M1	$M1a_{Contra\ Nod}$	IV	IV	IV	IV
	$M1a_{Pl\ Disem}$	IV	IV	IV	IV
	M1b	IV	IV	IV	IV

Sleep Disorders

Obstructive sleep apnea (OSA) is a sleep disorder found in adults and children. It is characterized by obstructive apnea or hypopnea; daytime symptoms such as fatigue, sleepiness, and poor concentration; and signs of disturbed sleep like snoring, restlessness, and resuscitative snorts. OSA has a significant impact of neurocognitive function and plays a role in other medical conditions. OSA has been associated with hypertension, cardiovascular disease, atrial fibrillation, congestive heart failure, and stroke [17]. There is a higher incidence of these comorbidities in the elderly [18]. The prevalence of sleep disorders increases with age, with the elderly population between 70 and 80 years having an incidence almost twice that for people younger than 40 years. Traditional risk factors include obesity, neck circumference, snoring, and BMI. The elderly population may not have the same risk factors, and the presentation of OSA may be atypical. This leads to underdiagnosis of OSA in aging patients [19].

There is speculation that the pathophysiology of OSA is different in the elderly population. Anatomic and physiologic changes that occur with aging may increase the risk for apnea in the elderly. Alterations to the pharynx are conducive to obstructive physiology. Elderly patients have an increase in parapharyngeal fat deposition, increased length of the soft palate, and a change in the bony structure of the pharynx. Diagnosis of OSA is based on symptoms and polysomnography. Polysomnography is considered the gold standard to diagnosis OSA. It is performed by monitoring the patient during a full night's sleep. OSA is diagnosed if 15 or more episodes of apnea, hypopnea, or respiratory effort-related arousals per hour of sleep (i.e., an apnea hypopnea index or respiratory disturbance index ≥15 events/h) occur in an asymptomatic patient or there are five or more obstructive apneic events per hour in a symptomatic patient [20].

CPAP (continuous positive airway pressure) is the standard treatment for OSA. Positive airway pressure splints the airway open to prevent upper airway collapse. Consistent utilization of nighttime CPAP yields reduced frequency of nighttime apnea, decreased daytime sleepiness, and improvement of quality of life. Surgical options to remodel the upper airway are considered when patients fail CPAP therapy or are intolerant to positive pressure.

References

1. Theodore PR, Jablons D. Chapter 18. Thoracic wall, pleura, mediastinum, & lung. In: Doherty GM, editor. CURRENT diagnosis & treatment: surgery. 13th ed. New York: McGraw-Hill; 2010.
2. Limmer KK, Kernstine KH, Grannis Jr FW, Weiss LM. Chapter 127. Overview. In: Sugarbaker DJ, Bueno R, Krasna MJ, Mentzer SJ, Zellos L, editors. Adult chest surgery. New York: McGraw-Hill; 2009.
3. Janssens JP. Aging of the respiratory system: impact on pulmonary function tests and adaptation to exertion. Clin Chest Med. 2005;26:469–84.
4. Crapo RO. Pulmonary-function testing. N Engl J Med. 1994; 331:25–30.
5. Jeffrey B. Halter, Joseph G. Ouslander, Mary E. Tinetti, Stephanie Studenski, Kevin P. High, Sanjay Asthana, editors. Hazzard's geriatric medicine and gerontology. 6th ed., McGraw-Hill.
6. National Asthma Education and Prevention Program. Expert panel report III: guidelines for the diagnosis and management of asthma. Bethesda: National Heart, Lung, and Blood Institute; 2007. NIH publication no. 08-4051. www.nhlbi.nih.gov/guidelines/asthma/asthgdln.htm.
7. Enright PL, McClelland RL, Newman AB, Gottlieb DJ, Lebowitz MD. Underdiagnosis and undertreatment of asthma in the elderly. Cardiovascular Health Study Research Group. Chest. 1999; 116(3):603–13.
8. Morris MJ. Difficulties with diagnosing asthma in elderly. Chest. 1999;116(3), 591–3.
9. Stein PD, et al. Clinical characteristics of patients with acute pulmonary embolism: data from PIOPED II. Am J Med. 2007;120(10):871–9.
10. Silverstein M, Heit J, Mohr D, Petterson T, O'Fallon W, Melton L. Trends in the incidence of deep vein thrombosis and pulmonary embolism: a 25-year population-based study. Arch Intern Med. 1998;158:585–93.
11. Meehan TP, Chua-Reyes JM, Tate J, et al. Process of care performance, patient characteristics, and outcomes in elderly patients hospitalized with community-acquired or nursing home-acquired pneumonia. Chest. 2000;117:1378.
12. Heffner JE. Infection of the pleural space. Clin Chest Med. 1999;20:607. General review of parapneumonic effusions and empyema with a discussion of the value of biochemical tests to guide drainage decisions.
13. Marik PE. Aspiration pneumonitis and aspiration pneumonia. N Engl J Med. 2001;344:665–71.
14. Alberg AJ, Samet JM. Epidemiology of lung cancer. Chest. 2003;123(1 Suppl):21S.
15. Janssen-Heijnen ML, Schipper RM, Razenberg PP, et al. Prevalence of co-morbidity in lung cancer patients and its relationship with treatment: a population-based study. Lung Cancer. 1998;21: 105–13.
16. Pallis AG, et al. EORTC Elderly Task Force and Lung Cancer Group and International Society for Geriatric Oncology (SIOG) experts' opinion for the treatment of non-small-cell lung cancer in an elderly population. Ann Oncol. 2010;21(4):692–706.
17. Richert A, Ansarin K, Baran AS. Sleep apnea and hypertension: pathophysiologic mechanisms. Semin Nephrol. 2002;22(1): 71–7.
18. Young T, Shahar E, Nieto FJ, Redline S, Newman AB, Gottlieb DJ, et al. Predictors of sleep-disordered breathing in community-dwelling adults: the Sleep Heart Health Study. Arch Intern Med. 2002;162(8):893–900.
19. Butt M, Dwivedi G, Khair O, Lip GY. Obstructive sleep apnea and cardiovascular disease. Int J Cardiol. 2010;139(1):7–16.
20. Thurnheer R, Wraith PK, Douglas NJ. Influence of age and gender on upper airway resistance in NREM and REM sleep. J Appl Physiol. 2001;90(3):981–8.

Renal Function in the Elderly

4

Dirk C. Johnson and Lewis J. Kaplan

Introduction

Structural and functional changes occur within the renal parenchyma with advancing age [1, 2]. These changes have been well characterized and allow the elaboration of estimation formulae that are ubiquitous in electronic medical records and laboratory profiles [3]. Understanding how these predictable changes in structure and function impact laboratory profiling, medication dosing, nutritional support, fluid prescription, and decisions regarding renal support techniques for acute kidney injury or acute renal failure is essential for clinicians who care for the injured or ill elderly.

Renal Biomass and Aging

Advancing age predictably reduces both renal size and functional biomass. All aspects of renal biomass are reduced in size; parenchymal loss involved both the cortex and medulla but appears to spare the collecting tubules and renal pelvis [1]. Biomass reduction also involves lean body mass, and there are well-chronicled reductions in muscle mass and proportionate increases in adipose mass in health; of course, disproportionate increases in adipose mass are observed in the clinically severely obese. Nonetheless, reduced lean body mass reduces the measured serum creatinine (Scr) with advancing age [4, 5]. The reduction in Scr from reduced lean body mass renders interpretation of Scr with reduced renal biomass difficult to interpret during critical illness.

D.C. Johnson, MD
Department of Surgery, Yale New Haven Hospital,
Yale University School of Medicine, 330 Cedar Street, BB-310, 2080602, New Haven, CT 06520, USA
e-mail: dirk.johnson@yale.edu

L.J. Kaplan, MD, FACS, FCCM, FCCP (✉)
Department of Surgery, Section of Trauma, Surgical Critical Care and Surgical Emergencies, Yale University School of Medicine, 330 Cedar Street, BB-310, New Haven, CT 06520-8062, USA
e-mail: lewis.kaplan@yale.edu, andrea.barada@yale.edu

Reduced renal biomass limits the ability to clear creatinine. Thus, an individual with reduced lean body mass may have a normal Scr as creatinine is less readily cleared. Alternatively, an elderly individual with a low Scr likely has severe protein-calorie malnutrition as the only way to have a low Scr is to have severely reduced lean body mass in the setting of reduced renal clearance ability. Since fluid resuscitation may also acutely dilute Scr, knowledge of an individual's baseline Scr is essential, as assumptions regarding renal function are fraught with peril when renal function is not normal [6, 7]. Relatedly, using published estimates of renal function such as Cockroft-Gault that is based on gender, age, ideal weight, and a measured Scr are likely inaccurate during acute illness.

Since Scr is also a reflection of plasma volume, thirst may exert a strong influence on the evaluation of renal function. Thirst sensing is reduced in the elderly [8, 9]. Reduced thirst sensation is likely related to reduced hindbrain visceral sensory flow receptor competency, impaired lamina terminalis (osmoreceptor region that resides in the wall of the 3rd ventricle that lacks a blood–brain barrier) responsivity, reduced angiotensin II elaboration (related to reduced renal biomass), cultural norms, and psychogenic influences [8, 10–12]. Additionally, the cingulate cortex is involved in thirst sensing and may be impaired with aging, especially in the setting of stroke [13, 14]. Hypertension also decreases thirst via baroreceptor-mediated reductions in the renin-angiotensin system. Both economic hardship and illnesses such as Alzheimer's and dementia may significantly impair medication compliance, allowing hypertension to exist unchecked. Hormonal influences either support (orexin) or retard (atrial natriuretic peptide, glucagon-like peptide-1) thirst, and their elaboration may be impacted by age [15, 16]. Furthermore, as advancing age reduces mobility through chronic illness including major axial joint arthritis, cerebrovascular accidents, dementia, and Alzheimer's, the ability to satisfy perceived thirst may be reduced as well. Therefore, the elderly individual hosts multiple competing influences that generally reduce thirst sensation and thirst satisfaction.

J.A. Yelon, F.A. Luchette (eds.), *Geriatric Trauma and Critical Care*,
DOI 10.1007/978-1-4614-8501-8_4, © Springer Science+Business Media New York 2014

These influences generally leave the acutely injured or ill geriatric patient ill equipped to manage intravascular volume deficits related to infection, vasodilatation, or hemorrhage. The clinician should be aware that the elderly may present with a volume deficit that includes the intravascular and intracellular as well as extravascular/extracellular spaces due to impaired thirst sensing and satisfaction. Therefore, the resuscitative fluid prescription may be larger than anticipated. Additionally, hypotension may occur earlier than anticipated due to reduced intravascular volume and the reduced ability to compensate for vasodilating influences such as sepsis, severe sepsis, or septic shock. Such knowledge may also inform clinicians with regard to the timing of fluids as opposed to vasopressors.

Evaluation of Renal Function

The principal means of evaluating renal function in clinical practice are as follows: urinalysis and urine microscopy, BUN, Scr, BUN/Scr ratio, urine electrolytes, fractional excretion of sodium (Fe_{Na}) or urea (FEUN), 24-h creatinine clearance ($CrCl_{24}$), eGFR, and urinary biomarkers. A detailed discussion regarding the use of urine microscopy is outside of the scope of this chapter.

Urinalysis

This simple bedside assay is rather useful in a variety of fashions. With regard to renal function, assessment of urine specific gravity and pH is helpful in the context of plasma osmolarity and pH. One must determine whether the renal response is appropriate or inappropriate for a given state. One expects that an intact renal system would preserve the ability to both concentrate and dilute urine in an appropriate fashion. For example, an individual with dehydration should not have dilute urine.

Similarly, an impaired renal biomass would lose the ability to concentrate or dilute urine. Such a condition is identified in the post-ATN kidney where the kidney functions as a "pass-through" mechanism with the tonicity of urine approximating that of plasma. Urine in this state generally has a specific gravity of 1.010 and establishes a condition known as isosthenuria. Individuals with "high output renal failure" have such a condition and must be evaluated for unexpected dehydration.

Injured kidneys may shed casts of the tubular system and these are readily apparent on microscopic examination of urine from such patients; renal tubular epithelial cells may also be readily identified. Similarly, renal inflammation may recruit WBC that are also noted but are identified generally in the absence of bacteria; when bacteria are present, cystitis or pyelonephritis must also be considered and is aided by urine culture and evaluation of the clinical circumstance. Urine casts may be useful in differentiating ATN from prerenal azotemia in that ATN generally demonstrates renal tubular cell casts, granular casts, and muddy brown or mixed cellular casts. In contradistinction, those with intravascular volume deficit-associated AKI generally demonstrate either no casts or hyaline or fine granular casts. A scoring system to help differentiate these two has been articulated as well [2].

BUN, Scr, and BUN/Scr Ratio

The paired evaluation of blood urea nitrogen (BUN) with Scr is well entrenched in modern medicine. This evaluation tool may be valid prior to medical therapy, but hospital-based therapy may render interpretation difficult or misleading. For instance, nutritional supplementation may artificially raise the BUN while not impacting the Scr establishing a ration that exceeds the classic cutoff of 20:1 that purportedly indicates prerenal azotemia. In the elderly in particular, reductions in lean body mass may artificially depress the Scr leading to the inappropriate diagnosis of dehydration when it is not present. Alternatively, an increase in Scr from both decreased lean body mass and renal biomass may elevate the Scr impeding the diagnosis of dehydration when it is truly present. Accordingly, in the elderly, the BUN/Scr ratio as well as their individual values may be less reliable than in their more youthful counterparts.

Urine Electrolytes

One modality to aid in the evaluation of renal function as well as plasma volume is the assessment of urine electrolytes. It is important to recognize that there are no fixed normal concentrations as they will change with both dietary intake and the volume of generated urine. In particular, the urinary sodium (U_{Na}) has excellent fidelity in illuminating the renal response to the patient's intravascular volume status and mean arterial pressure. In the absence of a diuretic, a low U_{Na} (<20 mEq/L) indicates intravascular volume depletion, and a high U_{Na} (>40 mEq/L) indicates the absence of depletion [17]. Note that a high U_{Na} does not indicate whether there is any additional volume recruitable cardiac performance to be garnered. Other electrolytes may be assessed including potassium and chloride but are of less utility in general practice than U_{Na}.

Fractional Excretion of Sodium (Fe_{Na}) or Urea Nitrogen (FEUN)

These measures purport to better enable the clinician to determine whether there is intravascular volume depletion or an intrarenal condition such as acute tubular necrosis (ATN) by creating a ratio of U_{Na}, urinary creatinine, plasma sodium, and plasma creatinine such that

$$Fe_{Na} = (U_{Na} \times P_{Cr} / U_{Cr} \times P_{Na}) \times 100$$

In general, Fe_{Na} is < 1 % with plasma volume depletion, congestive heart failure, and acute glomerulonephritis but is > 1 % with bilateral ureteric obstruction and ATN; values commonly exceed 3 % with ATN [18]. Fe_{Na} validity is degraded by the presampling administration of diuretics [19]. In that case, the FEUN may be more useful as urea excretion is believed to be more dependent on passive forces but is controversial [19–21].

Relatedly, the FEUN may be calculated in a fashion similar to that of Fe_{Na} where FEUN is represented by the formula:

$$FEUN = (U_{Ur} \times P_{Cr} / U_{Cr} \times P_{Ur}) \times 100$$

A FEUN < 35 % is consistent with the diagnosis of decreased plasma volume [21, 22]. In some studies, FEUN outperforms Fe_{Na} in differentiating between acute renal failure due to prerenal azotemia and that due to ATN.

24-Hour Creatinine Clearance ($CrCl_{24}$)

This measure is perhaps the most sensitive indicator of renal function in that it relies on a 24-h collection of urine that is kept on ice to retard degradation. The 24-h nature of this test accounts for any diurnal or therapy-driven variations in clearance that would be inherent to a spot or 2-h assessment [23]. This assay also allows the clinician to determine whether the patient's native renal function exceeds or fails to reach the clearance that can be achieved by intermittent or continuous renal replacement therapy. The major disadvantage is the time required for collection and the need to keep the entire volume of urine on ice.

eGFR

This ubiquitous measure accompanies every laboratory profile that measures Scr and is accompanied by descriptors of age, gender, and race but does not require height and weight [24]. The currently reported eGFR is derived from multiple studies to replace the eGFR derived from the Modified Diet in Renal Disease (MDRD) calculation in patients where the actual GFR exceeds 60 mL/min per 1.73 m² body surface area [25]. The original MDRD calculation employs age, creatinine, albumin, urea, gender, and ethnicity in its calculation; a 4-variable modification also exists [25]. The eGFR calculation is represented by

$$GFR = 141 \times \min(Scr / \kappa, 1) \alpha \times \max(Scr / \kappa, 1) - 1.209 \times 0.993 \; Age \times 1.018 [\text{if female}] \times 1.159 [\text{if black}]$$

where Scr is serum creatinine (mg/dL), κ is 0.7 for females and 0.9 for males, α is −0.329 for females and −0.411 for males, min indicates the minimum of Scr/κ or 1, and max indicates the maximum of Scr/κ or 1 [26].

This test is primarily used as a screening tool to readily follow the trend in renal function and will be useful over time as the patient ages. Cutoffs for eGFR have been articulated to help categorize the stage of renal failure [3–5]; stages 1 and 2 are applied to renal function estimates when there is a structural abnormality that is present – otherwise a eGFR of 60–89 is not considered abnormal [26]. eGFR is inaccurate in multiple conditions including but not limited to acute renal failure, age < 18, pregnancy, edematous states, severe protein-calorie malnutrition, muscle wasting diseases, critical illness, and following extremity amputation [27, 28].

Urinary Biomarkers

Since Scr and the measures explored above are insensitive and inaccurate in determining early AKI to perhaps enable early therapy that might change the seemingly invariate mortality rate associated with this injury, a more sensitive marker would be ideal in clinical practice. A variety of biomarkers including kidney injury molecule-1 (KIM-1), *N*-acetyl-β-D-glucosaminidase (NAG), trefoil factor 3, cyanuric acid, cystatin C, monocyte chemotactic peptide-1, netrin-1, and IL-18 have been proposed as sensitive indicators of renal injury or failure. A KIM-1 assay is available but currently remains restricted to research applications. Only urinary neutrophil gelatinase-associated lipocalin (NGAL) has been made commercially available for clinical application [29, 30]. Of note, sepsis-associated-AKI patients have been noted to have higher urinary NGAL levels compared to those with AKI from other causes [31]. In research undertakings, a combination of biomarkers to establish a profile outperforms any single entity in detecting acute kidney injury after cardiac surgery, and current thinking supports establishing a panel-based profile rather than relying on a single marker to identify AKI.

Limitations in Renal Function Assessment

Recall that the kidney has multiple functions that span, in part, regulation of salt and water concentration, blood pressure, red blood cell production, as well as nitrogenous metabolic product and waste clearance. In general, clinicians only regularly assess those related to salt and water clearance, with a lesser assessment (indirectly) of nitrogenous metabolic product and waste handling. Less frequently, in-depth assessments are undertaken (including on rare occasion, renal blood flow), but there is little assessment, if ever, in the clinical arena of hormone function (endocrine, autocrine, or paracrine). Similarly, renal replacement therapy is generally limited to nonhormonal functions as well. Thus, assessment of renal function is limited at best.

Epidemiology of Acute Kidney Injury and Acute Renal Failure

An accurate analysis of the epidemiology of acute kidney injury and acute renal failure is hampered by a wide variety of definitions that describe each of these entities. For example, acute renal failure in many clinical investigations has been defined as a doubling of baseline Scr, an Scr > 2.0, the need for renal replacement therapy (based on clinician determination, not a proscribed protocol), tripling of Scr, as well as a function of changes in urine flow that is not necessarily coupled with a change in Scr. As a result, comparing across studies is difficult at best. Further complicating analysis is the fact that the term AKI is relatively new and many patients who were previously labeled as having ARF actually had Stage III AKI instead [32]. In a related fashion, many terms are used in the literature and describe the same process including acute or chronic renal insufficiency, compromise, or failure. Of course, an acute renal injury may also be a structural injury as a result of trauma. The increased use of CT scans in a wide variety of medical and surgical conditions may also influence the epidemiology of AKI and ARF by increasing the at-risk population to contrast and the well-described radiocontrast nephropathy (RCN) that may follow, especially in elderly patients with concomitant dehydration and diabetes [33]. The incidence of AKI has increased in recent years as has the survival rate of geriatric patients with renal insults [34]. New nephrotoxic medications, including immunosuppressives and chemotherapeutic agents, impact the number of patients who are at risk for and develop AKI or ARF [35–37]. Thus, the epidemiology of these two entities should be anticipated to be in flux, especially as the population ages [38]. Global access to, and delivery of, certain diagnostics and therapeutics may establish a geographically biased epidemiology for AKI and ARF as well. Thus, AKI and ARF may occur with disparate frequency in developed compared to developing nations.

Data on AKI and ARF epidemiology does exist for specific hospital domains, including most commonly the intensive care unit. In a fashion similar to that of sepsis and acute lung injury/acute respiratory distress syndrome, the incidence of AKI that does not require renal replacement therapy (RRT) is estimated to be 2,000–3,000 per million population per year [39]. In contrast, the estimates for AKI that does require RRT are 100-fold higher at 200–300 per million population per year. In order to put these numbers into perspective, 4–5 % of intensive care unit patients receive RRT, and as many as 66 % of intensive care unit patients will develop RIFLE classification-defined AKI [39]. In-hospital mortality strongly correlates with the maximum RIFLE class suffered during that episode of care, as well as with progression through each RIFLE stage of risk, injury, and failure [39, 40]. Despite therapy, RRT-requiring AKI carries a 50–60 % mortality rate with up to one in five sustaining permanent dialysis-dependent renal failures [39].

Certain patient populations may have a higher than population expected risk for AKI, including those suffering from sepsis or injury. In a large cohort of nearly 10,000 injured patients, the crude AKI incidence was 18.1 % with a greater than twofold increased mortality rate; advanced age, female gender, increased number of comorbid illnesses, and a greater illness severity all increased AKI risk [40]. Similarly, in a study of greater than 120,000 patients, 27.8 % of septic patients had a sepsis-related diagnosis; 42.1 % of septic patients developed AKI [41]. Sepsis-associated AKI patients were generally more ill, hypotensive, and tachycardic and demonstrated lower PaO_2/FIO_2 ratio and greater leukocytosis compared to those with AKI of non-septic etiologies. Increased ICU and hospital mortality as well as ICU length of stay was also observed in those with sepsis-associated AKI across all RIFLE categories [41]. These data have important implications for the elderly as they are well represented in the critically ill and injured patient populations. Specific efforts should be pursued at mitigating known risk factors to reduce the incidence and downstream sequelae of AKI in the elderly after critical injury or illness. In particular, AKI predisposes to chronic kidney disease, and the elderly with reduced GFR appear to be at greater risk for this progression than age-matched counterparts with normal GFR [34].

Etiology of Acute Kidney Injury and Acute Renal Failure

The etiology of AKI is complex and multifactorial [42]. Multiple etiologies for the genesis of AKI have been proposed, including, but not limited to, vasoconstriction, leukostasis, venous hypertension, apoptosis, and a disordered humoral factor milieu including hormones, growth factors, receptors, and intracellular signaling mechanisms. Therefore, multiple etiologies may lead to AKI or ARF. Most AKI appears to be a toxic phenomenon rather than purely a volume-based issue. This observation is easily understood as the RCN that occurs in the well-perfused and volume-loaded patient. Therefore, AKI may also not respond to plasma volume expansion with regard to hastening resolution.

Seemingly paradoxically, AKI may be worsened by excess volume loading as the excess salt and water (and likely starch in patients with sepsis) may lead to renal parenchymal edema and distorted organ pressure-volume relationships.

Unsurprisingly, therefore, both intra-abdominal hypertension and the abdominal compartment syndrome are increasingly cited as etiologies for AKI and ARF [43]. Several detailed investigations into these entities have been published for the interested reader [44, 45]. Of note, specific mention is made of intrarenal compartment syndrome that may result from renal parenchymal edema (tissue edema and venous hypertension) that may be only incompletely relieved (tissue edema persists) even after abdominal decompression. Thus, AKI may not dramatically or completely improve despite relief of the abdominal compartment syndrome. It is, however, clear that the renal structural and functional changes detailed above place the elderly patient at increased risk for AKI regardless of cause [46]. Nonetheless, acute kidney injury and acute renal failure all directly impact acid–base homeostasis.

Strong Ions, Acute Kidney Injury, and Acute Renal Failure

While acid–base balance has been traditionally taught using the Henderson-Hasselbalch approach, it is occasionally unwieldly as it is logarithmically based and requires the six "Bostonian rules" to account for chronicity and to provide correction of the derived data [47]. Recognizing that the human body is complex, this scheme works well in the clinical circumstance. An alternative to the imprecision of the Henderson-Hasselbalch approach has been articulated by Peter Stewart in 1983 that is termed the "strong ion" approach [48]. Strong ions are cations and anions dissociated from their ionic partners in an aqueous milieu in the physiologic pH range. This approach equates plasma ionic charge with pH through the influence of charge of water dissociation. A complete exploration of the intricacies of this approach is beyond the scope of this chapter. The interested reader is referred to one of several thorough reviews on this topic [49–52]. Nonetheless, this approach provides a concise framework to both teach acid–base physiology and as a platform from which to prescribe a fluid prescription.

In the strong ion approach, rendering the net plasma charge more positive is an alkalinizing influence, and reducing the net plasma positive charge is acidifying. Therefore, fluids may be categorized based on charge difference relative to human plasma and their anticipated impact on pH. Appropriate fluid selection is aided by understanding the patient's pre-fluid infusion pH. By way of example, if a patient has preexisting metabolic acidosis that is due to lactate from hypoperfusion, the choice of fluid may be irrelevant as plasma volume expansion should correct perfusion defects and result in lactic acid metabolism. However, if the acidosis is from organ failure, infusing an acidifying solution such as 0.9 % NSS may be maladaptive. Similarly, if the patient is metabolically alkalotic, then an acidifying solution is an intelligent approach and is well embraced in the concept of a chloride-responsive alkalosis; 0.9 % NSS is the most acidifying solution in common use and provides a gross excess of chloride relative to plasma. This approach has been used in a variety of settings including those focused specifically on the geriatric patient with excellent outcomes [53].

The strong ion approach has also been evaluated in terms of outcome prediction. The presence of unmeasured ions, a specific entity that is readily ascertained by that approach, correlates with increased mortality risk in diverse patient populations. These populations include those with major vascular injury, unselected but significantly injured patients, as well as pediatric patients [54–57]. Moreover, the specific fluid selected for resuscitation may drive unmeasured ion generation [58]. Unmeasured ions are known to accompany a host of critical illnesses including injury, renal failure, hepatic failure, and following cardiopulmonary bypass [50, 59–61]. Outcome modeling using this approach has not been specifically undertaken in the elderly but offers a potentially fertile domain for future investigation.

Conclusions

Predictable changes in renal function are to be expected with advancing age. The clinician should be cognizant of these expected changes as they may directly impact the evaluation of renal function, medication dosing, fluid selection, and the management of acute kidney injury and acute renal failure. Recognizing that acute kidney injury is a toxic process and not a preload-dependent phenomenon may reduce the common practice of plasma volume expansion for this increasingly recognized clinical entity. The articulation of renal biomarkers may better enable the bedside clinician to accurately identify elderly patients with a clinically inapparent renal injury and initiate therapy or protective strategies in an earlier time frame than was traditionally possible.

References

1. Pannarale G, Carbone R, Del Mastro G, et al. The aging kidney: structural changes. J Nephrol. 2010;23 Suppl 15:S37–40.
2. Perazella MA, Coca SG, Kanbay M, et al. Diagnostic value of urine microscopy for differential diagnosis of acute kidney injury in hospitalized patients. Clin J Am Soc Nephrol. 2008;3:1615–9.

3. Steffl JL, Bennett W, Olyaei AJ. The old and new methods of assessing kidney function. J Clin Pharmacol. 2012;52:63S–71.
4. Swaminathan R, Major P, Snieder H, et al. Serum creatinine and fat-free mass (lean body mass). Clin Chem. 2000;46:1695–6.
5. Baxmann AC, Ahmed MS, Marques NC, et al. Influence of muscle mass and physical activity on serum and urinary creatinine and serum cystatin C. Clin J Am Soc Nephrol. 2008;3:348–54.
6. Candela-Toha AM, Recio-Vazquez M, Delgado-Montero A, et al. The calculation of baseline serum creatinine overestimates the diagnosis of acute kidney injury in patients undergoing cardiac surgery. Nefrologia. 2012;32:53–8.
7. Bagshaw SM, Uchino S, Cruz D, et al. A comparison of observed versus estimated baseline creatinine for determination of RIFLE class in patients with acute kidney injury. Nephrol Dial Transplant. 2009;24:2739–44.
8. Phillips PA, Johnston CI, Gray L. Disturbed fluid and electrolyte homoeostasis following dehydration in elderly people. Age Ageing. 1993;22:S26–33.
9. Kenney WL, Chiu P. Influence of age on thirst and fluid intake. Med Sci Sports Exerc. 2001;33:1524–32.
10. Stachenfeld NS, DiPietro L, Nadel ER, et al. Mechanism of attenuated thirst in aging: role of central volume receptors. Am J Physiol. 1997;272:R148–57.
11. Johnson AK, Thunhorst RL. The neuroendocrinology of thirst and salt appetite: visceral sensory signals and mechanisms of central integration. Front Neuroendocrinol. 1997;18:292–353.
12. Thornton SN. Thirst and hydration: physiology and consequences of dysfunction. Physiol Behav. 2010;100:15–21.
13. Farrell MJ, Bowala TK, Gavrilescu M, et al. Cortical activation and lamina terminalis functional connectivity during thirst and drinking in humans. Am J Physiol Regul Integr Comp Physiol. 2011;301:R623–31.
14. Rodriguez GJ, Cordina SM, Vazquez G, et al. The hydration influence on the risk of stroke (THIRST) study. Neurocrit Care. 2009;10:187–94.
15. Fukunaka Y, Shinkai T, Hwang R, et al. The orexin 1 receptor (HCRTR1) gene as a susceptibility gene contributing to polydipsia-hyponatremia in schizophrenia. Neuromolecular Med. 2007;9:292–7.
16. Diepvens K, Haberer D, Westerterp-Plantenga M. Different proteins and biopeptides differently affect satiety and anorexigenic/orexigenic hormones in healthy humans. Int J Obes (Lond). 2008;32:510–8.
17. Strazzullo P, Barbato A, Vuotto P, et al. Relationships between salt sensitivity of blood pressure and sympathetic nervous system activity: a short review of evidence. Clin Exp Hypertens. 2001;23:25–33.
18. Sabiston DC, Townsend CM. Sabiston textbook of surgery: the biological basis of modern surgical practice. Philadelphia: Elsevier/Saunders; 2012.
19. Pepin MN, Bouchard J, Legault L, et al. Diagnostic performance of fractional excretion of urea and fractional excretion of sodium in the evaluations of patients with acute kidney injury with or without diuretic treatment. Am J Kidney Dis. 2007;50:566–73.
20. Carvounis CP, Nisar S, Guro-Razuman S. Significance of the fractional excretion of urea in the differential diagnosis of acute renal failure. Kidney Int. 2002;62:2223–9.
21. Fenske W, Stork S, Koschker AC, et al. Value of fractional uric acid excretion in differential diagnosis of hyponatremic patients on diuretics. J Clin Endocrinol Metab. 2008;93:2991–7.
22. Cecil RL, Goldman L, Schafer AI. Goldman's Cecil medicine. Philadelphia: Elsevier/Saunders; 2012.
23. McPherson RA, Pincus MR, Henry JB. Henry's clinical diagnosis and management by laboratory methods. Philadelphia: Saunders/Elsevier; 2007.
24. Rule AD, Rodeheffer RJ, Larson TS, et al. Limitations of estimating glomerular filtration rate from serum creatinine in the general population. Mayo Clin Proc. 2006;81:1427–34.
25. Prigent A. Monitoring renal function and limitations of renal function tests. Semin Nucl Med. 2008;38:32–46.
26. Brenner BM, Rector FC. Brenner & Rector's the kidney. Philadelphia: Saunders/Elsevier; 2008.
27. Stevens LA, Coresh J, Greene T, et al. Assessing kidney function – measured and estimated glomerular filtration rate. N Engl J Med. 2006;354:2473–83.
28. Baptista JP, Udy AA, Sousa E, et al. A comparison of estimates of glomerular filtration in critically ill patients with augmented renal clearance. Crit Care. 2011;15:R139.
29. Fassett RG, Venuthurupalli SK, Gobe GC, et al. Biomarkers in chronic kidney disease: a review. Kidney Int. 2011;80:806–21.
30. Siew ED, Ware LB, Ikizler TA. Biological markers of acute kidney injury. J Am Soc Nephrol. 2011;22:810–20.
31. Bagshaw SM, Bennett M, Haase M, et al. Plasma and urine neutrophil gelatinase-associated lipocalin in septic versus non-septic acute kidney injury in critical illness. Intensive Care Med. 2010;36:452–61.
32. Kellum JA. Acute kidney injury. Crit Care Med. 2008;36:S141–5.
33. Brown JR, Thompson CA. Contrast-induced acute kidney injury: the at-risk patient and protective measures. Curr Cardiol Rep. 2010;12:440–5.
34. Coca SG, Cho KC, Hsu CY. Acute kidney injury in the elderly: predisposition to chronic kidney disease and vice versa. Nephron Clin Pract. 2011;119 Suppl 1:c19–24.
35. Jacobson PA, Schladt D, Israni A, et al. Genetic and clinical determinants of early, acute calcineurin inhibitor-related nephrotoxicity: results from a kidney transplant consortium. Transplantation. 2012;93:624–31.
36. Kuypers DR. Immunotherapy in elderly transplant recipients: a guide to clinically significant drug interactions. Drugs Aging. 2009;26:715–37.
37. Haase M, Story DA, Haase-Fielitz A. Renal injury in the elderly: diagnosis, biomarkers and prevention. Best Pract Res Clin Anaesthesiol. 2011;25:401–12.
38. Del Giudice A, Aucella F. Acute renal failure in the elderly: epidemiology and clinical features. J Nephrol. 2012;25:S48–57.
39. Hoste EA, Schurgers M. Epidemiology of acute kidney injury: how big is the problem? Crit Care Med. 2008;36:S146–51.
40. Bagshaw SM, George C, Gibney RT, et al. A multi-center evaluation of early acute kidney injury in critically ill trauma patients. Ren Fail. 2008;30:581–9.
41. Bagshaw SM, George C, Bellomo R, et al. Early acute kidney injury and sepsis: a multicentre evaluation. Crit Care. 2008;12:R47.
42. Kinsey GR, Okusa MD. Pathogenesis of acute kidney injury: foundation for clinical practice. Am J Kidney Dis. 2011;58:291–301.
43. De Waele JJ, De Laet I, Kirkpatrick AW, et al. Intra-abdominal hypertension and abdominal compartment syndrome. Am J Kidney Dis. 2011;57:159–69.
44. Ronco C, Bellomo R, Kellum JA. Critical care nephrology. Philadelphia: Saunders/Elsevier; 2009.
45. Luckianow GM, Ellis M, Governale D, et al. Abdominal compartment syndrome: risk factors, diagnosis, and current therapy. Crit Care Res Pract. 2012;2012:908169.
46. Chronopoulos A, Rosner MH, Cruz DN, et al. Acute kidney injury in the elderly: a review. Contrib Nephrol. 2010;165:315–21.
47. Van Slyke DD. Some points of acid–base history in physiology and medicine. Ann N Y Acad Sci. 1966;133:5–14.
48. Stewart PA. Modern quantitative acid–base chemistry. Can J Physiol Pharmacol. 1983;61:1444–61.
49. Story DA. Bench-to-bedside review: a brief history of clinical acid–base. Crit Care. 2004;8:253–8.

50. Naka T, Bellomo R. Bench-to-bedside review: treating acid–base abnormalities in the intensive care unit–the role of renal replacement therapy. Crit Care. 2004;8:108–14.
51. Kaplan LJ, Kellum JA. Fluids, pH, ions and electrolytes. Curr Opin Crit Care. 2010;16:323–31.
52. Stewart PA, Kellum JA, Elbers PWG. Stewart's textbook of acid–base. Amsterdam: AcidBase.org; 2009.
53. Wilkes NJ, Woolf R, Mutch M, et al. The effects of balanced versus saline-based hetastarch and crystalloid solutions on acid–base and electrolyte status and gastric mucosal perfusion in elderly surgical patients. Anesth Analg. 2001;93:811–6.
54. Kaplan LJ, Kellum JA. Initial pH, base deficit, lactate, anion gap, strong ion difference, and strong ion gap predict outcome from major vascular injury. Crit Care Med. 2004;32:1120–4.
55. Zehtabchi S, Soghoian S, Sinert R. Utility of Stewart's strong ion difference as a predictor of major injury after trauma in the ED. Am J Emerg Med. 2007;25:938–41.
56. Corey HE, Vallo A, Rodriguez-Soriano J. An analysis of renal tubular acidosis by the Stewart method. Pediatr Nephrol. 2006;21:206–11.
57. Balasubramanyan N, Havens PL, Hoffman GM. Unmeasured anions identified by the Fencl-Stewart method predict mortality better than base excess, anion gap, and lactate in patients in the pediatric intensive care unit. Crit Care Med. 1999;27:1577–81.
58. Guidet B, Soni N, Della Rocca G, Kozek S, Vallet B, Annane D, James M. A balanced view of balanced solutions. Crit Care. 2012;14:325.
59. Martin M, Murray J, Berne T, et al. Diagnosis of acid–base derangements and mortality prediction in the trauma intensive care unit: the physiochemical approach. J Trauma. 2005;58:238–43.
60. Naka T, Bellomo R, Morimatsu H, et al. Acid–base balance in combined severe hepatic and renal failure: a quantitative analysis. Int J Artif Organs. 2008;31:288–94.
61. Liskaser F, Story DA, Hayhoe M, et al. Effect of pump prime on acidosis, strong-ion-difference and unmeasured ions during cardiopulmonary bypass. Anaesth Intensive Care. 2009;37:767–72.

5 Skin, Soft Tissue, and Wound Healing in the Elderly

David G. Greenhalgh

In the industrialize world the birth rate is down, and with modern healthcare people are living longer so that the elderly are occupying a much larger percentage of the population. US census results reveal that in 2010, 24 % of the population was greater than 55 years of age, and 13 % was greater than 65 years of age. These values are projected to be 31.1 % >55 years, 20.2 % >65 years, and 4.3 % >85 years in 2050 [1]. All practitioners are going to be exposed to more geriatric patients, so familiarity with skin problems will become essential knowledge. Not only are the elderly at greater risk for skin breakdown but they also have skin changes that alter their ability to heal. Many treatments for diseases in the elderly (steroids, chemotherapy, and radiation) impair tissue repair. Chronic wounds – diabetic, vascular, venous stasis, and pressure ulcers – are much more common in the geriatric population. Chronic wounds are a huge economic burden for today's healthcare and for the individual; they frequently accompany the person for the rest of his or her life. Pressure ulcers are considered a "never event" by governmental health agencies that, if they occur, may lead to loss of reimbursement. Since simple injuries often lead to major wounds that fail to heal, prevention efforts are essential to reduce the burden of chronic wounds in the elderly. While there are increased problems with healing in the elderly, their wounds can be treated and lead to successful outcomes. This chapter will review the factors that increase the risks for wounds in the elderly, describe the pathophysiology of chronic wounds, and discuss prevention and describe strategies for treating those wounds.

D.G. Greenhalgh, MD, FACS
Department of Surgery, University of California, Davis Medical Center, Shriners Hospitals for Children Northern California, 2425 Stockton Blvd., Sacramento, CA 95817, USA
e-mail: david.greenhalgh@ucmdc.ucdavis.edu

Skin Changes with Aging

The skin changes related to aging are well documented in the dermatology literature [2–7]. Typically, skin alterations due to aging are classified into "intrinsic" and "extrinsic" changes. *Intrinsic* changes are those that occur "within the body" as part of the normal aging process and are independent of environmental exposure. *Extrinsic* changes are those alterations that are induced by environmental forces – most notably the ultraviolet portion of the sunlight. While it is difficult to differentiate which factors are totally intrinsic versus extrinsic, it is clear that extrinsic factors accelerate the degenerative changes in the skin. Everyone is aware of the changes that occur in skin that is abused by sun exposure or just poor self-care. The skin becomes thinner, dryer, more wrinkled, sags, and has variable pigment changes. Clearly, sun exposure increases the risks of skin cancers of all types. While these changes will occur with aging, good skin care, especially protection from the sun, will slow these changes.

The structural changes of skin that occur with aging are well documented. The epidermis tends to become thinner with aging but thickens in response to ultraviolet light damage. The dermal-epidermal junction becomes flatter. The flattening of the normal rete pegs of the dermal-epidermal junction weakens the resistance to epithelial shear. In other words, the elderly are more prone to superficial wounds from minor shear forces. There are also significant changes to the normal skin adnexa – hair follicles, oil glands, sebaceous glands, and other dermal appendages. Sebaceous glands are decreased which leads to more dryness of the skin. In addition, there is decreased replacement of lipids in the stratum corneum which interferes with the normal barrier function of the epidermis. Hair follicles clearly change in many parts of the body. They heal more slowly and change in distribution. Clearly, male and female alopecia (baldness) is the most recognizable hair change, but hair follicles increase in size and decrease in density [6].

J.A. Yelon, F.A. Luchette (eds.), *Geriatric Trauma and Critical Care*,
DOI 10.1007/978-1-4614-8501-8_5, © Springer Science+Business Media New York 2014

The significance of the dermal appendage changes is that healing of superficial wounds is impaired. To heal a partial-thickness wound (such as a superficial burn or blister), the dermal appendages are required. Normally, reepithelialization takes place in two areas of the skin, the edge of normal skin and from dermal appendages [8]. At the edge of the wound, the basal cells of the bottom layer of the epidermis are stimulated to migrate across the wound by three factors: loss of cell-cell contact, stimulation by growth factors (epidermal growth factor, transforming growth factor-α, and keratinocyte growth factors 1 and 2), and contact with proteins of the exposed wound (fibronectins, collagen type 1). Migration from the original wound edge stops after around 1–2 cm in a full-thickness wound, and the remainder of the closure is by contraction. In a superficial wound, epithelial migration also occurs in the epithelial cells of the dermal appendages, especially hair follicles. The higher the hair follicle density in a wound, the faster it can reepithelialize. As an example, if a hair-bearing scalp is used as a split-thickness skin graft donor site, it will heal within 4–5 days. If the skin adnexa are sparse in number, such as occurs in a lower leg with impaired circulation, then healing may take weeks. Thus, the problem with the decreased density of dermal appendages in the elderly is that their ability to reepithelialize a wound is impaired. I have observed very superficial wounds in a hairless, elderly patient that never reepithelialize and thus are said to "convert" to full-thickness. They did not "convert" but instead had no ability to reepithelialize.

There are significant dermal changes in the skin due to aging. The dermis is also the main target of ultraviolet light damage [2]. With increasing age there is a decrease in dermal cells (macrophages, fibroblasts, mast cells) and a decrease in antigen-presenting cells (Langerhans cells) which results in a decrease in the immune function. The dermis becomes thinner and the collagen becomes less organized. The collagen molecules actually become larger but have more fragmentation and less orientation along lines of stress. The activation of matrix metalloproteinases by ultraviolet light exposure may contribute to these collagen molecule changes. This degradation in collagen is reflected in studies which demonstrate that the tensile strength of skin is decreased with age [9]. The dermal hydration decreases, and while the amount of elastin changes little, it becomes more fragmented. Thus, skin becomes less elastic, more wrinkled, and more prone to tearing or lacerations. Everyone knows that with aging comes looser skin that sags with gravity. While looser skin is considered undesirable in our society, it does benefit the healing of the elderly with small full-thickness wounds. These wounds heal by contraction so that the loose skin tends to not interfere with this process as it would in a younger person. Tension tends to interfere with wound contraction, so the process may be augmented with looser skin. Clearly, contraction can lead to contractures if it occurs over functional areas such as joints. Since looser skin allows for closure with less tension, the elderly have a lower risk for contracture. In other words, allowing a wound to contract may be an alternative to surgical repair.

Besides the actual structural changes to the skin, there is a generalized decrease in sensation, decreased vascularity, and impaired lymph flow with aging. The sensory changes occur in a distal to proximal fashion and are especially related to decreased cold/warm sensory abilities [10]. There are actual decreases in the density of thermal sensory receptors, and some suggest that there is a decrease in peripheral nerve density. Studies suggest that there is altered angiogenesis associated with decreased cutaneous vascular reactivity [2–7]. In response to sun damage, there may be an increased angiogenic response, but the new vessels are more disorganized and more prone to leaking proteins. With impaired lymph flow there is an increase in edema – which impairs healing. In addition, impaired lymphatic function decreases the ability to fight infections or contract wounds. There are obvious pigment changes that occur in skin with aging. Melanocytes decrease in numbers, but with ultraviolet light exposure, there are more spotty areas of hyperpigmentation. Many cells develop mutations that alter local areas leading to "age spots" such as keratoses and nevi. While not covered in this review, skin cancers increase with aging. All of these changes are accelerated with sun exposure. In addition, increased bruisability from the use of antiplatelet drugs or anticoagulants will often lead to pigment changes from the retained heme products.

Finally, changes beneath the skin contribute to the risk of skin injury in the elderly. There is a tendency to lose muscle mass from either decreased exercise or activity. Fat stores are often (but not always) reduced with aging. These changes are clearly accelerated with malnutrition – a factor that impairs wound repair. The significance of these changes is that the loss of padding tends to expose bony prominences to increased pressure and chronic breakdown. Incontinence of urine or stool increases the risk for maceration which increases the risk of shear injury. As people age, they become slower in their ability to respond to a dangerous situation. Their reflexes tend be slower so that they have more difficulty escaping an injury. I have observed many elderly patients who were unable to extinguish flaming clothing or escape scalding water. This slowing of reflexes and an impaired ability to respond to injury lead to more extensive and deeper wounds. We know from burn studies that the elderly have a much lower ability to tolerate large wounds, so a small injury can be fatal. Finally, people at the extremes of ages become more dependent on others for care. An unfortunate consequence of this unwanted dependency is that there is an increase in the risk for elderly abuse. One must always be wary if an injury does not fit the "story" of how it occurred. Just as for children, caregivers are obligated to report suspected abuse.

Diseases of the Elderly Affecting Wound Healing

Fortunately, healing processes remain fairly normal in healthy people until the extremes of ages. Since many elderly take good care of themselves, they tolerate surgery and minor injuries quite well. It is important to recognize, however, the factors or diseases that impair tissue repair. These inhibitors of wound healing affect all age groups, but they are, unfortunately, more common in the elderly population. One must be aware of these factors that may delay or prevent healing if he or she is planning surgery or treating a wound.

Malnutrition

Studies have shown for over 100 years that malnutrition impairs wound healing [11–14]. The impairment exists with total protein/calorie (marasmus) malnutrition or with protein (kwashiorkor) malnutrition. Simply, if one holds nutritional support at the time of wounding, a marked impairment in tensile strength will result within 1–2 weeks [15]. The clinical significance of malnutrition relates to the risks of complications with surgery such that if a patient has lost weight from a malignancy or from an inability to eat, then there is a much higher risk for dehiscence. The hidden side of this healing impairment is that altered healing could lead to a bowel anastomosis leak which in turn, may lead to an abscess. Since the metabolic reserve is reduced in the elderly, this complication of failing to heal often leads to sepsis, multiple organ dysfunction syndrome, and ultimately death. The clinician can reduce complications by assessing the nutritional status of the elderly and providing supplemental nutrition prior to surgery. In addition, an aggressive approach to perioperative nutrition may make the difference between normal healing without complications and a rocky course and ultimate death.

There are some vitamins and micronutrients that influence tissue repair. Vitamin C is essential for the hydroxylation of proline or lysine in the formation of normal procollagen triple helices [16]. When there is a deficiency, collagen is not properly produced, and people may suffer from scurvy. Since there is a balance between collagen formation and breakdown during the maturation phase of scar formation, recently healed wounds may break down. In addition, vitamin A has been found to augment tissue repair [17, 18]. Several minerals such as zinc [19, 20] and copper [20] are essential for normal healing, and when they are deficient, problems may result. We have noted that patients with subnormal copper levels have impaired healing of their burn wounds [21]. A deficiency in arginine may also lead to altered tissue repair [22].

Diabetes Mellitus

Diabetes mellitus is a major cause of healing problems in people of all ages [23–25]. Since the disease is seen more commonly in the elderly, it is important to know its impact on tissue repair. Some statistics are important to emphasize its impact on the development of chronic wounds. Twenty percent of hospital admissions in diabetes are related to wound healing problems. Twenty-five percent of diabetic patients will have a foot ulcer during their lifetimes, and 50 % of all nontraumatic amputations are related to diabetes mellitus. A common scenario is that a diabetic patient will not notice a pebble in their shoe due to their impaired sensation. This will create a small wound that goes unnoticed, and eventually a wound is noticed and not properly treated. When the patient finally seeks care, the wound is infected with purulence tracking up the fascial planes of the foot. This patient often presents with cellulitis or invasive infection that leads to an amputation.

Even if a wound is detected early, tissue repair is significantly impaired. As an example, Margolis reviewed several clinical trials that tested treatments for diabetic ulcers [26]. He collected the "controls" which received "standard" treatment. What he found was that only 31 % healed within 20 weeks of aggressive therapy. It is likely that the two-thirds that did not heal stayed open for the remainder of their lives. There are several reasons why tissue repair is impaired in patients with diabetes mellitus [23–25]. First of all, *peripheral vascular disease* is increased in this population. Diabetics not only suffer from *macrovascular* disease but also from *microvascular* disease where there is thickening of the capillary basement membrane. This *microvascular* disease leads to impaired delivery of oxygen and nutrients from an increase in edema which impairs diffusion. This process also impairs leukocyte migration into the wound. If the patient suffers from renal disease, healing is inhibited further by *uremia* and its resulting edema [27].

The second factor that contributes to alter healing in diabetes mellitus is its tendency to cause peripheral *neuropathy*. Loss of sensation progresses from distal to proximal in the extremity so that the feet are usually involved first. As stated earlier, people with neuropathic feet do not sense injury, and thus minor injuries tend to worsen or go unrecognized by the patient. We have recently reviewed our 10-year experience with diabetics who burn their feet [28]. It is common for them to walk outside on hot pavement or try to warm their "cold" feet with hot water or by placing them near space heaters. We admitted 68 patients with thermal injury to their feet during that period, and the incidence is increasing. As for other types of diabetic wounds, the patients admitted for burns to their feet tended to have prolonged hospital stays and frequent graft failure. Another often unrecognized consequence of neuropathy is that the foot loses its normal feedback to maintain the arch. The foot thus tends to flatten which leads to increased pressure on the first or second metatarsal head. The classic diabetic foot ulcer is a wound that is on the plantar surface on the first or second metatarsal head. The final consequence of neuropathy is that with loss of normal sympathetic innervation, the skin loses its ability to sweat and thus tends to dry and crack. These cracks may then be a site for infection.

There is an increased risk for infection for wounds that form in the diabetic patient. It is well known that hyperglycemia leads to an impaired ability to fight local infection. There are also studies that suggest that leukocyte migration and function is impaired. The impaired ability to fight infections predisposes diabetics to a higher risk for amputation. In addition, there are several metabolic factors that may contribute to impair healing that are covered in other reviews [25, 29]. One interesting concept is that hyperglycemia may lead to deposition of glucose by-products known as advanced glycosylation end-products (AGES) in the tissues. There are "receptors for advanced glycosylation end-products" (RAGES) that detect these products of hyperglycemia and stimulate an inflammatory response. One theory is that activation of RAGES may lead to the chronic inflammatory state ("metabolic syndrome") of diabetes mellitus and obesity [30]. This chronic inflammatory state may also contribute to impaired tissue repair.

Since healing is so impaired in diabetic patients, it is essential that prevention efforts are made to prevent a wound from developing. The Wound Healing Society has published guidelines for the treatment and prevention of diabetic wounds [31, 32]. All clinicians who treat diabetes mellitus should discuss the risks of foot ulcers with their patients. Diabetics should inspect their feet daily and be extremely careful with the care of their nails. Podiatrists are extremely helpful in these matters. Diabetics with neuropathy should always wear well-fitted shoes and be especially vigilant after the first few days of wearing new shoes. Any new wound should be treated aggressively and early. People with diabetes mellitus should always avoid walking outside while barefoot and never warm their insensate feet with any heated agent. Once a wound develops, they should be treated with something that "off-loads" the pressure point on the wound (metatarsal head). "Total contact casts" have been found to be effective [33]. Studies suggest that topical growth factors or skin substitutes may be effective, but they are extremely costly [34–36]. Vascular disease should be treated if present. Unfortunately, our success with treating these wounds is only marginal, so prevention is essential.

Therapies That Alter Wound Healing

Wound healing involves the recruitment and rapid proliferation of many different cell types. It makes sense, then, that any drug that impairs rapid proliferation of cells alters tissue repair. Unfortunately, the strategy for dealing with many diseases includes suppressing the inflammatory response, which also requires rapid proliferation of cells. *Steroids* have been known for decades to impair tissue repair, and their use should be minimized if possible to allow for better healing [37, 38]. The treatment of cancer also involves the killing of rapidly proliferating malignant cells, so it is also obvious that *chemotherapy agents* [39, 40] or *radiation* [41, 42] impairs tissue repair. With the advent of neoadjuvant therapy (chemotherapy and/or radiation) combined with surgery, it is clear that one must be extremely careful with the healing of these patients. One must optimize their nutritional status if they are to undergo these combined treatments. There are very few agents that augment healing in these situations, but vitamin A has been shown to at least partially reverse impairments due to steroids or radiation [17, 18]. Growth factors may also play a role in improving healing, but these are based on animal studies [43–49].

Neurologic Diseases

Neurologic diseases do not impair wound healing, but they do predispose the elderly to the risk of developing wounds. Dementia leads to forgetfulness and risky behavior that may lead to injury. The person may forget to turn off stoves or fail to practice safe techniques for self-care. People with dementia have a more difficult time with cleanliness and maintaining a diet and thus may not clean wounds and tend to be more malnourished. Neuropathies have previously been mentioned as a risk for many types of wounds. Any loss of sensation clearly predisposes a person to pressure sores since pain is the main warning sign of chronic pressure. Tremors may predispose the elderly to spills and an inability to quickly react to a dangerous situation. Incontinence may lead to maceration of the skin which in turn increases the risks for abrasions or tears with moving. Seizures are risky in people who cook or are around hot items since during the seizure, they will not react to an injury. People who seize while cooking or bathing frequently sustain very deep burns.

Problem Wounds of the Elderly

There are specific types of wounds that all practitioners must know about when treating the elderly. These wounds are relatively easy to prevent but are particularly difficult to treat once they are present. These chronic wounds are a significant burden to society in cost and interference with normal living. They may occur in any age group, but they are more common in the elderly. Since they are a major contributor to morbidity in the elderly, one must know how to diagnose and treat these problem wounds. The Wound Healing Society has recently published consensus guidelines in the prevention and treatment of these problem wounds which provide hundreds of references [50–55].

Pressure Ulcers

Pressure ulcers may develop at any age, but they are commonly manifested in the elderly as they develop reduced ability to move or after the development of neuropathy [50, 51, 56]. These wounds are found in around 10 % of inpatients. The pathophysiology is simple; any pressure on the skin and underlying tissues of greater than 30 mmHg that persists for a prolonged period of time can lead to enough ischemia to create a pressure ulcer. Normally, pressure produces pain which leads to a shift in the body to redistribute the pressure to another area. When we sleep we are constantly and subconsciously moving. Even intoxicated people will move to prevent these wounds. When people lose sensation, such as after paralysis, or when so ill that they are unable to move (such as in an intensive care unit), they are prone to pressure ulcers. Nurses play a major prevention role by repositioning patients from side to side. Not uncommonly, however, pressure ulcers develop where bony prominences create pressure. The classic sites are in the presacral region, the occiput, and on the heels. There are scoring systems that grade the severity of pressure ulcers that are useful for documentation. Pressure ulcers are staged as 1 when the skin is intact but just reddened for a prolonged period, 2 when the skin has been broken, 3 when the ulcer has become full-thickness, and 4 when the wound involves deeper tissues [56, 57]. The wound management becomes more difficult with increasing severity. The usefulness of this paradigm, however, has been recently challenged [58]. It is unclear of the relevance of a stage 1 ulcer, and the pathophysiology varies between stage 2 and stage 3 or 4 ulcers. Stage 2 ulcers occur because of damage from the "outside in" and higher-staged ulcers produced from the "inside out." Despite these limitations, the staging system is helpful for documentation and management strategies.

The factors that predispose the healthy elderly patient to pressure ulcers include the loss of padding with aging, malnutrition, loss of sensation, thinner skin, and incontinence. People with more fat are slightly more protected from development of skin breakdown. Like all wounds, prevention is essential with frequent repositioning of the patient, frequent inspection, maintaining normal nutrition, preventing maceration, and getting people out of bed. The Braden Score is the most commonly used screening method to determine the risk for pressure ulcers [59]. The score is based on six parameters: sensory perception, moisture, activity, mobility, nutrition, and friction/shear. Pressure ulcers have become such an important issue that they have been declared a "never event" that requires documentation and monitoring in hospitals. The Centers for Medicare and Medicaid Services (CMS) has set up guidelines that result in fines of up to $10,000 per day if compliance is lacking. As noted above, once a pressure ulcer develops, it is very difficult to heal. Clearly, one must eliminate pressure from that area, but it is often difficult to prevent people from bearing weight on bony protuberances. Studies suggest that growth factors may improve healing of pressure ulcers [60, 61]. Frequently, plastic surgeons will perform rotation flaps to try to cover these wounds, but once they develop they have a high incidence of recurrence.

Arterial Insufficiency Ulcers

These ulcers are the result of ischemia that results from vascular insufficiency [52, 53]. In fact, pure arterial insufficiency ulcers are rare, but usually tissue hypoxia contributes to the failure to heal in wounds caused by other etiologies. It is clear that hypoxia leads to impaired tissue repair. Since peripheral vascular disease is a major problem in the elderly (around 30 % of people over 75 years), it is important to remember that if a wound lacks blood supply (or oxygen), it will not heal. One of the major indicators for operating on peripheral vascular disease is for a "limb at risk" from failing to heal a wound. The elderly should have a proper assessment of their pulses if they have a wound that does not heal. Other signs of peripheral vascular disease include loss of hair, shiny and dry skin, mummified or black toes, devitalized soft tissue with a moist or dry crust, thickened toenails, purple skin color with dependency, and cool skin. As a general rule, if the region around the wound has a transcutaneous partial pressure of oxygen ($PtcO_2$) less than 40 mmHg, there will be difficulty with healing. If the level drops below 20 mmHg, then healing will not occur. Revascularization will often remedy this situation and allow for healing. All lower extremity wounds must be assessed for an adequate blood supply in order to treat them. Simple ankle/branchial indices are useful, but the assistance of Doppler studies is also beneficial. Vascular surgeons are experts in the evaluation and treatment of peripheral vascular disease and should be consulted as necessary (see Chap. 18). Prevention of arterial ulcers really involves all of the standard means of reducing atherosclerosis – cessation of smoking, reducing hyperlipidemia, exercise, and others. Unfortunately, once one leg requires revascularization of an ulcer, then there is a 20 % chance of the other leg developing an arterial insufficiency ulcer [62].

Venous Stasis Disease

These wounds are not a sole problem of the elderly but are important to discuss in this chapter. Advanced venous disease, manifested by edema, pigment changes (lipodermatosclerosis), and ulceration, affects 2.5 million people per year in the United States and cost around three billion dollars in 1997 healthcare dollars [54, 55, 63–66]. The pathophysiology for these ulcers is venous valvular insufficiency that usually results from deep venous thrombosis. The classic venous stasis ulcer occurs above the medial malleolus with a surrounding hyperpigmented region. As for all venous insufficiency, edema contributes to the problem. With a column of blood coursing from the heart to the feet while standing, there is a large amount of venous pressure that tends to interfere with capillary blood flow. The resulting increase in hydrostatic pressure leads to increased capillary leak and more edema. Any edema creates a greater distance for nutrients to diffuse from the capillaries to the cells and an increased risk for local hypoxia. Local capillary leaks tend to deposit fibrin which may lead to further hypoxia and impaired nutrient delivery or may "trap" leukocytes leading to persistent inflammation. The actual mechanism creating the cutaneous wound is not clearly known. There are many theories that need to be proven or disproven [67].

Venous ulcers tend to increase with advancing age but may occur in younger age groups with venous insufficiency. Once the ulcer develops it can be healed, but since the underlying venous hypertension persists, it tends to recur. Treatment is conceptually simple. The leg must be elevated to reduce venous pressure and edema. Compression plays a major role in healing by reducing edema. The "Unna boot" (fine mesh gauze with calamine lotion and zinc oxide) has been used with some success for years. Clinical studies suggest that growth factors [68–70] and biologic skin substitutes [71, 72] may help with closure, but there is no current treatment that has reduced recurrences. Surgery that interferes with venous backflow ("subfascial endoscopic perforator surgery") may be helpful [73, 74]. What is needed is some way of repairing venous valves, but this has not yet been accomplished.

Prevention

It is clear that prevention is by far better than treating a wound in the elderly. It is interesting that teaching prevention is helpful, but despite understanding prevention principles, people often do not follow them. People often take shortcuts or risks that lead to injury. The most effective prevention means is through regulations and legislation. Many laws have saved thousands of lives. An example is the law that requires all buildings to have smoke detectors. Voluntary efforts were only moderately successful in reducing fire-related deaths, but with the introduction of regulations requiring smoke detector use, deaths from fires have decreased markedly. The legislative efforts to reduce chronic wounds really do not exist. The intention of making pressure sores a "never event" that is reportable should at least make hospital personnel more aware of the risks of pressure sores. I am very doubtful that they will be eliminated.

Prevention efforts for the elderly should include close monitoring for the maintenance of adequate nutrition. Education and training about dangerous behaviors will also help. Their living environment should be made as safe as possible to reduce falls, the risk for burns, and other injuries. As the elderly lose the ability to manage themselves, especially with dementia, caregivers should be provided to at least monitor their well-being. The elderly must be educated that their reflexes may be slower so that they are less able to respond to a dangerous situation. I have treated many elderly patients who have placed logs onto fires "just as they had for years," but due to a slower response time, they could not react in time to prevent their clothes from catching on fire. Simple matters such as avoiding loose clothing over flames may reduce injury. Lowering water heater temperatures to 120 °F will prevent many accidental scald burns. As stated earlier, those people with neuropathies should have their feet checked on a regular basis. Simple actions such as these may prevent many lifelong wounds and potentially reduce deaths.

Outcomes for Wounds in the Elderly

It is known that the metabolic reserve of a person decreases with increasing age. This fact is best demonstrated in people with burns. The size of the burn wound that leads to a 50 % mortality based on age (LD50) decreases markedly with aging. A 15-year-old has a 50 % chance of surviving an 85 % total body surface area burn. However, the size of the cutaneous wound that leads to the "LD50" decreases rapidly with increasing age. The wound size that leads to a 50 % survival drops to 10–12 % in the elderly (>75 years). The likely reason for this inability to handle a large wound with increasing age is because the body has a decreased ability to handle the increased metabolic demand. It is as if the cells are "running on limited fuel" in the later stages of life. Clearly, the heart has a decreased ability to increase cardiac output compared to a teenager, and the same is true for other organ response to the injury. What this means is that a relatively minor wound may be the start of a cascade of complications leading to multiple organ failure and ultimately death. It is for all these reasons that prevention is so important.

Fortunately, people are taking better care of themselves, and more people are living to the 80s, 90s, and even over 100 years old. One must not assume that all individuals are the same at the same age. We all know relatively young people who have maintained their health and appear "older" than their stated age. There are just as many elderly who have lived well with managing their fitness. We have treated older patients who have tolerated moderate-sized burns who have done amazingly well. The elderly who have been able to avoid many of the risk factors for impaired healing (diabetes, peripheral vascular disease, malignancy) tend to be able to tolerate significant injuries. It is clear that with sound surgical principles of treating wounds, the elderly can heal their wounds with minimal disability.

References

1. U.S. Census Bureau. Statistical abstract of the United States. 2012. http://www.census.gov/compendia/statab/2012/tables/12s0009.pdf. Accessed 28 June 2012.
2. Gosain A, DiPietro LA. Aging and wound healing. World J Surg. 2004;28:321–6.
3. Zouboulis CC, Makrantonaki E. Clinical aspects and molecular diagnostics of skin aging. Clin Dermatol. 2011;29:3–14.
4. Ramos-e-Silva M, Boza JC, Cestari TF. Effects of age (neonates and elderly) on skin barrier function. Clin Dermatol. 2012;30:274–6.
5. Wulf HC, Sandby-Moller J, Kobayasi T, Gniadecki R. Skin aging and natural photoprotection. Micron. 2004;35:185–91.
6. Birch MP, Messenger JF, Messenger AG. Hair density, hair diameter and the prevalence of female pattern hair loss. Br J Dermatol. 2001;144:297–304.
7. Sharma R. Skin age testing criteria: characterization of human skin structures by 500 MHz MRI multiple contrast and image processing. Phys Med Biol. 2010;55:3959–79.
8. Greenhalgh DG. Chapter 46. Wound healing. In: Herndon D, editor. Total burn care. 3rd ed. Edinburgh: Saunders Elsevier, Inc; 2007. p. 578–95.
9. Sussman MD. Aging of connective tissue: physiologic properties of healing wounds in young and old rats. Am J Physiol. 1973;224:1167–71.
10. Guergova S, Dufour A. Thermal sensitivity in the elderly: a review. Ageing Res Rev. 2011;10:80–92.
11. Howes EL, Briggs H, Shea R. Effect of complete and partial starvation on the rate of fibroplasia in the healing wound. Arch Surg. 1933;26:846–58.
12. Rhoads JE, Fliegelman MT, Panzer LM. The mechanism of delayed wound healing in the presence of hypoproteinemia. JAMA. 1942;118:21–5.
13. Daly JM, Vars HM, Dudvich SJ. Effects of protein depletion on strength of colonic anastomoses. Surg Gynecol Obstet. 1972;134:15–21.
14. Irvin TT. Effects of malnutrition and hyperalimentation on wound healing. Surg Gynecol Obstet. 1978;146:33–7.
15. Greenhalgh DG, Gamelli RL. Immunomodulators and wound healing. J Trauma. 1987;27:510–4.
16. Bartlett MK, Jones CM, Ryan AE. Vitamin C and wound healing. I. Experimental wounds in guinea pigs. N Engl J Med. 1942;226:469–73.
17. Ehrlich HP, Hunt TK. Effects of cortisone and vitamin A on wound healing. Ann Surg. 1968;167:324–8.
18. Levenson SM, Gruber CA, Rettura G, Gruber DK, Demetriou AA, Seifter E. Supplemental vitamin A prevents the acute radiation-induced defect in wound healing. Ann Surg. 1984;200:494–512.
19. Pories WJ. Acceleration of healing with zinc oxide. Ann Surg. 1967;165:432–6.
20. Pinnell SR, Martin GR. The cross linking of collagen and elastin. Proc Natl Acad Sci U S A. 1968;61:708–14.
21. Liusuwan RA, Palmieri T, Warden N, Greenhalgh DG. Impaired healing due to copper deficiency in a pediatric burn: a case report. J Trauma. 2006;51:464–6.
22. Seifter E, Rettura G, Barbul A, Levenson SM. Arginine: an essential amino acid for injured rats. Surgery. 1978;84:224–30.
23. McMurry Jr JF. Wound healing with diabetes mellitus. Surg Clin North Am. 1984;64:769–78.
24. Goodson III WH, Hunt TK. Wound healing and the diabetic patient. Surg Gynecol Obstet. 1979;149:600–8.
25. Greenhalgh DG. Wound healing and diabetes mellitus. Clin Plast Surg. 2003;30:37–45.
26. Margolis DJ, Kantor J, Berlin JA. Healing of diabetic neuropathic foot ulcers receiving standard treatment. A meta-analysis. Diabetes Care. 1999;22:692–5.
27. Yue DK, McLennan S, Marsh M, Mai YW, Spaliviero J, Delbridge L, et al. Effects of experimental diabetes, uremia, and malnutrition on wound healing. Diabetes. 1987;36:295–9.
28. Barsun A, Sen S, Palmieri TL, Greenhalgh DG. A ten year review of lower extremity burns in diabetics: small burns that lead to major problems. J Burn Care Res. 2013;34(2):255–60.
29. Kamal K, Powell RJ, Sumpio BE. The pathobiology of diabetes mellitus: implications for surgeons. J Am Coll Surg. 1996;183:271–89.
30. Medzhitov R. Origin and physiological roles of inflammation. Nature. 2008;454:428–35.
31. Steed DL, Attinger C, Colaizzi T, Crossland M, Franz M, Harkless L, et al. Guidelines for the treatment of diabetic ulcers. Wound Repair Regen. 2006;14:680–92.
32. Steed DL, Attinger C, Brem H, Colaizzi T, Crossland M, Franz M, et al. Guidelines for the prevention of diabetic ulcers. Wound Repair Regen. 2008;16:169–74.
33. Armstrong DG, Nguyen HC, Lavery LA, van Schie CH, Boulton AJ, Harkless LB. Off-loading the diabetic foot: a randomized clinical trial. Diabetes Care. 2001;24:1019–22.
34. Steed DL, The Diabetic Ulcer Study Group. Clinical evaluation of recombinant human platelet-derived growth factor for the treatment of lower extremity diabetic ulcers. J Vasc Surg. 1995;21:71–81.
35. Embil JM, Papp K, Sibbald G, Tousignant J, Smiell JM, Wong B, Lau CY. Recombinant human platelet-derived growth factor-BB (becaplermin) for healing chronic lower extremity diabetic ulcers: an open-label clinical evaluation of efficacy. Wound Repair Regen. 2000;8:162–8.
36. Veves A, Falanga V, Armstrong DG, Sabolinski ML. Graftskin, a human skin equivalent, is effective in the management of noninfected neuropathic diabetic foot ulcers: a prospective, randomized multicenter clinical trial. Diabetes Care. 2001;24:290–5.
37. Howes EL, Plotz CM, Blunt JW, Ragan C. Retardation of wound healing by cortisone. Surgery. 1950;28:177–81.
38. Sandberg N. Time relationship between administration of cortisone and wound healing in rats. Acta Chir Scand. 1964;127:446–55.
39. Ferguson MK. The effects of antineoplastic agents on wound healing. Surg Gynecol Obstet. 1982;154:421–9.
40. Falcone RE, Napp JF. Chemotherapy and wound healing. Surg Clin North Am. 1984;64:779–95.
41. Reinisch JF, Puckett CL. Management of radiation wounds. Surg Clin North Am. 1984;64:795–802.
42. Luce EA. The irradiated wound. Surg Clin North Am. 1984;64:821–9.
43. Laato M, Heino J, Kahari VM, Niinikoski J, Gerdin B. Epidermal growth factor (EGF) prevents methylprednisolone-induced inhibition of wound healing. J Surg Res. 1989;47:354–9.
44. Pierce GF, Mustoe TA, Lingelbach J, Masakowski VR, Gramates P, Deuel TF. Transforming growth factor β reverses the glucocorticoid-induced wound healing deficit in rats: possible regulation in macrophages by platelet-derived growth factor. Proc Natl Acad Sci U S A. 1989;86:2229–33.
45. Beck LS, DeGuzman L, Lee WP, Xu Y, McFatridge LA, Amento EP. TGF-β1 accelerates wound healing: reversal of steroid-impaired healing in rats and rabbits. Growth Factors. 1991;5:295–300.

46. Lawrence WT, Sporn MB, Gorschboth C, Gorschboth C, Grotendorst GR. The reversal of an Adriamycin induced healing impairment with chemoattractants and growth factors. Ann Surg. 1986;203:142–7.
47. Mustoe TA, Purdy J, Gramates P, Deuel TF, Thomason A, Pierce GF. Reversal of impaired wound healing in irradiated rats by platelet-derived growth factor-BB. Am J Surg. 1989;158: 345–50.
48. Bernstein EF, Harisiadis L, Saloman G, Norton J, Sollberg S, Uitto J, et al. Transforming growth factor beta improves healing of radiation-impaired wounds. J Invest Dermatol. 1991;97:430–4.
49. Tattini C, Manchio J, Zaporojan V, Carderelli G, Bonassar L, Spangenberger A, Weinzbweig J. The role of TGF-β and FGF in the treatment of radiation-induced wounds using a novel drug delivery system. Plast Reconstr Surg. 2008;122:1036–45.
50. Whitney J, Phillips L, Aslam R, Barbul A, Gottrup F, Gould L, et al. Guidelines for the treatment of pressure ulcers. Wound Repair Regen. 2006;14:663–79.
51. Stechmiller JK, Cowan L, Whitney J, Phillips L, Aslam R, Barbul A, et al. Guidelines for the prevention of pressure ulcers. Wound Repair Regen. 2008;16:151–68.
52. Hopf HW, Ueno C, Aslam R, Burnard K, Fife C, Grant L, et al. Guidelines for the treatment of arterial insufficiency ulcers. Wound Repair Regen. 2006;14:693–710.
53. Hopf HW, Ueno C, Aslam R, Dardik A, Fife C, Grant L, et al. Guidelines for the prevention of arterial insufficiency ulcers. Wound Repair Regen. 2008;16:175–88.
54. Robson MC, Cooper DM, Aslam R, Gould LJ, Harding KG, Margolis DJ, et al. Guidelines for the treatment of venous ulcers. Wound Repair Regen. 2006;14:649–62.
55. Robson MC, Cooper DM, Aslam R, Gould LJ, Harding KG, Margolis DJ, et al. Guidelines for the prevention of venous ulcers. Wound Repair Regen. 2008;16:147–50.
56. Lyder CH. Pressure ulcer prevention and management. JAMA. 2003;289:223–6.
57. Bluestein D, Javaheri A. Pressure ulcers: prevention, evaluation, and management. Am Fam Physician. 2008;78:1186–94.
58. Sibbald RG, Krasner DL, Woo KY. Pressure ulcer staging revisited: superficial skin changes & deep pressure ulcer framework. Adv Skin Wound Care. 2011;24:571–80.
59. Braden BJ, Bergstrom NA. Clinical utility of the Braden scale for predicting pressure sore risk. Decubitus. 1989;2:44–51.
60. Mustoe TA, Cutler NR, Allman RM, Goode PS, Deuel TF, Prause JA, et al. A phase II study to evaluate recombinant platelet-derived growth factor-BB in the treatment of stage 3 and 4 pressure ulcers. Arch Surg. 1994;129:213–9.
61. Rees RS, Robson MC, Smiell JM, Perry BH. Becaplermin gel in the treatment of pressure ulcers: a phase II randomized double-blind, placebo-controlled study. Wound Repair Regen. 1999;7: 141–7.
62. Tarry WC, Walsh DB, Birkmeyer NJO, Fillinger MF, Zwolak RM, Cronenwett JL. Fate of the contralateral leg after infrainguinal bypass. J Vasc Surg. 1998;27:1039–48.
63. Gillespie DL. Venous ulcer diagnosis, treatment, and prevention of recurrences. J Vasc Surg. 2010;52:8S–14.
64. Robertson LEC, Fowkes F. Epidemiology of chronic venous disease. Phlebology. 2008;23:103–11.
65. Ruckley CV. Socioeconomic impact of chronic venous insufficiency and leg ulcers. Angiology. 1997;48:67–9.
66. Van den Oever RHB, Debbaut B, Simon I. Socio-economic impact of chronic venous insufficiency: an underestimated public health problem. Int Angiol. 1998;17:161–7.
67. Liu YC, Margolis DJ, Isseroff RR. Does inflammation have a role in the pathogenesis of venous ulcers? A critical review of the evidence. J Invest Dermatol. 2011;131:818–27.
68. DaCosta RM, Ribeiro J, Aniceto C, Mendes M. Randomized, double-blind, placebo-controlled, dose-ranging study of granulocyte-macrophage colony-stimulating factor in patients with chronic venous ulcers. Wound Repair Regen. 1999;7:17–25.
69. Falanga V, Eaglstein WH, Bucalo B, Katz MH, Harris B, Carson P. Topical use of human recombinant epidermal growth factor (h-EGF) in venous ulcers. J Dermatol Surg Oncol. 1992;18:604–6.
70. Robson MC, Phillips LG, Cooper DM, Odenheimer DJ, Parish LC, Jensen JL, Steed DL. The safety and effect of transforming growth factor-B2 for treatment of venous stasis ulcers. Wound Repair Regen. 1995;3:157–67.
71. Falanga V, Margolis D, Alvarez O, Auletta M, Maggiacomo F, Altman M. Rapid healing of venous ulcers and the lack of clinical rejection with an allogeneic cultured human skin equivalent. Human Skin Equivalent Investigators Group. Arch Dermatol. 1998;134:293–300.
72. Atillasoy E. The safety and efficacy of Graftskin (Apligraf) in the treatment of venous leg ulcers: a multicenter, randomized, controlled clinical trial. Wounds. 2000;12(Suppl A):20A–6.
73. Pierik EG, van Urk H, Hop WC, Wittens CH. Endoscopic versus open subfascial division of incompetent perforating veins in the treatment of venous leg ulceration: a randomized trial. J Vasc Surg. 1997;26:1049–54.
74. Sybrandy JE, van Gent WB, Pierik EG, Wittens CH. Endoscopic versus open subfascial division of incompetent perforating veins in the treatment of venous leg ulceration: long-term follow-up. J Vasc Surg. 2001;33:1028–32.

Immunologic

6

Jeffrey A. Claridge and Aman Banerjee

Introduction

The immune system is comprised of two mutually dependent cellular lines: an innate system and adaptive system. The innate system is the host's first line of defense and is largely responsible for orchestrating the appropriate response for a given pathogen. It consists of neutrophils, monocytes, dendritic cells, and natural killer cells. The adaptive system consists of B cells and T cells. These cells interact with the products of the innate immune system to recognize new pathogens, undergo clonal expansion, combat a multitude of pathogens, and revert to memory cells which can be reactivated rapidly upon reinfection. A decline in immune function with aging is shown in Table 6.1.

Aging of the Innate Immune System

Neutrophil

Neutrophils play a critical role in the acute inflammatory host response. These short-lived phagocytic cells are recruited from the peripheral blood via a gradient of chemokines and cytokines produced locally at the site of infection. Aging per se does not have a known affect on the number of neutrophils in the blood or the number of neutrophil precursors in the bone marrow [1]. Despite their preserved quantity most other aspects of neutrophil function are diminished such as phagocytosis and the generation of reactive oxygen species [2, 3]. There is conflicting data on the effect of aging on chemotaxis with some studies showing no effect [4, 5] and others demonstrating decreased chemotaxis [6–8].

J.A. Claridge, MD, MS, FACS (✉)
Department of Surgery, Division of Trauma, Critical Care, Burns, and Acute Care Surgery, MetroHealth Medical Center, Room H938A, Hamann Bldg 2500 MetroHealth Drive, Cleveland, OH 44109, USA

Northern Ohio Trauma System, Cleveland, OH, USA

Department of Surgery, Case Western Reserve University School of Medicine, Cleveland, OH, USA

Department of Surgery, MetroHealth Medical Center, Room H938A, Hamann Bldg 2500 MetroHealth Drive, Cleveland, OH 44109, USA
e-mail: jclaridge@metrohealth.org

A. Banerjee, MD
Department of Surgery, MetroHealth Medical Center, Room H938A, Hamann Bldg 2500 MetroHealth Drive, Cleveland, OH 44109, USA
e-mail: aman.banerjee@gmail.com

Table 6.1 Impact of aging on the immune system

Innate
Macrophage
Reduced phagocytic activity
Reduced generation of nitric oxide
Reduced generation of superoxide
Neutrophil
Reduced phagocytic activity
Reduced generation of superoxide
Dendritic cells
Reduced pinocytosis and endocytosis activity
Reduced phagocytosis of apoptotic cells
Impaired cellular migration
Natural killer cells
Increased total cell number
Reduced cytotoxic ability
Reduced cell proliferation after interleukin-2 exposure
Cytokines
Increased production of interleukin-6
Increased production of TNF-α
Increased production of IL-1β
Adaptive
T cells
Reduced naïve cell population
Increased memory cell population
B cells
Reduced antibody isotype switching
Reduced dendritic cell stimulation
Reduced naïve cell population
Increased memory cell population

J.A. Yelon, F.A. Luchette (eds.), *Geriatric Trauma and Critical Care*,
DOI 10.1007/978-1-4614-8501-8_6, © Springer Science+Business Media New York 2014

Macrophages

Macrophages have many integral functions in the innate immune system. They function as sentinels for microbes in tissue; through the release of effector molecules, they orchestrate the adaptive immune response and play an essential role in wound healing. Macrophages function as first responders to invading microbes. They reside in numerous tissues, such as Kupffer cells in the liver, microglia in the brain, osteoclasts in the bone, and undifferentiated monocytes in the blood. They detect pathogens by recognizing specific pathogen-associated molecular patterns (PAMPs) present on the microbes. They phagocytize invading bacteria, fungi, parasites, protozoa, and apoptotic cells and destroy them via both oxygen-dependent and oxygen-independent pathways [9].

Although the number of circulating blood monocytes in elderly and young subjects is similar, there is a significant decrease in macrophage precursors and macrophages in the bone marrow [10]. Macrophages in the elderly have reduced levels of MHC class II, which may contribute to poorer T-cell responses [11]. The macrophage's phagocytic function and its chemotactic ability are also diminished with age [12, 13]. Additionally, the ability of aged macrophages to destroy microbes via products of the respiratory burst is diminished; this impaired bactericidal capacity may increase the duration of infection in the elderly [14].

Natural Killer Cells

Natural killer cells (NK) are responsible for destroying host cells that have been compromised by tumor or viral infection. The number of NK cells increases with age; however, cytolytic activity and production of interferon-γ are decreased [15]. NK cells kill cells directly by releasing perforin and granzymes which activate caspases that induce apoptosis. The loss of cytotoxic ability is thought to occur as the result of decreased perforin secretion and production [16, 17]. Clinically, these NK cell deficits can result in an increased risk of infection, morbidity, and mortality in elderly patients [3, 18].

Dendritic Cells

Dendritic cells serve as a bridge between the innate and adaptive immune systems. Acting as antigen-presenting cells they capture microbes through phagocytosis, process extracellular and intracellular antigens, and migrate to lymphoid tissue to stimulate T cells. Dendritic cells also have a regulatory function as demonstrated by their production of type I interferons in response to viral infection and the TNF-α inducible nitric oxide synthase (iNOS) production to defend against bacterial infection [19, 20]. In addition to eliciting immune response, dendritic cells also provoke immunological tolerance by inducing deletion or anergy, thereby limiting autoimmunity [21, 22].

Aging dendritic cells generated from peripheral blood monocytes have been shown to be deficient in pinocytosis and endocytosis when presented with an antigen challenge [23]. Additionally, dendritic cells from aged patients have an impaired capacity to phagocytose apoptotic cells compared to those of younger patients. These cells also display impaired migration [24]. Phagocytosis of apoptotic cells produces an anti-inflammatory effect by inhibiting proinflammatory cytokines [25]. Clinically, the impaired uptake and inefficient removal of apoptotic cells by dendritic cells from aged patients may result in the inflammation and autoimmunity commonly seen with aging [12, 24].

Aging of the Adaptive Immune System

T Lymphocytes

T lymphocytes, also known as T cells, play a central role in cell-mediated immunity. These cells recognize and eliminate cells that have undergone viral or malignant transformation. T cells are differentiated from B cells and natural killer cells by their expression of a T-cell receptor (TCR) on their surface membrane; this receptor binds to antigen and CD3. Progenitor cells from the bone marrow migrate to the thymus where they undergo a highly selective elimination process based on the ability of the cell's TCR to recognize major histocompatibility proteins, degree of affinity for normal self antigens, and the magnitude and duration of TCR signaling [26]. There are primarily two types of naïve T cells that leave the thymus: CD4+ helper cells and CD8+ cytotoxic T cells.

T-cell responses are initiated in secondary lymphoid tissues by exposure to dendritic cells that present antigen. T cells that possess the specific antigen are then induced to proliferate and differentiate into effector cells that reenter the circulation from the lymph system and disseminate to the site of infection. After the infection is eradicated, the vast majority of the effector cells are destroyed with only a few cells remaining as long-lived memory cells [27].

Thymus involution reaches its maximal level at age 50. This involves the replacement of the lymphoid component and epithelial matrix of the thymus with fibrous and adipose tissue [28]. The net result of these changes is that generation of naïve T cells is severely compromised beginning at the age of 40 years [29–31]. Additionally, there is also a loss of diversity as a substantial shift from naïve T cell to memory T cell occurs, especially after age 65 for CD8+ T cells. Naïve CD4+ T-cell numbers are well maintained until age 70 after which their numbers begin to contract [32]. Elderly patients tend to rely on memory T cells for their primary T-cell response, which may result in compromised immune response following vaccination [33, 34].

B Lymphocytes

B lymphocytes, or B cells, mature in the bone marrow and function in the humoral immune response. During B-cell development genetic rearrangement of immunoglobulin light and heavy chains occurs to produce the antigen-binding region of the B-cell receptor (membrane-bound immunoglobulin). B cells that react with self-antigen are removed by a process of apoptosis or inactivation in the bone marrow [35]. At this point the B cell enters the peripheral blood and lymph circulation as mature naïve B cells, where antigen activation occurs. Further differentiation is dependent on activation by antigen and signaling from helper T cells [36]. Mature naïve B cells can become either plasma cells, which produce and secrete large quantities of antibodies or memory B cells, which are long-lived cells capable of responding to reactivation by the same antigen.

While the number of precursor B cells and peripheral B cells does not decline with aging, there is a shift toward more antigen-experienced B cells and fewer naïve B cells [37, 38]. There is also a diminished ability for antibody isotype switching resulting in a shift in antibody isotype from IgG to IgM [39]. Isotype switching maintains the same antigen specificity but changes the effector functions of the antibody. Additionally, B cells in elderly patients are less efficiently stimulated by dendritic cells than younger patients due to their relative deficiency in the expression of co-stimulatory molecules CD40 and CD27 [40, 41]. The net effect of these changes is that elderly patients are forced to rely on a B-cell repertoire which lacks optimal diversity and have a low affinity to antigens and are therefore less protective [42].

Inflamm-Aging: Age-Related Subclinical Chronic Inflammation

The aging immune system is characterized by a low-grade, chronic systemic inflammatory state sometimes referred to as "inflamm-aging" [43]. With aging, there is an increased production of proinflammatory cytokines such as interleukin 6 (IL-6), tumor necrosis factor-alpha (TNF-α), and IL-1β [44–47]. This subclinical inflammation may be caused by chronic stimulation of the innate immune system or by the inability of the immune system to eliminate certain pathogens [12].

Increased IL-6 levels are associated with lower muscle mass and strength in healthy elderly adults [48, 49]. Elevated levels of IL-6 and TNF-α have been shown to be associated with increased disability and mortality in community-dwelling elderly adults [48, 50, 51] and an overall increased inflammatory state.

Risk Factors for Infection

Chronic Obstructive Pulmonary Disorder (COPD)

The prevalence of COPD in the US population varies from 2.9 to 14.3 % depending on how COPD is defined [52]. COPD is characterized by airflow obstruction associated with chronic cough, dyspnea on exertion, wheezing, and expectoration [53]. It is the 4th cause of death for all patients 65 and older [54]. The causative agents associated with COPD are cigarette smoking, biomass exposure, and the resulting inflammatory response orchestrated by neutrophils, macrophages, and CD8+ T cells [55]. Exacerbations are common and become more frequent with increasing disease severity [56]. COPD has been shown to be an independent risk factor for developing pneumonia and pulmonary complications after thoracic surgery [57, 58]. Mucosal lesions of the tracheobronchial tree in the presence of mucous hypersecretion promote bacterial adhesion, colonization, and growth that then impede mucociliary clearance. These changes in the histology of the airway in patients with COPD increase the risk for pneumonia [59, 60].

The majority of cases of community-acquired pneumonia (CAP) in COPD patients are caused by *Streptococcus pneumoniae*, followed by *Chlamydia pneumoniae*, *Haemophilus influenzae*, *Legionella pneumophila*, *Streptococcus viridans*, *Coxiella burnetii*, and *Mycoplasma pneumoniae* [61]. COPD patients hospitalized with CAP have higher 30-day and 90-day mortality rates compared to patients without COPD [62].

Additionally, a study of elderly patients older than 65 years undergoing elective surgery for diverticulitis found that patients with COPD had significantly increased odds of developing pulmonary complications (OR 2.2, 95 % CI 1.94–2.50) that were associated with increased morbidity and mortality [63].

Diabetes Mellitus

Increasing age and diabetes work in concert to further weaken an elderly patient's response to infections. Diabetes is known to increase the risk of surgical site infection (SSI) and nosocomial infections [64–69]. These infectious complications occur in 20–23 % of all patients presenting with postoperative sepsis [70, 71]. Large population studies have concluded that diabetes mellitus increases the risk of cystitis, pneumonia, cellulitis, and tuberculosis [65, 72, 73]. Recent studies have described an association between perioperative and postoperative hyperglycemia with increased risk for an SSI [74–77]. Controlling hyperglycemia has been shown to reduce perioperative nosocomial and wound infections in diabetic patients [77–79].

The increased risk of infection in diabetics is the result of deficiencies in neutrophil and humoral function [80]. Neutrophil functions such as adhesion, chemotaxis, intracellular bactericidal activity, and phagocytosis are impaired [80–84]. Total IgG levels are lower in both uncontrolled diabetic patients [85] and insulin-treated diabetics but not those on oral medications [86]. Furthermore, diabetic patients are less likely to develop a protective antibody response following hepatitis B vaccination [87–89]. Revaccination with one to three additional doses of hepatitis B vaccine can safely increase the proportion of adults that achieve protective antibody levels [90]. The duration of protection against symptomatic and chronic hepatitis B virus infection has been shown to last for more than 22 years in healthy vaccine responders [91]; however, the duration of immunity among persons with diabetes is unknown. Data on vaccine response to influenza is less clear. Diabetic patients have fewer activated lymphocytes but no reduction in antibody response following influenza vaccination [92, 93].

Chronic Kidney Disease and End-Stage Renal Disease

The prevalence of chronic kidney disease in the United States is rising, up from 10 % in 1988–1994 to 13 % in 1999–2004, and is thought to be the result of the increased prevalence of diabetes, hypertension, and an aging population [94]. Infection is the second most common cause of death in patients with end-stage renal disease [95]. Rates of hospitalization for infection are higher for patients with chronic kidney disease for every major organ system than for patients without kidney disease [96, 97]. Chronic dialysis patients often fail to respond to standard vaccination protocols and may require augmented regimens to achieve a protective effect [98–100]. Despite being a high-risk group for infection, vaccination rates for influenza and pneumococcal pneumonia in end-stage renal patients are far lower than recommended [101, 102].

End-stage renal disease and its precursor chronic kidney disease are associated with marked systemic inflammation and diminished immune response [103, 104]. Cytokine dysregulation results from kidney dysfunction, as the kidney is the main route for elimination of cytokines [105, 106]. Uremia causes deficiencies of both the innate and adaptive immune systems [104, 107, 108]. Uremic patients have increased T-cell turnover and apoptosis which leads to a depletion of naïve and memory CD4+ and CD8+ T cells [109–111]. Reduced B-cell proliferation and antibody production are seen in uremic patients [112–114]. Uremia decreases the function of antigen-presenting dendritic cells [115, 116]. Phagocytic function in macrophages and neutrophils is also diminished [117, 118]. Aging further exacerbates these alterations in immune function.

Challenges in Diagnosing Infection in the Elderly

Elderly patients often do not present with pathognomonic signs and symptoms of infection [119, 120]. Cardinal markers of infection such as fever are often absent in older patients. Physiologic changes in the skin cause older patients to conserve less of the body heat they generate. As a result, many noninfected elderly patients fail to achieve a normal body temperature of 37 °C [121]. Nearly a third of patients over the age of 65 with infection have temperatures below the threshold of fever (38.3 °C), and by age 80 approximately 50 % of patients fail to reach this threshold [122–124].

Nonspecific symptoms such as change in mental status, decline in functional status, failure to thrive, loss of appetite, and incontinence can all be presenting signs of infection [125, 126]. Additionally, cognitive impairment can render older adults incapable of communicating their symptoms to providers. These nonspecific findings are also commonly seen in noninfectious diseases, making the diagnosis of infection in this population challenging.

Microbiology of Infection in the Elderly

Infectious diseases in the elderly are caused by a more diverse group of pathogens than in younger patients [126, 127]. Changes in microbiology may be related to age, comorbid disease, and environmental setting, e.g., community, long-term care, and hospital [60, 120, 128–131]. Long-term care residents are at great risk for infection [132]. There are more than 15,000 long-term nursing facilities serving approximately 1.5 million residents in the United States; of these residents 90 % are older than 65 years [133]. Antibiotic use is common among long-term care residents with durations that can vary dramatically from less than 10 days to greater than 90 days [134]. Low dose and prolonged use of antibiotics select for bacterial resistance [135, 136]. This practice has led to the emergence of highly resistant pathogens among residents at long-term care facilities, which impacts both empiric antibiotic selection and infection control during periodic hospitalizations [137–139].

Common Infections

Urinary Tract Infection

Urinary tract infections (UTI) account for 25 % of community-acquired bacterial infections and 30 % of infections from long-term nursing facilities [140]. Age-related changes contributing to increased risk of UTI include thinning of the mucopolysaccharide layer of the urinary epithelium and reduction in the Tamm-Horsfall protein (THP) in urine that covers type 1 fimbriae on gram-negative bacteria. THP reduces bacterial attachment and deterioration of bladder and urethral function [140–143].

E. coli is the most commonly isolated organism in urine from patients in both community and long-term care facilities. Gram-negative polymicrobial infections with multidrug-resistant organisms are more frequent in residents of long-term care facilities [143, 144]. Microbiologic differences are seen in diabetic patients where *E. coli* remains the most common causative agent, but to a lesser extent than in nondiabetic patients, greater proportions of Klebsiella species are reported [131, 145, 146]. Enterococci and *Staphylococcus* species are the most common gram-positive causative agents.

There is a high prevalence of asymptomatic bacteriuria in residents of long-term nursing facilities ranging from 15 to 30 % in men and 25–50 % in females [147]. It is not recommended to initiate antibiotic therapy for asymptomatic bacteriuria, as there is no improvement in survival rate and a tendency toward increased mortality secondary to adverse side effects and superinfection with resistant organisms is observed [148, 149].

The treatment of symptomatic UTI should be based on antimicrobial susceptibility testing. The selection of antibiotic agent is similar to that in the younger community dwelling population and should take into consideration the local antimicrobial resistance patterns [150].

In patients with a symptomatic uncomplicated UTI, the current recommendations for antibiotic duration are 3–7 days, whereas for more complicated UTI, 10–14 days is appropriate [151, 152]. Men with recurrent UTI require workup for chronic bacterial prostatitis, which could require 6–12 weeks of therapy [150]. For catheter-associated UTI, the Infectious Diseases Society of America suggests 7 days of treatment in patients who have a prompt response and 10–14 days in those who have a delayed response [153].

Respiratory Infections

Influenza and pneumonia ranks as the seventh leading cause of death for patients 65 years and older [54]. In addition to changes in the immune system, age-related changes in oral clearance, mucociliary clearance, respiratory muscle strength, cough reflexes, and lung structure increase the risk for pneumonia in the elderly [120].

A recent 2005 guidelines from the American Thoracic Society and Infectious Diseases Society of America added a new pneumonia category termed healthcare-associated pneumonias (HCAP). Hospital-acquired pneumonia (HAP) is defined as pneumonia that occurs 48 h or more after admission and was not present at the time of admission [154, 155]. In contrast, ventilator-associated pneumonia (VAP) arises more than 48–72 h after endotracheal intubation [155, 156]. HAP and VAP are distinctly different from HCAP which is defined as a pneumonia diagnosed in a patient subjected to one of the following conditions: hospitalized in an acute care hospital for 2 or more days within the past 90 days; residents of a nursing home or long-term care facility; treated with intravenous antibiotic therapy, chemotherapy, or wound care within the past 30 days; or received hemodialysis at either a hospital or outpatient clinic [157].

Several studies examining the etiology of community-acquired pneumonia (CAP) have shown *Streptococcus pneumoniae* to be the most common pathogen, accounting for 20–60 % of cases followed by *Haemophilus influenzae* (3–10 % of cases) [158, 159]. Other causative organisms include the atypical pathogens *Mycoplasma pneumoniae*, *Chlamydophila psittaci*, and *Legionella* species [160]. Pathogens associated with HAP, VAP, and HCAP differ from CAP, with multidrug-resistant gram-positive and gram-negative bacteria being more common [161].

Summary

An understanding of the aging immune system is vital for those caring for elderly patients sustaining trauma or undergoing emergency operation. The presentation of infection in the elderly may be subtle, yet early identification, source control, and treatment may improve survival. Appropriate use of antibiotics, based upon prior exposure, environment of residence, and likely organisms, is essential. The complex interplay of organ system disease, physiologic changes, and the effects of trauma requires astute attention to the details of the aging patient.

References

1. Chatta GS, Andrews RG, Rodger E, Schrag M, Hammond WP, Dale DC. Hematopoietic progenitors and aging: alterations in granulocytic precursors and responsiveness to recombinant human G-CSF, GM-CSF, and IL-3. J Gerontol. 1993;48(5):M207–12. Epub 1993/09/01.
2. Fortin CF, McDonald PP, Lesur O, Fulop Jr T. Aging and neutrophils: there is still much to do. Rejuvenation Res. 2008;11(5):873–82. Epub 2008/10/14.

3. Mahbub S, Brubaker AL, Kovacs EJ. Aging of the innate immune system: an update. Curr Immunol Rev. 2011;7(1):104–15. Epub 2011/04/05.
4. MacGregor RR, Shalit M. Neutrophil function in healthy elderly subjects. J Gerontol. 1990;45(2):M55–60. Epub 1990/03/01.
5. Biasi D, Carletto A, Dell'Agnola C, Caramaschi P, Montesanti F, Zavateri G, et al. Neutrophil migration, oxidative metabolism, and adhesion in elderly and young subjects. Inflammation. 1996;20(6): 673–81. Epub 1996/12/01.
6. Niwa Y, Kasama T, Miyachi Y, Kanoh T. Neutrophil chemotaxis, phagocytosis and parameters of reactive oxygen species in human aging: cross-sectional and longitudinal studies. Life Sci. 1989;44(22):1655–64. Epub 1989/01/01.
7. Antonaci S, Jirillo E, Ventura MT, Garofalo AR, Bonomo L. Non-specific immunity in aging: deficiency of monocyte and polymorphonuclear cell-mediated functions. Mech Ageing Dev. 1984;24(3):367–75. Epub 1984/03/01.
8. Fulop T, Larbi A, Douziech N, Fortin C, Guerard KP, Lesur O, et al. Signal transduction and functional changes in neutrophils with aging. Aging Cell. 2004;3(4):217–26. Epub 2004/07/23.
9. Verschoor CP, Puchta A, Bowdish DM. The macrophage. Methods Mol Biol. 2012;844:139–56. Epub 2012/01/21.
10. Ogawa T, Kitagawa M, Hirokawa K. Age-related changes of human bone marrow: a histometric estimation of proliferative cells, apoptotic cells, T cells, B cells and macrophages. Mech Ageing Dev. 2000;117(1–3):57–68. Epub 2000/08/26.
11. Zissel G, Schlaak M, Muller-Quernheim J. Age-related decrease in accessory cell function of human alveolar macrophages. J Investig Med. 1999;47(1):51–6. Epub 1999/03/11.
12. Weiskopf D, Weinberger B, Grubeck-Loebenstein B. The aging of the immune system. Transpl Int. 2009;22(11):1041–50. Epub 2009/07/25.
13. Plowden J, Renshaw-Hoelscher M, Engleman C, Katz J, Sambhara S. Innate immunity in aging: impact on macrophage function. Aging Cell. 2004;3(4):161–7. Epub 2004/07/23.
14. Plackett TP, Boehmer ED, Faunce DE, Kovacs EJ. Aging and innate immune cells. J Leukoc Biol. 2004;76(2):291–9. Epub 2004/03/25.
15. Borrego F, Alonso MC, Galiani MD, Carracedo J, Ramirez R, Ostos B, et al. NK phenotypic markers and IL2 response in NK cells from elderly people. Exp Gerontol. 1999;34(2):253–65. Epub 1999/06/11.
16. Rukavina D, Laskarin G, Rubesa G, Strbo N, Bedenicki I, Manestar D, et al. Age-related decline of perforin expression in human cytotoxic T lymphocytes and natural killer cells. Blood. 1998;92(7):2410–20. Epub 1998/09/25.
17. Hazeldine J, Hampson P, Lord JM. Reduced release and binding of perforin at the immunological synapse underlies the age-related decline in Natural Killer cell cytotoxicity. Aging Cell. 2012;11:751–9. Epub 2012/05/31.
18. Ogata K, An E, Shioi Y, Nakamura K, Luo S, Yokose N, et al. Association between natural killer cell activity and infection in immunologically normal elderly people. Clin Exp Immunol. 2001;124(3):392–7. Epub 2001/07/27.
19. Reis e Sousa C. Dendritic cells in a mature age. Nat Rev Immunol. 2006;6(6):476–83. Epub 2006/05/13.
20. Serbina NV, Salazar-Mather TP, Biron CA, Kuziel WA, Pamer EG. TNF/iNOS-producing dendritic cells mediate innate immune defense against bacterial infection. Immunity. 2003;19(1):59–70. Epub 2003/07/23.
21. Cools N, Ponsaerts P, Van Tendeloo VF, Berneman ZN. Balancing between immunity and tolerance: an interplay between dendritic cells, regulatory T cells, and effector T cells. J Leukoc Biol. 2007;82(6):1365–74. Epub 2007/08/23.
22. Nagy L, Szanto A, Szatmari I, Szeles L. Nuclear hormone receptors enable macrophages and dendritic cells to sense their lipid environment and shape their immune response. Physiol Rev. 2012;92(2):739–89. Epub 2012/04/27.
23. Agrawal A, Agrawal S, Cao JN, Su H, Osann K, Gupta S. Altered innate immune functioning of dendritic cells in elderly humans: a role of phosphoinositide 3-kinase-signaling pathway. J Immunol. 2007;178(11):6912–22. Epub 2007/05/22.
24. Agrawal A, Agrawal S, Gupta S. Dendritic cells in human aging. Exp Gerontol. 2007;42(5):421–6. Epub 2006/12/22.
25. Fadok VA, Bratton DL, Konowal A, Freed PW, Westcott JY, Henson PM. Macrophages that have ingested apoptotic cells in vitro inhibit proinflammatory cytokine production through autocrine/paracrine mechanisms involving TGF-beta, PGE2, and PAF. J Clin Invest. 1998;101(4):890–8. Epub 1998/03/21.
26. Singer AL, Koretzky GA. Control of T cell function by positive and negative regulators. Science. 2002;296(5573):1639–40. Epub 2002/06/01.
27. Sprent J, Tough DF. T cell death and memory. Science. 2001;293(5528):245–8. Epub 2001/07/14.
28. Kendall MD, Johnson HR, Singh J. The weight of the human thymus gland at necropsy. J Anat. 1980;131(Pt 3):483–97. Epub 1980/10/01.
29. Hakim FT, Memon SA, Cepeda R, Jones EC, Chow CK, Kasten-Sportes C, et al. Age-dependent incidence, time course, and consequences of thymic renewal in adults. J Clin Invest. 2005; 115(4):930–9. Epub 2005/03/19.
30. Goronzy JJ, Lee WW, Weyand CM. Aging and T-cell diversity. Exp Gerontol. 2007;42(5):400–6. Epub 2007/01/16.
31. Malaguarnera L, Ferlito L, Imbesi RM, Gulizia GS, Di Mauro S, Maugeri D, et al. Immunosenescence: a review. Arch Gerontol Geriatr. 2001;32(1):1–14. Epub 2001/03/17.
32. Goronzy JJ, Weyand CM. T cell development and receptor diversity during aging. Curr Opin Immunol. 2005;17(5):468–75. Epub 2005/08/16.
33. Schwab R, Szabo P, Manavalan JS, Weksler ME, Posnett DN, Pannetier C, et al. Expanded CD4+ and CD8+ T cell clones in elderly humans. J Immunol. 1997;158(9):4493–9. Epub 1997/05/01.
34. Naylor K, Li G, Vallejo AN, Lee WW, Koetz K, Bryl E, et al. The influence of age on T cell generation and TCR diversity. J Immunol. 2005;174(11):7446–52. Epub 2005/05/21.
35. Cooper MD, Alder MN. The evolution of adaptive immune systems. Cell. 2006;124(4):815–22. Epub 2006/02/25.
36. McHeyzer-Williams M, Okitsu S, Wang N, McHeyzer-Williams L. Molecular programming of B cell memory. Nat Rev Immunol. 2012;12(1):24–34. Epub 2011/12/14.
37. Frasca D, Blomberg BB. Aging affects human B cell responses. J Clin Immunol. 2011;31(3):430–5. Epub 2011/02/15.
38. Chong Y, Ikematsu H, Yamaji K, Nishimura M, Nabeshima S, Kashiwagi S, et al. CD27(+) (memory) B cell decrease and apoptosis-resistant CD27(−) (naive) B cell increase in aged humans: implications for age-related peripheral B cell developmental disturbances. Int Immunol. 2005;17(4):383–90. Epub 2005/02/23.
39. Frasca D, Diaz A, Romero M, Landin AM, Blomberg BB. Age effects on B cells and humoral immunity in humans. Ageing Res Rev. 2011;10(3):330–5. Epub 2010/08/24.
40. Aydar Y, Balogh P, Tew JG, Szakal AK. Age-related depression of FDC accessory functions and CD21 ligand-mediated repair of co-stimulation. Eur J Immunol. 2002;32(10):2817–26. Epub 2002/10/02.
41. Colonna-Romano G, Bulati M, Aquino A, Scialabba G, Candore G, Lio D, et al. B cells in the aged: CD27, CD5, and CD40 expression. Mech Ageing Dev. 2003;124(4):389–93. Epub 2003/04/26.
42. Kogut I, Scholz JL, Cancro MP, Cambier JC. B cell maintenance and function in aging. Semin Immunol. 2012;24(5):342–9.
43. Franceschi C, Bonafe M, Valensin S, Olivieri F, De Luca M, Ottaviani E, et al. Inflamm-aging. An evolutionary perspective on

immunosenescence. Ann N Y Acad Sci. 2000;908:244–54. Epub 2000/07/27.
44. Alvarez-Rodriguez L, Lopez-Hoyos M, Munoz-Cacho P, Martinez-Taboada VM. Aging is associated with circulating cytokine dysregulation. Cell Immunol. 2012;273(2):124–32. Epub 2012/02/10.
45. Forsey RJ, Thompson JM, Ernerudh J, Hurst TL, Strindhall J, Johansson B, et al. Plasma cytokine profiles in elderly humans. Mech Ageing Dev. 2003;124(4):487–93. Epub 2003/04/26.
46. O'Mahony L, Holland J, Jackson J, Feighery C, Hennessy TP, Mealy K. Quantitative intracellular cytokine measurement: age-related changes in proinflammatory cytokine production. Clin Exp Immunol. 1998;113(2):213–9. Epub 1998/08/26.
47. Roubenoff R, Harris TB, Abad LW, Wilson PW, Dallal GE, Dinarello CA. Monocyte cytokine production in an elderly population: effect of age and inflammation. J Gerontol A Biol Sci Med Sci. 1998;53(1):M20–6. Epub 1998/02/19.
48. Reuben DB, Cheh AI, Harris TB, Ferrucci L, Rowe JW, Tracy RP, et al. Peripheral blood markers of inflammation predict mortality and functional decline in high-functioning community-dwelling older persons. J Am Geriatr Soc. 2002;50(4):638–44. Epub 2002/05/02.
49. Ferrucci L, Penninx BW, Volpato S, Harris TB, Bandeen-Roche K, Balfour J, et al. Change in muscle strength explains accelerated decline of physical function in older women with high interleukin-6 serum levels. J Am Geriatr Soc. 2002;50(12):1947–54. Epub 2002/12/11.
50. Roubenoff R, Parise H, Payette HA, Abad LW, D'Agostino R, Jacques PF, et al. Cytokines, insulin-like growth factor 1, sarcopenia, and mortality in very old community-dwelling men and women: the Framingham Heart Study. Am J Med. 2003;115(6):429–35. Epub 2003/10/18.
51. Ferrucci L, Harris TB, Guralnik JM, Tracy RP, Corti MC, Cohen HJ, et al. Serum IL-6 level and the development of disability in older persons. J Am Geriatr Soc. 1999;47(6):639–46. Epub 1999/06/12.
52. Mannino DM. COPD: epidemiology, prevalence, morbidity and mortality, and disease heterogeneity. Chest. 2002;121(5 Suppl):121S–6. Epub 2002/05/16.
53. Rennard SI. COPD: overview of definitions, epidemiology, and factors influencing its development. Chest. 1998;113(4 Suppl):235S–41. Epub 1998/04/29.
54. Heron M. Deaths: leading causes for 2007. Natl Vital Stat Rep. 2011;59(8):1–95. Epub 2011/09/29.
55. Singanayagam A, Joshi PV, Mallia P, Johnston SL. Viruses exacerbating chronic pulmonary disease: the role of immune modulation. BMC Med. 2012;10:27. Epub 2012/03/17.
56. Hurst JR, Vestbo J, Anzueto A, Locantore N, Mullerova H, Tal-Singer R, et al. Susceptibility to exacerbation in chronic obstructive pulmonary disease. N Engl J Med. 2010;363(12):1128–38. Epub 2010/09/17.
57. Agostini P, Cieslik H, Rathinam S, Bishay E, Kalkat MS, Rajesh PB, et al. Postoperative pulmonary complications following thoracic surgery: are there any modifiable risk factors? Thorax. 2010;65(9):815–8. Epub 2010/09/02.
58. Sliedrecht A, den Elzen WP, Verheij TJ, Westendorp RG, Gussekloo J. Incidence and predictive factors of lower respiratory tract infections among the very elderly in the general population. The Leiden 85-plus Study. Thorax. 2008;63(9):817–22.
59. Jansen HM, Sachs AP, van Alphen L. Predisposing conditions to bacterial infections in chronic obstructive pulmonary disease. Am J Respir Crit Care Med. 1995;151(6):2073–80. Epub 1995/06/01.
60. Herrero FS, Olivas JB. Microbiology and risk factors for community-acquired pneumonia. Semin Respir Crit Care Med. 2012;33(3):220–31. Epub 2012/06/22.
61. Torres A, Dorca J, Zalacain R, Bello S, El-Ebiary M, Molinos L, et al. Community-acquired pneumonia in chronic obstructive pulmonary disease: a Spanish multicenter study. Am J Respir Crit Care Med. 1996;154(5):1456–61. Epub 1996/11/01.
62. Restrepo MI, Mortensen EM, Pugh JA, Anzueto A. COPD is associated with increased mortality in patients with community-acquired pneumonia. Eur Respir J. 2006;28(2):346–51. Epub 2006/04/14.
63. Sheer AJ, Heckman JE, Schneider EB, Wu AW, Segal JB, Feinberg R, et al. Congestive heart failure and chronic obstructive pulmonary disease predict poor surgical outcomes in older adults undergoing elective diverticulitis surgery. Dis Colon Rectum. 2011;54(11):1430–7. Epub 2011/10/08.
64. Hruska LA, Smith JM, Hendy MP, Fritz VL, McAdams S. Continuous insulin infusion reduces infectious complications in diabetics following coronary surgery. J Card Surg. 2005;20(5):403–7. Epub 2005/09/13.
65. Shah BR, Hux JE. Quantifying the risk of infectious diseases for people with diabetes. Diabetes Care. 2003;26(2):510–3. Epub 2003/01/28.
66. Shilling AM, Raphael J. Diabetes, hyperglycemia, and infections. Best Pract Res Clin Anaesthesiol. 2008;22(3):519–35. Epub 2008/10/04.
67. Fietsam Jr R, Bassett J, Glover JL. Complications of coronary artery surgery in diabetic patients. Am Surg. 1991;57(9):551–7. Epub 1991/09/11.
68. Angarita FA, Acuna SA, Torregrosa L, Tawil M, Escallon J, Ruiz A. Perioperative variables associated with surgical site infection in breast cancer surgery. J Hosp Infect. 2011;79(4):328–32. Epub 2011/11/08.
69. Latham R, Lancaster AD, Covington JF, Pirolo JS, Thomas Jr CS. The association of diabetes and glucose control with surgical-site infections among cardiothoracic surgery patients. Infect Control Hosp Epidemiol. 2001;22(10):607–12. Epub 2002/01/05.
70. NICE-SUGAR Study Investigators, Finfer S, Chittock DR, Su SY, Blair D, Foster D, et al. Intensive versus conventional glucose control in critically ill patients. N Engl J Med. 2009;360(13):1283–97. Epub 2009/03/26.
71. Stegenga ME, Vincent JL, Vail GM, Xie J, Haney DJ, Williams MD, et al. Diabetes does not alter mortality or hemostatic and inflammatory responses in patients with severe sepsis. Crit Care Med. 2010;38(2):539–45. Epub 2009/10/24.
72. Muller LM, Gorter KJ, Hak E, Goudzwaard WL, Schellevis FG, Hoepelman AI, et al. Increased risk of common infections in patients with type 1 and type 2 diabetes mellitus. Clin Infect Dis. 2005;41(3):281–8. Epub 2005/07/12.
73. Dooley KE, Chaisson RE. Tuberculosis and diabetes mellitus: convergence of two epidemics. Lancet Infect Dis. 2009;9(12):737–46. Epub 2009/11/21.
74. Ramos M, Khalpey Z, Lipsitz S, Steinberg J, Panizales MT, Zinner M, et al. Relationship of perioperative hyperglycemia and postoperative infections in patients who undergo general and vascular surgery. Ann Surg. 2008;248(4):585–91. Epub 2008/10/22.
75. Ata A, Lee J, Bestle SL, Desemone J, Stain SC. Postoperative hyperglycemia and surgical site infection in general surgery patients. Arch Surg. 2010;145(9):858–64. Epub 2010/09/22.
76. Furnary AP, Zerr KJ, Grunkemeier GL, Starr A. Continuous intravenous insulin infusion reduces the incidence of deep sternal wound infection in diabetic patients after cardiac surgical procedures. Ann Thorac Surg. 1999;67(2):352–60; discussion 60–2. Epub 1999/04/10.
77. Golden SH, Peart-Vigilance C, Kao WH, Brancati FL. Perioperative glycemic control and the risk of infectious complications in a cohort of adults with diabetes. Diabetes Care. 1999;22(9):1408–14. Epub 1999/09/10.

78. Zerr KJ, Furnary AP, Grunkemeier GL, Bookin S, Kanhere V, Starr A. Glucose control lowers the risk of wound infection in diabetics after open heart operations. Ann Thorac Surg. 1997; 63(2):356–61. Epub 1997/02/01.
79. Pomposelli JJ, Baxter 3rd JK, Babineau TJ, Pomfret EA, Driscoll DF, Forse RA, et al. Early postoperative glucose control predicts nosocomial infection rate in diabetic patients. JPEN J Parenter Enteral Nutr. 1998;22(2):77–81. Epub 1998/04/07.
80. Koh GC, Peacock SJ, van der Poll T, Wiersinga WJ. The impact of diabetes on the pathogenesis of sepsis. Eur J Clin Microbiol Infect Dis. 2012;31(4):379–88. Epub 2011/08/02.
81. van Oss CJ, Border JR. Influence of intermittent hyperglycemic glucose levels on the phagocytosis of microorganisms by human granulocytes in vitro. Immunol Commun. 1978;7(6):669–76. Epub 1978/01/01.
82. Perner A, Nielsen SE, Rask-Madsen J. High glucose impairs superoxide production from isolated blood neutrophils. Intensive Care Med. 2003;29(4):642–5. Epub 2003/01/29.
83. Andersen B, Goldsmith GH, Spagnuolo PJ. Neutrophil adhesive dysfunction in diabetes mellitus; the role of cellular and plasma factors. J Lab Clin Med. 1988;111(3):275–85. Epub 1988/03/01.
84. Delamaire M, Maugendre D, Moreno M, Le Goff MC, Allannic H, Genetet B. Impaired leucocyte functions in diabetic patients. Diabet Med. 1997;14(1):29–34. Epub 1997/01/01.
85. Liberatore Jr RR, Barbosa SF, Alkimin MG, Bellinati-Pires R, Florido MP, Isaac L, et al. Is immunity in diabetic patients influencing the susceptibility to infections? Immunoglobulins, complement and phagocytic function in children and adolescents with type 1 diabetes mellitus. Pediatr Diabetes. 2005;6(4):206–12. Epub 2006/01/05.
86. Farid NR, Anderson J. Immunoglobulins and complement in diabetes mellitus. Lancet. 1973;2(7820):92. Epub 1973/07/14.
87. Bouter KP, Diepersloot RJ, Wismans PJ, Gmelig Meyling FH, Hoekstra JB, Heijtink RA, et al. Humoral immune response to a yeast-derived hepatitis B vaccine in patients with type 1 diabetes mellitus. Diabet Med. 1992;9(1):66–9. Epub 1992/01/01.
88. Pozzilli P, Arduini P, Visalli N, Sutherland J, Pezzella M, Galli C, et al. Reduced protection against hepatitis B virus following vaccination in patients with type 1 (insulin-dependent) diabetes. Diabetologia. 1987;30(10):817–9. Epub 1987/10/01.
89. Ficicioglu C, Mikla S, Midilli K, Aydin A, Cam H, Ergin S. Reduced immune response to hepatitis B vaccine in children with insulin dependent diabetes. Acta Paediatr Jpn. 1995;37(6):687–90. Epub 1995/12/01.
90. Mast EE, Weinbaum CM, Fiore AE, Alter MJ, Bell BP, Finelli L, et al. A comprehensive immunization strategy to eliminate transmission of hepatitis B virus infection in the United States: recommendations of the Advisory Committee on Immunization Practices (ACIP) Part II: immunization of adults. MMWR Recomm Rep. 2006;55(RR-16):1–33; quiz CE1–4. Epub 2006/12/13.
91. Leuridan E, Van Damme P. Hepatitis B and the need for a booster dose. Clin Infect Dis. 2011;53(1):68–75. Epub 2011/06/10.
92. Pozzilli P, Gale EA, Visalli N, Baroni M, Crovari P, Frighi V, et al. The immune response to influenza vaccination in diabetic patients. Diabetologia. 1986;29(12):850–4. Epub 1986/12/01.
93. Diepersloot RJ, Bouter KP, Beyer WE, Hoekstra JB, Masurel N. Humoral immune response and delayed type hypersensitivity to influenza vaccine in patients with diabetes mellitus. Diabetologia. 1987;30(6):397–401. Epub 1987/06/01.
94. Coresh J, Selvin E, Stevens LA, Manzi J, Kusek JW, Eggers P, et al. Prevalence of chronic kidney disease in the United States. JAMA. 2007;298(17):2038–47. Epub 2007/11/08.
95. Excerpts from the United States Renal Data System 1998 Annual Data Report. Am J Kidney Dis. 1998;32(2 Suppl 1):S1–162. Epub 1998/09/19.
96. Collins AJ, Foley RN, Chavers B, Gilbertson D, Herzog C, Johansen K, et al. United States Renal Data System 2011 annual data report: atlas of chronic kidney disease & end-stage renal disease in the United States. Am J Kidney Dis. 2012;59(1 Suppl 1):A7, e1–420. Epub 2011/12/30.
97. James MT, Laupland KB, Tonelli M, Manns BJ, Culleton BF, Hemmelgarn BR, et al. Risk of bloodstream infection in patients with chronic kidney disease not treated with dialysis. Arch Intern Med. 2008;168(21):2333–9. Epub 2008/11/26.
98. Martin P, Friedman LS. Chronic viral hepatitis and the management of chronic renal failure. Kidney Int. 1995;47(5):1231–41. Epub 1995/05/01.
99. Pesanti EL. Immunologic defects and vaccination in patients with chronic renal failure. Infect Dis Clin North Am. 2001;15(3):813–32. Epub 2001/09/26.
100. McGrath LJ, Kshirsagar AV, Cole SR, Wang L, Weber DJ, Sturmer T, et al. Influenza vaccine effectiveness in patients on hemodialysis: an analysis of a natural experiment. Arch Intern Med. 2012;172(7):548–54. Epub 2012/04/12.
101. Naqvi SB, Collins AJ. Infectious complications in chronic kidney disease. Adv Chronic Kidney Dis. 2006;13(3):199–204. Epub 2006/07/04.
102. Gilbertson DT, Unruh M, McBean AM, Kausz AT, Snyder JJ, Collins AJ. Influenza vaccine delivery and effectiveness in end-stage renal disease. Kidney Int. 2003;63(2):738–43. Epub 2003/03/13.
103. Carrero JJ, Stenvinkel P. Inflammation in end-stage renal disease–what have we learned in 10 years? Semin Dial. 2010;23(5):498–509. Epub 2010/11/03.
104. Girndt M, Sester U, Sester M, Kaul H, Kohler H. Impaired cellular immune function in patients with end-stage renal failure. Nephrol Dial Transplant. 1999;14(12):2807–10. Epub 1999/11/26.
105. Descamps-Latscha B, Herbelin A, Nguyen AT, Zingraff J, Jungers P, Chatenoud L. Immune system dysregulation in uremia. Semin Nephrol. 1994;14(3):253–60. Epub 1994/05/01.
106. Carrero JJ, Yilmaz MI, Lindholm B, Stenvinkel P. Cytokine dysregulation in chronic kidney disease: how can we treat it? Blood Purif. 2008;26(3):291–9. Epub 2008/04/19.
107. Girndt M, Sester M, Sester U, Kaul H, Kohler H. Molecular aspects of T- and B-cell function in uremia. Kidney Int Suppl. 2001;78:S206–11. Epub 2001/02/13.
108. Vaziri ND, Pahl MV, Crum A, Norris K. Effect of uremia on structure and function of immune system. J Ren Nutr. 2012;22(1):149–56. Epub 2011/12/28.
109. Matsumoto Y, Shinzato T, Amano I, Takai I, Kimura Y, Morita H, et al. Relationship between susceptibility to apoptosis and Fas expression in peripheral blood T cells from uremic patients: a possible mechanism for lymphopenia in chronic renal failure. Biochem Biophys Res Commun. 1995;215(1):98–105. Epub 1995/10/04.
110. Moser B, Roth G, Brunner M, Lilaj T, Deicher R, Wolner E, et al. Aberrant T cell activation and heightened apoptotic turnover in end-stage renal failure patients: a comparative evaluation between non-dialysis, haemodialysis, and peritoneal dialysis. Biochem Biophys Res Commun. 2003;308(3):581–5. Epub 2003/08/14.
111. Yoon JW, Gollapudi S, Pahl MV, Vaziri ND. Naive and central memory T-cell lymphopenia in end-stage renal disease. Kidney Int. 2006;70(2):371–6. Epub 2006/06/02.
112. Smogorzewski M, Massry SG. Defects in B-cell function and metabolism in uremia: role of parathyroid hormone. Kidney Int Suppl. 2001;78:S186–9. Epub 2001/02/13.
113. Pahl MV, Gollapudi S, Sepassi L, Gollapudi P, Elahimehr R, Vaziri ND. Effect of end-stage renal disease on B-lymphocyte subpopulations, IL-7, BAFF and BAFF receptor expression. Nephrol Dial Transplant. 2010;25(1):205–12. Epub 2009/08/18.

114. Beaman M, Michael J, MacLennan IC, Adu D. T-cell-independent and T-cell-dependent antibody responses in patients with chronic renal failure. Nephrol Dial Transplant. 1989;4(3):216–21. Epub 1989/01/01.
115. Lim WH, Kireta S, Leedham E, Russ GR, Coates PT. Uremia impairs monocyte and monocyte-derived dendritic cell function in hemodialysis patients. Kidney Int. 2007;72(9):1138–48. Epub 2007/08/31.
116. Lim WH, Kireta S, Russ GR, Coates PT. Uremia impairs blood dendritic cell function in hemodialysis patients. Kidney Int. 2007;71(11):1122–31. Epub 2007/03/23.
117. Alexiewicz JM, Smogorzewski M, Fadda GZ, Massry SG. Impaired phagocytosis in dialysis patients: studies on mechanisms. Am J Nephrol. 1991;11(2):102–11. Epub 1991/01/01.
118. Massry S, Smogorzewski M. Dysfunction of polymorphonuclear leukocytes in uremia: role of parathyroid hormone. Kidney Int Suppl. 2001;78:S195–6. Epub 2001/02/13.
119. Metlay JP, Schulz R, Li YH, Singer DE, Marrie TJ, Coley CM, et al. Influence of age on symptoms at presentation in patients with community-acquired pneumonia. Arch Intern Med. 1997;157(13):1453–9. Epub 1997/07/14.
120. Meyer KC. Lung infections and aging. Ageing Res Rev. 2004;3(1):55–67. Epub 2004/05/28.
121. Gomolin IH, Aung MM, Wolf-Klein G, Auerbach C. Older is colder: temperature range and variation in older people. J Am Geriatr Soc. 2005;53(12):2170–2. Epub 2006/01/10.
122. High KP. Infection as a cause of age-related morbidity and mortality. Ageing Res Rev. 2004;3(1):1–14. Epub 2004/05/28.
123. Roghmann MC, Warner J, Mackowiak PA. The relationship between age and fever magnitude. Am J Med Sci. 2001;322(2):68–70. Epub 2001/08/29.
124. Norman DC. Fever in the elderly. Clin Infect Dis. 2000;31(1):148–51. Epub 2000/07/29.
125. Chassagne P, Perol MB, Doucet J, Trivalle C, Menard JF, Manchon ND, et al. Is presentation of bacteremia in the elderly the same as in younger patients? Am J Med. 1996;100(1):65–70. Epub 1996/01/01.
126. Gavazzi G, Krause KH. Ageing and infection. Lancet Infect Dis. 2002;2(11):659–66. Epub 2002/11/01.
127. Yoshikawa TT. Epidemiology and unique aspects of aging and infectious diseases. Clin Infect Dis. 2000;30(6):931–3. Epub 2000/07/06.
128. Marrie TJ. Community-acquired pneumonia in the elderly. Clin Infect Dis. 2000;31(4):1066–78. Epub 2000/10/26.
129. Molinos L, Clemente MG, Miranda B, Alvarez C, del Busto B, Cocina BR, et al. Community-acquired pneumonia in patients with and without chronic obstructive pulmonary disease. J Infect. 2009;58(6):417–24. Epub 2009/03/31.
130. Ronald A. The etiology of urinary tract infection: traditional and emerging pathogens. Am J Med. 2002;113(Suppl 1A):14S–9. Epub 2002/07/13.
131. Lye WC, Chan RK, Lee EJ, Kumarasinghe G. Urinary tract infections in patients with diabetes mellitus. J Infect. 1992;24(2):169–74. Epub 1992/03/01.
132. High KP, Bradley SF, Gravenstein S, Mehr DR, Quagliarello VJ, Richards C, et al. Clinical practice guideline for the evaluation of fever and infection in older adult residents of long-term care facilities: 2008 update by the Infectious Diseases Society of America. Clin Infect Dis. 2009;48(2):149–71. Epub 2008/12/17.
133. Smith PW, Bennett G, Bradley S, Drinka P, Lautenbach E, Marx J, et al. SHEA/APIC guideline: infection prevention and control in the long-term care facility. Am J Infect Control. 2008;36(7):504–35. Epub 2008/09/13.
134. Daneman N, Gruneir A, Newman A, Fischer HD, Bronskill SE, Rochon PA, et al. Antibiotic use in long-term care facilities. J Antimicrob Chemother. 2011;66(12):2856–63. Epub 2011/09/29.
135. Levy SB. Antibiotic resistance: consequences of inaction. Clin Infect Dis. 2001;33 Suppl 3:S124–9. Epub 2001/08/29.
136. Guillemot D, Carbon C, Balkau B, Geslin P, Lecoeur H, Vauzelle-Kervroedan F, et al. Low dosage and long treatment duration of beta-lactam: risk factors for carriage of penicillin-resistant Streptococcus pneumoniae. JAMA. 1998;279(5):365–70. Epub 1998/02/12.
137. Parish A, Holliday K. Long-term care acquired urinary tract Infections' antibiotic resistance patterns and empiric therapy: a pilot study. Geriatr Nurs. 2012;33:473–8. Epub 2012/07/04.
138. van Buul LW, van der Steen JT, Veenhuizen RB, Achterberg WP, Schellevis FG, Essink RT, et al. Antibiotic use and resistance in long term care facilities. J Am Med Dir Assoc. 2012;13(6):568.e1–e13. Epub 2012/05/12.
139. Yoshikawa TT, Norman DC. Approach to fever and infection in the nursing home. J Am Geriatr Soc. 1996;44(1):74–82. Epub 1996/01/01.
140. Richards CL. Urinary tract infections in the frail elderly: issues for diagnosis, treatment and prevention. Int Urol Nephrol. 2004;36(3):457–63. Epub 2005/03/24.
141. Herrmann V, Palma P, Geo MS, Lima RS. Urinary tract infections: pathogenesis and related conditions. Int Urogynecol J Pelvic Floor Dysfunct. 2002;13(3):210–3. Epub 2002/07/26.
142. Pfisterer MH, Griffiths DJ, Schaefer W, Resnick NM. The effect of age on lower urinary tract function: a study in women. J Am Geriatr Soc. 2006;54(3):405–12. Epub 2006/03/23.
143. Htwe TH, Mushtaq A, Robinson SB, Rosher RB, Khardori N. Infection in the elderly. Infect Dis Clin North Am. 2007;21(3):711–43, ix. Epub 2007/09/11.
144. Yoshikawa TT, Nicolle LE, Norman DC. Management of complicated urinary tract infection in older patients. J Am Geriatr Soc. 1996;44(10):1235–41. Epub 1996/10/01.
145. Brauner A, Flodin U, Hylander B, Ostenson CG. Bacteriuria, bacterial virulence and host factors in diabetic patients. Diabet Med. 1993;10(6):550–4. Epub 1993/07/01.
146. Hansen DS, Gottschau A, Kolmos HJ. Epidemiology of Klebsiella bacteraemia: a case control study using Escherichia coli bacteraemia as control. J Hosp Infect. 1998;38(2):119–32. Epub 1998/04/02.
147. Nicolle LE. Urinary tract infection in long-term-care facility residents. Clin Infect Dis. 2000;31(3):757–61. Epub 2000/10/06.
148. Nicolle LE, Bradley S, Colgan R, Rice JC, Schaeffer A, Hooton TM, et al. Infectious Diseases Society of America guidelines for the diagnosis and treatment of asymptomatic bacteriuria in adults. Clin Infect Dis. 2005;40(5):643–54. Epub 2005/02/17.
149. Nicolle LE. Asymptomatic bacteriuria: review and discussion of the IDSA guidelines. Int J Antimicrob Agents. 2006;28 Suppl 1:S42–8. Epub 2006/07/11.
150. Nicolle LE. Urinary tract infections in the elderly. Clin Geriatr Med. 2009;25(3):423–36. Epub 2009/09/22.
151. Vogel T, Verreault R, Gourdeau M, Morin M, Grenier-Gosselin L, Rochette L. Optimal duration of antibiotic therapy for uncomplicated urinary tract infection in older women: a double-blind randomized controlled trial. CMAJ. 2004;170(4):469–73. Epub 2004/02/19.
152. Lutters M, Vogt-Ferrier NB. Antibiotic duration for treating uncomplicated, symptomatic lower urinary tract infections in elderly women. Cochrane Database Syst Rev. 2008(3):CD001535. Epub 2008/07/23
153. Hooton TM, Bradley SF, Cardenas DD, Colgan R, Geerlings SE, Rice JC, et al. Diagnosis, prevention, and treatment of catheter-associated urinary tract infection in adults: 2009 International Clinical Practice Guidelines from the Infectious Diseases Society of America. Clin Infect Dis. 2010;50(5):625–63. Epub 2010/02/23.

154. Niederman MS. Guidelines for the management of respiratory infection: why do we need them, how should they be developed, and can they be useful? Curr Opin Pulm Med. 1996;2(3):161–5. Epub 1996/05/01.
155. Tablan OC, Anderson LJ, Besser R, Bridges C, Hajjeh R, CDC, et al. Guidelines for preventing health-care – associated pneumonia, 2003: recommendations of CDC and the Healthcare Infection Control Practices Advisory Committee. MMWR Recomm Rep. 2004;53(RR-3):1–36. Epub 2004/03/30.
156. Craven DE, Kunches LM, Kilinsky V, Lichtenberg DA, Make BJ, McCabe WR. Risk factors for pneumonia and fatality in patients receiving continuous mechanical ventilation. Am Rev Respir Dis. 1986;133(5):792–6. Epub 1986/05/01.
157. American Thoracic Society, Infectious Diseases Society of America. Guidelines for the management of adults with hospital-acquired, ventilator-associated, and healthcare-associated pneumonia. Am J Respir Crit Care Med. 2005;171(4):388–416. Epub 2005/02/09.
158. Bartlett JG, Mundy LM. Community-acquired pneumonia. N Engl J Med. 1995;333(24):1618–24. Epub 1995/12/14.
159. File TM. Community-acquired pneumonia. Lancet. 2003; 362(9400):1991–2001. Epub 2003/12/20.
160. Thiem U, Heppner HJ, Pientka L. Elderly patients with community-acquired pneumonia: optimal treatment strategies. Drugs Aging. 2011;28(7):519–37. Epub 2011/07/05.
161. Falcone M, Venditti M, Shindo Y, Kollef MH. Healthcare-associated pneumonia: diagnostic criteria and distinction from community-acquired pneumonia. Int J Infect Dis. 2011;15(8): e545–50. Epub 2011/05/28.

7 Hematologic Changes with Aging

Peter E. Fischer, Thomas G. DeLoughery, and Martin A. Schreiber

Introduction

The population of patients experiencing injury is changing. As the "baby boomer" generation grows older, age 65 and over men and women are expected to represent nearly 20 % of the total population [1]. With this population comes a unique challenge following injury. The death rate following injury is higher in this older population than any other age group [2]. Falls are a substantial component of the injury profile, and it is estimated that almost one third of adults age 65 and older fall each year [3]. Knowledge of age-related changes in the hematologic system is crucial to the care of this distinct cohort following injury.

Anemia

The overall rate of anemia increases significantly in patients over the age of 60 and is thought to be a normal consequence of aging. Large studies of men and women over the age of 65 show decreased hemoglobin levels with age [4–6]. This was first thought to be secondary to iron-deficiency anemia, but further studies revealed iron deficiency to be found in only a small subset of the population [7]. Further studies have linked the steady decline in blood hemoglobin levels not to the previously believed nutritional elements but rather to decreased stem cell proliferation. Lipschitz showed a relative reduction of bone marrow normoblasts without a decrease in progenitor cells suggesting a decrease in stem cell proliferation [8]. There is a compensatory rise in serum erythropoietin levels to compensate for this anemia [9]. However, these changes are not enough to effectively compensate. Some more recent studies [10] did not reveal an age-related anemia in healthy older adults but did show increased incidence of anemia in the aged population suffering from various medical problems. It is this older patient with multiple medical problems that is most likely to present to the trauma physician. Therefore, the physician should expect some level of baseline anemia.

Bone Marrow Changes

Within the bone marrow lies the hematopoietic stem cell. This cell is responsible for replenishing all cell types of the blood. The bone marrow itself, as well as the stem cells, undergoes changes with aging that can make the body less responsive to hematologic insults. For example, the increased incidence of myeloproliferative disorders with age is thought to be secondary to age-related changes of the stem cell [11]. The architecture of the bone marrow shows a significant decline in cellularity with advancing age. Hematopoietic tissue, which usually occupies 40–60 % of the bone marrow space in young adults, subsequently drops to only 20–40 % of the mass in older adults. The space remaining is occupied by fat. The stem cell is dependent on this marrow environment for efficient function. Bones from older mice show a decreased repopulation of cells after being implanted into younger mice likely secondary to the structural changes [12]. Similar results are shown when marrow from old and young mice is implanted into young mice. The younger marrow assumes the majority of the production burden [13]. The reduced cellularity of bone marrow with aging could be secondary to a proinflammatory state associated with increased age. Age-related inflammation has been shown to cause a decrease in P-selectin

P.E. Fischer, MD, MS (✉)
Department of Surgery, Carolinas Medical Center, 1000 Blythe Blvd., MEB 6, Charlotte, NC 28203, USA
e-mail: peter.fischer@carolinashealthcare.org

T.G. DeLoughery, MD
Department of Medicine, Oregon Health and Science University, 3181 SW Sam Jackson Park Road, L611, Portland, OR 97239, USA
e-mail: delought@ohsu.edu

M.A. Schreiber, MD, FACS
Department of Surgery, Oregon Health and Science University, 3181 SW Sam Jackson Park Road, L611, Portland, OR 97239, USA
e-mail: schreibm@ohsu.edu

J.A. Yelon, F.A. Luchette (eds.), *Geriatric Trauma and Critical Care*,
DOI 10.1007/978-1-4614-8501-8_7, © Springer Science+Business Media New York 2014

expression which is the surface adhesion molecule responsible for populating bone marrow with hematopoietic stem cells and thus making it more difficult for the stem cells to populate the older more fat-laden marrow [14]. The increase in adipose tissue of the bone marrow is also a negative regulator of the bone marrow environment [15]. These structural changes seen in the marrow with aging have a negative impact on the responsiveness of the stem cell, and the body is less able to repopulate cell lines after injury.

Response to Hemorrhage

One of the most important factors to consider in the aging population is their hematologic response to hemorrhage. As stated above, the bone marrow and the hematopoietic stem cell both have diminished function with advancing age and as a result have a decreased ability to adapt to a hematologic insult. The debate of whether the hematopoietic system undergoes any major changes with aging in the normal individual continues without resolution [16]. However, chemotherapy has proven that the hematologic system does not recover as fast in older individuals. Treatment of older patients with chemotherapy results in more life-threatening myelosuppression and treatment-related deaths than their younger counterparts [17, 18]. The hematologic system of elderly patients exhibits an impaired ability to recover following insult. The recovery of the total red cell mass after hemorrhage is also decreased in the older population. Boggs and Patrene showed that although anemia was more profound in older mice, it was not secondary to a decrease in the red cell mass but rather an expansion in the plasma volume. The overall survival of the red cell was also no different in the older mice. However, when the older mice were subjected to hemorrhage reducing the hematocrit to a nadir of 25 %, the recovery was much slower and reflected a difference in erythropoiesis rather than plasma volume equilibration [19]. This slower return to pre-trauma hematocrit can have negative consequences. Wu showed that even mild degrees of preoperative anemia resulted in higher rates of postoperative morbidity and mortality in older patients [20]. While we do not advocate unnecessary transfusions because of the negative impact of blood transfusion in the trauma population, it is important for the physician to understand that an older individual will have a slower recovery from a low hematocrit than their younger counterparts with potential associated morbidity.

Hypercoagulability Associated with Aging

In the acute injury setting, the trauma surgeon is likely more concerned about a hypocoagulable state. This is often seen in the older population secondary to the medications commonly prescribed to this cohort. However, after the initial injury it is important to understand that elderly patients tend to be hypercoagulable at baseline, and this may put them at risk for a number of complications. Age is an important risk factor for the development of deep venous thrombosis in the ICU following trauma as well as other thromboembolic events including myocardial infarction and pulmonary emboli [21]. The physiologic reasons for this hypercoagulable state are multifactorial and best understood in the cardiovascular population. Thrombotic cardiovascular disease is known to increase with age [22]. Besides the atherosclerotic changes of the vascular endothelium seen with advanced age, hemostatic systems including platelets, coagulation, and fibrinolytic factors all show age-associated changes that result in a relative hypercoagulable state. Platelet, factor VII, and factor VIII activity are all enhanced with increasing age. In an epidemiologic study of an industrial population of over 3,000 individuals, Balleisen et al. showed an increase in factor VII and factor VIII with age and a significant surge in women after menopause [23]. Mari also showed increased levels of factor VII in centenarians suggesting an increased coagulation response [24]. One might surmise that if these natural procoagulant factors increase with age, then proportional rises in natural anticoagulants including protein C and protein S might also occur to achieve normality. However, Sagripanti did not find this to be true [25]. The age-related genetic mechanism responsible for increased procoagulant factor levels also results in increased production of protein C and protein S but at a slower rate, resulting in the proportional rise of the procoagulant factors [26]. The increased platelet activity accompanying advanced age is likely related to three separate yet related changes [27]. First, the number of prostacyclin receptors decreases with aging and subsequently downgrades their inhibitory response on platelet aggregation [28]. Second, there appears to be an age-related increase in platelet transmembrane signaling (phosphoinositide turnover) or second messenger accumulation resulting in increased platelet activity [29]. Finally, there is increased production of von Willebrand factor with age resulting in increased platelet activity [30].

The fibrinolytic system also contributes to the hypercoagulable state associated with aging. There is a prolongation of the euglobulin lysis time [31] as well as an increase in plasminogen activator inhibitor-1 (PAI-1), which specifically inhibits both tissue-type and urokinase-type plasminogen activators [32]. Higher levels of PAI-1 have been noted in mouse models of aging. Takeshita et al. showed increased levels of PAI-1 mRNA expression and PAI-1 plasma antigen in a rapidly aging mouse model compared with normal controls. This finding implies a decrease in fibrinolysis and increased risk of thromboembolic events with advanced age [33]. One of the most interesting findings concerning PAI-1 is its increased production in times of stress. Stress (as seen following trauma and critical illness) results in increased production of glucocorticoids through the hypothalamic-pituitary-adrenal axis. These glucocorticoids have been shown to induce PAI-1 expression [34]. Furthermore, this stress-induced expression is even more profound in aged mice [35].

Medication of an Aged Population That Affects the Hematologic System

While not a natural change with aging, any discussion of the changes in the hematologic system with age, especially related to trauma, would be remiss not to mention the common medications that are prescribed. Antiplatelet therapy with aspirin or platelet ADP antagonists (clopidogrel, prasugrel, or ticagrelor) is common in the older trauma population. It is estimated that 50 million Americans are on aspirin therapy [36], and 29 million are prescribed clopidogrel or similar agents [37]. Pre-injury treatment with these drugs has been shown to increase trauma mortality especially with head injury [38, 39]. Aspirin inhibits platelet cyclooxygenase-1, which then blocks thromboxane A2 generation and subsequently inhibits platelet function. Clopidogrel-like drugs work by inhibiting the ADP-dependent mechanism of platelet aggregation. Both aspirin and ADP antagonists are reversed by platelet transfusion. Laboratory studies indicate that while one pheresis unit (6 random units) can reverse the aspirin defect, 2 pheresis units may be needed for ADP antagonists [40].

Desmopressin also has been shown to improve platelet function in the presence of these antiplatelet agents. Ranucci showed improved platelet function from 48 to 71 % by thromboelastography (TEG) with desmopressin therapy [41]. However, more clinical trials need to be performed before desmopressin should be included in antiplatelet reversal protocols.

There is increasing interest in using point-of-care assays such as VerifyNow to guide reversal therapy for antiplatelet agents. Bansal showed that many patients allegedly on antiplatelet agents had normal platelet function, and Bachelani showed that these assays may help guide platelet therapy [42, 43]. More widespread use of this type of laboratory testing may help avoid unnecessary transfusion and result in more efficient reversal of antiplatelet agents.

One of the leading medical indications for anticoagulation in the older population is atrial fibrillation. The prevalence of atrial fibrillation is steadily increasing [44], and it is estimated that by 2030, four million people in the USA will suffer from it [45]. While studies have shown that over a lifetime the benefit of reduced stroke rate with anticoagulation for atrial fibrillation does outweigh the bleeding risk, in an acutely injured patient, anticoagulation can be life-threatening. Warfarin acts by antagonizing vitamin K and thus inhibiting the vitamin K-dependent coagulation factors II, VII, IX, and X [46]. Pre-trauma treatment with warfarin has been associated with worse outcomes especially in patients with intracranial injury [47]. Rapid reversal protocols utilizing fresh frozen plasma (FFP) have been shown to reduce further bleeding and improve outcomes [39]. While traditional reversal relies on the transfusion of FFP and the administration of vitamin K, the process can be lengthy due to the time needed to thaw the plasma and infuse the product. Another issue is that substantial amounts of FFP are required for adequate reversal (15–20 ml/kg). The large volume of blood products may be detrimental to patients at risk for congestive heart failure.

Prothrombin complex concentrates (PCCs) contain variable concentrations of factors II, VII, IX, and X. Currently, due to the concern of thrombosis, only 3-factor concentrates containing minimal factor VII are currently available in the USA, but 4-factor concentrates are approved in Europe and Canada. PCCs are FDA approved for use in patients with hemophilia B. PCCs have several advantages over fresh frozen plasma. They are readily available and do not require infusion of large volumes of fluid. They are virally inactivated and have a reduced risk of causing transfusion-related acute lung injury. Reported uses include reversal of vitamin K antagonists, surgical procedures in hemophiliacs, cardiopulmonary bypass, and massive bleeding. PCCs have been associated with more rapid normalization of the INR compared to FFP, decreased incidence of hematoma enlargement, and improved neurologic outcomes in patients with anticoagulant-associated intracerebral hemorrhage [48] (Box 7.1).

Our current approach to reversing warfarin is to give PCC along with 1 mg of recombinant factor VIIa as a source of factor VII plus vitamin K for long-term warfarin reversal (Box 7.2). In the future when 4-factor PCCs are approved, these will become the product of choice for reversing warfarin [49].

Newer anticoagulant agents including dabigatran (direct thrombin inhibitor), rivaroxaban (factor Xa inhibitor), and apixaban (factor Xa inhibitor) are now being used in the elderly population. These drugs have advantages over warfarin in that they do not require lab monitoring, and they have much less drug interactions and no food interactions. All these agents have been shown to be equally or more effective than warfarin with respect to stroke prevention and safer with respect to intracranial hemorrhage complications. They are all options for stroke prevention in atrial fibrillation [50]. In addition, both dabigatran and rivaroxaban have been shown to be equal to warfarin in the therapy of venous thrombosis [51]. At this time there are no direct reversal agents for these new drugs. However, animal studies have suggested that PCC may be effective at halting bleeding, and at our institution, we use PCC + rVIIa combination for bleeding with these new agents [52, 53].

Box 7.1 OHSU Anticoagulation Reversal Protocol

Definition of bleeding:

Minor bleeding – any clinically overt sign of hemorrhage (including imaging) that is associated with a <5 g/dl decrease in the hemoglobin concentration or <15 % decrease in the hematocrit felt by the clinician to be related to anticoagulation

Major bleeding – intracranial hemorrhage or a ≥5 g/dl decrease in the hemoglobin concentration or a ≥15 % absolute decrease in the hematocrit resulting in hemodynamic compromise or compression of a vital structure and felt by the clinician to be related to anticoagulation

Antiplatelet agents

Aspirin

Minor – desmopressin 0.3 mcg/kg × 1

Major – platelet transfusion

Clopidogrel (Plavix®)

Minor – desmopressin 0.3 mcg/kg × 1

Major – platelet transfusion, consider two units if life- or brain-threatening bleeding

Prasugrel (Effient®)

Minor – desmopressin 0.3 mcg/kg × 1

Major – platelet transfusion, consider two units if life- or brain-threatening bleeding

Ticagrelor (Brilinta®)

Minor – desmopressin 0.3 mcg/kg × 1

Major – platelet transfusion, consider two units if life- or brain-threatening bleeding

Sustained release aspirin/dipyridamole (Aggrenox®)

Minor – desmopressin 0.3 mcg/kg × 1

Major – platelet transfusion

Abciximab (ReoPro®)

Major – platelet transfusion

Eptifibatide (Integrilin®)

Minor – desmopressin 0.3 mcg/kg × 1

Major bleeding reversal: platelet transfusions plus infusion of 10 units of cryoprecipitate

Tirofiban (Aggrastat®)

Minor – desmopressin 0.3 mcg/kg × 1

Major bleeding reversal: platelet transfusions plus infusion of 10 units of cryoprecipitate

Heparin and heparin-like agents

Standard heparin

Time since last heparin dose	Dose of protamine
<30 min	1 unit/100 units of heparin
30–60 min	0.5–0.75 units/100 units of heparin
60–120 min	0.375–0.5 units/100 units of heparin
>120 min	0.25–0.375 units/100 units of heparin

Infusion rate should not exceed 5 mg/min. Maximum dose is 50 mg per dose

Low molecular weight heparin

Reversal of bleeding: protamine (works just as well with LMWH as heparin) – if within 4 h of dose, give 1 mg of protamine for each 1 mg of enoxaparin or 100 units of dalteparin and tinzaparin. Repeat one-half dose of protamine in 4 h. If 4–8 h after dose, give 0.5 mg for each 1 mg of enoxaparin or 100 units of dalteparin and tinzaparin.

Fondaparinux (Arixtra®)

Major bleeding reversal – protamine ineffective, rVIIa (90 mcg/kg) may be of use

Dabigatran (Pradaxa®)

Reverse if patient shows signs of bleeding and had an elevated aPTT >40 s

1. Profilnine (factor IX complex) 4,000 units (50 units/kg for patients under 80 kg) *plus* 1 mg of rfVIIa

Rivaroxaban (Xarelto®)

Reverse if patient shows signs of bleeding and has an INR >1.5

1. Profilnine (factor IX complex) 4,000 units (50 units/kg for patients under 80 kg) *plus* 1 mg of rfVIIa

Thrombolytic therapy

Reversal: immediate infusions of equivalent of 6–8 units of platelets (or one platelet pheresis product), 2 units of plasma, and 10 units of cryoprecipitate. No value in infusing antifibrinolytic agents

Box 7.2 OHSU Warfarin Reversal Protocol

For patients who present with warfarin and demonstrated ICH with an INR >1.45

1. Profilnine 4,000 units
   (a) 50 units/kg for patients under 80 kg
2. 1 mg of rfVIIa
3. 10 mg vitamin K slow IV infusion
4. INR check after infusions
   (a) If still >1.5 repeat with 2,000 units dosing

Rationale:

Profilnine – replenishment of factors II, IX, and X depleted by warfarin

rfVIIa – replenishment of factor VII depleted by warfarin

Vitamin K – longer-term warfarin reversal

Conclusion

Considering the complexity of the hematologic system, its function is very well preserved as an individual ages, but the trauma physician needs to be aware of the slight changes that impact the older injured patient. An older patient will likely present with a lower baseline hemoglobin. It will be more difficult for the patient to recover from any hemorrhage secondary to the bone marrow and hematopoietic stem cell changes that are part of normal aging. After the initial injury, the older patient will return to their slightly hypercoagulable state which is important to consider in their recovery. Finally, with the prescribing practices in the USA, the older patient may be on certain medications that affect the hematologic system and can have negative impacts on their post-injury recovery.

References

1. MacKenzie EJ, Fowler CJ. Epidemiology. In: Feliciano DV, Moore EE, Mattox KL, editors. Trauma. 6th ed. New York: McGraw Hill; 1996. p. 26–32.
2. Kannus P, Parkkari J, Koshkinen S, Niemi S, Palvanen M, Jarvinen M, Vuori I. Fall-induced injuries and deaths among older adults. JAMA. 1999;281:1895–9.
3. Alexander BH, Rivara FP, Wolf ME. The cost and frequency of hospitalization for fall-related injuries in older adults. Am J Public Health. 1992;82:1020–3.
4. Hill RD. The prevalence of anemia in the over-65's in a rural practice. Practitioner. 1967;217:963–7.
5. Myers MA, Saunders CRG, Chalmers DG. The hemoglobin level of fit elderly people. Lancet. 1968;292:261–3.
6. McLennan WJ, Andrews VGR, Macleod C, Caird FL. Anemia in the elderly. Q J Med. 1973;42:1–13.
7. Gershoff SN, Brusis OA, Hipolito VN, Huber AM. Studies of the elderly in Boston. The effects of iron fortification on moderately anemic people. Am J Clin Nutr. 1977;30:226–34.
8. Lipschitz DA, Udupa KB, Milton KY, Thompson CO. Effect of age on hematopoiesis in man. Blood. 1984;63:502–9.
9. Ershler WB, Sheng S, McKelvey J, Artz AS, Denduluri N, Tecson J, et al. Serum erythropoietin and aging: a longitudinal analysis. J Am Geriatr Soc. 2005;53:1360–5.
10. Brightwell RF, Crawford GP, Cale JB, Pedler PJ, Bittles AH. Ageing and the haematological profiles of an Australian Community. Ann Hum Biol. 1998;25:1–10.
11. Deschler B, Lubbert M. Acute myeloid leukemia: epidemiology and etiology. Cancer. 2006;107:2099–107.
12. Hotta T, Hirabayashi N, Utsumi M, Murate T, Yamada H. Age-related changes in the function of hemopoietic stroma in mice. Exp Hematol. 1980;8:933–6.
13. Harrison DE. Long-term erythropoietic repopulating ability of old, young, and fetal stem cells. J Exp Med. 1983;157:1496–504.
14. Gross L. Mechanisms of aging in bone marrow stem cells. PLoS Biol. 2007;5:e215.
15. Woolthuis C, deHaan G, Huls G. Aging of hematopoietic stem cells: intrinsic changes or micro-environment effects? Curr Opin Immunol. 2011;23:512–7.
16. Pinto A, De Filippi R, Frigeri F, Corazzelli G, Normanno N. Aging and the hemopoietic system. Crit Rev Oncol Hematol. 2003;48:S3–12.
17. Balducci L, Lyman GH. Patients aged ≥70 are at high risk for neutropenic infection and should receive hemopoietic growth factors when treated with moderately toxic chemotherapy. J Clin Oncol. 2000;18:3558–85.
18. Gaynor E, Dahlberg S, Fisher R. Factors affecting reduced survival of the elderly with intermediate and high-grade lymphoma: an analysis of SWOG-8516 (INT 0067). Proc Am Soc Clin Oncol. 1994;13:370.
19. Boggs DR, Patrene KD. Hematopoiesis and the aging III: anemia and a blunted erythropoietic response to hemorrhage in aged mice. Am J Hematol. 1985;19:327–38.
20. Wu W, Schifftner TL, Henderson WG, Eaton CB, Poses RM, Uttley G, et al. Preoperative hematocrit levels and postoperative outcomes in older patients undergoing noncardiac surgery. JAMA. 2007;297:2481–7.
21. Gearhart MM, Luchette FA, Proctor MC, Lutomski DM, Witsken C, James L, et al. The risk assessment profile score identifies trauma patients at risk for deep vein thrombosis. Surgery. 2000;128:631–40.
22. Tracy RP, Bovill EG. Thrombosis and cardiovascular risk in the elderly. Arch Pathol Lab Med. 1992;116:1307–12.
23. Balleisen L, Bailey J, Epping PH, Schulte H, van de Loo J. Epidemiological study on factor VII, factor VIII and fibrinogen in an industrial population: I. Baseline data on the relation to age, gender, body-weight, smoking, alcohol, pill-using, and menopause. Thromb Haemost. 1985;54:475–9.
24. Mari D, Mannucci PM, Coppola R, Bottaso B, Bauer KA, Rosenburg RD. Hypercoagulability in centenarians: the paradox of successful aging. Blood. 1995;85:3144–9.
25. Sagripanti A, Capri A. Natural anticoagulants, aging, and thromboembolism. Exp Gerontol. 1998;33:891–6.
26. Sakkin PA, Cushman M, Psaty BM, Kuller LH, Bajaj SP, Sabharwal AK, et al. Correlates of antithrombin, protein C, protein S, and TFPI in a healthy elderly cohort. Thromb Haemost. 1998;80:134–9.
27. Zahavi J, Jones NAG, Leyton J, Dubiel M, Kakkar VV. Enhanced in vivo "platelet reaction" in old healthy individuals. Thromb Res. 1980;17:329–36.
28. Modesti PA, Fortini A, Abbate R, Gensini GF. Age related changes of platelet prostacyclin receptors in humans. Eur J Clin Invest. 1985;15:204–8.
29. Bastyr III EJ, Kadrofske MM, Vink AI. Platelet activity and phosphoinositide turnover increases with advancing age. Am J Med. 1990;88:601–6.
30. Conlan MG, Folsom AR, Finch A, Davis CE, Sorlie P, Marucci G, et al. Associations of factor VIII and von Willebrand factor with age, race, sex, and risk factors for atherosclerosis. The Atherosclerosis Risk in Communities (ARIC) Study. Thromb Haemost. 1993;70:380–5.

31. Abbate R, Prisco D, Rostagno C, Boddi M, Gensini GF. Age-related changes in the hemostatic system. Int J Clin Lab Res. 1993; 23:1–3.
32. Yamamoto K, Takeshita K, Kojima T, Takamatsu J, Saito H. Aging and plasminogen activator inhibitor-1 (PAI-1) regulation: implication in the pathogenesis of thrombotic disorders in the elderly. Cardiovasc Res. 2005;66:276–85.
33. Yamamoto K, Takeshita K, Shimokawa T, Yi H, Isobe K, Loskutoff DJ, et al. Plasminogen activator inhibitor-1 is a major stress-related gene: implications for stress-induced thrombosis in aged individuals. Proc Natl Acad Sci U S A. 2002;99:890–5.
34. Konkle BA, Schuster SJ, Kelly MD, Harjes K, Hassestt DE, Bohrer M, et al. Plasminogen activator inhibitor-1 messenger RNA expression is induced in rat hepatocytes in vivo by dexamethasone. Blood. 1992;79:2636–42.
35. Yamamoto K, Loskutoff DJ. Fibrin deposition in tissues from endotoxin-treated mice correlates with decreases in the expression of urokinase-type but not tissue-type plasminogen activator. J Clin Invest. 1996;97:2440–51.
36. Pignone M, Anderson GK, Binns K, Tilson HH, Weisman SM. Aspirin use among adults aged 40 and older in the United States: results of a national survey. Am J Prev Med. 2007;32:403–7.
37. Clinton P, et al. Pharma Exec 50. May 2010. http://pharmexec.findpharma.com/pharmexec/data/articlestandard//pharmexec/222010/671415/article.pdf. Accessed 8/1/2012.
38. Ohm C, Mina A, Howells G, Bair H, Bendick P. Effects of antiplatelet agents on outcomes for elderly patients with traumatic intracranial hemorrhage. J Trauma. 2055;58:518–22.
39. Ivascu FA, Howells GA, Junn FS, Bair HA, Bendick PJ, Janczyk RJ. Predictors of mortality in trauma patients with intracranial hemorrhage on preinjury aspirin or clopidogrel. J Trauma. 2008;65: 785–8.
40. Thiele T, Sumnig A, Hron G, Muller C, Althaus K, Schroeder HW, et al. Platelet transfusion for reversal of dual antiplatelet therapy in patients requiring urgent surgery: a pilot study. J Thromb Haemost. 2012;10:968–71.
41. Ranucci M, Nano G, Pazzaglia A, Bianchi P, Casana R, Tealdi DG. Platelet mapping and desmopressin reversal of platelet inhibition during emergent carotid endarterectomy. J Cardiothorac Vasc Anesth. 2007;21:851–4.
42. Bansal V, Fortlage D, Lee J, Doucet J, Potenza B, Coimbra R. A new clopidogrel (Plavix) point-of-care assay: rapid determination of antiplatelet activity in trauma patients. J Trauma. 2011;70:65–9.
43. Bachelani AM, Bautz JT, Sperry JL, Corcos A, Zenati M, Billiar TR, et al. Assessment of platelet transfusion for reversal of aspirin after traumatic brain injury. Surgery. 2011;150:836–43.
44. Feinberg WM, Blackshear JL, Laupacis A, Kronmal R, Hart RG. Prevalence, age distribution, and gender of patients with atrial fibrillation. Analysis and implications. Arch Intern Med. 1995;155: 469–73.
45. Go AS, Hylek EM, Phillips KA, Chang Y, Henault LE, Selby JV, et al. Prevalence of diagnosed atrial fibrillation in adults: national implications for rhythm management and stroke prevention: the AnTicoagulation and Risk Factors in Atrial Fibrillation (ATRIA) Study. JAMA. 2001;285:2370–5.
46. Ageno W, Gallus AS, Witkowsky A, Crowther M, Hylek EM, Palareti G, American College of Chest Physicians. Oral anticoagulant therapy and prevention of thrombosis, 9th ed: American College of Physicians Evidence-Based Clinical Practice Guidelines. Chest. 2012;141:e44s–88.
47. Mina AA, Bair HA, Howells GA, Bendick PJ. Complications of preinjury warfarin use in the trauma patient. J Trauma. 2003; 54:842–7.
48. Kuwashiro T, Yasaka M, Itabashi R, Nakagaki H, Miyashita F, Naritomi H, et al. Effect of prothrombin complex concentrate on hematoma enlargement and clinical outcome in patients with anticoagulant-associated intracerebral hemorrhage. Cerebrovasc Dis. 2001;31:170–6.
49. Sarode R, Matevosyan K, Bhagat R, Rutherford C, Madden C, Beshay JE. Rapid warfarin reversal: a 3-factor prothrombin complex concentrate and recombinant factor VIIA cocktail for intracerebral hemorrhage. J Neurosurg. 2012;116:491–7.
50. DeLoughery TG. Practical aspects of the oral new anticoagulants. Am J Hematol. 2011;86:586–90.
51. Furie KL, Goldstein LB, Albers GW, Khatri P, Neyens R, Turakhia MP, et al. Oral antithrombotic agents for the prevention of stroke in nonvalvular atrial fibrillation: a science advisory for healthcare professionals from the American Heart Association/American Stroke Association. Stroke. 2012;43:3442–53.
52. Pragst I, Zeitler SH, Doerr B, Kaspereit FJ, Herzog E, Dickneite G, et al. Reversal of dabigatran anticoagulation by prothrombin complex concentrate (Beriplex P/N) in a rabbit model. J Thromb Haemost. 2012;10(9):1841–8.
53. Fukuda T, Honda Y, Kamisato C, Morishima Y, Shibano T. Reversal of anticoagulant effects of edoxaban, an oral, direct factor Xa inhibitor, with haemostatic agents. Thromb Haemost. 2012;107:253–9.

Geriatric Psychology and the Injured Elderly

8

Robert D. Barraco, Anne M. Yawman, and Joshua Gish

Introduction

Cognitive and other psychological disorders adversely affect outcomes in the hospitalized elderly [1]. This has also been demonstrated in those with orthopedic injury [2–5]. Functional impairment (ADL, IADL), cognitive impairment, and a history of cognitive deterioration have been associated with in-hospital mortality in critically ill patients. Dependence in activities of daily living and moderate-to-severe cognitive impairment are independent risk factors for in-hospital mortality [6]. Studies in the trauma literature are few and far between. Conflicting results seem to be related to inaccuracy in the diagnoses of dementia and delirium [7]. In the following pages, we will discuss the essentials of several neuropsychiatric disorders prevalent in the geriatric trauma patient.

Cognitive Disorders/Dementia

The DSM-IV describes dementia as the development of multiple cognitive deficits that include memory impairment and at least one of the following:

- Aphasia
- Apraxia
- Agnosia
- Disturbance in executive functioning

The cognitive deficits must be sufficiently severe to cause impairment in occupational or social functioning and represent a decline from a previous higher level of functioning. If the deficits only occur during the course of delirium, the diagnosis of dementia should not be made. Both may be diagnosed if the dementia is present at times when the delirium is not present [8].

Dementia is often moderate to severe by the time it is diagnosed. Overall, women exhibit dementia and cognitive impairment more often than males. Alzheimer's disease is more common in women and vascular dementia is more common in men.

People with dementia were more likely to be admitted for fractured femurs, lower respiratory tract infections, urinary tract infections, and head injuries than people without dementia. Mean length of stay for admissions for people with dementia was 16.4 days as opposed to those without dementia. People with dementia were more likely than those without to be readmitted within 3 months for another multi-day stay. Mortality rates and transfers to nursing home care were higher for people with dementia than for people without dementia. These outcomes were more pronounced in younger people with dementia [1].

Types of Dementia

There are many different types of dementia. In this section, we will focus on the most common types of dementia encountered in the geriatric trauma patient. Table 8.1 summarizes the most common types that are discussed in the following pages.

Alzheimer's disease is the most common type of dementia with up to 50–70 % of cases. Vascular dementia can have

R.D. Barraco, MD, MPH, FACS, FCCP (✉)
Department of Surgery, Lehigh Valley Health Network, 1240 S Cedar Crest Blvd, Suite 308, Allentown, PA 18103, USA
e-mail: robert_d.barraco@lvhn.org

A.M. Yawman, MD
Department of Geriatric Medicine, Lehigh Valley Hospital Network, 17th & Chew Streets, 7017, Allentown, PA 18105, USA
e-mail: anne_m.yawman@lvhn.or

J. Gish, MD
General Surgery Resident, Lehigh Valley Health Network, 1240 S Cedar Crest Blvd, Suite 308, PGY 4, Allentown, PA 18103, USA
e-mail: joshua_s.gish@lvhn.org

J.A. Yelon, F.A. Luchette (eds.), *Geriatric Trauma and Critical Care*,
DOI 10.1007/978-1-4614-8501-8_8,

Table 8.1 Comparison of common types of dementia

	Alzheimer's	Lewy body	Frontal lobe	Vascular
% of cases	50	20	<10	20
Pathology	Neurofibrillary tangles	Lewy bodies in cortex and amygdala	Degeneration of frontal regions	Varied vascular
Distinct Features	Progressive memory loss	Parkinson-like symptoms; hallucinations; transient loss of consciousness	Behavioral and personality changes	Varied depending on location
Specific medical treatment	Cholinesterase inhibitors and memantine	No specific treatment; cholinesterase inhibitors for cognitive symptoms; Parkinson's meds for motor symptoms	No specific treatment; Alzheimer's meds may worsen symptoms	No specific treatment

a number of different etiologies and is the second most common behind Alzheimer's disease. Frontal lobe dementia and Lewy body dementia will also be discussed here.

Alzheimer's Disease

Alzheimer's disease (AD) is progressive and irreversible and eventually leads to death [9]. At least 5.4 million people in the United States are affected. It is the sixth leading cause of death in adults. One in eight adults age 65 and over and half of those 85 and over have the disease. Direct costs for caring for patients with Alzheimer's disease is $200 billion dollars, of which $140 billion is paid by Medicare and Medicaid. By the year 2050, over $1 trillion dollars will be spent on Alzheimer's disease [10].

Neurofibrillary tangles and neuritic plaques are the characteristic lesions in the brain with Alzheimer's disease. Beta-amyloid protein is present in these lesions and may play a central role in the disease as may a deficit of acetylcholine and cholinergic areas [11, 12]. A history of head trauma as well as vascular disease increases the risk of Alzheimer's disease. Clinical features include progressive memory loss, impairment of language, visuospatial ability, and executive function. As in most dementias, behavioral and psychotic symptoms may occur.

Lewy Body Dementia

Lewy body dementia is characterized by Parkinson-like symptoms, recurrent visual hallucinations, neuroleptic sensitivity, fluctuating cognition, falls or syncope, and a transient loss of consciousness. Lewy body dementia may account for up to 20 % of dementia in the United States, affecting up to 1.3 million people. Only 30–50 % of cases are accurately diagnosed [13].

Hallmark lesions are protein deposits known as Lewy bodies. These deposits are located in the cortex and amygdala in Lewy body dementia, as opposed to Parkinson's, where the deposits are in the brainstem and substantia nigra.

Both the cholinergic and dopaminergic systems are severely disrupted in this disease. Other causes for cognitive decline in the setting of Parkinsonism should be excluded with testing.

Frontal Lobe Dementias

Frontotemporal dementias are a heterogeneous group of disorders that involve degeneration of different regions of the frontal and temporal lobes. Behavioral and personality changes may predominate over cognitive deficits in the clinical picture. These include a loss of personal or social awareness, a lack of insight, inappropriate and stereotyped behaviors, aggression, distraction, a loss of inhibitions, apathy, or extroverted behavior. Some cases involve language and aphasia as primary characteristics. The majority of cases of this group of disorders occur in those under 65 years old.

As this is a group of disorders, the pathophysiology is not well understood.

The cognitive, neuropsychiatric, and behavioral symptoms depend on the regions of the brain involved. Though beginning as a regional process, as the disease progresses, the atrophy and pathology become more generalized.

Vascular Dementia

The term vascular dementia applies to many vascular causes of dementia, including multi-infarct dementia and small vessel disease. About one-fifth of all cases of dementia are vascular. Many of the same things that put one at risk for cardiovascular disease also put one at risk for vascular dementia. These include diabetes, hypercholesterolemia, hyperhomocysteinemia, hypertension, cigarette smoking, and physical inactivity. The effects of these risk factors may vary depending on the type of vascular dementia. Some types are related to specific gene mutations but are rare.

The presenting symptoms and signs will depend on the location of the lesions. Left hemisphere lesions usually cause language problems, and right hemisphere lesions generally cause visuospatial problems. The course may be stepwise, either with abrupt declines or more insidious. Memory or mood complaints are common in both vascular and Alzheimer's disease. Recognition memory is often preserved in vascular dementia, not in Alzheimer's. Isolated psychotic symptoms, apathy, and higher cortical disturbance with intact memory may also be vascular dementia.

Cognitive Screening Tests

Dementia is characterized by an acquired and persistent deficit in cognitive domains that interferes with daily functioning. One must first rule out potentially reversible cognitive deficits due to underlying disorders. Laboratory and imaging tests should be done as indicated. Disorders that can mimic dementia include depression, delirium, anticholinergic medications, and toxic metabolic encephalopathy. We will discuss this further in our final section of this chapter.

There are several standardized screening tests for cognitive impairment. One of the oldest and most well known is the Mini-Mental State Examination (MMSE) [14]. It is a brief, 30-point questionnaire which takes about 10 minutes to complete. It can be used to evaluate a patient at a point in time and then repeated to check response to treatment. Categories assessed are orientation to time and place, registration, attention and calculation, recall, language, repetition, and complex commands. A score of 25 or greater is normal. Scores of 21–24, 10–20, and ≤9 indicate mild, moderate, and severe cognitive impairment, respectively. Adjustments may need to be made to the raw score for educational level and age.

The Mini-Cog is a quick and simple method of screening for cognitive dysfunction [15]. It takes about 3–5 minutes to complete. It consists of three-item recall and clock drawing. Clock drawing was used to clarify scores when memory was intermediate. Recall of none of three items signified dementia. Recall of one or two items signified dementia when accompanied by an abnormal clock drawing test. Recall of all three items was considered normal. When compared to the MMSE, the Mini-Cog had better sensitivity at 99 % and correctly classified the greatest percentage (96 %) of subjects. Its diagnostic value was not influenced by education or language [15].

The Montreal Cognitive Assessment (MoCA) is a one-page 30-point test that takes about 10 minutes to complete [16]. The domains assessed are short-term memory recall, visuospatial abilities, executive functions, attention, concentration and working memory, language, and orientation to time and place. MoCA may be better for mild cognitive impairment and early dementias as well as other neurological disorders that affect younger patients such as Huntington's and Parkinson's diseases [17–21].

The Saint Louis University Mental Status Examination (SLUMS) is an alternative to the MMSE. In fact, in a large study comparing the two tests, SLUMS was able to better detect mild neurocognitive disorder [22]. Sensitivity and specificity of the two tests are comparable. The test takes about 10 minutes to administer and includes a clock drawing test.

Overview of Treatments

Since the focus of this chapter is the effects of neuropsychological problems on the geriatric trauma patient, treatments of dementia will be addressed briefly. Practitioners should discuss these with the geriatricians and pharmacists. However, treatment of the symptoms that influence our care of the trauma patient will be discussed in more detail.

Alzheimer's disease had several FDA-approved drug therapies. The cholinesterase inhibitors and memantine are used to address cognitive symptoms. Patients may survive as long as 20 years with Alzheimer's disease but many patients succumb in the early or middle stages of the disease.

Lewy body dementia has no FDA-approved treatment. As there are cholinergic losses and relationship with Alzheimer's disease, cholinesterase inhibitors were found to have a role and have become standard treatment for cognitive symptoms [23]. Low doses of Parkinson's medications, i.e., levodopa, may help motor symptoms, but caution must be used as higher doses can worsen neuropsychiatric symptoms. Average duration of illness is 5–7 years but with much variability.

Frontal lobe dementias have no specific treatments or cures. Not all cases have the same underlying pathology. Cholinesterase inhibitors and memantine may worsen behavioral and psychological symptoms. Long-term care is necessary as the average duration between onset of illness and death is 7 years.

There are no specific treatments for vascular dementia. Control of vascular risk factors is primary. Behavioral and psychological features are treated as necessary.

Behavioral and psychological symptoms including depression occur in the majority of patient with dementia. Psychological symptoms include delusions, hallucinations, paranoia, anxiety, and apathy. Behavioral symptoms include wandering, aggression, hostility, insomnia, inappropriate eating, and abnormal sexual behaviors [24].

Non-pharmacological strategies should be employed in all acute care facilities and are the first-line therapies for behavioral and psychological symptoms in dementia. These consist of environmental and behavioral interventions such as regularly scheduled routines for meals, sleep, and bathing. Reorientation with a clearly visible clock and calendar is indicated. Caregivers should use clear instructions and make frequent eye contact with patients. Sensory impairments, such as vision and hearing loss, should be minimized. These will be addressed in more depth in the section on delirium.

Pharmacological interventions are variable depending on the type of dementia. When medication is necessary, neuropsychiatric symptoms in many dementias have been treated with antipsychotics. Atypical antipsychotics may be better than typical [25]. Quetiapine has been used for psychosis in Parkinsonian syndromes [26]. However, there are concerns regarding the use of these agents. First-generation antipsychotics produce more extrapyramidal symptoms. The second-generation antipsychotics have had a "black box" warning label added by the US Food and Drug Administration for a small but statistically significant increase in cerebrovascular events and death. The older antipsychotics also carry an increased risk of death [27]. In fact, a recent cohort study looking at over 75,000 elderly nursing home patients using antipsychotics found that haloperidol had a higher risk of dying when compared with risperidone [28]. Quetiapine users had a decreased risk of dying. A dose–response relation was noted with all drugs but quetiapine.

Patients with dementia may have a paradoxical agitation when given benzodiazepines and tricyclic antidepressants have unwanted anticholinergic effects. Mood stabilizers, especially SSRIs, may help neuropsychiatric features of frontotemporal dementias.

Cholinesterase inhibitors have been used for neuropsychiatric symptom treatment of Alzheimer's disease and vascular dementias since cholinergic deficiency also appears to be involved in their development [29]. However, when used in frontotemporal dementias, they may worsen these symptoms.

Neuropsychiatric symptoms in Lewy body dementias can be challenging to treat medically. Older antipsychotic drugs may cause worsening of symptoms and neuroleptic malignant syndrome in Lewy body dementias. As mentioned previously, newer antipsychotics seem to be more beneficial. Benzodiazepines, anticholinergics, and some antidepressants may cause sedation, motor impairment, or confusion. Medications for Parkinsonian symptoms may also worsen confusion, delusions, and hallucinations in higher doses.

In summary, the bottom line is that first-line therapies for neuropsychiatric and behavioral symptoms should be nonpharmacological and medications should be used judiciously and with caution. As the principle of geriatric pharmacological intervention states, "start low, go slow but go." But in this case, only go if you have to.

Delirium

Definition and Epidemiology

Delirium is a transient, reversible syndrome of impairment of consciousness, attention, and perception in the setting of a medical condition that is acute and fluctuating. The roots of the word are Latin with the term coined by Celsus and included in his work De Medicina. Taking the term apart, "de" is Latin for "away from" and "lira" is the Latin term for "furrow in a field." So putting it together, it means "going off track." [30]

Delirium occurs in 60 % of hospitalized frail-elderly patients [31]. One study found that 89 % of survivors of stupor or coma progressed to delirium [32]. Similarly, in the general surgical population, the incidence of delirium is about 37–46 % and postoperative delirium has been described to occur in 10–60 % of patients [33, 34]. Again, the range in incidence of postoperative delirium depends on the type of surgery and the population studied. For example, the incidence of delirium was found to be 65 % after femoral neck fracture repair [35–37]. Approximately seven out of ten surgical intensive care and trauma intensive care patients experience delirium [38].

There are three subtypes of delirium: hyperactive, hypoactive, and mixed. To be diagnosed with hyperactive delirium, the patient must exhibit three or more of the following: hypervigilance, restlessness, fast and/or loud speech, anger, irritability, combativeness, impatience, uncooperativeness, laughing, swearing, singing, euphoria, easy startling, distractibility, nightmares, persistent thoughts, and wandering. For hypoactive, the most difficult to identify, the patient must exhibit four or more of the following: unawareness, lethargy, decreased alertness, decreased motor activity, staring, sparse and/or slow speech, and apathy [39]. Mixed, which is the most common subtype, has features of both.

Delirium has been shown to increase mortality when other factors are controlled for. Studies have shown that the mortality rate at whatever interval studied and in whatever population was significantly higher. Mortality rates range from 8 to 1 % in hospitalized inpatients, 34–15 % 6-month mortality after ICU stay, and 11–3 % 90-day mortality in med-surg patients [31, 40, 41].

The costs of delirium can be staggering, ranging from $38 billion to $152 billion per year in a study of healthcare costs [42]. Though patients with delirium survived fewer days than those without, they had significantly higher adjusted costs, over 2.5 times the costs of patients without delirium. Costs attributable to delirium were $16,303 to $64,421 per patients.

Causes and Risk Factors

The causes and risk factors are many. Temporal relationship to clinical events is an important clue to cause. For example, exposure to midazolam is an independent and potentially modifiable risk factor for the transitioning to delirium [38]. So delirium arising after administration of midazolam would point to the drug as the cause.

The cause may also be determined by the clinical situation or condition. Potentially life-threatening conditions that

Table 8.2 Causes of delirium

Categories	Examples
*I*nfectious	Encephalitis, meningitis, pneumonia, urinary tract infection
*W*ithdrawal	Alcohol, sedative-hypnotics
*A*cute metabolic	Acidosis, alkalosis, electrolyte disturbances, hepatic or renal failure
*T*rauma	Heat stroke, burns, surgery
*C*NS pathology	Hemorrhage, seizures, stroke, tumors, vasculitis, hydrocephalus
*H*ypoxia	Hypoxia from cardiac or pulmonary cause, anemia, carbon monoxide poisoning, hypotension
*D*eficiencies	Vitamin B_{12}, niacin, thiamine
*E*ndocrinopathies	Disorders of glucose, cortisol, thyroid, and parathyroids
*A*cute vascular	Hypertensive encephalopathy, shock
*T*oxins or drugs	Medications, toxins
*H*eavy metals	Lead, manganese, mercury

cause delirium can be remembered by the mnemonic WHHHHIMPS. They are Wernicke's disease; hypoxia; hypoglycemia; hypertensive encephalopathy; hyperthermia or hypothermia; intracerebral hemorrhage; meningitis/encephalitis; poisoning, either exogenous or iatrogenic; and status epilepticus.

Other risk factors can be divided into potentially modifiable and nonmodifiable. Nonmodifiable risk factors include dementia or cognitive impairment, age over 65, chronic renal or hepatic disease, multiple comorbidities, and a history of delirium, stroke, neurological disease, falls, or gait disorder. Potentially modifiable risk factors include surgery pain, intercurrent illness, acute neurological diseases, medications, immobilization even by catheters or restraints, sensory impairment of hearing or vision, metabolic derangements, environment, emotional distress, and sustained sleep deprivation. The categories of causes can be remembered by the mnemonic I WATCH DEATH. Table 8.2 explains the mnemonic.

Dementia as a risk factor was discussed in the previous section. Two studies help accentuate its importance. Wahlund and Bjorlin in 1999 found that approximately 70 % of elderly patients admitted to a specialized delirium ward had either dementia or mild cognitive impairment [43]. In a study of total joint replacement patients, all demented patients postoperatively developed delirium, compared with 31.8 % in the non-demented patients [37].

Age is another risk factor for delirium. One study suggests this relationship is linear after age 65. In mechanically ventilated patients, the probability of developing delirium increased by 2 % for each year over 65 [44].

Hypoxia is a well-known risk factor for delirium. Not only poor oxygenation but also poor oxygen delivery, i.e., anemia, can contribute to delirium [45, 46]. Hypoxia can come from many causes, even obstructive sleep apnea [47].

Table 8.3 Objective tests to diagnose delirium

Cognitive Test for Delirium (CTD)
Confusion Assessment Method (CAM and Confusion Assessment Method for the Intensive Care Unit(CAM-ICU)
Confusional State Evaluation (CSE)
Delirium Assessment Scale (DAS)
Delirium Detection Score (DDS)
Delirium Index (DI)
Delirium Rating Scale and Delirium Rating Scale-revised-98 (DRS)
Delirium Severity Scale (DSS)
Delirium Symptom Interview (DSI)
Memorial Delirium Assessment Scale (MDAS)
Short Portable Mental Status Questionnaire (SPMSQ)

Many medications have the capacity to cause delirium. This is especially true of those with psychoactive effects and those with anticholinergic affects. There appears to be a direct relationship between a drug's anticholinergic properties and the development of delirium [48–50]. A study by Han et al. found that exposure to anticholinergic agents was an independent risk factor for the development of delirium and an increased symptom severity [51].

Dr. Mark Beers created the first Beers' Criteria list in 1991with a consensus panel of experts. It has been updated several times, most recently in 2012. The list identifies medications or classes of medication that are potentially inappropriate that one should avoid in all older adults, in older adults with certain diseases and syndromes that the drugs listed can exacerbate, and medications to be used with caution in older adults [52]. The drugs which contribute to delirium are on this list. All practitioners caring for the elderly must be aware of this list and utilize it to the benefit of their patients. The most recent update of the criteria will be used as an educational tool and a quality measure.

Postoperative pain is an independent predictor of delirium after surgery [34]. Narcotic agents may cause delirium as well [53]. Some opioids may be more likely to cause delirium than others, with the data on meperidine being the most consistent [54].

Diagnosis and Screening

Delirium is unrecognized in many cases. Numbers in the literature range from 65 to 84 % of cases that go undiagnosed. Delirium can mimic many other mental illnesses. A cornerstone of diagnosis is looking for the underlying causes and correcting modifiable ones.

There are a host of objective diagnostic and screening tests for delirium in the literature (Table 8.3). In December 2008, the Canadian Agency for Drugs and Technologies in Health published a review of evidence-based guidelines on diagnostic tests for delirium. They reviewed the 2006

Canadian Coalition for Seniors' Mental Health (CCSMH) published evidence-based guidelines for the assessment and treatment of delirium, the 2006 British Geriatrics Society and the Royal College of Physicians' evidence-based delirium guidelines, and the 2007 delirium guidelines for general hospitals by Swiss and French physicians [55–58]. They concluded that early assessment for delirium is needed in hospitalized elderly patients. This early detection of risk factors may prevent delirium and its complication. Physicians and nurses must be trained to recognize delirium and educated in the use of validated screening and diagnostic tools. They suggested that the Confusion Assessment Method be used for screening and diagnosis and the Diagnostic and Statistical Manual of Mental Disorders (DSM-IV) criteria be used to confirm the diagnosis.

In 2010, the National Clinical Guideline Centre of Britain published its clinical guideline titled "Delirium: Diagnosis, Prevention and Management." As to screening and diagnosis, they recommended screening for behavioral changes at presentation and daily during hospital admission. If indicators of delirium are identified, they recommend that a healthcare professional who is trained and competent in the diagnosis of delirium carry out a clinical assessment based on the DSM-IV criteria or Confusion Assessment Method short version (short CAM) to confirm the diagnosis. The CAM-ICU should be used when patients are intubated in the ICU or recovery room postoperatively [59].

Since the CAM and CAM-ICU have been recommended in these evidence-based reviews, we will discuss them here. The Confusion Assessment Method was unveiled in 1990 and the Confusion Assessment Method-ICU in 2001 [60, 61]. Both have a sensitivity of 94–100 %, a specificity of 89–95 %, and high inter-rater reliability [62].

The CAM has a long and a short version. The long version is comprehensive and screens for nine clinical features. The short version focuses on the four features that have the greatest discriminatory ability to detect delirium from other cognitive disorders (Fig. 8.1).

The CAM-ICU addresses the same four areas as the short version CAM. It was developed by Ely et al. at Vanderbilt. It takes less than 2 minutes to complete and can be given to intubated patients. The process is shown in Fig. 8.1.

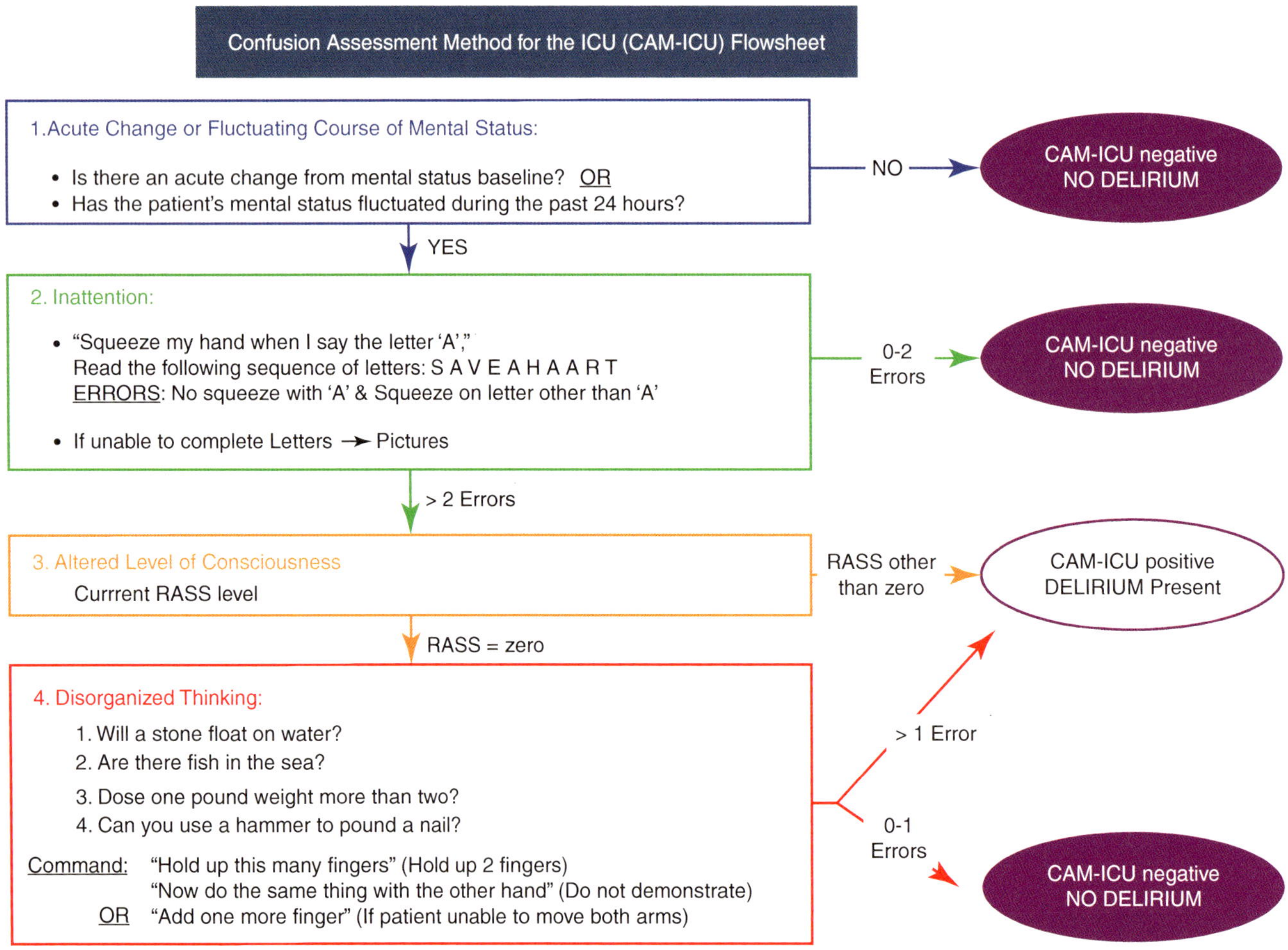

Fig. 8.1 Confusion Assessment Method for the ICU (CAM-ICU) flow sheet

Prevention and Treatment

In the case of delirium, prevention is truly the best medicine. The National Clinical Guideline Centre of Britain addressed prevention in its clinical guideline titled "Delirium: Diagnosis, Prevention and Management." [59] The following paragraphs are a summary of the findings of the review supplemented by additional sources as indicated.

Delirium can be difficult to recognize and treat. People at risk for delirium should be under the care of an interdisciplinary team that is "trained and competent in delirium prevention." It would be best if the team were familiar to the patient at risk. Patients at risk should remain with the same caregivers and not change units unless necessary. A tailored multicomponent program should be administered which includes environmental change and non-pharmacological interventions. Rather than recommend a particular program, they chose to focus on the elements that should be addressed. They are detailed below. The early assessment of risk is key to this process.

Changes to ensure good sleep patterns include changes to the method of carrying out clinical care. Nursing and medical procedures should be avoided during sleep periods. This includes administration of medication as is possible. Noise should be reduced to a minimum during these times as well.

Attention must be paid to medications themselves. Utilization of a tool such as the Beers' Criteria list mentioned earlier will help identify medications placing the patient at risk and suggest substitutes. Including a pharmacist on the interdisciplinary team can help.

Closely assessing for and correcting hypoxia are essential. The same is true for infection. Occult infection can present as delirium. Infection control procedures including reducing use of catheters are important.

Any sensory impairment that can be improved or resolved should be addressed. Removing impacted earwax and ensuring the availability and use of working hearing and visual aids are among the interventions that can reduce risk.

Lack of or impaired mobility is another risk factor that can be addressed. Early postoperative mobilization should be encouraged whenever possible. Assistive devices should be readily available. Even those who cannot walk should be encouraged to perform active range-of-motion exercises. Physical therapy or rehabilitation medicine can help as part of the interdisciplinary team.

Dehydration and constipation can be detrimental risk factors. Appropriate hydration can be maintained by oral, subcutaneous, or intravenous fluids depending on the status of the patient. Consult as necessary for patients with comorbidities such as heart or renal failure. A bowel regimen should be used with a stepwise approach for prophylaxis and treatment.

Nutrition must be maintained. Dentures should be properly fitting and available when needed.

Pain must be assessed by whatever means appropriate. Pain management should be undertaken if not already in place. Pain medication should be reviewed if already being administered.

Environmental and practice changes can address cognitive impairment and/or disorientation. Steps include appropriate lighting, clear signage, and easily visible clocks and calendars. As mentioned earlier, clear communication with eye contact should be the norm when dealing with these patients. Frequent reorientation and reassurance can help. Regular visits from family and friends and activities to stimulate cognition, such as reminiscing, have a positive impact as well.

When patients become agitated or a danger to themselves or others, verbal and nonverbal techniques should be used to de-escalate the situation. When these techniques fail, pharmacological interventions should be considered for short-term use. Haloperidol or olanzapine is recommended in the NICE Guideline. Again, per the geriatric medication mantra, "start low, go slow but go." Cautiously titrate to symptoms. Particular caution must be used with antipsychotics for those with Parkinson's-type diseases or Lewy body dementia if they are to be used at all.

One example of an algorithm for prevention and treatment was published by Maldonado in Critical Care Clinics 2008 [63]. Recommendations for the pharmacological treatment begin with assessing current medications and discontinuing inappropriate ones. If possible, only use benzodiazepines or barbiturates for CNS-depressant withdrawal, i.e., alcohol withdrawal, or when other recommended agents have failed and sedation is needed to prevent harm.

For the correction of central anticholinergic syndrome, consider acetylcholinesterase inhibitors. Serotonin antagonists (e.g., ondansetron) can be used to control serotonin elevations usually associated with hypoactive delirium.

Consider changing narcotics from morphine and meperidine to fentanyl or hydromorphone. Sleep can be promoted by melatonin or its agonists.

Choice and dose of agents differ depending on the type of delirium. For hyperactive delirium, low to moderate dose (<20 mg/24 h) haloperidol can be used after ascertaining there are no significant electrolyte abnormalities and other medications that prolong QTc or cardiac conditions. Haloperidol must be discontinued if QTc is prolonged to >25 % of baseline or >500 ms. Atypical antipsychotics should be considered in cases where haloperidol is contraindicated or not desirable. Maldonado suggests there is better evidence for risperidone and quetiapine and limited data for olanzapine, aripiprazole, and perospirone. Clozapine and ziprasidone should be avoided.

For hypoactive delirium, dopamine antagonists may have a place given the excess dopamine theory. Haloperidol may be used but in very low doses, 0.25 to 1 mg/24 h. If atypical antipsychotics are used, ones with low sedative properties should be used, like risperidone, unless sleep pattern is at issue. In cases of extreme psychomotor retardation or catatonia without agitation or psychosis, psychostimulant or conventional dopamine agonists can be of use.

Depression

Epidemiology

Depression in the elderly is under-recognized and under-treated. Almost one in five older adults who commit suicide have visited a physician within 24 h of their death, 41 % visited within 1 week of their suicide, and three-quarters of the elderly who commit suicide visited a physician within a month before their death [64, 65]. The incidence of major depression in the community of elderly is reported up to 1 in 20. This increases to 11.5 % in the hospitalized elderly and 13.5 % of those receiving home healthcare [66]. It is estimated that five million elderly have some symptoms of a depressive disorder [67]. There is a gender difference with the rate of depression higher for elderly women than men [68]. Depression also lowers life expectancy in this age group.

Periods of feeling blue, sad, or unhappy are normal. When these feelings persist and interfere significantly with the ability to function, they become abnormal. Major depressive disorder is diagnosed by DSM-IV-TR criteria when five (or more) of the symptoms in Table 8.4 have been present during the same 2-week period and represent a change from previous functioning [8]. At least one of the symptoms is (1) depressed mood or (2) loss of interest or pleasure. These symptoms must cause clinically significant distress or impairment in social, occupational, or other important areas of functioning. They cannot be a part of mixed episode and cannot be caused by the physiological effects of a substance or other general medical condition or better accounted for by bereavement.

Subclinical depression or minor depressive disorder is even more common. This is defined in the DSM-IV-TR as having 2–4 of the aforementioned depressive symptoms for major depressive disorder. The symptoms must be present for 2 weeks. There must be no history of major depressive disorder. The presentation of subclinical depression may be even more clouded in the elderly. Patients may present with new medical complaints, exacerbation of existing conditions, and a preoccupation with their health.

Many changes in life and function can increase the risk of or worsen depression. Chronic pain, poor health from multiple illnesses, loss of independence, children moving away, and death of a spouse or loved one are just some of the factors contributing to the increased risk. Physical illnesses can cause or increase the risk of depression.

Table 8.4 Symptoms of depression

1. Depressed mood most of the day, nearly every day, as indicated by either subjective report or observation made by others
2. Markedly diminished interest or pleasure in all, or almost all, activities most of the day, nearly every day
3. Significant weight loss when not dieting or significant gain, or decrease or increase, in appetite nearly every day
4. Insomnia or hypersomnia nearly every day
5. Psychomotor agitation or retardation nearly every day
6. Fatigue or loss of energy nearly every day
7. Feelings of worthlessness or excessive or inappropriate guilt (which may be delusional) nearly every day (not merely self-reproach or guilt about being sick)
8. Diminished ability to think or concentrate, or indecisiveness, nearly every day (either by subjective account or as observed by others)
9. Recurrent thoughts of death (not just fear of dying), recurrent suicidal ideation without a specific plan, or a suicide attempt or specific plan for committing suicide

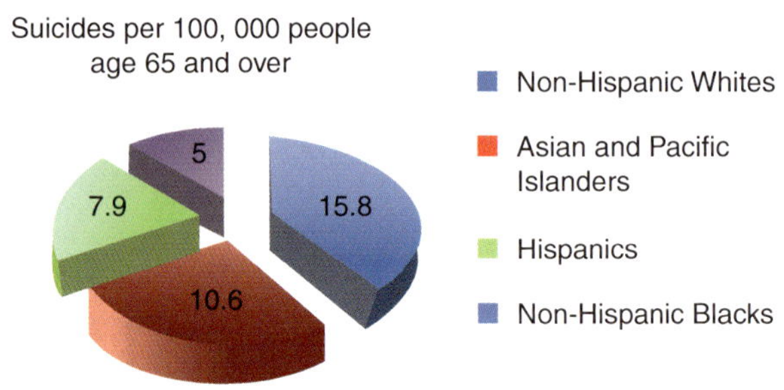

Fig. 8.2 Suicides per 100,000 people age 65 and over

Dementia, thyroid disease, cancer, and stroke, to name a few, can increase the risk of depression. After a stroke, 25–50 % develop depression within 2 years [69]. About 20–30 % of those with Alzheimer's disease are diagnosed with depression. Half of Parkinson's patients have or have had depression [70]. Various medications can also cause symptoms of depression. Healthcare providers, as well as older adults, can incorrectly assume that depression is normal and an acceptable response to these serious illnesses and life hardships [71, 72].

Suicide can be a tragic manifestation of depression. Taking one's own life is disproportionately represented as a cause of death in older Americans. While they make up only 12 % of the US population, people age 65 and older accounted for 16 % of suicide deaths in 2004 [73]. The suicide rate for those age 65 and over is 14.3 of every 100,000 compared to 11 per 100,000 in the general population [73]. Suicide rates increase with age, and suicide rates differ by race (Fig. 8.2). Non-Hispanic white men age 85 and older were most likely to die by suicide. They had a rate of 49.8 suicide deaths per 100,000 persons in that age group. Guns, overdose, and asphyxiation are the most common mechanisms for suicide in the elderly. Older adults are more likely to use lethal means and make fewer attempts per completed suicide.

Factors that increase the risk for suicide are different in older adults. They tend to be more socially isolated [74]. They are more likely to have seen a physician prior to their suicide as mentioned earlier [65, 66]. The highest rates of suicide in the elderly are for those who are divorced or widowed. Future factors such as growth in the numbers of the elderly population, health status, availability of and access to care, and attitudes about aging and suicide will affect suicide rates in this age group.

Risk factors for suicide are present in more than 90 % of older adults who commit suicide. They include depression or other mental disorders, a personal or family history, stressful life events, prior personal or family history of suicide attempt, family violence, guns in the home, incarceration, or exposure to suicidal behavior even in media figures [75]. Substance abuse, the subject of the final section of this chapter, is a contributing factor to successful suicides in all populations.

Assessment and Screening

Assessment of depression can be challenging. The elderly present differently than younger patients. They are less likely to voice emotions or guilt. The elderly tend to minimize or deny depressed mood. They may be preoccupied with somatic symptoms. Cognitive deficits can be marked. They tend to have more anxiety, agitation, and psychosis and other conditions may mask the depression.

The Geriatric Depression Scale (Table 8.5) is widely used to screen for depression [76]. A short form is available as well as apps for the iPhone and Droid. A score of 6–9 on the short form suggests depression and ten or greater is always indicative of depression. As mentioned earlier, the criteria for diagnosing depression is the same as they are in the general population. The aforementioned criteria can be found in the DSM-IV-TR. An easy mnemonic to remember is SIG E CAPS. It stands for sleep, interest, guilt, energy, concentration, appetite, psychomotor changes, and suicidality. The vegetative symptoms of sleep, energy, appetite, and psychomotor changes can occur in other medical conditions. They do not discriminate depression. The psychological symptoms of interest, guilt, concentration, and suicidality are more reliable in teasing out the diagnosis of depression.

Table 8.5 Geriatric Depression Scale (GDS)

Choose the best answer for how you felt this past week.		
Circle one		
1. Are you basically satisfied with your life?	yes	NO
2. Have you dropped many of your activities and interests?	YES	no
3. Do you feel that your life is empty?	YES	no
4. Do you often get bored?	YES	no
5. Are you hopeful about the future?	yes	NO
6. Are you bothered by thoughts you can't get out of your head?	YES	no
7. Are you in good spirits most of the time?	yes	NO
8. Are you afraid that something bad is going to happen to you?	YES	no
9. Do you feel happy most of the time?	yes	NO
10. Do you often feel helpless?	YES	no
11. Do you often get restless and fidgety?	YES	no
12. Do you prefer to stay at home, rather than going out and doing new things?	YES	no
13. Do you frequently worry about the future?	YES	no
14. Do you feel you have more problems with memory than most?	YES	no
15. Do you think it is wonderful to be alive now?	yes	NO
16. Do you often feel downhearted and blue?	YES	no
17. Do you feel pretty worthless the way you are now?	YES	no
18. Do you worry a lot about the past?	YES	no
19. Do you find life very exciting?	yes	NO
20. Is it hard for you to get started on new projects?	YES	no
21. Do you feel full of energy?	yes	NO
22. Do you feel that your situation is hopeless?	YES	no
23. Do you think that most people are better off than you are?	YES	no
24. Do you frequently get upset over little things?	YES	no
25. Do you frequently feel like crying?	YES	no
26. Do you have trouble concentrating?	YES	no
27. Do you enjoy getting up in the morning?	yes	NO
28. Do you prefer to avoid social gatherings?	YES	no
29. Is it easy for you to make decisions?	yes	NO
30. Is your mind as clear as it used to be?	yes	NO
*Count number of CAPITALIZED (depressed) answers		
Score: _____ (number of "depressed" answers)		
Norms		
Normal 5 ± 4		
Mildly depressed 15 ± 6		
Very depressed 23 ± 5		

Treatment

Depression in the elderly should be treated, even when accompanying other illnesses. Left untreated, depression can worsen the outcome of the other illnesses. The decreased ability to metabolize drugs and an increased sensitivity to drug side effects make treatment challenging. To lessen the risk of adverse events from treatment medications, the mantra "start low, go slow but go" is effective. Drugs with anticholinergic effects and excessive sedation should be avoided as they can cause confusion and falls among the adverse events. At times, these side effects can be useful to treat symptoms. For example, a patient with significant weight loss and insomnia may benefit from a sedating medication that increases appetite. Those at risk for suicide should be treated aggressively as inpatients.

Electroconvulsive therapy (ECT) may work well when medical therapy has failed or in patients with Parkinson's disease, high suicide risk, or psychotic features. It is very effective in the short term. Though there can be high relapse rates, drug therapy can reduce relapses.

Nonmedical treatments are useful and synergistic with medical therapy. Individual psychotherapy, interpersonal therapy, and cognitive-behavioral therapy can be used in this population.

Substance Abuse

Epidemiology

Substance abuse and alcoholism are issues that are often overlooked in the elderly. While it is true that the proportion of people who abuse substances decreases with senescence, the truth is that about 1 % of elders do abuse alcohol and up to 16 % of elders engage in heavy drinking (more than two drinks a day for men or one drink a day for women) [77, 78]. This number is expected to increase as the baby boomer generation reaches old age since they have had greater exposure and less stigmata associated with use of alcohol and other substances compared to other age cohorts [79].

Alcoholic elders can be divided into two broad groups – early-onset and late-onset alcoholics. Early-onset users, comprising two-thirds of alcoholic elders, have started using alcohol early in life and have adjusted to their state over time. They have had their first alcohol-related problem in their third or fourth decade of life. Late-onset users begin abusing substances in their middle ages, often after a significant life event such as the death of a spouse or loss of a job [78]. In particular, widows are at a greater risk for increasing drinking, even though women tend to drink less than men at all ages [77]. In general, the late-onset users have achieved a higher level of social class than the early-onset users.

Aging brings a change in the body's ability to metabolize alcohol in a multitude of ways. Lean muscle mass decreases, decreasing total body water and thus decreasing the volume of distribution, and increasing the blood alcohol level for a given amount of imbibed alcohol. The liver is slower at metabolizing ethanol due to decreased hepatic blood flow and decreased enzymatic activity. Brain cells also decline in number with age and increase the risk of delirium – either from intoxication or withdrawal. In addition, the risk of falling carries with it much more dire consequences in the elderly. Inhibition of antidiuretic hormone results in urinary incontinence and a free water deficit. Changes in the proportions of gastric cells also predispose the elderly to gastritis [78]. The overall deleterious effects of alcohol use are thus accentuated in the elderly.

Diagnosis and Screening

The stigmata of alcoholism, substance abuse, and withdrawal syndromes are often confused with other conditions endemic in the geriatric patient population such as dementia and delirium; thus, it is important to screen patients for at-risk behavior. Perhaps the simplest and most widely used device is the CAGE questionnaire. This consists of four questions: (1) Have you ever felt that you should Cut down on your drinking? (2) Have people Annoyed you when criticizing your drinking? (3) Have you ever felt bad or Guilty about your drinking? (4) Have you ever had a drink first thing in the morning (an Eye-opener) to steady your nerves or get rid of a hangover? With a cutoff score of 2, this test has a sensitivity of 0.48 and a specificity of 0.99 in geriatric patients. This test has been modified to test for substance abuse, as well with good results [80]. Additionally, several comorbid conditions are common with alcoholism such as depression, insomnia, grief, anxiety, psychosis, and dementia and are worth screening for in alcoholics [77].

Treatment

Treatment for elders can consist of pharmacological interventions as well as counseling interventions. Benzodiazepines are the most commonly used pharmacological intervention, although in the elderly, the potential for adverse effects is heightened. Daytime somnolence, ataxia, and cognitive impairment are all potential adverse effects of benzodiazepine use. Hallucinations can be treated with antipsychotics. Disulfiram should be continued if it has successfully treated alcoholism in the past; however, the elderly have decreased tolerance for the disulfiram/ethanol interaction, and thus, it should be started with caution in the elderly. Naltrexone can be used to curb cravings [78]. Brief interventions that follow the FRAMES method (giving Feedback, assigning Responsibility, offering Advice, giving a Menu of methods to cut down drinking, expressing Empathy, and encouraging Self-efficacy) have proven to be effective [78].

Summary/Differentiating Features/Impact on Care

Cognitive and psychological disorders can have a significant impact not only on the care of the trauma patient but on the incidence of trauma. The following summary consists of quick references and figures that address major areas of this chapter (see Tables 8.6, 8.7, 8.8, 8.9 and Fig. 8.3).

Table 8.6 Summary table comparing cognitive tests

	Comparison of cognitive tests			
	MMSE	Mini-Cog	SLUMS	MoCA
Test	30-point questionnaire	3-item recall and clock drawing	30-point questionnaire	30-point questionnaire
Time to complete (min)	10	3–5	10	10
What makes it special?	Can adjust for educational level and age	Better sensitivity than MMSE and not influenced by age or level	Better at detecting mild neurocognitive disorder	Better for mild, early, and Huntington's/Parkinson's

Table 8.7 Summary table of comparison of disorders

Comparison of conditions			
	Dementia	Delirium	Depression
Central feature	Memory loss	Confusion	Sadness
Onset	Masked	Acute	Slow
Course	Chronic	Fluctuating	Episodic, possibly chronic
Consciousness	Normal	Altered	Normal
Attention	Normal	Diminished	Possibly diminished
Hallucinations	Rare	Common	Not common
Psychomotor	No	Yes	No

Table 8.8 Summary table of depression screening: GDS short

Geriatric Depression Scale (GDS) short form scoring instructions		
Instructions: Score 1 point for each bolded answer. A score of 5 or more suggests depression		
1. Are you basically satisfied with your life?	Yes	**No**
2. Have you dropped many of your activities and interests?	**Yes**	No
3. Do you feel that your life is empty?	**Yes**	No
4. Do you often get bored?	**Yes**	No
5. Are you in good spirits most of the time?	Yes	**No**
6. Are you afraid that something bad is going to happen to you?	**Yes**	No
7. Do you feel happy most of the time?	Yes	**No**
8. Do you often feel helpless?	**Yes**	No
9. Do you prefer to stay at home rather than going out and doing things?	**Yes**	No
10. Do you feel that you have more problems with memory than most?	**Yes**	No
11. Do you think it is wonderful to be alive now?	Yes	**No**
12. Do you feel worthless the way you are now?	**Yes**	No
13. Do you feel full of energy?	Yes	**No**
14. Do you feel that your situation is hopeless?	**Yes**	No
15. Do you think that most people are better off than you are?	**Yes**	No

Table 8.9 Summary of substance abuse screening and brief intervention

CAGE questionnaire
1. Have you ever felt that you should Cut down on your drinking?
2. Have people Annoyed you when criticizing your drinking?
3. Have you ever felt bad or Guilty about your drinking?
4. Have you ever had a drink first thing in the morning (an Eye-opener) to steady your nerves or get rid of a hangover?
Brief substance abuse intervention outline: FRAMES method
Giving Feedback
Assigning Responsibility
Offering Advice
Giving a Menu of methods to cut down drinking
Expressing Empathy
Encouraging Self-efficacy

CAM-ICU Worksheet

Feature 1: Acute Onset or Fluctuating Course	Score	Check here if Present
Is the pt different than his/her baseline mental status? OR Has the patient had any fluctuation in mental status in the past 24 hours as evidenced by fluctuation on a sedation scale (i.e., RASS), GCS, or previous delirium assessment?	Either question Yes →	☐
Feature 2: Inattention		
<u>Letters Attention Test</u> (See training manual for alternate **Pictures**) <u>Directions</u>: Say to the patient, *"I am going to read you a series of 10 letters. Whenever you hear the letter 'A,' indicate by squeezing my hand."* Read letters from the following letter list in a normal tone 3 seconds apart. **S A V E A H A A R T** **Errors are counted when patient fails to squeeze on the letter "A" and when the patient squeezes on any letter other than "A."**	Number of Errors >2 →	☐
Feature 3: Altered Level of Consciousness		
Present if the Actual RASS score is anything other than alert and calm (zero)	RASS anything other than zero →	☐
Feature 4:Disorganized Thinking		
<u>**Yes/No Questions**</u> (See training manual for alternate set of questions) 1. Will a stone float on water? 2. Are there fish in the sea? 3. Does one pound weigh more than two pounds? 4. Can you use a hammer to pound a nail? **Errors are counted when the patient incorrectly answers a question.** <u>**Command**</u> Say to patient: "Hold up this many fingers" (Hold 2 fingers in front of patient) "Now do the same thing with the other hand" (Do not repeat number of fingers)*If pt is unable to move both arms, for 2nd part of command ask patient to "Add one more finger" **An error is counted if patient is unable to complete the entire command.**	Combined number of errors >1→	☐

Overall CAM-ICU **Feature 1 plus 2 and either 3 or 4 present = CAM-ICU positive**	**Criteria Met →** **Criteria Not Met →**	☐ **CAM-ICU Positive (Delirium Present)** ☐ **CAM-ICU Negative (No Delirium)**

Fig. 8.3 Summary figure (Reproduced, with permission, from E. Wesley Ely, MD, MPH)

References

1. Draper B, Karmel R, Gibson D, Peut A, Anderson P. The Hospital Dementia Services Project: age differences in hospital stays for older people with and without dementia. Int Psychogeriatr. 2011;23(10):1649–58. Epub 2011 Sep 9.
2. Fisher AA, Srikusalanukul W, Davis MW, Smith PN. Clinical profiles and risk factors for outcomes in older patients with cervical and trochanteric hip fracture: similarities and differences. J Trauma Manag Outcomes. 2012;6(1):2.
3. Björkelund KB, Hommel A, Thorngren KG, Lundberg D, Larsson S. Factors at admission associated with 4 months outcome in elderly patients with hip fracture. AANA J. 2009;77(1):49–58.
4. Givens JL, Sanft TB, Marcantonio ER. Functional recovery after hip fracture: the combined effects of depressive symptoms, cognitive impairment, and delirium. J Am Geriatr Soc. 2008;56(6):1075–9. Epub 2008 Apr 18.
5. Holmes J, House A. Psychiatric illness predicts poor outcome after surgery for hip fracture: a prospective cohort study. Psychol Med. 2000;30(4):921–9.
6. Bo M, Massaia M, Raspo S, Bosco F, Cena P, Molaschi M, Fabris F. Predictive factors of in-hospital mortality in older patients admitted to a medical intensive care unit. J Am Geriatr Soc. 2003;51(4):529–33.
7. Grossman MD, Miller D, Scaff DW, Arcona S. When is an elder old? effect of preexisting conditions on mortality in geriatric trauma. J Trauma. 2002;52:242–6.
8. American Psychiatric Association. Diagnostic and statistical manual of mental disorders IV, text revision. Washington, D.C.: American Psychiatric Association; 2000.
9. Cummings JL. Alzheimer's disease. N Engl J Med. 2004;351(1):56–67.
10. Alzheimer's Association. 2012 Alzheimer's disease facts and figures. Alzheimers Dement. 2012;8:131–68.
11. Selkoe DJ. Aging, amyloid, and Alzheimer's disease: a perspective in honor of Carl Cotman. Neurochem Res. 2003;28:1705–13.
12. Francis PT. Neuroanatomy/pathology and the interplay of neurotransmitters in moderate to severe Alzheimer disease. Neurology. 2005;65:S5–9.
13. Lewy Body Dementia Association, Inc. Publications for Professionals Fact Sheet 2010. http://www.lbda.org/sites/default/files/2010-Fact-Sheet-EC.pdf.
14. Folstein MF, Folstein SE, McHugh PR. "Mini-mental state". A practical method for grading the cognitive state of patients for the clinician. J Psychiatr Res. 1975;12(3):189–98.
15. Borson S, Scanlan J, Brush M, Vitaliano P, Dokmak A. The mini-cog: a cognitive 'vital signs' measure for dementia screening in multi-lingual elderly. Int J Geriatr Psychiatry. 2000;15(11):1021–7.
16. Nasreddine ZS, Phillips NA, Bédirian V, Charbonneau S, Whitehead V, Collin I, Cummings JL, Chertkow H. The montreal cognitive assessment (MoCA): a brief screening tool for mild cognitive impairment. J Am Geriatr Soc. 2005;53:695–9.
17. Hoops S, et al. Validity of the MoCA and MMSE in the detection of MCI and dementia in Parkinson disease. Neurology. 2009;73(21):1738–45.
18. Videnovic A, et al. The Montreal Cognitive Assessment as a screening tool for cognitive dysfunction in Huntington's disease. Mov Disord. 2010;25(3):401–4.
19. Gagnon JF, et al. The montreal cognitive assessment: a screening tool for mild cognitive impairment in REM sleep behavior disorder. Mov Disord. 2010;25(7):936–40.
20. Smith T, et al. The montreal cognitive assessment: validity and utility in a memory clinic setting. Can J Psychiatry. 2007;52(5):329–32.
21. Nazeem S, et al. Montreal cognitive assessment performance in patients with Parkinson's disease with "normal" global cognition according to mini- mental state examination score. J Am Geriatr Soc. 2009;57(2):304–8.
22. Tariq SH, Tumosa N, Chibnall JT, Perry 3rd MH, Morley JE. Comparison of the Saint Louis University mental status examination and the mini-mental state examination for detecting dementia and mild neurocognitive disorder–a pilot study. Am J Geriatr Psychiatry. 2006;14:900–10.
23. McKeith IG, Dickson DW, Lowe J, et al. Diagnosis and management of dementia with Lewy bodies: third report of the DLB consortium. Neurology. 2005;65:1863–72.
24. Tariot PN. Treatment of agitation in dementia. J Clin Psychiatry. 1999;60 Suppl 8:11–20.
25. Carson S, McDonagh MS, Peterson K. A systematic review of the efficacy and safety of atypical antipsychotics in patients with psychological and behavioral symptoms of dementia. J Am Geriatr Soc. 2006;54:354–61.
26. McManus DQ, Arvanitis LA, Kowalcyk BB. Quetiapine, a novel anti- psychotic: experience in elderly patients with psychotic disorders. Seroquel Trial 48 Study Group. J Clin Psychiatry. 1999; 60:292–8.
27. Schneeweiss S, Setoguchi S, Brookhart A, Dormuth C, Wang PS. Risk of death associated with the use of conventional versus atypical antipsychotic drugs among elderly patients. CMAJ. 2007; 176(5):627–32.
28. Huybrechts KF, Gerhard T, Crystal S, Olfson M, Avorn J, Levin R, Lucas JA, Schneeweiss S. Differential risk of death in older residents in nursing homes prescribed specific antipsychotic drugs: population based cohort study. BMJ. 2012;344:e977. doi:10.1136/bmj.e977.
29. Feldman H, Gauthier S, Hecker J, et al. Efficacy of donepezil on maintenance of activities of daily living in patients with moderate to severe Alzheimer's disease and the effect of caregiver burden. Am J Geriatr Soc. 2003;51:737–44.
30. Lindesay J. The concept of delirium. Dement Geriatr Cogn Disord. 1999;10(5):310–4.
31. Francis J, Martin D, Kapoor WN. A prospective study of delirium in hospitalized elderly. JAMA. 1990;263(8):1097–101.
32. McNicoll L, et al. Delirium in the intensive care unit: occurrence and clinical course in older patients. J Am Geriatr Soc. 2003; 51(5):591–8.
33. Dyer CB, Ashton CM, Teasdale TA. Postoperative delirium. A review of 80 primary data- collection studies. Arch Intern Med. 1995;155(5):461–5.
34. Vaurio LE, et al. Postoperative delirium: the importance of pain and pain management. Anesth Analg. 2006;102(4):1267–73.
35. Gustafson Y, et al. Acute confusional states in elderly patients treated for femoral neck fracture. J Am Geriatr Soc. 1988; 36(6):525–30.
36. Marcantonio ER, et al. Delirium is independently associated with poor functional recovery after hip fracture. J Am Geriatr Soc. 2000;48(6):618–24.
37. Wacker P, et al. Post-operative delirium is associated with poor cognitive outcome and dementia. Dement Geriatr Cogn Disord. 2006; 21(4):221–7.
38. Pandharipande P, Cotton BA, Shintani A, Thompson J, Pun BT, Morris Jr JA, Dittus R, Ely EW. Prevalence and risk factors for development of delirium in surgical and trauma intensive care unit patients. J Trauma. 2008;65(1):34–41.

39. Liptzin B, Levkoff SE. An empirical study of delirium subtypes. Br J Psychiatry. 1992;161:843–5.
40. Ely EW, et al. Delirium as a predictor of mortality in mechanically ventilated patients in the intensive care unit. JAMA. 2004; 291(14):1753–62.
41. Pompei P, et al. Delirium in hospitalized older persons: outcomes and predictors. J Am Geriatr Soc. 1994;42(8):809–15.
42. Leslie DL, et al. One-year health care costs associated with delirium in the elderly population. Arch Intern Med. 2008;168(1):27–32.
43. Wahlund L, Bjorlin GA. Delirium in clinical practice: experiences from a specialized delirium ward. Dement Geriatr Cogn Disord. 1999;10(5):389–92.
44. Pandharipande P, et al. Lorazepam is an independent risk factor for transitioning to delirium in intensive care unit patients. Anesthesiology. 2006;104(1):21–6.
45. Joosten E, Lemiengre J, Nelis T, Verbeke G, Milisen K. Is anaemia a risk factor for delirium in an acute geriatric population? Gerontology. 2006;52(6):382–5. Epub 2006 Aug 17.
46. Aldemir M, Ozen S, Kara IH, Sir A, Baç B. Predisposing factors for delirium in the surgical intensive care unit. Crit Care. 2001;5(5):265–70. Epub 2001 Sep 6.
47. Whitney JF, Gannon DE. Obstructive sleep apnea presenting as acute delirium. Am J Emerg Med. 1996;14(3):270–1.
48. Tune L, et al. Association of anticholinergic activity of prescribed medications with postoperative delirium. J Neuropsychiatry Clin Neurosci. 1993;5(2):208–10.
49. Tune LE. Anticholinergic effects of medication in elderly patients. J Clin Psychiatry. 2001;62 Suppl 21:11–4.
50. Tune LE, Egeli S. Acetylcholine and delirium. Dement Geriatr Cogn Disord. 1999;10(5):342–4.
51. Han L, et al. Use of medications with anticholinergic effect predicts clinical severity of delirium symptoms in older medical inpatients. Arch Intern Med. 2001;161(8):1099–105.
52. American Geriatrics Society 2012 Beers Criteria Update Expert Panel. American Geriatrics Society Updated Beers Criteria for potentially inappropriate medication use in older adults. J Am Geriatr Soc. 2012;60(4):616–31.
53. Gaudreau JD, et al. Opioid medications and longitudinal risk of delirium in hospitalized cancer patients. Cancer. 2007;109(11): 2365–73.
54. Fong HK, Sands LP, Leung JM. The role of postoperative analgesia in delirium and cognitive decline in elderly patients: a systematic review. Anesth Analg. 2006;102(4):1255–66.
55. Chatsis V, Cunningham J. Diagnostic tests for delirium: a review of the clinical evidence of accuracy and reliability. Ottawa: Canadian Agency for Drugs and Technologies in Health (CADTH); 2008.
56. Canadian Coalition for Seniors' Mental Health. National Guidelines for Seniors' Mental Health: the assessment and treatment of delirium. Toronto: Canadian Coalition for Seniors' Mental Health; 2006. Available: http://www.ccsmh.ca/en/projects/delirium.cfm. Accessed 6 Nov 2008.
57. British Geriatrics Society and Royal College of Physicians. The prevention, diagnosis and management of delirium in older people: national guidelines. In: Concise guidance to good practice, No. 6. London: Royal College of Physicians; 2006. Available: http://www.rcplondon.ac.uk/pubs/contents/e8b55299-11c0-4953-994b-e56f137a2215.pdf. Accessed 6 Nov 2008.
58. Michaud L, Bula C, Berney A, Camus V, Voellinger R, Stiefel F, et al. Delirium: guidelines for general hospitals. J Psychosom Res. 2007;62(3):371–83.
59. Delirium: diagnosis, prevention and management [Internet]. NICE Clinical Guidelines, No. 103. National Clinical Guideline Centre (UK). London: Royal College of Physicians (UK); 2010.
60. Inouye SK, et al. Clarifying confusion: the confusion assessment method. A new method for detection of delirium. Ann Intern Med. 1990;113(12):941–8.
61. Ely EW, et al. Evaluation of delirium in critically ill patients: validation of the confusion assessment method for the intensive care unit (CAM-ICU). Crit Care Med. 2001;29(7):1370–9.
62. Waszynski CM. The confusion assessment method (CAM). Hartford Institute for Geriatric Nursing, consultGeriRN.org, Clinical Resources. Try this: best practices in nursing care to older adults. Issue Number 13, Revised 2007.
63. Maldonado JR. Delirium in the acute care setting: characteristics. Diagnosis and treatment. Crit Care Clin. 2008;24:657–722.
64. Conwell Y, Brent D. Suicide and aging. I: patterns of psychiatric diagnosis. Int Psychogeriatr. 1995;7(2):149–64.
65. Conwell Y. Suicide in later life: a review and recommendations for prevention. Suicide Life Threat Behav. 2001;31(Suppl):32–47.
66. Hybels CF, Blazer DG. Epidemiology of late-life mental disorders. Clin Geriatr Med. 2003;19:663–96.
67. Alexopoulos GS. Mood disorders. In: Sadock BJ, Sadock VA, editors. Comprehensive textbook of psychiatry, vol. 2. 7th ed. Baltimore: Williams and Wilkins; 2000.
68. Dew MA, Whyte EM, Lenze EJ, et al. Recovery from major depression in older adults receiving augmentation of antidepressant pharmacotherapy. Am J Psychiatry. 2007;164:892–9.
69. Carota A, Berney A, Aybek S, et al. A prospective study of predictors of post stroke depression. Neurology. 2005;64:428–33.
70. Ravina B, Camicioli R, Como PG, et al. The impact of depressive symptoms in early Parkinson disease. Neurology. 2007;69: 342–7.
71. Depression Guideline Panel. Depression in primary care: volume 1. Detection and diagnosis. Clinical practice guideline, number 5. AHCPR Publication No. 93–0550. Rockville: Agency for Health Care, Policy and Research; 1993.
72. Lebowitz BD, Pearson JL, Schneider LS, Reynolds III CF, Alexopoulos GS, Bruce ML, Conwell Y, Katz IR, Meyers BS, Morrison MF, Mossey J, Niederehe G, Parmelee P. Diagnosis and treatment of depression in late life. Consensus statement update. JAMA. 1997;278(14):1186–90.
73. Centers for Disease Control and Prevention, National Center for Injury Prevention and Control. Web-based Injury Statistics Query and Reporting System (WISQARS) [online]. 2005 . Available from URL: www.cdc.gov/ncipc/wisqars. Accessed 31 Jan 2007.
74. Rowe JL, Conwell Y, Shulberg HC, et al. Social support and suicidal ideation in older adults using home healthcare services. Am J Geriatr Psychiatry. 2006;14:758–66.
75. National Institute of Mental Health, Health and Education, Publications. http://www.nimh.nih.gov/health/publications/suicide-in-the-us-statistics-and-prevention/index.shtml. NIH Publication No. 06 - 995 4594.
76. Yesavage JA. The use of rating depression series in the elderly. In: Poon LW, editor. Clinical memory assessment of older adults. Washington, D.C.: American Psychological Association; 1986.
77. Stern TA, et al. Massachusetts General Hospital comprehensive clinical psychiatry: expert consult – online and print, chapter 70. Philadelphia: Mosby/Elsevier, p. 963–71.
78. Menninger JA. Assessment and treatment of alcoholism and substance-related disorders in the elderly. Bull Menninger Clin. 2002;66(2):166–83.
79. Graham K, Schmidt G. The effects of drinking on health of older adults. Am J Drug Alcohol Abuse. 1998;24(3):465–81.
80. Hinkin CH, et al. Screening for drug and alcohol abuse among older adults using a modified version of the CAGE. Am J Addict. 2001;10(4):319–26.

Health-Care Economics and the Impact of Aging on Rising Health-Care Costs

9

Preston B. Rich and Sasha D. Adams

Trends in US Health-Care Spending

With a gross domestic product (GDP) of $15 trillion, the US' economy is the largest in the world, representing 20 % of all global economic activity. Currently, US health-care costs represent a larger percentage of this GDP than any other developed nation in the Organisation for Economic Co-operation and Development (OECD) and result in the highest national per capita spending ($8,233) in the world [1]. Historically, US health-care expenditures have progressively outpaced growth in real income and have consistently exceeded GDP expansion by an average of 2.5 % since 1975 [2] (CMS). US health-care spending has grown from $27.1 billion (5.3 % of GDP) in the pre-Medicare era of 1960 to $2.6 trillion in 2010 (17.6 % of GDP). Over the same period, the percentage of health-care costs paid for by the US government (federal and state) has progressively increased such that public sources now account for nearly 50 % of all payments [3].

Looking forward, economists project that health-care costs will continue to increase at a rate of 4–7 % per annum (forecasts are highly dependent on public policy and legislative action), a rate that if unabated will expand health-care spending as a percentage of GDP to 30 % by 2035 and will eventually exceed 50 % of all US economic transactions in aggregate by 2080. Federal financing of health care is already facing profound shortfalls, with Medicare Part A payments currently exceeding committed payroll tax revenue. If Medicare costs continue to grow at contemporary rates, the Trust Fund assets will be depleted by 2017. Given simple economics, it is evident that the rising costs of health care may represent the single greatest threat to the economic security of the US population.

Key Drivers of Health-Care Spending

There is growing consensus that the disproportionate rise in health-care costs is unsustainable and must be controlled given realistic expectations for associated growth in GDP. While the major factors that contribute to cost acceleration can be reasonably well identified and agreed upon, there is more controversy regarding the relative magnitude and economic importance of the various components. The aging of the baby boomer generation is commonly thought to be a major driving force for the increase in overall health-care expenditures. However, despite the increasing proportion of the elderly and the higher per capita spending incurred by this group, most economists attribute only about 3 % of the cumulative increase in health-care spending to this one driver.

Health care as a commodity is effectively a surrogate for the underlying associated values, which are the quality of health itself and the desire to maximize both individual and collective welfare. There is little doubt that in many cases, health-care spending and resource allocation can be directly translated into the development of productive technological developments, the prolongation of life, the relief of suffering, and a measurable improvement in the quality of health. However, cost, quality, and well-being are not always directly related. From the perspective of economic efficiency and the appropriate allocation of scarce resources, this nonlinear relationship necessitates the distribution of our scarce resources within the broader context of efficacy, cost-effectiveness, comparative analysis, and efficiency.

P.B. Rich, MD, MBA, FACS (✉)
Division of Acute Care Surgery, Department of Surgery, University of North Carolina at Chapel Hill, 4008 Burnett-Womack Clinical Sciences Bldg, Chapel Hill, NC 27516-7228, USA
e-mail: prich@med.unc.edu

S.D. Adams, MD, FACS
Division of Acute Care Surgery, Department of Surgery, University of North Carolina, 4008 Burnett Womack Bldg, Campus 7228, Chapel Hill, NC 27599-7228, USA
e-mail: sasha_adams@med.unc.edu

J.A. Yelon, F.A. Luchette (eds.), *Geriatric Trauma and Critical Care*,
DOI 10.1007/978-1-4614-8501-8_9,

Technology

As the USA has transitioned from its manufacturing-based industrial revolution to an economy that is 80 % service oriented, Americans have grown accustomed to rapid disruptive innovation and the development of advanced technological breakthroughs that fundamentally alter the structure and function of markets. In no sector is this phenomenon more evident than in health care. The development of new drugs, devices, services, procedures, and applications not only impacts current treatment paradigms but in many cases also expands possible treatments to new populations. Technological advances often outpace our ability to adequately study their effectiveness, and evidence-based strategies designed to rationally apply them are often replaced by their rapid and unsystematic adoption with unpredictable incorporation into medical practice.

Although the potential exists for innovative technological advancements to decrease the cost of health care by reducing hospitalization or avoiding associated morbidity, most experts agree that the majority of medical technological developments significantly increase the costs of health care [4]. Even when cost reductions are possible, technology expansion and application into broader populations has the net effect of increasing spending. While measuring the direct financial impact of technology can be difficult, the cost contribution of technology on health-care spending can be estimated as the cost residual that remains after accounting for more readily measurable drivers. Using this methodology, the Congressional Budget Office (CBO) estimates that approximately 50 % of the growth in US health-care costs can be attributed to technology, making it the single greatest contributor to health spending, [5]. It is reasonable to predict that desirable technologies will continue to be developed in the future, perhaps at an even greater pace, further complicating our decisions regarding allocation of our limited resources [2].

Insurance

Although health insurance was initially conceived as a mechanism to reduce the financial impact of catastrophic illness, its role has expanded in attempts to make all types of health care financially accessible and available to the population. As health-care costs have continued to rise, the amount of out-of-pocket expenses paid by the end user has almost inversely decreased [6, 7]. Although causality in this relationship is difficult to directly establish, a classic experiment conducted by the RAND Corporation from 1974 to 1982 provided strong evidence that reductions in coinsurance lead to more people using health services and more services used per person [8]. On the other hand, cost-sharing reduced the use of both inappropriate and appropriate medical services. Whereas this effect had minimal consequences on the health status of the majority of people enrolled in the study, for those who were poor and suffered chronic illnesses, the reduction in health utilization was harmful. The CBO concluded that between 5 and 20 % of the increase in health costs can be attributed to the progressive expansion of more extensive health-care coverage. One economist estimates that the insurance expansion represented by the institution of Medicare in 1965 may explain nearly half of the increase in health-care spending that occurred between 1950 and 1990 [2, 9].

Other Costs

As medical care and its financial components become more complex, so must the infrastructure that sustains it. While the administrative costs required to deliver health care can be difficult to accurately capture and gauge comprehensively, few would argue that the associated expenditures are rising. Historical estimates attribute 3–10 % of rising costs simply to increases in administrative and support functions in the sector. The CBO found that administrative costs have increased approximately 7 % year over year between the 1995 and 2005 fiscal years.

The role of medical malpractice liability on escalating health costs relates both to the measurable impact of rising insurance costs paid by providers and the less quantifiable but arguably more significant contribution of increased costs related to the practice of "defensive medicine." Because malpractice premiums constitute only 1–2 % of US health-care expenditures, the projected 6 % direct reduction in premiums that would likely result from tort reform would be expected to have only a modest impact on total expenditures [10]. This larger potential issue is also the most controversial – the notion that health-care costs are driven dramatically higher by medical practice that may overutilize medical resources solely to reduce the chance of litigation. Several studies designed to address this issue have provided disparate results, and the relationship between malpractice liabilities and global health-care costs remains in large part unanswered [2].

Because health and wellness are desired states of being, health care as their market-based surrogate is also a desired service. As personal income rises, one's ability to pay for a variety of health-care services increases. Health care is a normal good, such that aggregate demand for it increases as income increases. Furthermore, because there are few substitutes available to replace it, health care exhibits significant price elasticity of its demand function. Consumers are fairly price insensitive, and this effect is further magnified by the relative disengagement of payment and services that occurs from the interposition of third-party intermediaries. A high per capita income in the USA is often cited as one of the key factors that contribute to our comparatively high health-care costs. The true magnitude of this effect is a matter of debate, but economists have estimated the elasticity of US health care at approximately 0.2, meaning that for every 10 % increase in real income, associated health expenditures can be anticipated to rise by 2 % [11].

Chronic Disease and Disability

In the USA, health-care resources are not distributed equally among the population. To the contrary, the sickest 5 % of the US population accounted for nearly half of all health spending in 2008 and 2009, and just 30 % of the population account for nearly 90 % of aggregate US health expenditures. The elderly are disproportionately represented among this top decile of spenders, comprising 13.2 % of the population, but 42.9 % of the heaviest consumers. Not surprisingly, chronic diseases are more prevalent in the older population, and their presence increases and maintains the elevated costs of health care in this portion of the population [12].

Chronic diseases, which affect older adults disproportionately, are the leading cause of death and disability in the USA, and modifiable conditions such as obesity and smoking are the most significant contributors [13]. In aggregate, the treatment of chronic diseases accounts fully for 75 % of US health-care costs [12, 14]. In the USA, approximately 80 % of individuals over age 65 have at least one chronic condition, and 50 % have at least two [14]. The ten most prevalent chronic disease diagnoses account for nearly one-third of national hospital charges. Of these, the Agency for Healthcare Research and Quality (AHRQ) identified five as sources of potentially preventable hospitalizations given exposure to appropriate health modification strategies and preventive health measures (coronary artery disease, congestive heart failure, diabetes, chronic obstructive pulmonary disease, and asthma). The economic costs of chronic disease are cumulative; treating patients with one chronic condition (25 % of the US population) costs twice as much as treating those without chronic disease. Treating patients who suffer from multiple comorbid conditions costs up to seven times as much as does treating patients burdened by only one chronic condition [13, 15].

In addition to the increasing incidence of chronic disease, the aging process is associated with increasing disability secondary to sarcopenia or progressive loss of muscle mass. Approximately 45 % of Americans over age 65 are sarcopenic, with approximately 20 % of the US population being functionally disabled [16]. When the prevalence of disability and the estimated increased cost for each individual are multiplied by the increasing number of older Americans, the economic burden of sarcopenia alone is estimated at $18.5 billion [16].

The rise in obesity in the USA has been particularly problematic and costly to the US health-care system. Obesity rates in the USA are now the highest in the world and have dramatically increased in all age groups over the last decade [13, 17]. For adults, the obesity rate (BMI >30) has tripled since 1960 while the incidence of morbid obesity (BMI >40) has risen sixfold. Because obesity raises the associated risks of major comorbidities such as cancer, stroke, coronary artery disease, and diabetes, the impact of its effect on health is essentially magnified. In real terms, the relative cost of obesity was $1,429 per year (42 %) higher than caring for the nonobese population in 2006 [18]. When combined with its prevalence, this high cost translated into $147 billion annually by 2008, or roughly 21 % of US health spending – a cost that has now surpassed that associated with smoking [19]. As obesity rates continue to increase in the future, one can expect continued increases in associated chronic diseases and related health costs.

End-of-Life Care

Elderly patients undergoing elective or emergent surgical procedures experience significantly more 30-day serious morbidity and higher mortality when compared to younger patients [20]. Often, the perioperative care of the aging occurs in either a medical or surgical intensive care unit (ICU), and elderly patients account for approximately 50 % of all ICU admissions and nearly 60 % of all ICU days [21]. Intensive care accounts for 20–30 % of overall hospital care costs in the USA, which was approximately $62 billion in 1992 [22]. Of the patients treated in the top decile of expensive hospitalizations which included ICU care, 20 % (2 % of all hospitalizations requiring ICU care) died within 3 months [22]. The elderly account for more than 70 % of all in-hospital deaths according to the Healthcare Cost and Utilization Project (HCUP). The average hospital cost for a stay that ended in death was $23,000, which is 2.7 times higher than for a patient discharged alive.

Health-Care Pricing

Some estimates attribute between 10 and 20 % of rising health costs to higher price trends prevalent in the health-care sector [HCCI]. While data patterns clearly support a progressive and significant rise in prices over time, an adequate analysis of their relationship to true cost is more challenging. Complicating these conclusions is lack of an effective and concurrent measure of comparative effectiveness and the impact of economic externalities. Because increases in technology tend to be associated with higher prices, it is unclear how much of a given price rise represents simple price inflation versus a marker of improved care that may be associated with increased quality or even global reductions in total economic cost. It is plausible that some higher prices may generate cost reductions if the higher price yields even higher benefits from downstream-associated effects such as increased comparative effectiveness, superior diagnostic quality reducing unnecessary procedures, the avoidance of high-cost care such as hospital admissions or readmissions, or a subsequent decrease in the development or severity of chronic illnesses and conditions.

Market Failures in the Health-Care Sector

The US health system has become increasingly complex, particularly from an economic perspective, as its overarching structure has progressively evolved from a fundamentally free-market system into a mixed system that incorporates components of both free-market forces and the command attributes marked by government intervention that are common in many European health-care systems. While Americans typically regard the US health system as a free-market economy, various interventions, including the introduction of third-party payer systems such as private health insurance and the development and expansion of government-sponsored programs like Medicare, Medicaid, and SCHIP, have generated many instances of what economists would refer to as "market failures" endemic in our system.

A market is a place, real or virtual, where sellers and buyers meet to execute transactions. Free markets exhibit qualities of perfect competition, where each and every participant is considered a "price taker," and no party possess the unilateral power to influence the price of a product it either buys or sells. Prices are determined by the laws of supply and demand, where a single price exists whereby the marginal benefit of obtaining one more unit exactly equals the marginal cost required to produce that one additional unit. This price, determined simultaneously by the market participants, is the only price that will effectively "clear" the market. Such a "perfect" market demonstrates "Pareto efficiency," whereby no single market participant can benefit further by additional transactions without simultaneously disadvantaging another member.

Perfectly competitive markets demonstrate several key features that are each necessary to permit the ongoing efficiency of the marketplace:

1. An infinite number of market participants must be present and willing to both buy and produce a product at the market clearing price
2. There must be no barriers to exit or entry; any willing participant can freely enter or exit the market
3. All buyers and sellers must possess perfect information about the prices, quality, and nature of the products represented in the market
4. In zero transaction costs, buyers and sellers can incur no costs associated with the buying or selling of goods or services
5. Firms will exhibit profit maximization whereby they strive to produce and sell products at a price where their marginal costs exactly equal their marginal benefit
6. Products in the market must be homogeneous, without variation across various suppliers. When one or more of these conditions are not met, market failure occurs, and the allocation of goods and services in a given marketplace is not economically efficient

In practice, market failures occur commonly and are often associated with information asymmetries, noncompetitive markets, the existence of significant barriers to entry for new participants, and what are known as principal-agent concerns problems, as occur with moral hazard, conflicts of interests, and misaligned financial incentives. Many would argue that the current system of health-care delivery in the USA suffers from frequent and significant market failures that fundamentally alter its economics and contribute greatly to health disparities, inefficient allocation of scarce resources, and escalating costs that do not represent true market clearing prices and alter the nature of the relationship between supply and demand.

Information Asymmetry

An efficient and free market is highly dependent upon the presence of perfect and inclusive information being readily available to both buyers and sellers about all marketable goods and services transacted upon. Comprehensive information permits market participants to ascertain value, such that decisions about marginal cost and utility can result in an optimal and efficient clearing price. Perhaps in no situation is information asymmetry as apparent as in health care. The practice of medicine is a highly specialized and difficult-to-understand field, often with the superimposed potential for life-and-death outcomes, and aggravated by marked time-pressure constraints that preclude adequate information gathering. This extreme and almost universal asymmetry of information causes severe market failures, with the result often being inefficient resource allocation and price deflections.

Physicians as Agents

Information asymmetry in health care produces an unusual relationship between market participants; patients rely on their providers to act as their advocate, or agent, with licensure and professional codes of conduct as quality control measures. However, because physicians also serve as market suppliers with financial motives to provide goods and services, the potential for market failure is always present. This issue may result in supplier-induced demand, whereby providers allocate resources based on the potential for personal financial gain rather than to simply satisfy the health needs of a population.

Barriers to Entry

In the 1960s, the American Medical Association (AMA) sought to restrict the supply of health-care providers by introducing the requirement that physicians become licensed to practice medicine. While this practice sought to ensure a basic standard of competence in the health field, it also restricted the supply of practitioners. In the early 1970s, a report from the Graduate Medical Education National Advisory Committee (GMENAC) predicted an excess of physicians by the year 2000 if medical school and residency positions continued to increase. There was a voluntary moratorium on growth of medical schools, and eventually a federal freeze on GME positions in 1997. These decisions were based on projections of US population growth that were in fact underestimates of actual growth and did not take into account the increasing specialization of the physician workforce, both of which have led to an increasing shortage of physicians in the face of a rapidly aging population. The shortage has therefore led to reduced competition in the marketplace and an influx of physicians from alternate educational paths [23].

Moral Hazard

The occurrence of illness is an unpredictable and costly event. Insurance markets have been developed in an attempt to mitigate this inhomogeneous risk and to financially prepare a priori for the uncertainty inherent in health and the human condition. By distributing risk among a population-based risk pool, the impact of individual unpredictability is diffused throughout a larger absorptive base. However, having insurance impacts an individual's behavior through what a phenomenon economists call moral hazard. Because health-care costs are paid by a third party, regardless of actual cost, insurance tends to induce an overconsumption of health-care resources by the end user. Similarly, health-care providers are subject to moral hazard as well; since prescribed treatments are known to be covered, insurance may induce the over-allocation of health care. Both phenomena create market inefficiency and can result in the overutilization of scarce resources, which is a major driver of rising health costs.

Adverse Selection

Insurance providers would ideally accurately price risk into individual insurance premiums to appropriately match cost with utilization. Because information is imperfect, risk assessment is necessarily incomplete. When premiums are set uniformly to reflect an "average" population-based aggregate risk, cost burden is unequal; the sickest users of health care pay less than their actual incurred costs, while the healthiest pay a disproportionately high cost for the goods and services they receive. In such a situation, the healthiest often forgo insurance and accept their lower perceived risk. This "adverse selection" results in only the sickest being insured at relatively underpriced premiums. Attempts to counteract this effect by pricing tiered premiums based on relative risk stratification result in very high health-care costs borne by the greatest consumers of health care, effectively undermining the theoretical advantages of a distributed insurance pool.

Imperfect Competition

A free market is dependent upon the presence of large numbers (infinite in theory) of buyers and sellers, none having the individual power to influence supply, demand, or clearing prices. The last decade has witnessed the progressive consolidation of the health sector, with hospitals growing into health delivery systems and insurance carriers merging together in attempts to maximize efficiency through the leveraging of economies of both scale and scope. Consolidation can lead to the development of regional monopolies, which possess the capability of influencing market conditions whereby individual entities set price, effectively becoming "price makers" rather than "price takers." All of these trends have had the effect of reducing competition and altering the dynamic equilibria of supply and demand, generating inefficient allocation of resources and producing incentive for the escalation of health-care prices.

Externalities

In economics, externalities are unmeasured transaction spillover effects that represent either costs or benefits of a given market that are not reflected in the price of goods or services. Externalities reflect inefficiencies in a marketplace and can either be positive or negative. Immunization is a classic example of a positive externality in health care. Most consumers purchase vaccinations for the tangible personal benefit of specific disease prevention. However, vaccination provides not only the consumer with benefit but also others in the population who enjoy a reduced chance of infection because the vaccinated can no longer spread the disease. This provides an important degree of social benefit (an externality) that is unmeasured on the individual transaction scale. Because the total benefit is in actuality a combination of individual benefit and the marginal social benefit (which is however unmeasured), society will underestimate the true demand and therefore under-allocate vaccinations. This effect will in turn incur a cost to society. Because of the tremendously complex matrix and inherent interrelatedness of both benefits and costs in health care, externalities are common sources of market failures.

Aging of the US Population

As the world enters the twenty-first century, the majority of developed nations face pronounced structural alterations in their demographic profiles marked by a progressive and sustained shift toward an older population. The world's population is aging more rapidly than at any time in our past, a global effect driven primarily by a relative reduction in fertility rate combined with a prolongation in life expectancy [24]. According to the United Nations Population Division (UNPD), the number of individuals over the age of 65 will outnumber those under age five for the first time in human history. The life increases in life expectancy seen in Organisation for Economic Co-operation and Development (OECD) countries are indeed profound; populations in developed nations can be demonstrated to increase their life expectancy by one full day out of every four. Globally, life expectancy has increased 3 months per year consistently since 1840 with no evidence of a plateau occurring [25].

An important corollary of the relative expansion of the aging demographic is the simultaneous relative and absolute contraction of the employed labor force which contributes capital for societal consumption. As the leading edge of the expanded baby boomer cohort enters retirement age and produces an increased demand for goods and services, a reduced labor force is left behind to generate the required supply. In 1970, there were 5.3 workers for every postproduction retiree; currently, there are 4.6, and it is predicted that the ratio will decline to 2.6 workers per pensioner [24, 26]. As the trend toward decreasing fertility and increasing life expectancy alters the demographic landscape for the foreseeable future, the imbalance between economic supply and demand from a population perspective will become even more extreme [14].

Despite implementation of the comprehensive government-sponsored Medicare program in 1965, associated deductibles, co-payments, and uncovered services generate a significant financial burden on the expanding aging cohort of Americans. As both demand and costs continue to increase, the individual economic impact of health care on American seniors will become increasingly significant. Assuming current insurance structure but projecting a systematic *reduction* in recent trends in cost escalation, the yearly out-of-pocket expense for Americans over age 65 will more than double over the next several decades, while the median real income will grow much more slowly [27]. As costs grow disproportionately to income, the percentage of real income required to maintain the current levels of health-care service utilization will increase significantly from 10–20 %. The percentage of senior Americans that spend more than one-fifth of their income on health care will increase to 45 % by 2040 [27]. Projections will be more dire for American seniors if cost containment is not achieved and if employers eliminate current levels of retiree health benefits.

Conclusion

National health-care expenditures constitute a substantial and continuously expanding component of the US economy. In the context of a complex and rapidly evolving health delivery system, costs are rising at an unsustainable rate and widespread market failures are exacerbating disparities in the efficient allocation of our scarce resources. A meticulous analysis of health-care spending patterns combined with an objective assessment of need can shed important light on how to best restrain rising health-care costs while simultaneously providing appropriate high-quality care.

Systematically identifying and characterizing the relatively small group of individuals that accounts for the largest percentage of US health spending may facilitate the introduction of targeted interventions into key areas where their impact may be most profound. Changing demographics, an increasing incidence of chronic disease and progressive disability, rapid technological advances, and systemic market failures in the health-care sector combine to drive exponential cost expansion and a comprehensive multidisciplinary approach will become increasingly necessary to balance the delicate relationship between our constrained supply and increasing demand.

In a consensus statement by the Council on Scientific Affairs of the American Medical Association, the authors declared that "one of the most important tasks that the medical community faces is to prepare for the problems in caring for the elderly" [28]. As the USA moves deeper into the twenty-first century, encumbered by rising national deficits and a cumulative debt that may soon exceed GDP, it is clear that any plan to achieve sustainable quality care for our aging population will necessarily require seamless integration into an overarching strategy for our nation's entire health-care system and the broader economy as a whole.

References

1. OECD health data 2012. www.oecd.org.
2. Schieber SJ, et al. Social Security Advisory Board. The unsustainable cost of health care. 2009. www.ssab.gov.

3. National Health Expenditure Projections 2011-2021: forecast summary. Centers for Medicare & Medicaid Services. www.cms.gov.
4. Fuchs VR. Health care for the elderly: how much? Who will pay for it? Stanford Med Rev. 1999;1(1).
5. Newhouse J. Medical care costs: how much welfare loss? J Econ Perspect. 1992;6(3):3–21.
6. Henry J. Kaiser Family Foundation. Trends in health care costs and spending. Menlo Park: Henry J. Kaiser Family Foundation; 2009. www.kff.org.
7. Henry J. Kaiser Family Foundation. Health care costs: a primer. Key information on health care costs and their impact. Menlo Park: Henry J. Kaiser Family Foundation; 2009. www.kff.org.
8. Brook RH, Ware JE, Rogers WH, et al. The effect of co-insurance on the health of adults. The Rand Corporation. Dec 1984.
9. Finkelstein Amy. The Aggregate effects of health insurance: evidence from the introduction of medicare. NBER working paper. 2005. www.nber.org.
10. Paik M, Black BS, Hyman DA, et al. Will Tort reform bend the cost curve? Evidence from Texas. J Empirical Leg Stud. 2012;9(2): 173–216.
11. Su L, Deborah C. Price and income elasticity of the demand for health insurance and health care services: a critical review of the literature. Mathematica Policy Research, Inc. 2006. www.mathematica-mpr.com.
12. Cohen SB, Yu W. Agency for Healthcare Research and Quality (AHRQ) Statistical Brief. The concentration and persistence in the level of health expenditures over time: estimates for the US Population, 2008-2009. 2012.
13. Ehrlich E, Kofke-Egger H, Udow-Phillips M. Health care cost drivers: chronic disease, comorbidity, and health risk factors in the US and Michigan. Ann Arbor: Center for Healthcare Research & Transformation; 2010. www.chrt.org.
14. Centers for Disease Control and Prevention (CDC). Public health and aging: trends in aging – United States and worldwide. MMWR Morb Mortal Wkly Rep. 2003;52(6):101–6. www.cdc.gov.
15. Stanton MW, Rutherford MK. The high concentration of U.S. health care expenditures. Rockville: Agency for Healthcare Research and Quality (AHRQ); 2005.
16. Janssen I, Shepard DS, Katzmarzyk PT, et al. The healthcare costs of sarcopenia in the United States. J Am Geriatr Soc. 2004; 52:80–5.
17. Ogden CL, Carroll MD, Kit BK, et al. Prevalence of obesity in the United States, 2009-2010. NCHS Data Brief. 2012;(82). www.cdc.gov.
18. Finkelstein EA, Trogdon JG, Cohen JW, et al. Annual medical spending attributable to obesity: payer- and service-specific estimates. Health Aff. 2009;28(5):w822–31. www.cdc.gov.
19. Cawley J, Meyerhoefer C. The medical care costs of obesity: an instrumental variables approach. J Health Econ. 2012;31(1):219–30.
20. Ingraham AM, Cohen ME, Raval MV. Variation in quality of care after emergency general surgery procedures in the elderly. J Am Coll Surg. 2011;212:1039–48.
21. Menaker J, Scalea TM. Geriatric care in the surgical intensive care unit. Crit Care Med. 2010;38(9):S452–9.
22. Yu W, Ash AS, Levinsky NG, et al. Intensive care unit use and mortality in the elderly. J Gen Intern Med. 2000;15:97–102.
23. Sheldon GF, Ricketts TC, Charles A, et al. The global health workforce shortage: role of surgeons and other providers. Adv Surg. 2008;42:63–85.
24. Lee R, Mason A, Cotlear A. Some economic consequences of global aging. HNP discussion paper. The World Bank. 2010. www.worldbank.org. Topics: Health Nutrition & Population, Research: HNP Discussion Papers.
25. U.S. Census Bureau. Statistical abstract. 2012. www.census.gov.
26. Coggan P. Falling short special report. People in rich countries are living longer. Without big reforms they will not be able to retire in comfort. The Economist. 9 Apr 2011.
27. Johnson RW, Mommaerts C. Will health care costs bankrupt aging boomer? Washington, DC: The Urban Institute; 2010. www.urban.org.
28. Council on Scientific Affairs. American Medical Association white paper on elderly health. Arch Intern Med. 1990;150(12):2459–72.
29. Aging and the Health Care Workforce. Today's research on aging. Issue 19, June 2010. Population Reference Bureau. www.prb.org. PRB News: Today's Research on Aging.
30. Health Care Cost and Utilization Report: 2010. Health Care Cost Institute. 2012. www.healthcostinstitute.org.

Operative Risk Stratification

10

Gary T. Marshall and Andrew B. Peitzman

Introduction

The elderly are the most rapidly enlarging segment of the population due to the combined effects of the "baby boom," the population growth during the two decades after World War II, and the increase in life expectancy; this increased life span has become the burden of chronic disease and disability [1]. These trends in the aging of the population have resulted in parallel growth in the number of patients undergoing operation, with elderly patients comprising a significant percentage of the surgical workload [2]. Over 20 % of elderly patients undergoing surgery develop in-hospital complications, primarily involving the cardiovascular, neurologic, and pulmonary systems [3]. These complications significantly affect outcomes, with a substantial increase in-hospital length of stay. Over twice as many patients will be discharged to a skilled nursing facility or nursing home than those elderly patients without complications, often due to a reduced ability to perform activities of daily living. Complications result in a significant reduction in physical functioning, mental, and emotional health when compared to the general elderly population [4]. In addition, in-hospital complications result in substantially increased costs [5]. Need for operation has increased in the very elderly, with patients over the age of 80 making up a growing percentage of operative patients. These patients are more likely to undergo emergency operations with associated higher surgical risk. In this population one in five will experience complications, leading to mortality in 25 %, with comorbid illness playing a greater role in outcome than age. The increase in mortality associated with complications is even more dramatic, and thus their avoidance even more important [6, 7]. Many of these risk factors can be identified during the preoperative period, allowing the surgeon to employ strategies for their avoidance, and proper counseling of patients and families.

G.T. Marshall, MD
Department of Surgery, University of Pittsburgh Medical Center, 200 Lothrop Street, PUH F1266.2, Pittsburgh, PA 15203, USA

Department of Surgery, New York University, 550 First Avenue, 15 S 14, New York, NY 10016, USA
e-mail: marshallgt@upmc.edu, gtmarshall@me.com, gary.marshall@nyumc.org

A.B. Peitzman, MD (✉)
Department of Surgery, University of Pittsburgh Medical Center, 200 Lothrop Street F-1281, UPMC-Presbyterian, Pittsburgh, PA 15213, USA
e-mail: peitzmanab@upmc.edu

General Evaluation

History and Physical

Preoperative assessment of the elderly patient, similar to any patient, begins with a careful and thorough history. The history is the most expedient and sensitive method to determine the presence of comorbid conditions, and the extent to which these conditions limit the patient. The importance of this phase cannot be overstated. Pay special attention to cardiac, pulmonary, renal, and neurologic conditions, as these are most likely to impact management in the operating room and the perioperative period. In addition, preoperative interventions may help limit the impact of these comorbidities. The use of medications and supplements should be sought in detail. This allows appropriate management in both the perioperative and postoperative periods. Finally, signs and symptoms of activity-limiting cardiac and pulmonary conditions should be investigated.

The effects and extent of comorbid illness can be determined during the physical examination. Pay special attention to both cognitive and physical function in the elderly, as limitations in these areas predict postoperative complications. In the emergency situation with the obtunded or demented patient, the physical examination may be the only perioperative evaluation possible. The signs of significant cardiac, pulmonary, or hepatic dysfunction can be readily observed when present. Surgical scars can provide a basic

J.A. Yelon, F.A. Luchette (eds.), *Geriatric Trauma and Critical Care*,
DOI 10.1007/978-1-4614-8501-8_10, © Springer Science+Business Media New York 2014

surgical history. The stigmata of malnutrition and frailty can be easily identified.

After completing the history and physical, a general sense of the operative and perioperative risks has usually been determined; history and physical alone can determine fitness for surgery in up to 96 % of patients [8]. At this point, the remainder of the assessment will be determined by those comorbid conditions identified during the history and physical as well as the urgency of operation. The remainder of the evaluation discussed below will attempt to describe optimal evaluation of the geriatric patient. Emergency surgery rarely allows a complete assessment, but the information gleaned to this point will guide the remainder of the preoperative evaluation.

Basic Labs and Tests

The laboratory assessment and basic testing should be determined by the history of comorbid conditions, symptoms experienced by the patient, findings on physical examination, and the use of certain medications. Laboratory assessment in the healthy, asymptomatic patient has little value. The presence of abnormalities is low, and these findings rarely alter the intraoperative management of patients [9–11]. Despite these observations, numerous laboratory assessments are frequently ordered in geriatric patients. Each of these common tests will be addressed, with attention paid to their indications and implications in the geriatric patient (Table 10.1).

Table 10.1 Recommendations for preoperative testing in elderly patients

Test	Indications and implications
BUN and Cr	Recommended for all geriatric patients [12, 13]
	Should be used for all elderly patients to determine creatinine clearance for dosage adjustment of medications [13]
	Cr clearance is determined by Cr, patient age, and weight [14]
	Cr > 2.0 mg/dL is predictive of cardiac complications [15]
	Diabetes, hypertension, cardiovascular disease, and medications including diuretics, ACE inhibitors, and NSAIDS increase likelihood of abnormality
Electrolytes	Useful in patients with known renal disease, use of diuretics, ACE inhibitors, or other medications with renal effects [13]
Serum glucose	Patients with diabetes or obesity [16]
Albumin	Recommended for all geriatric patients for nutritional screening [12, 13]
Hemoglobin and hematocrit	Reasonable for all geriatric patients, especially those over 80 years [12, 13]
	Recommended when history and physical suggest anemia [16], tachycardia, or conjunctival pallor on exam
	History of anemia, extreme fatigue, cancer, renal disease, cardiovascular disease, or respiratory illness
	Recommended when significant blood loss and transfusion anticipated
	30-day postoperative mortality increases with each percentage point deviation in hematocrit from normal value [17]
White blood cell	Not indicated for screening, but usually part of CBC
	Helpful when signs of infection or myeloproliferative disorder are present [13]
Platelet count	Useful in patients with history of bruising, bleeding, or history of bleeding with surgery [13]
Coagulation studies	Indicated for history of bleeding or anticoagulant use
	Useful when even small amounts of blood loss will result in severe complications
	Malnutrition, malabsorption, or liver disease should prompt assessment [13]
Urinalysis	Indicated in the presence of suspected urinary tract infection or diabetes [13, 16]
EKG	Recommended for [12, 13, 18–21]
	History of heart disease, prior MI, arrhythmias, peripheral vascular disease, cerebrovascular disease, CHF, diabetes, renal disease, or pulmonary disease
	History of cardiotoxic medication exposure
Chest X-ray	Not recommended for routine screening
	Recommended for
	History of pulmonary disease including smoking history
	History of stable cardiopulmonary disease when age over 70
	Possible ICU admission to establish baseline [13]
Echocardiogram	Indicated for patients with dyspnea of unknown origin, current or prior heart failure with worsening dyspnea, or other change in clinical status [18]

Medications and Supplements

General Considerations

A thorough medication history should be sought from all patients. This includes prescription medications and indication, over-the-counter medications, vitamins, and herbal supplements. Over 80 % of elder adults take at least one medication, and one-third take at least five medications. This becomes especially prevalent in those 75–85 years of age. Compounding potential adverse events related to medications, nearly half of all elders use at least one over-the-counter medication, and nearly half use some sort of dietary supplement [22]. Polypharmacy can be defined by either the absolute number of drugs taken or the use of medications without appropriate indication or the use of duplicate medications. Inappropriate prescribing may be present in half of older adults, and contributes to cognitive impairment, falls, incontinence, and impairment [23]. All unnecessary medications should be discontinued in the perioperative period.

When considering medication use in the perioperative period, consider the potential for withdrawal from the medication, potential progression of disease while the medication is not administered, and the potential for interactions with anesthetic agents. Abrupt discontinuation of medications may lead to complications from withdrawal syndromes which include selective serotonin reuptake inhibitors (SSRIs), beta-blockers, clonidine, statins, and corticosteroids. Other drugs such as tricyclic antidepressants, benzodiazepines, MAO inhibitors, and antipsychotics are generally deemed safe in the perioperative period and need not be discontinued. ACE inhibitors and angiotensin receptor blockers should be continued unless the only indication is for hypertension and this is well controlled [24]. Drug therapy may be predictive of postoperative complications, but withholding of regular medications, especially those used to treat cardiovascular disease, also increases complications. The rate of complications, especially cardiac, increases with the time the patient is off the medication. All essential medications discontinued at the time of surgery should be resumed as soon as safely possible during the postoperative period [25].

Beta-Blockers

Recent enthusiasm for the use of perioperative beta-blockade has been tempered by the findings from a large-scale study which demonstrated that despite significant reduction in cardiac events and myocardial infarction, an increase in both stroke and death in patients treated with metoprolol was observed [26]. The current recommendations for perioperative beta-blocker therapy are:

1. Beta-blockers should be continued in patients undergoing surgery who are receiving beta-blockers for approved indications.
2. Beta-blockers titrated to heart rate and blood pressure are indicated in patients undergoing vascular surgery with high risk due to coronary artery disease or the presence of ischemia on preoperative testing.
3. Beta-blockers titrated to heart rate and blood pressure are reasonable for patients in whom cardiac disease is discovered in preoperative evaluation or who have high cardiac risk based on the presence of more than one risk factor undergoing intermediate-risk surgery [18].

Statins

Numerous studies of perioperative statin use in patients undergoing noncardiac surgery and coronary artery bypass grafting have been conducted, and the majority of these have shown that statins are beneficial in surgical patients, with reduction in mortality and myocardial infarction. Long-term mortality may also be improved by the use of statins in the perioperative setting. The current recommendations for the use of statins are:

1. Statin therapy should be continued in all patients currently taking statin medications.
2. Statin use is reasonable in patients undergoing vascular procedures.
3. Statin use should be considered in patients undergoing intermediate-risk procedures when at least one clinical risk factor is present [18].
4. Statins should be initiated as soon as possible in any patient who has an acute coronary event postoperatively.
5. It is reasonable to continue use for at least 72 h in those patients receiving statins for perioperative use only [27].

Corticosteroids

Steroids should be continued when possible during the perioperative period. Withholding these drugs for 36–48 h before surgery is predictive of the need for stress dose steroids due to hypotension. When the routine dose of steroids is continued during the perioperative period, patients do not require stress doses of steroids. Stress dose steroid use is only required when patients are being treated for primary failure of the hypothalamic-pituitary-adrenal axis [28].

Supplements

The use of supplements by patients has been found in 30 % of the surgical population, and use is increasing. These same studies have found that 70 % of the patients taking these preparations failed to disclose their use during the preoperative assessment unless specifically asked. Excessive bleeding, myocardial infarction, excessive and inadequate anesthesia, or interference with needed therapeutic drugs have been documented for these supplements [29]. These supplements have various durations of effect, but the safest measure is to discontinue use 7 days prior to surgery when possible and be aware of the potential complications so they may be managed adequately [24] (Table 10.2).

Mental Status and Cognitive Function Assessment

Dementia and Cognitive Impairment

Cognitive impairment and dementia are increasingly prevalent in the elderly population. Cognitive impairment without dementia is estimated to occur in 22 % of patients age 71 or older. This prevalence is greater than that of dementia. Prominent subtypes include prodromal Alzheimer's disease, cerebrovascular disease, stroke, and adverse effect of medication. These findings are significant, as 12 % of the patients found to have cognitive impairment will progress to dementia annually. More importantly, mortality increases from 8 % in the cognitive impairment without dementia to 11 % in the group with dementia [30]. The prevalence of dementia among persons older than 71 years is 14 %. The prevalence increases dramatically with age in this group, from 5 % in those aged 71–79 years, to 37 % in the over 90 cohort [31], and to greater than 40 % in those 100 years or older [32].

Table 10.2 Effects of common herbal medicine

Herb	Pharmacologic effects	Effects	Time to discontinue
Echinacea (purple coneflower root)	Activation of cell-mediated immunity	Allergic reaction, immunosuppression with long-term use	No data
Ephedra (ma huang)	Increase in heart rate and blood pressure	Complications related to its increased sympathetic effects: stroke, myocardial infarction, dysrhythmia Interacts with MAO inhibitors	At least 24 h preop
Garlic (ajo)	Inhibition of platelet aggregation (can be irreversible); increase in fibrinolysis	Increase in risk of bleeding, particularly when combined with other platelet inhibitors	At least 7 days preop
Gingko (silver apricot, duck foot tree)	Inhibition of platelet activating factor	Increase in risk of bleeding, particularly when combined with other platelet inhibitors	At least 36 h preop
Ginseng	Inhibition of platelet aggregation (can be irreversible); lowering of blood glucose	Increase in risk of bleeding; may decrease efficacy of warfarin; hypoglycemia	At least 7 days preop
Kava (intoxicating pepper)	Sedation	May increase sedative effects of anesthetics; potential for addiction and withdrawal	At least 24 h preop
St John's wort (Hypercium, amber, goat weed)	Inhibition of neurotransmitter reuptake	Induction of cytochrome P450 enzymes (effects, warfarin, cyclosporine, steroids, protease inhibitors)	At least 5 days preop
Valerian (vandal root, all heal)	Sedation	May increase sedative effects of anesthetics; potential for withdrawal	No data

Modified from Ang-Lee et al. [29]

The presence of cognitive impairment dramatically increases postoperative complications and negatively influences short- and long-term outcome. Baseline cognitive impairment and dementia are strong predictors for delirium in the postoperative period [33–36], and thus increase the risk of postoperative functional decline [33] and mortality [36].

During the preoperative evaluation the presence and severity of cognitive impairment should be documented if possible. Numerous tests have been developed to screen for cognitive impairment, including the Mini-Mental State Examination (MMSE), the Memory Impairment Screen (MIS), and the Mini-Cog. These tests have shown a wide range in sensitivity and specificity, and more importantly for the acute care surgeon, the time and training required to administer ranges from 1.5 to 17 min [37]. The Mini-Cog, a brief screen that employs 3-item recall and a clock drawing task, has sensitivity and specificity of 99 and 96 % and can be administered in 3 min. This strikes the best balance between accuracy and ease of administration in the acute setting [38].

Delirium

The incidence of delirium has been reported at 5–52 % in a number of studies including a broad selection of surgical patients [39]. The usual onset is 2 days following operation and persists an average of 4 days [36]; the occurrence of delirium results in increased length of stay in the hospital [36, 40, 41]. Patients are also more likely to experience functional decline and impairment in the performance of activities of daily living [33]. This results in a higher likelihood of discharge to a skilled nursing or rehabilitation facility [36, 40]. Finally, mortality rates are increased for both in hospital [41] and the months following discharge [36, 40, 42].

Table 10.3 Risk factors for postoperative delirium [33–36, 39–45]

General: age > 70, cognitive impairment and dementia, depression, alcohol use, severe comorbid disease, frailty, polypharmacy, and use of psychotropic medications
Illness related: renal disease, anemia, hypoxia, prior stroke
Metabolic: electrolyte disturbances, malnutrition, fluid losses
Functional: functional impairment, visual and hearing impairment, institutional residence
Procedure and hospitalization related: blood loss, hypotension, transfusion, sleep deprivation, inadequate pain control

With its profound impact on morbidity and mortality, identification and prediction of postoperative delirium has been the subject of numerous studies. It is hoped that with identification of patients at risk, measures may be taken to mitigate delirium and prevent its consequences.

Once risk factors for delirium have been identified, those that can be corrected should (Table 10.3). In the postoperative period, numerous medications have been identified which contribute to delirium and should be avoided. These include meperidine, benzodiazepines, antihistamines, and anticholinergics. Opiates should be used with caution, but pain must be adequately controlled, as this too is a risk factor for delirium [46, 47]. Some studies have shown that preoperative geriatrics consultation has been helpful to reduce the incidence of delirium. Other small trials of prophylactic antipsychotic administration have had promising but conflicting results, and their use cannot be advocated at this time [48].

Depression

The incidence of depression in those aged 71 or greater is estimated to be over 11 %, based on the presence of major or minor depressive symptoms or current treatment for depression. Dementia and pain perception are associated with increased incidence [49]. Other risk factors for depression in the elderly are disability, new medical illness, poor overall health, and bereavement [50]. In studies of patients undergoing cardiac surgery, depression has been identified as a risk factor for mortality [51]. Preoperative depression is also associated with a longer recovery time due to delayed recovery in activities of daily living (ADL) and instrumental activities of daily living (IADL) [52]. Screening for depression may be accomplished using a variety of tools. The Patient Health Questionnaire-2 (PHQ-2) is a simple and reliable screening tool for depression in the elderly. Two questions are asked in this survey. First, "In your entire life, have you ever had a time when you felt sad, blue, depressed, or down for most of the time for at least 2 weeks?" Second, "In your entire life, have you ever had a time, lasting at least 2 weeks, when you didn't care about the things that you usually cared about or when you didn't enjoy the things that you usually enjoyed?" A positive response to either of these questions is suggestive of depression, with 100 % sensitivity and 77 % specificity [53]. When positive, the patient should be referred for evaluation when time and the patient's medical condition allow.

Substance Abuse

A 2005–2006 epidemiologic study on the use of alcohol and drugs of abuse demonstrated that 60 % of adults over age 50 used alcohol in the year prior to the survey, 2.6 % used marijuana, and 0.41 % used cocaine [54]. Furthermore, at-risk and binge drinking is also prevalent in the elderly population, with 13 % of men and 8 % of women reporting at-risk drinking, and 14 % of men and 3 % of women reporting binge drinking [55]. The effects of preoperative alcohol use include increased risk of pneumonia, sepsis, surgical site infection (SSI) and wound disruption, and longer length of stay. With the exception of SSI, all of these factors are associated with increased mortality [56]. Exposure to alcohol may also increase the stress response to surgery and increase morbidity [57].

All patients should be screened for alcohol misuse. A simple tool is the CAGE questionnaire. This involves four questions, and a positive answer to one or more is suggestive of alcohol abuse (Table 10.4).

When identified, patients with at-risk alcohol history should be supplemented with folic acid and thiamine (100 mg) daily. Care protocols should include frequent assessment for withdrawal and appropriate medications or alcohol administered to avoid withdrawal in the postoperative period.

Table 10.4 CAGE screening for alcohol abuse [58, 59]

C	Have you ever felt you should *C*ut down on your alcohol or drug use?
A	Have you been *A*nnoyed by people criticizing your alcohol or drug use?
G	Have you felt *G*uilty about your drinking or drug use?
E	Do you need to use alcohol or drugs early in the morning (*E*ye-opener) to calm your nerves?

Nutritional Evaluation

Malnutrition is prevalent in the elderly and has a major impact outcome in surgery. Overall, malnutrition is present in 22.8 % of the elderly, ranging from 5.8 % in community dwelling elders to over 50 % in patients in rehabilitation. Another 46 % of elders are at risk for malnutrition [60]. In the surgical patient, malnutrition is a risk factor for multiple complications, generally related to infection and poor wound healing, and for increased length of stay [61]. During the preoperative evaluation the patient's height and weight should be documented. In addition, serum albumin and prealbumin levels should be obtained [12, 13]. The occurrence of any significant unintentional weight loss should be sought. Risk factors for severe malnutrition and related complications include serum albumin <3.0 g/dL BMI <20 kg/m^2, prealbumin <10 mg/dL, or unintentional weight loss of >10 % in 6 months [62–66]. The presence of any of these should prompt full nutritional assessment, and when possible a strategy to treat deficits in the perioperative period devised.

Cardiac Evaluation

The cardiac evaluation of the geriatric patient is an essential part of the initial assessment when time permits. Major cardiac complications occur in 2 % of patients aged 50 years or greater [15]. The incidence of adverse cardiac events increases with age [67]. Emergency operation is associated with a significantly increased risk of postoperative cardiac complications [68]. Other risk factors include high-risk procedures, history of congestive heart failure, history of ischemic heart disease, history of cerebrovascular disease, treatment with insulin, and preoperative serum Cr >2.0 mg/dL. These risk factors are additive in their prediction of cardiac events [15]. Hospital mortality is 15–25 % after perioperative myocardial infarction, and the risk of death persists for at least 6 months following operation [69]. The current ACC/AHA recommendations (Fig. 10.1) for cardiac evaluation should be followed in geriatric patients.

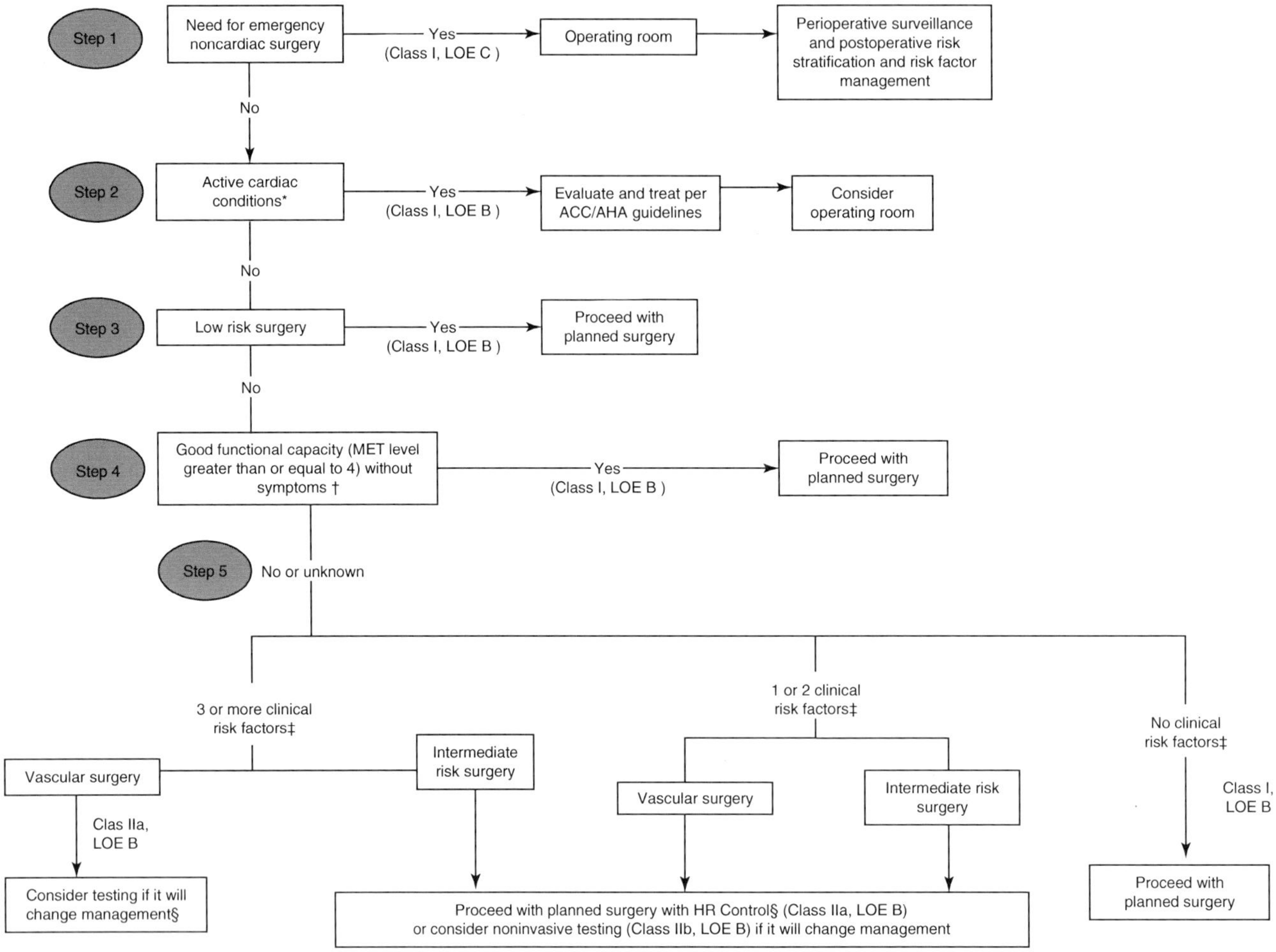

Fig. 10.1 Approach to cardiac evaluation and care prior to noncardiac (Fleisher et al. [118]). †See Class III recommendations in Section 5.2.3. Noninvasive Stress Testing. §Noninvasive testing may be considered before surgery in specific patients with risk factors if it will change management. ‡See Table 3 for estimated MET level equivalent

Pulmonary Evaluation

Pulmonary complications occur as frequently as cardiac complications in the postoperative period. Recent studies report an incidence of 2.7–5 % of patients will experience respiratory complications after non-thoracic surgery [70–73]. Postoperative respiratory complications are associated with a higher risk of myocardial infarction, pneumonia, renal failure, thromboembolic complications, or death. The cost of pulmonary complications is greater than any other adverse events, in part due to an increased length of hospital stay [74]. During the preoperative assessment, risk factors for pulmonary complications should be identified. Risk factors may be either patient or procedure related. Table 10.5 shows identified risk factors. Preoperative spirometry is not helpful to predict postoperative complications [75].

When high-risk patients are identified, several strategies may be employed for risk reduction. These include lung expansion techniques such as incentive spirometry, intermittent

Table 10.5 Risk factors for pulmonary complications following surgery [70–77]

Patient related	Procedure related
Advanced age	Emergency surgery
ASA class II or higher	Abdominal surgery (upper>lower)
Functional dependence	Aortic aneurysm repair
Chronic obstructive pulmonary disease	Non-resective thoracic surgery
Congestive heart failure	Neurosurgery
Serum albumin <3.5 g/dL	General anesthesia
History of smoking	Head and neck surgery
Obstructive sleep apnea	Prolonged surgery
Alcohol use	Vascular surgery
Preoperative anemia	Perioperative transfusion
Preoperative hypoxia	Perioperative nasogastric tube use
Blood urea nitrogen > 30 mg/dL	
Recent pneumonia	
Weight loss >10 % in prior 6 months	

positive pressure breathing, continuous positive airway pressure, and chest physiotherapy [76]. Preoperative inspiratory muscle training using individualized combinations of these techniques has been shown to reduce pulmonary complications in patients with concomitant coronary artery bypass surgery [78]. With regard to the anesthetic, residual neuromuscular blockade predicts postoperative complications, and longer-acting agents such as pancuronium should be avoided [79]. When possible, nerve blocks for regional anesthesia are less likely to cause complications than general anesthetic [76]. Laparoscopic techniques may have some value in limiting pulmonary complications when compared to open techniques. Nasogastric tubes should be used selectively, as routine use is associated with increased complications. Following celiotomy, continuous positive airway pressure and the use of epidural analgesia are shown to reduce complications [74]. Of note, preoperative smoking cessation has only been shown to reduce complications when done 1–2 months prior to surgery [75, 80–82].

Functional Status Determination

The patient's functional status should be determined during the preoperative evaluation. The ADL index involves functional independence in six areas: bathing, dressing, transferring, feeding, continence, and toileting [83]. A simple screening tool involves the following four questions: "Can you get out of bed yourself?" "Can you dress yourself?" "Can you make your own meals?" and "Can you do your own shopping?" [84]. A negative response to any question should prompt a more thorough evaluation of functional capacity, and the deficits should be documented. Other limitations should be documented, such as deficits in vision and hearing, as well as the use of assistive devices. A history of falls should be documented [12]. Physical disability can be assessed using the timed "Up & Go" test. A patient is instructed to rise from a chair, without using arms, and possibly walk 10 ft, turn, return to the chair, and sit down. A time greater than 15 s is suggestive of a high risk for falls [85, 86].

Poor functional status and impaired mobility are associated with postoperative delirium [40], surgical site infections due to methicillin-resistant *Staphylococcus aureus* [87], discharge to another level of care [88], and mortality [6, 83]. Preoperative functional status is also predictive of the time to postoperative recovery following abdominal surgery [52].

Frailty

Frailty is defined as a state of reduced physiologic reserve associated with increased susceptibility to disability [83]. Frailty manifests as age-related vulnerability to stressors secondary to this decrease in physiologic reserve and limits the maintenance of homeostasis. While similar in some ways to normal aging, it is a distinct entity [89]. Impairments associated with the frailty syndrome include sarcopenia, functional decline, neuroendocrine dysregulation, and immune impairment occurring in combination. The associated risk with the syndrome as a whole predicts poor outcomes greater than any single component, and no single component explains the entire spectrum of the manifestations. A physical phenotype was first defined in 2001; however, there is strong evidence to support additional domains to the model (Table 10.6). These include cognitive impairment, chronic diseases, and disability [90]. The overall prevalence of frailty in the United States ranges from 7 to 12 %. The prevalence increases with age, from 3.2 % in those age 65–70 years to over 25 % in the group aged 85–89 years. Frailty is more common in women across all ages [91, 92].

Table 10.6 Frailty phenotype [92]

Frailty criteria	Measurement
Shrinkage	Loss of 10 or more pounds in the last year
Weakness	Decreased grip strength (<20 % by gender and BMI)
Exhaustion	Self-reported "exhaustion," poor energy, or endurance
Slowness	Slow walking (lowest 20 % by age and gender)
Low activity	Low weekly energy expenditure: lowest 20 %
	Males: <383 kcal/week
	Females: <270 kcal/week
1 point for each criteria met	
0–1 = not frail	
2–3 = intermediate frail or pre-frail	
4–5 = frail	

Confusion over the exact definition and characteristics of frailty has resulted in the development of multiple definitions and screening tools. A Frailty Index was developed using the Comprehensive Geriatric Assessment (FI-CGA), which included measurements of impairment, disability, and comorbidity, which were scored and summed as a Frailty Index [93]. Although reliable and predictive of adverse outcomes, it is time consuming and not readily applied to the acute care surgery patients. The Canadian Study of Health and Aging Frailty Index involves up to 70 deficits, which is again a powerful predictive tool, but not widely used in clinical practice [94]. Regardless of the method used to screen for frailty, it is clear that it has a significant impact on the incidence of complications, mortality, and institutionalization [88, 95]. Once identified, the presence of frailty can help the surgeon counsel patients and families appropriately and modify the interventions proposed to minimize complications. Exercise and rehabilitation may also improve functional state [96]. When combined with physical exercise, nutritional interventions have also shown an improvement in functional abilities [97].

Table 10.7 Modified Frailty Index criteria [99]

History of diabetes mellitus	Functional status 2 (not independent in 30 days prior to surgery)	History of COPD or pneumonia
History of congestive heart failure	History of hypertension requiring medication	History of transient ischemic attack or stroke
History of myocardial infarction	History of peripheral vascular disease or rest pain	History of stroke with neurologic deficit
History of prior cardiac surgery or percutaneous intervention	History of impaired sensorium	

One of the most widely used assessments tools for defining frailty is the operational definition proposed by Fried. This involves five areas of physical performance shown in Table 10.6. The presence of frailty as defined by this method was predictive of falls, worsening mobility, and disability in activities of daily living, hospitalization, and death [92]. When this same method was applied to surgical patients, frailty increased risks for postoperative complications, with an odds ratio of 2.06 in the intermediate-frail group and 2.54 in frail patients. Length of stay was increased as well. Finally, discharge to a skilled- or assisted-living facility was increased, odds ratio of 3.16 in the intermediate group and 20.48 in the patients after operation [98].

Another tool which may be more easily applied in the acute setting is the Modified Frailty Index (MFI). This index system was created by the comparing the 70-item Canadian Study on Health and Aging Frailty Index with data from the National Surgical Quality Improvement Project (NSQIP) data set. The items included are shown in Table 10.7. One point is given for each feature present, and the total, divided by the number of variables for which the patient had data, produced results from 0 to 11, increasing frailty with higher total. In patients over age 60, undergoing emergency general surgery, the score was predictive of mortality, with a tenfold increase in mortality at the extremes of age. The incidence of infections also rose as the MFI increased. The benefits of this system include rapid application through history and physical, ease of employment in the acute setting, and the lack of requirement for any specialized equipment [99].

Patient Preferences, Counseling, and Advance Directives

Determination of Competency

Physicians must legally and ethically obtain informed consent from their patients before undertaking any procedure. The conditions that result in impaired decision capacity are common in the elderly patient, and the surgeon must be aware of their presence and skilled in evaluating that capacity. Conditions known to impact decision-making capacity include cognitive impairment, stroke [100], and psychiatric conditions such as schizophrenia, depression, or bipolar disorder. The general requirements for decision-making capacity are the ability to express a choice, understand pertinent information, understand the consequences of the procedure and those of foregoing treatment, and to be able to reason about these choices [101].

No single test has been shown to correlate with decision-making capacity. The Mini-Mental State Examination (MMSE) has been shown to correlate with this capacity, but without definite cutoff scores to determine capacity, although very-low (<19) and very-high (>23) scores predict absence or presence of capacity, respectively [102]. When the patient is deemed incompetent to make health-related decisions and an advance directive is not in place, the physician must seek substituted judgment, usually from a family member. Although the order may vary from state to state, the usual order is the spouse, adult children, parents, siblings, and other relatives [101].

Counseling Patients

Three things are usually taken into consideration as patients consider treatment options: treatment burden, treatment outcome, and the likelihood of the possible outcomes. When outcome is likely to be favorable, patients are typically willing to tolerate a greater treatment burden; however, this diminishes as outcomes show only marginal benefit. Quality-of-life outcomes such as prolongation of inevitable death, dependence on machinery, functional dependence, and excessive fatigue and pain are cited as important factors in patient's decisions. Nonmedical concerns, such as becoming a burden on the family or society, also influence these decisions [103]. Preparation for death, both by the family and the patient, is valued and important to the family and patient; however, physicians tend to place less emphasis on this aspect of end-of-life care. Patients appreciate being told the expected course of their disease, the symptoms they will experience, the time course, and what can be done for them. Finally, a sense of life completion is desired by patients, and adequate, timely communication may allow this to mature [104, 105]. Achieving the last of these goals may be difficult for the acute care surgeon. Our practice, by its nature, frequently encounters patients in a situation that is a clear departure from their usual state of health. While those patients receiving palliative care are aware that they are terminally ill, the patient suffering an acute catastrophic event has not had the luxury of time for preparation.

Advance Directives and DNR Orders in the Operating Room

According to Medicare data, nearly one-third of Americans underwent surgery during the last year of their life. Further, 18 % underwent procedures in the last month of life and 8 % during the last week of life [106]. The acute care surgeon must understand issues surrounding end-of-life care, especially the application of advance directives and "do not resuscitate" orders. The application of DNR orders and advance directives in the operating room was initially met with significant resistance [107]. Prior to the 1990s, policies for handling these directives were rare, and the usual practice was to suspend the DNR order in the OR and the immediate postoperative period. Forcing patients to give up their autonomy to qualify for surgery drew criticism [108, 109]. This led to the policy of "required reconsideration," meaning that the patient or surrogate, surgeon, and anesthesiologist must discuss and review the advance directive together. This was formalized by the American Society of Anesthesiologists (ASA) in 1993. Following this discussion, the DNR order could be formally rescinded with the patient's informed consent; it could be left in place, specifying the patient's goals of care; or it could be left in place with a detailed list of exactly what procedures the patient would allow [110]. The American College of Surgeons (ACS) echoed the views of the ASA. In their statement, they also stated that the automatic reversal of DNR status in the OR removed the patient from appropriate participation in the decision process and that inappropriate management in the perioperative setting might result [111].

As many as 15 % of patients with DNR orders will undergo surgery, either related to their preexisting illness or for treatment of unrelated conditions [112]. The procedures offered may be intended to either prolong life or ease suffering and improve quality of life. Many of these procedures fall within the scope of acute care surgery, and examples may include the repair of pathologic fractures, tracheostomy and feeding tube placement, treatment of bowel obstruction, vascular access, or a wide variety of others [110, 113]. A study of patients with DNR orders in place showed that the presence of the order did not affect the likelihood that patients would undergo the procedure considered. In only 18 % of the patients was the DNR order reversed. Half of the patients undergoing surgery with a DNR order in place were discharged from the hospital, and 44 % were alive 2 months following hospital discharge [113].

A Practical Approach to Working with Patients

When a patient presents for surgery with a DNR order in place, the physician must not only consider the risks and benefits of the specific procedure but also take the time to learn the values and goals of treatment for the patient. Communication is the key to resolving the complexities surrounding perioperative resuscitation. When discussions occur, the provider may learn the patient's rationale for the DNR order. Frequently, the patient is far more concerned with the quality of life after CPR, not before. When the surgeon understands the goals and fears of the patient, a contingency plan can be developed and implemented. Looking into these concerns may show that the patient is afraid of a long stay in the ICU or of losing independence, not wanting to spend the remainder of his life in a nursing home. By learning these fears, the surgeon and care team may adjust therapy and form appropriate plans. Surrogate decision makers and the anesthesiologist should be included in these discussions [114]. The addition of the surrogate will assist in ensuring that patient's wishes are respected, as it is not infrequent that the surrogate and the patient may not share the same goals and decisions [115]. During these discussions three options are available: rescinding the DNR order, providing limited resuscitation using a procedure-directed DNR order, and providing resuscitation with a goal-directed order.

The first option is to rescind the DNR order and provide full resuscitation regardless of clinical circumstances. This avoids the question of determining what exactly constitutes resuscitation, which may prove difficult during anesthesia. In addition, it frees the treating team to act in the event of an easily reversible or iatrogenic arrest, such as an arrhythmia on induction of anesthesia. Chances for an acceptable quality of life are better during these witnessed events [116], and care may be withdrawn later if the outcome in unfavorable. Despite all of the concern for ethics, this is a viable and appropriate course of action so long as the patient is involved in the decision.

A procedure-directed DNR order may be developed by the patient and surgeon. In this type of order, patients may specify which procedures and interventions for which they will and will not give consent. This is appealing to some patients, as they prefer the control of being able to dictate exactly which procedures will and, more importantly, will not be performed. This imitates the type of orders most commonly employed on hospital wards. The patient may be presented with a list of possible interventions. Frequently included items are intubation, postoperative ventilation, CPR, defibrillation, vasoactive drugs, and placement of invasive monitoring devices. When adapting these lists and preparing for the OR environment, interventions deemed mandatory for anesthesia are discussed with the patient, as they may not be refused [111]. Despite these procedure-specific orders being clear and easily understood, they do not allow for all the clinical circumstances which may arise, or those that may be difficult to document and define preoperatively [117].

The final approach to DNR orders in the OR is to take a goal-directed approach. In this scenario, the physician is left to determine which specific procedures should be performed in the event of cardiac arrest or instability. To supplant his own judgment for that of the patient, the surgeon must know the patient's concerns regarding resuscitation and outcome. Are they worried about pain, neurologic damage, loss of independence, or the need for further surgery and procedures? By knowing the answers to these questions, the physician is able to respond appropriately. For example, if a patient sustains an arrhythmia on induction that requires brief support with CPR, it would be administered, as outcome is likely to conform to the patient's wishes. Conversely, if the patient experiences a massive intraoperative myocardial infarction and arrest, CPR could be withheld, also supporting the patient's values. This approach to DNR is perhaps the most in line with preserving patient autonomy and allowing values held by the patient to be considered. The translation from theory to practice is not quite as easy. First, the surgeon and patient must understand each other, and this requires time that is not always present in emergency situations. In addition, the person responding to the arrest situation should be the same person who had the discussion with the patient. Clearly this is not the case for patients on hospital wards, but the OR, better than other places, provides for this continuity in care. When the continuity of care cannot be preserved, or when the trust required between patient and surgeon is not present, it is best to rely on a procedure-directed approach. When the goal-directed approach is taken, documentation in the medical record is essential. This will usually take the form of a descriptive narrative, detailing the conversations that have occurred and the preferences the patient has expressed for goals of care [111, 117].

References

1. Centers for Disease Control and Prevention (CDC). Trends in aging – United States and worldwide. MMWR Morb Mortal Wkly Rep. 2003;52(6):101–4, 106.
2. Etzioni DA, Liu JH, O'Connell JB, Maggard MA, Ko CY. Elderly patients in surgical workloads: a population-based analysis. Am Surg. 2003;69(11):961–5.
3. Leung JM, Dzankic S. Relative importance of preoperative health status versus intraoperative factors in predicting postoperative adverse outcomes in geriatric surgical patients. J Am Geriatr Soc. 2001;49(8):1080–5.
4. Manku K, Leung JM. Prognostic significance of postoperative in-hospital complications in elderly patients. II. Long-term quality of life. Anesth Analg. 2003;96(2):590–4, table of contents.
5. Dimick JB, Chen SL, Taheri PA, Henderson WG, Khuri SF, Campbell Jr DA. Hospital costs associated with surgical complications: a report from the private-sector National Surgical Quality Improvement Program. J Am Coll Surg. 2004;199(4):531–7.
6. Hamel MB, Henderson WG, Khuri SF, Daley J. Surgical outcomes for patients aged 80 and older: morbidity and mortality from major noncardiac surgery. J Am Geriatr Soc. 2005;53(3):424–9.
7. Rubinfeld I, Thomas C, Berry S, et al. Octogenarian abdominal surgical emergencies: not so grim a problem with the acute care surgery model? J Trauma. 2009;67(5):983–9.
8. Wilson ME, WIlliams NB, Baskett PJ, Bennett JA, Skene AM. Assessment of fitness for surgical procedures and the variability of anaesthetists' judgments. Br Med J. 1980;280(6213):509–12.
9. Turnbull JM, Buck C. The value of preoperative screening investigations in otherwise healthy individuals. Arch Intern Med. 1987;147(6):1101–5.
10. Kaplan EB, Sheiner LB, Boeckmann AJ, et al. The usefulness of preoperative laboratory screening. JAMA. 1985;253(24):3576–81.
11. Munro J, Booth A, Nicholl J. Routine preoperative testing: a systematic review of the evidence. Health Technol Assess. 1997; 1(12):i–iv; 1–62.
12. McGory ML, Kao KK, Shekelle PG, et al. Developing quality indicators for elderly surgical patients. Ann Surg. 2009; 250(2):338–47.
13. Woolger JM. Preoperative testing and medication management. Clin Geriatr Med. 2008;24(4):573–83, vii.
14. Stevens LA, Coresh J, Greene T, Levey AS. Assessing kidney function – measured and estimated glomerular filtration rate. N Engl J Med. 2006;354(23):2473–83.
15. Lee TH, Marcantonio ER, Mangione CM, et al. Derivation and prospective validation of a simple index for prediction of cardiac risk of major noncardiac surgery. Circulation. 1999;100(10):1043–9.
16. Smetana GW, Macpherson DS. The case against routine preoperative laboratory testing. Med Clin North Am. 2003;87(1):7–40.
17. Wu WC, Schifftner TL, Henderson WG, et al. Preoperative hematocrit levels and postoperative outcomes in older patients undergoing noncardiac surgery. JAMA. 2007;297(22):2481–8.
18. Fleischmann KE, Beckman JA, Buller CE, et al. 2009 ACCF/AHA focused update on perioperative beta blockade. J Am Coll Cardiol. 2009;54(22):2102–28.
19. Liu LL, Dzankic S, Leung JM. Preoperative electrocardiogram abnormalities do not predict postoperative cardiac complications in geriatric surgical patients. J Am Geriatr Soc. 2002;50(7): 1186–91.
20. van Klei WA, Bryson GL, Yang H, Kalkman CJ, Wells GA, Beattie WS. The value of routine preoperative electrocardiography in predicting myocardial infarction after noncardiac surgery. Ann Surg. 2007;246(2):165–70.
21. Correll DJ, Hepner DL, Chang C, Tsen L, Hevelone ND, Bader AM. Preoperative electrocardiograms: patient factors predictive of abnormalities. Anesthesiology. 2009;110(6):1217–22.
22. Qato DM, Alexander GC, Conti RM, Johnson M, Schumm P, Lindau ST. Use of prescription and over-the-counter medications and dietary supplements among older adults in the United States. JAMA. 2008;300(24):2867–78.
23. Hanlon JT, Schmader KE, Ruby CM, Weinberger M. Suboptimal prescribing in older inpatients and outpatients. J Am Geriatr Soc. 2001;49(2):200–9.
24. Whinney C. Perioperative medication management: general principles and practical applications. Cleve Clin J Med. 2009;76 Suppl 4:S126–32.
25. Kennedy JM, van Rij AM, Spears GF, Pettigrew RA, Tucker IG. Polypharmacy in a general surgical unit and consequences of drug withdrawal. Br J Clin Pharmacol. 2000;49(4):353–62.
26. Devereaux PJ, Yang H, Yusuf S, et al. Effects of extended-release metoprolol succinate in patients undergoing non-cardiac surgery (POISE trial): a randomised controlled trial. Lancet. 2008;371 (9627):1839–47.
27. Biccard BM, Sear JW, Foex P. Statin therapy: a potentially useful peri-operative intervention in patients with cardiovascular disease. Anaesthesia. 2005;60(11):1106–14.
28. Marik PE, Varon J. Requirement of perioperative stress doses of corticosteroids: a systematic review of the literature. Arch Surg. 2008;143(12):1222–6.
29. Ang-Lee MK, Moss J, Yuan CS. Herbal medicines and perioperative care. JAMA. 2001;286(2):208–16.
30. Plassman BL, Langa KM, Fisher GG, et al. Prevalence of cognitive impairment without dementia in the United States. Ann Intern Med. 2008;148(6):427–34.

31. Plassman BL, Langa KM, Fisher GG, et al. Prevalence of dementia in the United States: the aging, demographics, and memory study. Neuroepidemiology. 2007;29(1–2):125–32.
32. Corrada MM, Brookmeyer R, Paganini-Hill A, Berlau D, Kawas CH. Dementia incidence continues to increase with age in the oldest old: the 90+ study. Ann Neurol. 2010;67(1):114–21.
33. Rudolph JL, Inouye SK, Jones RN, et al. Delirium: an independent predictor of functional decline after cardiac surgery. J Am Geriatr Soc. 2010;58(4):643–9.
34. Rudolph JL, Jones RN, Levkoff SE, et al. Derivation and validation of a preoperative prediction rule for delirium after cardiac surgery. Circulation. 2009;119(2):229–36.
35. Marcantonio ER, Goldman L, Mangione CM, et al. A clinical prediction rule for delirium after elective noncardiac surgery. JAMA. 1994;271(2):134–9.
36. Robinson TN, Raeburn CD, Tran ZV, Angles EM, Brenner LA, Moss M. Postoperative delirium in the elderly: risk factors and outcomes. Ann Surg. 2009;249(1):173–8.
37. Holsinger T, Plassman BL, Stechuchak KM, Burke JR, Coffman CJ, Williams Jr JW. Screening for cognitive impairment: comparing the performance of four instruments in primary care. J Am Geriatr Soc. 2012;60(6):1027–36.
38. Borson S, Scanlan J, Brush M, Vitaliano P, Dokmak A. The mini-cog: a cognitive 'vital signs' measure for dementia screening in multi-lingual elderly. Int J Geriatr Psychiatry. 2000;15(11):1021–7.
39. Dasgupta M, Dumbrell AC. Preoperative risk assessment for delirium after noncardiac surgery: a systematic review. J Am Geriatr Soc. 2006;54(10):1578–89.
40. Brouquet A, Cudennec T, Benoist S, et al. Impaired mobility, ASA status and administration of tramadol are risk factors for postoperative delirium in patients aged 75 years or more after major abdominal surgery. Ann Surg. 2010;251(4):759–65.
41. Ansaloni L, Catena F, Chattat R, et al. Risk factors and incidence of postoperative delirium in elderly patients after elective and emergency surgery. Br J Surg. 2010;97(2):273–80.
42. Monk TG, Weldon BC, Garvan CW, et al. Predictors of cognitive dysfunction after major noncardiac surgery. Anesthesiology. 2008;108(1):18–30.
43. Noimark D. Predicting the onset of delirium in the post-operative patient. Age Ageing. 2009;38(4):368–73.
44. Demeure MJ, Fain MJ. The elderly surgical patient and postoperative delirium. J Am Coll Surg. 2006;203(5):752–7.
45. Leung JM, Tsai TL, Sands LP. Brief report: preoperative frailty in older surgical patients is associated with early postoperative delirium. Anesth Analg. 2011;112(5):1199–201.
46. Clegg A, Young JB. Which medications to avoid in people at risk of delirium: a systematic review. Age Ageing. 2011;40(1):23–9.
47. Marcantonio ER, Juarez G, Goldman L, et al. The relationship of postoperative delirium with psychoactive medications. JAMA. 1994;272(19):1518–22.
48. Flinn DR, Diehl KM, Seyfried LS, Malani PN. Prevention, diagnosis, and management of postoperative delirium in older adults. J Am Coll Surg. 2009;209(2):261–8, quiz 294.
49. Steffens DC, Fisher GG, Langa KM, Potter GG, Plassman BL. Prevalence of depression among older Americans: the Aging Demographics and Memory Study. Int Psychogeriatr. 2009; 21(5):879–88.
50. Cole MG, Dendukuri N. Risk factors for depression among elderly community subjects: a systematic review and meta-analysis. Am J Psychiatry. 2003;160(6):1147–56.
51. Blumenthal JA, Lett HS, Babyak MA, et al. Depression as a risk factor for mortality after coronary artery bypass surgery. Lancet. 2003;362(9384):604–9.
52. Lawrence VA, Hazuda HP, Cornell JE, et al. Functional independence after major abdominal surgery in the elderly. J Am Coll Surg. 2004;199(5):762–72.
53. Li C, Friedman B, Conwell Y, Fiscella K. Validity of the Patient Health Questionnaire 2 (PHQ-2) in identifying major depression in older people. J Am Geriatr Soc. 2007;55(4):596–602.
54. Blazer DG, Wu LT. The epidemiology of substance use and disorders among middle aged and elderly community adults: national survey on drug use and health. Am J Geriatr Psychiatry. 2009; 17(3):237–45.
55. Blazer DG, Wu LT. The epidemiology of at-risk and binge drinking among middle-aged and elderly community adults: National Survey on Drug Use and Health. Am J Psychiatry. 2009;166(10): 1162–9.
56. Nath B, Li Y, Carroll JE, Szabo G, Tseng JF, Shah SA. Alcohol exposure as a risk factor for adverse outcomes in elective surgery. J Gastrointest Surg. 2010;14(11):1732–41.
57. Tonnesen H, Kehlet H. Preoperative alcoholism and postoperative morbidity. Br J Surg. 1999;86(7):869–74.
58. Berks J, McCormick R. Screening for alcohol misuse in elderly primary care patients: a systematic literature review. Int Psychogeriatr. 2008;20(6):1090–103.
59. McGrath A, Crome P, Crome IB. Substance misuse in the older population. Postgrad Med J. 2005;81(954):228–31.
60. Kaiser MJ, Bauer JM, Ramsch C, et al. Frequency of malnutrition in older adults: a multinational perspective using the mini nutritional assessment. J Am Geriatr Soc. 2010;58(9):1734–8.
61. Schiesser M, Kirchhoff P, Muller MK, Schafer M, Clavien PA. The correlation of nutrition risk index, nutrition risk score, and bioimpedance analysis with postoperative complications in patients undergoing gastrointestinal surgery. Surgery. 2009;145(5): 519–26.
62. Hickson M. Malnutrition and ageing. Postgrad Med J. 2006;82(963):2–8.
63. Gibbs J, Cull W, Henderson W, Daley J, Hur K, Khuri SF. Preoperative serum albumin level as a predictor of operative mortality and morbidity: results from the National VA Surgical Risk Study. Arch Surg. 1999;134(1):36–42.
64. Corti MC, Guralnik JM, Salive ME, Sorkin JD. Serum albumin level and physical disability as predictors of mortality in older persons. JAMA. 1994;272(13):1036–42.
65. Souba WW. Nutritional support. N Engl J Med. 1997;336(1):41–8.
66. Volkert D, Berner YN, Berry E, et al. ESPEN guidelines on enteral nutrition: geriatrics. Clin Nutr. 2006;25(2):330–60.
67. Davenport DL, Ferraris VA, Hosokawa P, Henderson WG, Khuri SF, Mentzer Jr RM. Multivariable predictors of postoperative cardiac adverse events after general and vascular surgery: results from the patient safety in surgery study. J Am Coll Surg. 2007;204(6):1199–210.
68. Kumar R, McKinney WP, Raj G, et al. Adverse cardiac events after surgery: assessing risk in a veteran population. J Gen Intern Med. 2001;16(8):507–18.
69. Devereaux PJ, Goldman L, Cook DJ, Gilbert K, Leslie K, Guyatt GH. Perioperative cardiac events in patients undergoing noncardiac surgery: a review of the magnitude of the problem, the pathophysiology of the events and methods to estimate and communicate risk. CMAJ. 2005;173(6):627–34.
70. McAlister FA, Bertsch K, Man J, Bradley J, Jacka M. Incidence of and risk factors for pulmonary complications after nonthoracic surgery. Am J Respir Crit Care Med. 2005;171(5):514–7.
71. Johnson RG, Arozullah AM, Neumayer L, Henderson WG, Hosokawa P, Khuri SF. Multivariable predictors of postoperative respiratory failure after general and vascular surgery: results from the patient safety in surgery study. J Am Coll Surg. 2007;204(6):1188–98.
72. Arozullah AM, Daley J, Henderson WG, Khuri SF. Multifactorial risk index for predicting postoperative respiratory failure in men after major noncardiac surgery. The National Veterans Administration Surgical Quality Improvement Program. Ann Surg. 2000;232(2):242–53.

73. Canet J, Gallart L, Gomar C, et al. Prediction of postoperative pulmonary complications in a population-based surgical cohort. Anesthesiology. 2010;113(6):1338–50.
74. Smetana GW. Postoperative pulmonary complications: an update on risk assessment and reduction. Cleve Clin J Med. 2009;76 Suppl 4:S60–5.
75. Smetana GW, Lawrence VA, Cornell JE. Preoperative pulmonary risk stratification for noncardiothoracic surgery: systematic review for the American College of Physicians. Ann Intern Med. 2006;144(8):581–95.
76. Qaseem A, Snow V, Fitterman N, et al. Risk assessment for and strategies to reduce perioperative pulmonary complications for patients undergoing noncardiothoracic surgery: a guideline from the American College of Physicians. Ann Intern Med. 2006;144(8):575–80.
77. Arozullah AM, Khuri SF, Henderson WG, Daley J. Development and validation of a multifactorial risk index for predicting postoperative pneumonia after major noncardiac surgery. Ann Intern Med. 2001;135(10):847–57.
78. Hulzebos EH, Helders PJ, Favie NJ, De Bie RA, Brutel de la Riviere A, Van Meeteren NL. Preoperative intensive inspiratory muscle training to prevent postoperative pulmonary complications in high-risk patients undergoing CABG surgery: a randomized clinical trial. JAMA. 2006;296(15):1851–7.
79. Berg H, Roed J, Viby-Mogensen J, et al. Residual neuromuscular block is a risk factor for postoperative pulmonary complications. A prospective, randomised, and blinded study of postoperative pulmonary complications after atracurium, vecuronium and pancuronium. Acta Anaesthesiol Scand. 1997;41(9):1095–103.
80. Moller AM, Villebro N, Pedersen T, Tonnesen H. Effect of preoperative smoking intervention on postoperative complications: a randomised clinical trial. Lancet. 2002;359(9301):114–7.
81. Thomsen T, Tonnesen H, Moller AM. Effect of preoperative smoking cessation interventions on postoperative complications and smoking cessation. Br J Surg. 2009;96(5):451–61.
82. Lindstrom D, Sadr Azodi O, Wladis A, et al. Effects of a perioperative smoking cessation intervention on postoperative complications: a randomized trial. Ann Surg. 2008;248(5):739–45.
83. Robinson TN, Eiseman B, Wallace JI, et al. Redefining geriatric preoperative assessment using frailty, disability and co-morbidity. Ann Surg. 2009;250(3):449–55.
84. Lachs MS, Feinstein AR, Cooney Jr LM, et al. A simple procedure for general screening for functional disability in elderly patients. Ann Intern Med. 1990;112(9):699–706.
85. Podsiadlo D, Richardson S. The timed "Up & Go": a test of basic functional mobility for frail elderly persons. J Am Geriatr Soc. 1991;39(2):142–8.
86. Panel on Prevention of Falls in Older Persons, American Geriatrics Society and British Geriatrics Society. Summary of the Updated American Geriatrics Society/British Geriatrics Society clinical practice guideline for prevention of falls in older persons. J Am Geriatr Soc. 2011;59(1):148–57.
87. Chen TY, Anderson DJ, Chopra T, Choi Y, Schmader KE, Kaye KS. Poor functional status is an independent predictor of surgical site infections due to methicillin-resistant Staphylococcus aureus in older adults. J Am Geriatr Soc. 2010;58(3):527–32.
88. Robinson TN, Wallace JI, Wu DS, et al. Accumulated frailty characteristics predict postoperative discharge institutionalization in the geriatric patient. J Am Coll Surg. 2011;213(1):37–42; discussion 42–4.
89. Fedarko NS. The biology of aging and frailty. Clin Geriatr Med. 2011;27(1):27–37.
90. Abellan van Kan G, Rolland Y, Houles M, Gillette-Guyonnet S, Soto M, Vellas B. The assessment of frailty in older adults. Clin Geriatr Med. 2010;26(2):275–86.
91. Xue QL. The frailty syndrome: definition and natural history. Clin Geriatr Med. 2011;27(1):1–15.
92. Fried LP, Tangen CM, Walston J, et al. Frailty in older adults: evidence for a phenotype. J Gerontol A Biol Sci Med Sci. 2001; 56(3):M146–56.
93. Jones DM, Song X, Rockwood K. Operationalizing a frailty index from a standardized comprehensive geriatric assessment. J Am Geriatr Soc. 2004;52(11):1929–33.
94. Rockwood K, Song X, MacKnight C, et al. A global clinical measure of fitness and frailty in elderly people. CMAJ. 2005;173(5):489–95.
95. Lee DH, Buth KJ, Martin BJ, Yip AM, Hirsch GM. Frail patients are at increased risk for mortality and prolonged institutional care after cardiac surgery. Circulation. 2010;121(8):973–8.
96. Bergman H, Ferrucci L, Guralnik J, et al. Frailty: an emerging research and clinical paradigm – issues and controversies. J Gerontol A Biol Sci Med Sci. 2007;62(7):731–7.
97. Clegg A, Young J. The frailty syndrome. Clin Med. 2011;11(1): 72–5.
98. Makary MA, Segev DL, Pronovost PJ, et al. Frailty as a predictor of surgical outcomes in older patients. J Am Coll Surg. 2010;210(6):901–8.
99. Farhat JS, Velanovich V, Falvo AJ, et al. Are the frail destined to fail? Frailty index as predictor of surgical morbidity and mortality in the elderly. J Trauma Acute Care Surg. 2012;72(6):1526–30; discussion 1530–1.
100. Silveira MJ, Kim SY, Langa KM. Advance directives and outcomes of surrogate decision making before death. N Engl J Med. 2010;362(13):1211–8.
101. Appelbaum PS. Clinical practice. Assessment of patients' competence to consent to treatment. N Engl J Med. 2007; 357(18):1834–40.
102. Karlawish JH, Casarett DJ, James BD, Xie SX, Kim SY. The ability of persons with Alzheimer disease (AD) to make a decision about taking an AD treatment. Neurology. 2005;64(9): 1514–9.
103. Fried TR, Bradley EH. What matters to seriously ill older persons making end-of-life treatment decisions?: A qualitative study. J Palliat Med. 2003;6(2):237–44.
104. Steinhauser KE, Christakis NA, Clipp EC, et al. Preparing for the end of life: preferences of patients, families, physicians, and other care providers. J Pain Symptom Manage. 2001;22(3):727–37.
105. Steinhauser KE, Christakis NA, Clipp EC, McNeilly M, McIntyre L, Tulsky JA. Factors considered important at the end of life by patients, family, physicians, and other care providers. JAMA. 2000;284(19):2476–82.
106. Kwok AC, Semel ME, Lipsitz SR, et al. The intensity and variation of surgical care at the end of life: a retrospective cohort study. Lancet. 2011;378(9800):1408–13.
107. Truog RD, Waisel DB. Do-not-resuscitate orders: from the ward to the operating room; from procedures to goals. Int Anesthesiol Clin. Summer 2001;39(3):53–65.
108. Truog RD. "Do-not-resuscitate" orders during anesthesia and surgery. Anesthesiology. 1991;74(3):606–8.
109. Cohen CB, Cohen PJ. Do-not-resuscitate orders in the operating room. N Engl J Med. 1991;325(26):1879–82.
110. Ewanchuk M, Brindley PG. Perioperative do-not-resuscitate orders – doing 'nothing' when 'something' can be done. Crit Care. 2006;10(4):219.
111. Truog RD, Waisel DB, Burns JP. DNR in the OR: a goal-directed approach. Anesthesiology. 1999;90(1):289–95.
112. Margolis JO, McGrath BJ, Kussin PS, Schwinn DA. Do not resuscitate (DNR) orders during surgery: ethical foundations for institutional policies in the United States. Anesth Analg. 1995;80(4): 806–9.

113. Wenger NS, Greengold NL, Oye RK, et al. Patients with DNR orders in the operating room: surgery, resuscitation, and outcomes. SUPPORT Investigators. Study to Understand Prognoses and Preferences for Outcomes and Risks of Treatments. J Clin Ethics. 1997 Fall;8(3):250–7.
114. Caruso LJ, Gabrielli A, Layon AJ. Perioperative do not resuscitate orders: caring for the dying in the operating room and intensive care unit. J Clin Anesth. 2002;14(6):401–4.
115. Coppolino M, Ackerson L. Do surrogate decision makers provide accurate consent for intensive care research? Chest. 2001;119(2):603–12.
116. Taffet GE, Teasdale TA, Luchi RJ. In-hospital cardiopulmonary resuscitation. JAMA. 1988;260(14):2069–72.
117. Waisel DB. Perioperative do-not-resuscitate orders. Curr Opin Anaesthesiol. 2000;13(2):191–4.
118. Fleisher LA, et al. Correction. J Am Coll Cardiol. 2008;52:794–7.

Part II

Surgical Emergencies in the Elderly

11 Appendicitis

Michael F. Ditillo and Kimberly A. Davis

Introduction

Surgical emergencies encompass a wide range of pathology, and they often present diagnostic and therapeutic challenges to the acute care surgeon. In elderly patients, age-related changes in anatomy and physiology, coupled with preexisting medical conditions, often alter the presentation of common surgical problems and their management and can have a profound impact on outcomes. As the population of aged patients increases globally, it is essential for surgeons to understand how the aging process impacts all facets of patient care, from their initial presentation and work-up to their recovery. Appendicitis epitomizes this challenging situation.

History

The first description of the vermiform appendix was made by the physician-anatomist Berengarion Da Carpi in 1521 [1]. In 1711, Lorenz Heister became the first person to describe appendicitis when he speculated that a perforation of the appendix with an adjacent abscess may have been caused by inflammation of the appendix itself [2]. Francois Melier described six cases of appendicitis on autopsy and was the first to propose the possibility of removing the appendix as a treatment strategy in 1827 [2–4]. Caludius Amyand performed the first appendectomy in 1735. He reported a case of an 11-year-old boy who presented with a scrotal hernia and a fistula. Upon exploration, he identified the appendix which had been perforated by a pin and performed an appendectomy as part of the hernia repair [5]. Nearly 150 years have passed before Lawson Tait in London presented the first successful transabdominal appendectomy for gangrenous appendix in 1880. In 1886, Reginald Fitz became the first person to describe the natural history of the inflamed appendix, to advocate for the surgical removal of the appendix, and to coin the term "appendicitis." In 1889, Charles McBurney presented his case series of surgically treated appendicitis and described the anatomic landmark that now bears his name. In the 1890s, Sir Frederick Treves advocated conservative management of acute appendicitis followed by appendectomy after the infection had subsided; unfortunately, his youngest daughter developed perforated appendicitis and later died from such treatment [6–12].

M.F. Ditillo, DO • K.A. Davis, MD, MBA (✉)
Department of Surgery, Section of Trauma,
Surgical Critical Care and Surgical Emergencies,
Yale School of Medicine, 330 Cedar Street, BB 310,
P.O. Box 208062, New Haven, CT 06520-8062, USA
e-mail: michael.ditillo@yale.edu; kimberly.davis@yale.edu

Epidemiology

Appendicitis continues to be one of the most common causes of acute abdominal pain. It is commonly thought to be a disease of younger patients. One of every 15 persons (7 %) will develop acute appendicitis during their lifetime. The peak incidence of appendicitis occurs between the second and third decades. Appendicitis is more uncommon in extremes of age (<5 years old, >50 years old). The relative risk of developing appendicitis in patients greater than 50 years of age has been estimated to be 2 % for men and 3 % for women. Overall, 5–10 % of all cases of appendicitis occur in patients >60 years old, representing approximately 5 % of all elderly patients presenting with an acute abdomen [13–19]. The incidence of geriatric appendicitis appears to be increasing, which is likely due to increasing life expectancy and a larger proportion of elder individuals in our society [20–22].

It has been noted that there is wide variation in the rate of appendicitis between countries. Appendicitis is relatively more common in industrialized nations, where diets consisting of greater percentages of highly refined foods low in dietary fiber are the norm. The rate of appendicitis is

J.A. Yelon, F.A. Luchette (eds.), *Geriatric Trauma and Critical Care*,
DOI 10.1007/978-1-4614-8501-8_11, © Springer Science+Business Media New York 2014

lower in developing nations, where the typical agrarian diet consists of less refined and more high-fiber foods [23, 24]. It is postulated that low-fiber diets lead to hard stools and higher colonic pressures which aid in the development of fecaliths. These fecaliths act as obstructing agents within the appendiceal lumen forming a closed loop obstruction and eventual appendicitis. However, case-controlled studies of fiber intake and appendicitis have been inconclusive. The etiologic significance of diet is not clear; however, the remarkable variation in the geographic distribution of appendicitis strongly implies a dietary role in its pathophysiology.

Pathophysiology

The development of appendicitis appears similar to that of other inflammatory processes involving hollow visceral organs. A common theory to explain the inciting event which leads to inflammation is appendiceal luminal obstruction [25–30]. Appendiceal obstruction may be caused by fecaliths, lymphoid hyperplasia, benign or malignant tumors, and infectious processes. Luminal obstruction leads to an increase in endoluminal and intramural pressure, resulting in occlusion of the venules in the appendiceal wall, and stasis of lymphatic flow. As vascular and lymphatic occlusion progress, the wall of the appendix becomes ischemic. This allows invasion of the appendiceal wall by enteric bacteria. The inflammation of the appendiceal wall is followed by perforation and the development of a contained abscess or generalized peritonitis. Aerobic organisms predominate early in the course, while mixed flora is more common in late appendicitis. Common organisms include *Escherichia coli* and *Bacteroides fragilis* [31, 32]. The mechanism of luminal obstruction varies with patient's age. In the young, lymphoid follicular hyperplasia due to infection is thought to be the main cause. In older patients, luminal obstruction is more likely to be caused by fibrosis, fecaliths, or neoplasia (carcinoid, adenocarcinoma, or mucocele).

It has been proposed that elderly patients have anatomic and physiologic changes which predispose them to a more rapid progression of their appendicitis [27, 33, 34]. Thorbjarnarson and Loehr noted that in the elderly, the lumen of the appendix is often narrowed or obliterated, the mucosa is thin, minimal amounts of lymphoid tissue are present, and there is fibrous and fatty infiltration of the wall, resulting in the attenuation of appendiceal wall strength [21]. In addition, as patients age, the blood supply can be affected by atherosclerosis, predisposing to ischemia. Consequently, even mild increases in endoluminal pressure, which are typically seen in early appendicitis, may lead to perforation in elderly patients.

Presentation

The diagnosis of appendicitis is often made clinically. Abdominal pain is the most common clinical symptom of appendicitis and is found in nearly all confirmed cases [35]. The clinical presentation of acute appendicitis is often a collection of "classic" signs and symptoms which include right lower quadrant abdominal pain (at McBurney's point, defined as the point over the right side of the abdomen that is 1/3 the distance from the anterior superior iliac spine to the umbilicus), anorexia, nausea, and vomiting. In this "classic" presentation, the patient complains of abdominal pain as the first symptom, which typically starts as periumbilical and migrates to the right lower quadrant. This pattern is seen in 50–90 % of patients with appendicitis [35–37]. Nausea and vomiting, when they occur, usually follow the onset of pain. Fever and leukocytosis follow later in the course of illness. Low-grade fever up to 101.0 °F (38.3 °C) may be present [35, 38–41].

Unfortunately, in many patients, the initial presentation is atypical or nonspecific. Because the early signs and symptoms of appendicitis are often subtle, patients and clinicians may downplay their importance. It is generally held that approximately 25 % of patients with appendicitis present with atypical signs and symptoms. The symptoms of appendicitis can vary depending upon the location of the appendix, as it has no anatomically fixed position. It originates below the terminal ileum in either the dorsomedial location from the cecal fundus or directly beside the ileal orifice. The appendix may lie in the pelvis, or behind the cecum, terminal ileum, or the ascending colon. The danger with atypical presentation is that it may lead to a delay in diagnosis, and this delay will allow progression of inflammation until perforation occurs. Three factors associated with atypical presentation are extremes of age, pregnancy, and other medical conditions which interfere with diagnosis (i.e., Crohn's disease).

The clinical presentation of appendicitis in the elderly is often the same as in younger adults. Several authors have demonstrated similarity between the presenting complaints, signs, and symptoms of older versus younger patients with appendicitis [14, 33, 42]. It remains more difficult to diagnose appendicitis in elderly patients, perhaps due to the increased scope of the differential diagnosis of acute abdominal pain in the elderly. Errors in diagnosis occur in 30 % of patients older than 50, as compared to only 8 % of those patients younger than 50 despite similar presenting complaints, temperature, and leukocyte count in these patients [42, 43].

One fact that is consistent in the literature is that elderly patients present for evaluation later in the disease process than their younger counterparts. This delay in presentation also correlated with a significantly increased rate of perforation, when compared to young patients [43–46]. When sorting through this data, it appears that elderly patients with acute appendicitis do not in fact present differently from younger patients, but are more likely to present later in the disease process due to delays or errors in diagnosis. Thus, their presentation is more consistent with gangrenous or perforated appendicitis.

Diagnosis

To aid in the clinical diagnosis of acute appendicitis, several scoring systems have been proposed. Of these, the Alvarado score is the most widely used [47, 48]. The Alvarado scale assigns a score to each of the following diagnostic elements: migratory right iliac fossa pain (1 point), anorexia (1 point), nausea/vomiting (1 point), right lower quadrant tenderness (2 points), rebound tenderness in the right lower quadrant (1 point), temperature >37.5 °C (1 point), and leukocytosis (2 points). The points are additive and the total score used to guide management. A patient with a score of 0–3 is considered low risk of appendicitis and could be discharged with advice to return if there was no improvement in symptoms. A patient with a score of 4–6 would be admitted for observation and serial abdominal examinations. If the score remains unchanged at 12 h, operative intervention is recommended. Male patients with a score of 7–9 would proceed to appendectomy. A female patient should undergo diagnostic laparoscopy with appendectomy if indicated by the intraoperative findings [47, 48]. In validation studies, the Alvarado score had a sensitivity of 95 % for appendicitis with a score greater than 7 and overall accuracy of 83 % [49–52]. Konan et al. looked at Alvarado scoring in elderly patients. They found that no patient with acute appendicitis had an Alvarado score below 3 (sensitivity = 100 %, specificity = 75 %, accuracy = 88 %), and all patients with a score above 7 had appendicitis (sensitivity = 71 %, specificity = 100 %, accuracy = 85 %) [53].

Several other scoring systems have been described as well. A systematic review of several published scoring systems by Liu et al. identified a diagnostic sensitivity of 53–99 % and specificity of 30–99 % [52]. In general, scoring systems can aid clinical judgment, and they have the potential to improve specificity leading to lower false-positive rates in diagnosis of acute appendicitis. However, scoring systems cannot definitively determine or exclude the possibility of appendicitis.

Over the last several decades, there has been increasing use of imaging modalities such as ultrasonography and computed tomography in the diagnosis of acute appendicitis. Although the increased use of imaging has decreased the rate of negative appendectomies [54–56], diagnostic imaging is unnecessary when the clinical diagnosis of appendicitis is certain. However, imaging should be performed when the diagnosis of appendicitis is suspected or unclear, which is often the case in elderly patients.

Ultrasound is generally considered to be reliable for identifying acute appendicitis, but cannot be trusted to rule it out. It has little added value when the clinical presentation is clear [57]. Ultrasonographic findings of appendicitis include an immobile noncompressible tubular structure with a wall thickness >6 mm (Fig. 11.1a–c). The structure is tender during palpation with the ultrasound probe (sonographic

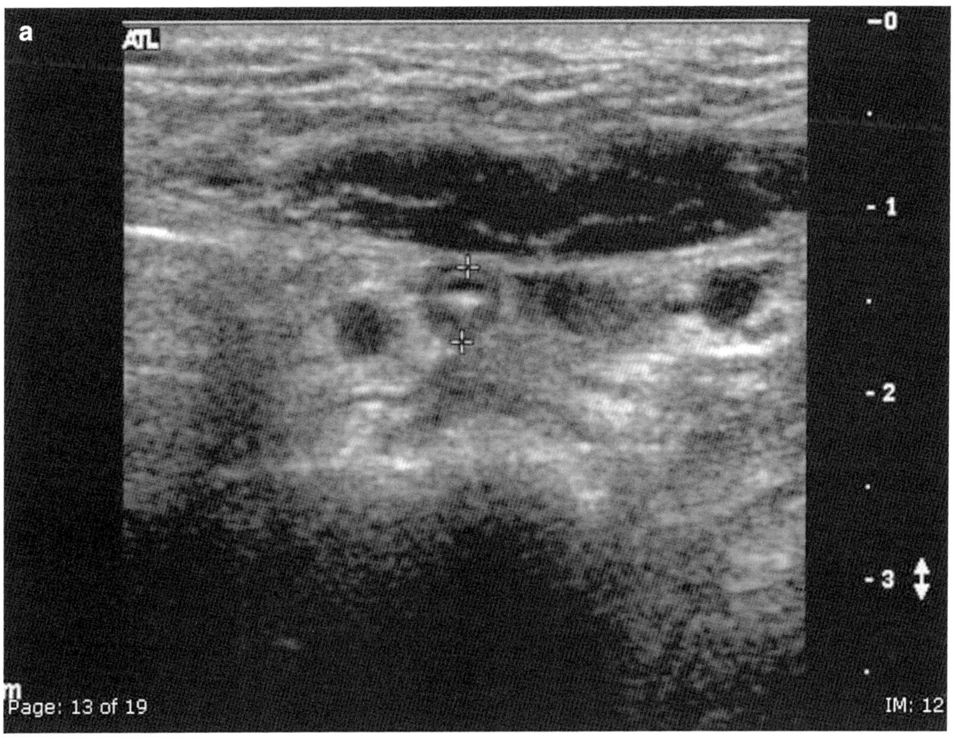

Fig. 11.1 (**a**) Ultrasound demonstrating a noncompressible tubular structure on ultrasound, with a transverse diameter of >6 mm, consistent with acute appendicitis. (**b**) Ultrasound demonstrating a longitudinal view of a noncompressible tubular structure with thickened walls consistent with acute appendicitis. (**c**) Endoluminal fecalith on ultrasound

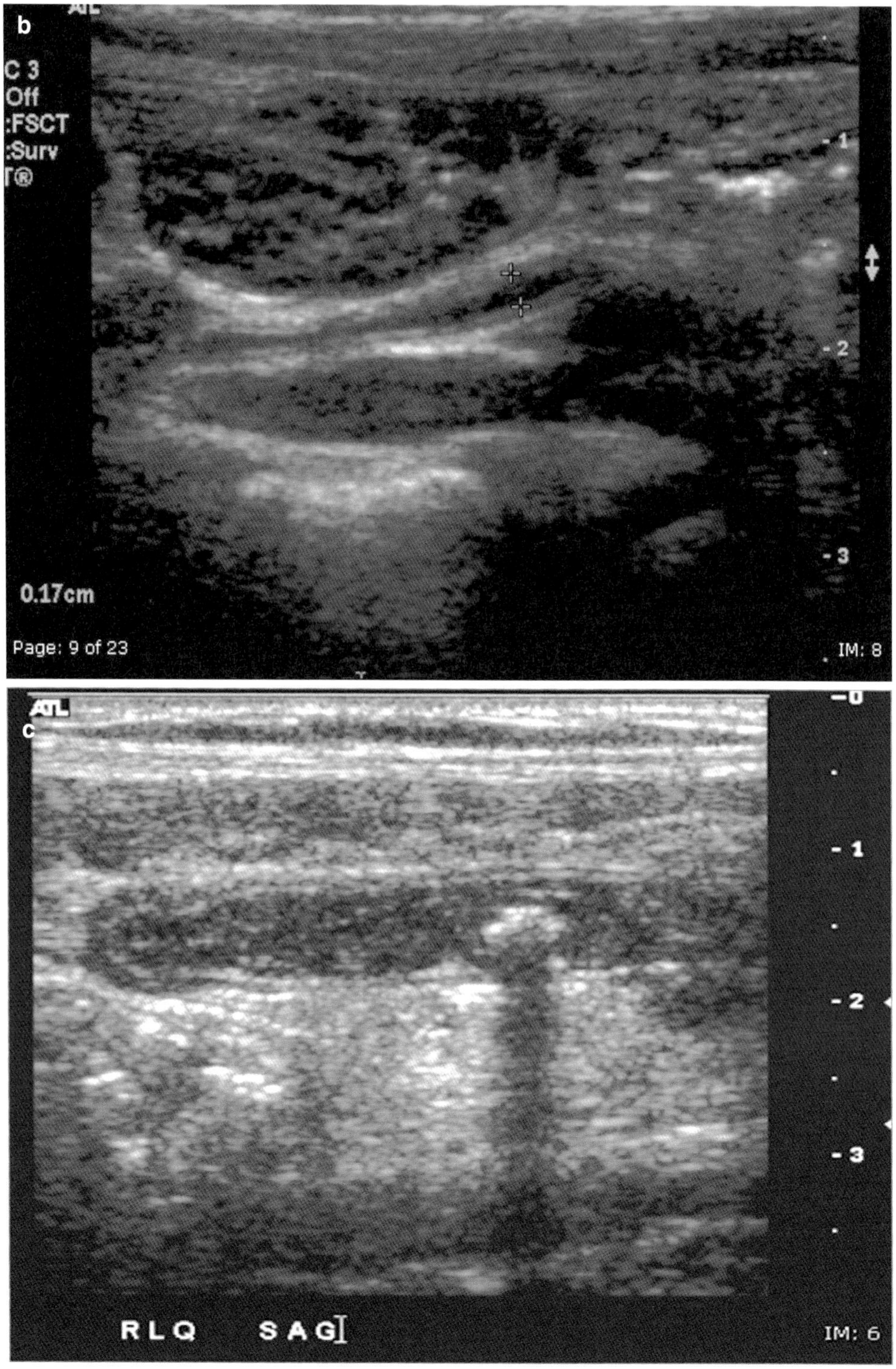

Fig. 11.1 (continued)

McBurney's sign). Additional supporting findings include an appendicolith, a transverse diameter of ≥6 mm, and fluid in the appendiceal lumen [35, 57–59].

The sensitivity and specificity of ultrasound in the diagnosis of appendicitis ranged from 35 to 98 % and 71 to 98 %, respectively. The main advantages of ultrasound are its lack of radiation, the rapidity of results, and lack of contrast agents. The disadvantages of ultrasonography are its limited ability to diagnose other pathologic processes that may be occurring. In addition, the accuracy of ultrasound is operator dependent, and it may be difficult to image patients with obesity or with a large amount of overlying bowel gas. Currently,

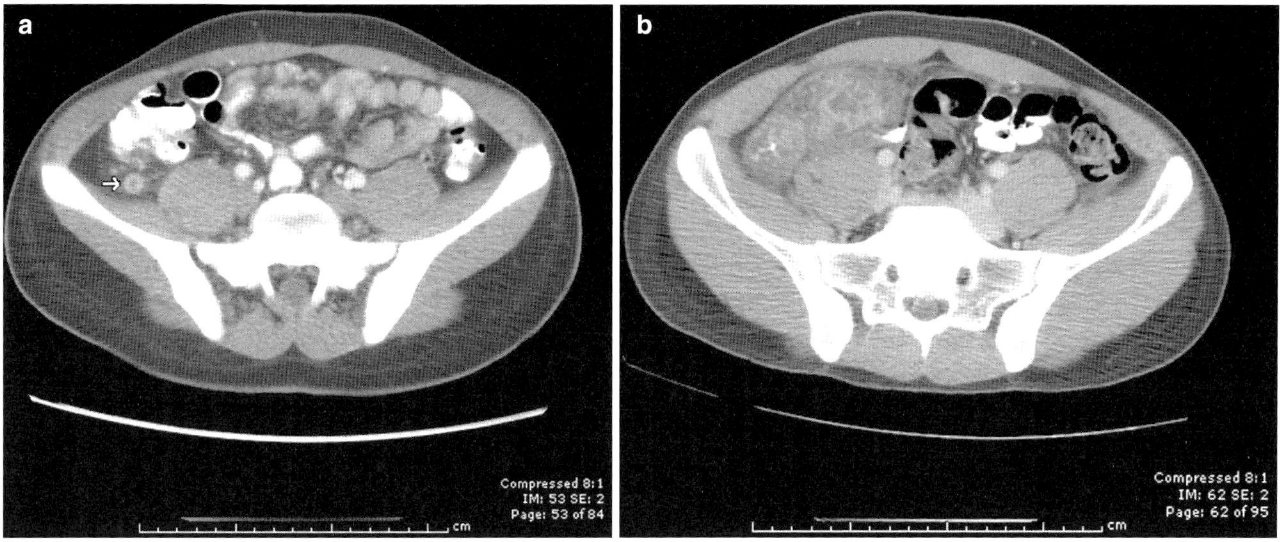

Fig. 11.2 (**a**) A target sign on CT scan of the abdomen and pelvis consistent with acute appendicitis. (**b**) Periappendiceal inflammation suspicious for perforated appendicitis

there are no studies focusing on the use of ultrasound in the diagnosis of appendicitis in elderly patients [35, 58–60].

Computed tomography of the abdomen and pelvis is frequently used in the radiographic diagnosis of appendicitis (Fig. 11.2a, b). CT findings of appendicitis include a nonfilling appendix that is thick walled and inflamed (appendix wall ≥7 mm), fat stranding around the appendix secondary to inflammatory changes, with or without periappendiceal fluid. A target sign with an appendicolith may be identified in 30 % of cases.

In a recently published study, Pooler et al. demonstrated that CT had a high sensitivity and specificity in elderly patients in whom the diagnosis of appendicitis was suspected. The overall diagnostic accuracy of CT is >99 %. This study also showed that despite a lower overall rate of acute appendicitis when compared to younger patients, the sensitivity and specificity of CT in elderly patients with clinically suspected appendicitis are statistically comparable to that of younger patients (sensitivity of 100 %, specificity of 99 %) [61]. This is the first study of its kind specifically examining the diagnostic performance of CT in an elderly population. Hui et al. also reported CT sensitivity of 91 % in elderly patients in whom appendicitis was clinically suspected [62].

Treatment

The goals of therapy for acute appendicitis should be timely diagnosis followed by prompt surgical intervention. Traditional surgical teaching has accepted a negative appendectomy rate of up to 20 % in patients diagnosed by clinical criteria. With advances in imaging technology, the acceptable negative appendectomy rate has been reduced to 10 %. It is well established that patients often delay seeking medical attention, causing the diagnosis of appendicitis to be difficult. This is especially true in elderly patients [35, 43–46, 53–60, 63]. The elderly tend to have a diminished inflammatory response, resulting in a less remarkable history and physical examination. For these reasons, older patients often delay seeking medical care, and as a result, they have a considerably higher rate of perforation at the time of presentation [44–46].

Whether open or laparoscopic techniques are used, surgical intervention remains the mainstay of treatment. In open appendectomy, a right lower quadrant incision should be the incision of choice. It has been shown that paramedian and vertical midline incisions, which might be used to explore patients in whom a definitive diagnosis has not been reached, are associated with higher postoperative infectious complications [46, 64].

Laparoscopic appendectomy can be used successfully in the elderly population and results in decreased length of stay, decrease postoperative complications, and decreased mortality for older patients with both perforated and nonperforated appendicitis [65–67].

There are a handful of circumstances in which appendectomy should be delayed. Patients who present early in their course of appendicitis will typically undergo immediate appendectomy. However, if a patient presents with a longer duration of symptoms (>72 h), they will likely have advanced appendicitis. These patients will often have a palpable mass on physical exam, and imaging studies may show a phlegmon or abscess. Operative intervention in patients with a long duration of symptoms and a phlegmon is associated with increased morbidity, due to dense adhesions and inflammation. Appendectomy under these circumstances will often require extensive dissection and may lead to injury of adjacent structures. Complications such as a postoperative abscess or enterocutaneous fistula may occur, necessitating an ileocolectomy or cecostomy. Because of these potential complications, a nonoperative approach can be considered if the patient is to be clinically stable. Many of these patients will respond to nonoperative management since the inflammatory process has already been "walled off." Nonoperative management includes antibiotics, intravenous fluids, and bowel rest [68–71]. Repeat imaging may be necessary to document resolution of the phlegmon or progression to abscess formation.

If imaging studies demonstrate an abscess, CT- or ultrasound-guided drainage can be performed percutaneously [71–73]. Patients who have an abscess are ideal candidates for percutaneous drainage along with antibiotics, IV fluids, and bowel rest. This allows inflammation to subside, sometimes negating the need for extended bowel resection, such as ileocecectomy. This approach to appendiceal abscesses results in a decrease in morbidity and shorter lengths of stay [70, 74, 75]. Patients should be closely monitored in the hospital during this time. Treatment failure includes bowel obstruction, sepsis, or persistent pain, fever, or leukocytosis and requires immediate appendectomy. If fever, tenderness, and leukocytosis improve, diet can be slowly advanced. Patients are discharged home when clinical parameters have normalized.

More than 80 % of patients who present with a "walled-off" appendiceal process and undergo nonoperative management can be spared an appendectomy at the time of initial presentation. Traditionally, an interval appendectomy has been recommended for these patients 6–8 weeks after treatment [76]. The reason for this is to prevent recurrent appendicitis [77, 78] and to exclude neoplasms (such as carcinoid, adenocarcinoma, mucinous cystadenoma, and cystadenocarcinomas) [79, 80]. The need for interval appendectomy has been debated, with some studies suggesting that interval appendectomy is unnecessary [81, 82]. Kaminski et al., in a retrospective review of 1,012 patients treated nonoperatively for acute appendicitis, reported that 864 patients did not undergo interval appendectomy [81]. Of those 864 patients, only 39 (4.5 %) required an appendectomy at a median follow-up of 4 years. A meta-analysis of 61 observational studies in which a phlegmon or an appendiceal abscess was present found that immediate surgery was associated with higher morbidity than nonsurgical treatment. After successful nonsurgical treatment, a malignancy was detected in 1.2 % of cases, and recurrent appendicitis developed in 7.4 % of cases (95 %, CI 3.7–11.1) [82]. In the case of elderly patients, one must weigh the benefit of interval appendectomy against the risk of surgical intervention. Colonoscopy should be considered prior to appendectomy in patients over 50 who have not had a recent colonoscopy to rule out concurrent colonic pathology necessitating resection.

Outcomes

Despite improvements in the diagnosis and management of geriatric surgical patients, morbidity and mortality for appendicitis remain high. Morbidity rates between 28 and 60 % and mortality rates as high as 10 % are all significantly higher than younger patients. One explanation for this is that typically, geriatric patients with appendicitis tend to have an increased prehospital delay seeking medical attention which correlates with an increased rate of perforation. Whether young or old, patients with perforated appendicitis have increased lengths of hospital stay, an increased number of wound infections, and an increased number of hospital-acquired infections of all types (urinary tract, pneumonia). Patients with perforated appendicitis also have an increased rate of intra-abdominal septic complication, which, when coupled with the preexisting medical conditions often seen in elderly patients, leads to a high mortality for these patients [42–46, 63, 64, 83].

Malignancy and Mucocele

Cancer of the appendix is an uncommon finding, occurring in approximately 1 % of appendectomy specimens, and accounts for roughly 0.5 % of intestinal neoplasms. Carcinoid tumors are the most common, comprising over 50 % of appendiceal neoplasms. As is the case with other carcinoid tumors arising in the intestines, appendiceal carcinoids can secrete serotonin and other vasoactive substances. These substances are responsible for the carcinoid syndrome, which is characterized by episodic flushing, diarrhea, wheezing, and right-sided valvular heart disease. Nearly all appendiceal carcinoids are found retrospectively after an operation for acute appendicitis, and the majority of those are located at the tip of the appendix [84, 85].

Surgical management for appendiceal carcinoids is a subject of some debate. Since the vast majority is discovered incidentally in an appendectomy specimen done for other reasons, a decision must be made whether or not to return the patient to the operating room for a right colectomy. Tumor size is an important determinant of the need for further surgery [86]. Small appendiceal carcinoids (<1 cm) are often considered benign; however, regional metastases and/or deep invasion has been reported in tumors between 1 and 2 cm. For patients with tumors ≥2 cm, the 5-year mortality from appendiceal carcinoid is ~30 %, whereas with a 1 cm appendiceal tumors, there is a 5 % mortality rate at 5 years [87].

Whether a colectomy should be performed in some patients with smaller tumors is unclear. There is limited evidence on which to make clear recommendations for a right hemicolectomy in patients with a diagnosis of appendiceal carcinoid <2 cm. Hemicolectomy is advocated for tumors >2 cm, tumors at the base of the appendix, and incompletely resected tumor. For tumors <2 cm, if there is mesoappendiceal invasion, lymphovascular invasion, and intermediate- to high-grade tumors, and in patients with mixed histology (goblet cell carcinoid, adenocarcinoid) or with obvious mesenteric nodal involvement, some authors recommend right hemicolectomy. Others disagree and consider that appendectomy alone is adequate for tumors <2 cm, even with mesoappendiceal invasion. For carcinoids less than 1 cm in size and those between 1.0 and 1.9 cm without evidence of mesoappendiceal invasion or nodal involvement, simple appendectomy alone is adequate [87–91].

In contrast to other appendiceal neoplasms, the majority of patients with adenocarcinomas present with symptoms consistent with acute appendicitis. Patients can also present with ascites, generalized abdominal pain, or an abdominal mass. Appendiceal adenocarcinomas fall into one of three separate histologic types: the most common is the mucinous type and intestinal or colonic type (which closely mimics adenocarcinomas found in the colon) and the least common, signet ring cell adenocarcinoma [92–94].

In general, the optimal treatment for most appendiceal adenocarcinomas is a right colectomy, although this is debated. Some authors advocate a simple appendectomy for adenocarcinomas that are confined to the mucosa or well-differentiated lesions that invade no deeper than the submucosa. Although this distinction can be difficult to make intraoperatively, a more common scenario is the unexpected finding of an adenocarcinoma when the surgical report of an appendectomy specimen is finalized. In such cases, a right colectomy need not be pursued for appendiceal adenocarcinomas that are confined to the mucosa or well-differentiated lesions that invade no deeper than the submucosa [95]. The role of adjuvant chemotherapy or radiation for adenocarcinoma of the appendix is unknown. The rarity of this disease has precluded the performance of randomized studies, and few institutions see sufficient numbers of patients to report series of homogeneously treated patients.

The term appendiceal mucocele refers to any lesion that is characterized by a distended, mucus-filled appendix. It may be either a benign or malignant condition. The course and prognosis of appendiceal mucoceles are related to their histologic subtypes which include mucosal hyperplasia, simple or retention cysts, mucinous cystadenomas, and mucinous cystadenocarcinomas. Mucoceles that are due to hyperplasia, or that arise from an accumulation of mucus distal to an obstruction in the appendiceal lumen, even if they rupture, are benign and do not recur. Benign appendiceal mucoceles are usually asymptomatic. They may be diagnosed after appendectomy, or more commonly, they are found incidentally on a CT scan done for another purpose. In contrast, mucoceles that develop from true neoplasms (cystadenomas or cystadenocarcinomas) when ruptured can lead to intraperitoneal spread and the clinical picture of pseudomyxoma peritonei.

Surgical resection should be pursued, even for a benign-appearing appendiceal mucocele, since lesions that appear to be benign on imaging studies may harbor an underlying cystadenocarcinoma [96–99]. A right hemicolectomy is indicated in patients with a complicated mucocele with involvement of the terminal ileum or cecum. If there is no evidence of peritoneal disease and the final pathology shows a cystadenocarcinoma, a right colectomy could be considered to remove lymph nodes; however, the chance of nodal spread is quite small. An acceptable approach (assuming negative resection margins) is observation alone. If, on the other hand, there is evidence of peritoneal disease at laparoscopy, then the procedure should be converted to an open laparotomy for debulking.

It is important to remember the association between appendiceal mucoceles and other tumors involving the GI tract, ovary, breast, and kidney [100, 101]. This possibility should be evaluated either preoperatively or intraoperatively.

Conclusions

Appendicitis is uncommon in elderly patients. However, when it does occur, elderly patients have poor outcomes. Delays in presentation and more rapid progression of disease contribute to poor outcomes. Elderly patients with significant comorbidities are less likely to tolerate the increased risk of complications associated with advanced disease. It is of the utmost importance that when an elderly patient presents to the hospital with abdominal pain, appendicitis be considered as a possible diagnosis. Rapid evaluation and management is important, and delay in treatment should be minimized whenever possible.

References

1. Deaver JB. Appendicitis. 3rd ed. Philadelphia: P Blakiston's Son & Co.; 1905.
2. Major RH. Classic descriptions of disease. 3rd ed. Springfield: Charles C. Thomas; 1945.
3. DeMoulin D. Historical notes on appendicitis. Arch Chir Neerl. 1975;27:97–102.
4. Meade RH. The evolution of surgery for appendicitis. Surgery. 1964;55:741–52.
5. Amyand C. Of an inguinal rupture, with a pin in the appendix caeci, incrusted with stone; and some observations on wounds in the guts. Philos Trans R Soc Lond. 1736;39:329–36.

6. Williams GR. Presidential address: a history of appendicitis. Ann Surg. 1983;197:495–506.
7. Fitz RH. Perforating inflammation of the vermiform appendix: with special reference to its early diagnosis and treatment. Am J Med Sci. 1886;92:321–46.
8. Brooks SM. McBurney's point: the story of appendicitis. New York: AS Barnes & Co; 1969.
9. Klingensmith W. Establishment of appendicitis as a surgical entity. Tex State J Med. 1959;55:878–82.
10. McBurney C. Experience with early operative interference in cases of disease of the vermiform appendix. NY Med J. 1889; 50:676–84.
11. McBurney C. The incision made in the abdominal wall in cases of appendicitis, with a description of a new method of operation. Ann Surg. 1894;20:38–43.
12. Bernays AC, Heidelberg MD. My recent work in appendicectomy. Med Rec. 1898;53:478–82.
13. Norman DC, Yoshikawa TT. Intraabdominal infections in the elderly. J Am Geriatr Soc. 1983;31:677–84.
14. Peltokallio P, Jauhiainen K. Acute appendicitis in the aged patient. Arch Surg. 1970;100:140–3.
15. Yusuf MF, Dunn E. Appendicitis in the elderly: learn to discern the untypical picture. Geriatrics. 1979;34:73–9.
16. Andersson A, Bergdahl L. Acute appendicitis in patients over sixty. Am Surg. 1978;44:445–7.
17. Addiss DG, Shaffer N, Fowler BS, Tauxe RV. The epidemiology of appendicitis and appendectomy in the United States. Am J Epidemiol. 1990;135:910–25.
18. Graffeo CS, Counselman FL. Appendicitis. Emerg Med Clin North Am. 1996;14:653–71.
19. Lau WY, Fan ST, Yiu TF, Chu KW, Lee JMH. Acute appendicitis in the elderly. Surg Gynecol Obstet. 1985;161:157–606.
20. Smithy WB, Wexner SD, Dailey TH. The diagnosis and treatment of acute appendicitis in the aged. Dis Colon Rectum. 1986;29: 170–3.
21. Thorbjarnarson B, Loehr WJ. Acute appendicitis in patients over the age of sixty. Surg Gynecol Obstet. 1967;125:1277–80.
22. Basta M, Morton NE, Mulvihill JJ, Radovanovic Z, Radojicic C, Marinkovic D. Inheritance of acute appendicitis: familial aggregation and evidence of polygenic transmission. Am J Hum Genet. 1990;46:377–82.
23. Burkitt DP. The aetiology of appendicitis. Br J Surg. 1971; 58:695–9.
24. Walker ARP, Walker BF. Appendectomy in South African interethnic school pupils. Am J Gastroenterol. 1987;82:219–22.
25. Lamer AJ. The aetiology of appendicitis. Br J Hosp Med. 1988;39: 540–2.
26. Miranda R, Johnston AD, O'Leary JP. Incidental appendectomy: frequency of pathologic abnormalities. Am Surg. 1980;46:355.
27. Arnbjörnsson E, Bengmark S. Obstruction of the appendix lumen in relation to pathogenesis of acute appendicitis. Acta Chir Scand. 1983;149:789.
28. Nitecki S, Karmeli R, Sarr MG. Appendiceal calculi and fecaliths as indications for appendectomy. Surg Gynecol Obstet. 1990;171:185.
29. Butler C. Surgical pathology of acute appendicitis. Hum Pathol. 1981;12:870.
30. Chang AR. An analysis of the pathology of 3003 appendices. Aust N Z J Surg. 1981;51:169–78.
31. Bennion RS, Baron EJ, Thompson Jr JE, et al. The bacteriology of gangrenous and perforated appendicitis – revisited. Ann Surg. 1990;211:165.
32. Lau WY, Teoh-Chan CH, Fan ST, et al. The bacteriology and septic complication of patients with appendicitis. Ann Surg. 1984; 200:576.
33. Freund HR, Rubinstein E. Appendicitis in the aged. Is it really different? Am Surg. 1984;50:573–6.
34. Paajanen H, Kettunen J, Kostiainen S. Emergency appendectomies in patients over 80 years. Am Surg. 1994;60:950–3.
35. Lee SL, Walsh AJ, Ho HS. Computed tomography and ultrasonography do not improve and may delay the diagnosis and treatment of acute appendicitis. Arch Surg. 2001;136:556.
36. Birnbaum BA, Wilson SR. Appendicitis at the millennium. Radiology. 2000;215:337.
37. Chung CH, Ng CP, Lai KK. Delays by patients, emergency physicians, and surgeons in the management of acute appendicitis: retrospective study. Hong Kong Med J. 2000;6:254.
38. Ricci MA, Trevisani MF, Beck WC. Acute appendicitis: a 5-year review. Am Surg. 1991;57:301–5.
39. Siberman VA. Appendectomy in a large metropolitan hospital: retrospective review of 1013 cases. Am J Surg. 1981;142:615–8.
40. Berry Jr J, Malt RA. Appendicitis near its centenary. Ann Surg. 1984;200:567–75.
41. Pieper R, Kager L, Nasman P. Acute appendicitis: a clinical study of 1018 cases of emergency appendectomy. Acta Chir Scand. 1982;48:51–62.
42. Nguyen BT, Nguyen BT, Thompson JS. Comparison of appendectomy at a Veterans Administration Medical Center and affiliated university hospital. Nebr Med J. 1991;76:35–8.
43. Owens BJ, Hamit HF. Appendicitis in the elderly. Ann Surg. 1978;187:392–6.
44. Horattas MC, Guyton DP, Wu D. A reappraisal of appendicitis in the elderly. Am J Surg. 1990;160:291–3.
45. Kraemer M, Franke C, Ohmann C, Yang Q, for the Acute Abdominal Pain Study Group. Acute appendicitis in late adulthood: incidence, presentation, and outcome. Results of a prospective multicenter acute abdominal pain study and a review of the literature. Langenbecks Arch Surg. 2000;385:470–81.
46. Lee JFY, Leow CK, Lau WY. Appendicitis in the elderly. Aust N Z J Surg. 2000;70:593–6.
47. Alvarado A. A practical score for the early diagnosis of acute appendicitis. Ann Emerg Med. 1986;15:557.
48. Kalan M, Talbot D, Cunliffe WJ, Rich AJ. Evaluation of the modified Alvarado score in the diagnosis of acute appendicitis: a prospective study. Ann R Coll Surg Engl. 1994;76:418.
49. Hong JJ, Cohn SM, Ekeh AP, et al. A prospective randomized study of clinical assessment versus computed tomography for the diagnosis of acute appendicitis. Surg Infect (Larchmt). 2003;4:231.
50. Denizbasi A, Unluer EE. The role of the emergency medicine resident using the Alvarado score in the diagnosis of acute appendicitis compared with the general surgery resident. Eur J Emerg Med. 2003;10:296.
51. Singh K, Gupta S, Pargal P. Application of Alvarado scoring system in diagnosis of acute appendicitis. JK Sci. 2008;10:84.
52. Liu JL, Wyatt JC, Deeks JJ, et al. Systematic reviews of clinical decision tools for acute abdominal pain. Health Technol Assess. 2006;10:1.
53. Konan A, Hayran M, Kılıç YA, et al. Scoring systems in the diagnosis of acute appendicitis in the elderly. Ulus Travma Acil Cerrahi Derg. 2011;17(5):396–400.
54. Stroman DL, Bayouth CV, Kuhn JA, et al. The role of the computed tomography in the diagnosis of acute appendicitis. Am J Surg. 1999;178:485–9.
55. SCOAP Collaborative, Cuschieri J, Florence M, et al. Negative appendectomy and imaging accuracy in the Washington State Surgical Care and Outcomes Assessment Program. Ann Surg. 2008;248:557.
56. Rao PM, Rhea JT, Novelline RA, Mostafavi AA, McCabe CJ. Effect of computed tomography of the appendix on treatment of patients and use of hospital resources. N Engl J Med. 1998;338:141–6.
57. Lee SL, Ho HS. Ultrasonography and computed tomography in suspected acute appendicitis. Semin Ultrasound CT MR. 2003; 24:69.

58. van Randen A, Bipat S, Zwinderman AH, et al. Acute appendicitis: meta-analysis of diagnostic performance of CT and graded compression US related to prevalence of disease. Radiology. 2008;249:97–106.
59. Flum DR, McClure TD, Morris A, Koepsell T. Misdiagnosis of appendicitis and the use of diagnostic imaging. J Am Coll Surg. 2005;201:933.
60. Wagner PL, Eachempati SR, Soe K, et al. Defining the current negative appendectomy rate: for whom is preoperative computed tomography making an impact? Surgery. 2008;144:276.
61. Pooler BD, Lawrence EM, Pickhardt PJ. MDCT for suspected appendicitis in the elderly: diagnostic performance and patient outcome. Emerg Radiol. 2012;19(1):27–33. doi:10.1007/s10140-011-1002-3.
62. Hui TT, Major KM, Avital I, Hiatt JR, Margulies DR. Outcome of elderly patients with appendicitis—effect of computed tomography and laparoscopy. Arch Surg. 2002;137:995–8.
63. Ditillo MF, Dziura JD, Rabinovici R. Is it safe to delay appendectomy in adults with acute appendicitis? Ann Surg. 2006;244:656–60.
64. Gurleyik G, Gurleyik E. Age-related clinical features in older patients with acute appendicitis. Eur J Emerg Med. 2003;10:200–3.
65. Paranjape C, Dalia S, Pan J, Horattas M. Appendicitis in the elderly: a change in the laparoscopic era. Surg Endosc. 2007;21:777–81.
66. Guller U, Hervey S, Purves H, et al. Laparoscopic versus open appendectomy: outcomes comparison based on a large administrative database. Ann Surg. 2004;239:43.
67. Harrell AG, Lincourt AE, Novitsky YW, et al. Advantages of laparoscopic appendectomy in the elderly. Am Surg. 2006;72:474.
68. Skoubo-Kristensen E, Hvid I. The appendiceal mass: results of conservative management. Ann Surg. 1982;196:584.
69. Nitecki S, Assalia A, Schein M. Contemporary management of the appendiceal mass. Br J Surg. 1993;80:18.
70. Oliak D, Yamini D, Udani VM, et al. Initial nonoperative management for periappendiceal abscess. Dis Colon Rectum. 2001;44:936.
71. Bagi P, Dueholm S. Nonoperative management of the ultrasonically evaluated appendiceal mass. Surgery. 1987;101:602.
72. Jeffrey Jr RB, Federle MP, Tolentino CS. Periappendiceal inflammatory masses: CT-directed management and clinical outcome in 70 patients. Radiology. 1988;167:13.
73. Gee D, Babineau TJ. The optimal management of adult patients presenting with appendiceal abscess: "conservative" vs immediate operative management. Curr Surg. 2004;61:524.
74. Brown CV, Abrishami M, Muller M, Velmahos GC. Appendiceal abscess: immediate operation or percutaneous drainage? Am Surg. 2003;69:829.
75. Siewert B, Raptopoulos V. CT of the acute abdomen: findings and impact on diagnosis and treatment. AJR Am J Roentgenol. 1994;163:1317.
76. Nguyen DB, Silen W, Hodin RA. Interval appendectomy in the laparoscopic era. J Gastrointest Surg. 1999;3:189.
77. Eriksson S, Tisell A, Granström L. Ultrasonographic findings after conservative treatment of acute appendicitis and open appendicectomy. Acta Radiol. 1995;36:173.
78. Hansson J, Körner U, Khorram-Manesh A, et al. Randomized clinical trial of antibiotic therapy versus appendicectomy as primary treatment of acute appendicitis in unselected patients. Br J Surg. 2009;96:473.
79. Blair NP, Bugis SP, Turner LJ, MacLeod MM. Review of the pathologic diagnoses of 2,216 appendectomy specimens. Am J Surg. 1993;165:618.
80. Deans GT, Spence RA. Neoplastic lesions of the appendix. Br J Surg. 1995;82:299.
81. Kaminski A, Liu IL, Applebaum H, et al. Routine interval appendectomy is not justified after initial nonoperative treatment of acute appendicitis. Arch Surg. 2005;140:897.
82. Andersson RE, Petzold MG. Nonsurgical treatment of appendiceal abscess or phlegmon: a systematic review and meta-analysis. Ann Surg. 2007;246:741.
83. Franz MG, Norman J, Fabri PJ. Increased morbidity of appendicitis with advancing age. Am Surg. 1995;61(1):40–4.
84. Hesketh KT. The management of primary adenocarcinoma of the vermiform appendix. Gut. 1963;4:158.
85. Connor SJ, Hanna GB, Frizelle FA. Appendiceal tumors: retrospective clinicopathologic analysis of appendiceal tumors from 7,970 appendectomies. Dis Colon Rectum. 1998;41:75.
86. Moertel CG, Weiland LH, Nagorney DM, Dockerty MB. Carcinoid tumor of the appendix: treatment and prognosis. N Engl J Med. 1987;317:1699.
87. Boudreaux JP, Klimstra DS, Hassan MM, et al. The NANETS consensus guideline for the diagnosis and management of neuroendocrine tumors: well-differentiated neuroendocrine tumors of the jejunum, ileum, appendix, and cecum. Pancreas. 2010;39:753–66.
88. Landry CS, Woodall C, Scoggins CR, et al. Analysis of 900 appendiceal carcinoid tumors for a proposed predictive staging system. Arch Surg. 2008;143:664.
89. Ponka JL. Carcinoid tumors of the appendix. Report of thirty-five cases. Am J Surg. 1973;126:77.
90. Syracuse DC, Perzin KH, Price JB, et al. Carcinoid tumors of the appendix. Mesoappendiceal extension and nodal metastases. Ann Surg. 1979;190:58.
91. Mullen JT, Savarese DM. Carcinoid tumors of the appendix: a population-based study. J Surg Oncol. 2011;104:41.
92. Ito H, Osteen RT, Bleday R, et al. Appendiceal adenocarcinoma: long-term outcomes after surgical therapy. Dis Colon Rectum. 2004;47:474.
93. Cerame MA. A 25-year review of adenocarcinoma of the appendix. A frequently perforating carcinoma. Dis Colon Rectum. 1988;31:145.
94. Turaga KK, Pappas SG, Gamblin TC. Importance of histologic subtype in the staging of appendiceal tumors. Ann Surg Oncol. 2012;19:1379–85.
95. Hata K, Tanaka N, Nomura Y, et al. Early appendiceal adenocarcinoma. A review of the literature with special reference to optimal surgical procedures. J Gastroenterol. 2002;37:210.
96. Stocchi L, Wolff BG, Larson DR, Harrington JR. Surgical treatment of appendiceal mucocele. Arch Surg. 2003;138:585.
97. Nitecki SS, Wolff BG, Schlinkert R, Sarr MG. The natural history of surgically treated primary adenocarcinoma of the appendix. Ann Surg. 1994;219:51.
98. Rutledge RH, Alexander JW. Primary appendiceal malignancies: rare but important. Surgery. 1992;111:244.
99. Lo NS, Sarr MG. Mucinous cystadenocarcinoma of the appendix. The controversy persists: a review. Hepatogastroenterology. 2003;50:432.
100. Mangram AJ, Horan TC, Pearson ML, et al. Guideline for prevention of surgical site infection, 1999. Hospital Infection Control Practices Advisory Committee. Infect Control Hosp Epidemiol. 1999;20:250.
101. Schropp KP, Kaplan S, Golladay ES, et al. A randomized clinical trial of ampicillin, gentamicin and clindamycin versus cefotaxime and clindamycin in children with ruptured appendicitis. Surg Gynecol Obstet. 1991;172:351.

Biliary

12

Ali Salim and Marko Bukur

Introduction

As the Western population continues to age and life expectancy continues to increase, the elderly population will account for an escalating amount of health-care expenditure. As health-care providers, we must find ways to contain costs while simultaneously optimizing the care of this special patient population. The most common cause of abdominal pain that requires surgical evaluation and treatment in the elderly is related to gallstones [1]. This is largely due to the fact that the incidence of cholelithiasis, particularly the symptomatic variant, increases with age [2] ranging from 20 to 80 % [3, 4]. Early recognition is important due to the fact that elderly patients will often present with complicated biliary disease compared to young patients [5, 6]. Delays in treatment often lead to poor outcomes associated with increased use of resources.

Biliary Physiology and Age-Related Pathophysiologic Changes

Normal biliary secretion is an intricate, multi-step process that serves several homeostatic functions. Bile is necessary for absorption of dietary cholesterol and fats, including the fat-soluble vitamins. Bile is also the final pathway for excretion of endogenous cholesterol along with drug and heavy metal metabolites. Hepatocytes secrete bile into the canalicular spaces that eventually coalesce to form the complex intrahepatic biliary tree before exiting the liver as the right and left hepatic ducts. The average volume secreted by the human liver is approximately 600 mL/day [7]. Bile is isoosmolar with plasma and is composed predominately of water (97 %) and bile acids (2 %) with the remainder being phospholipids, cholesterol, and bile pigments [8]. Cholesterol is insoluble in water and requires a fine balance of bile acids and phospholipids to allow formation of mixed micelles that are non-lithogenic.

The hepatic ducts join to form the common hepatic duct which is of variable length depending on the location of the cystic duct. The gallbladder acts as a storage organ for bile between meals. The mucosa of the gallbladder actively reabsorbs water resulting in a bile that is concentrated [9]. After eating, the gallbladder normally empties 75 % of the bile into the digestive tract. Bile acids are then reabsorbed in the ileum and recycled to the liver via the enterohepatic circulation.

In the elderly patient, there are three factors that lead to an increased incidence of gallstones. They include an altered composition of hepatic bile, increased cholesterol nucleation, and decreased gallbladder motility [10]. There are several age-related changes that lead to changes in bile salt composition. With aging, there is a corresponding decrease in bile salt synthesis [11]. This decreased synthesis can alter the balance in the mixed micelles that will lead to nucleation of cholesterol crystals and eventual stone formation. There is also an increased incidence of bactobilia in the elderly largely due to decreased biliary motility. These bacteria produce enzymes that will lead to deconjugation of bile salts and promote sludge and formation of calculi [10]. Finally, senescent alterations in biliary protein concentration can lead to increased bile lithogenicity.

Changes in cholesterol metabolism are also responsible for increased formation of calculi. There is an increased relative quantity of cholesterol present in the bile of older patients. This leads to nucleation of cholesterol crystals as they become insoluble in the aqueous bile and serve as a nidus for stone formation [10]. Finally, there are multiple factors that lead to altered motility of the gallbladder with

A. Salim, MD, FACS
Department of Surgery, Cedars-Sinai Medical Center,
8700 Beverly Blvd., Suite 8215-NT, Los Angeles, CA 90048, USA
e-mail: ali.salim@cshs.org

M. Bukur, MD, FACS (✉)
Department of Surgery, Cedars-Sinai Medical Center,
8635 West 3rd Street, Suite 650W, Los Angeles, CA 90048, USA
e-mail: marko.bukur@cshs.org

J.A. Yelon, F.A. Luchette (eds.), *Geriatric Trauma and Critical Care*,
DOI 10.1007/978-1-4614-8501-8_12, © Springer Science+Business Media New York 2014

aging such as decreased physical activity, decreased responsiveness to cholecystokinin, and comorbidities such as diabetes mellitus [10–12]. Taken together, all of these changes related to aging lead to an increased propensity for gallstone formation and their subsequent pathologic sequelae.

Perioperative Considerations

The expected mortality for elective cholecystectomy is less than 0.1 %; however, the rate rises in the elderly. The presence of comorbidities, decreased physiologic reserve, and delays in seeking medical care result in the need for emergent operative intervention. Elderly patients that undergo appropriate perioperative evaluation and elective operation have outcomes that are similar to younger counterparts [13]. Therefore, perhaps the greatest impact the treating surgeon can have is to make a timely diagnosis and not delay operation in appropriately selected patients. Geriatric patients should be appropriately risk stratified in conjunction with the patient's primary physician and anesthesiologist.

Major risk factors for cardiopulmonary-related morbidity can be assessed with minimal ancillary testing by assessing the patient's pre-illness level of activity using metabolic equivalents (MET) [14], ASA score [15], or Goldman cardiac risk profile [16]. For those patients that require more intensive cardiac evaluation, well-established guidelines from the American College of Cardiology are available [14].

Careful perioperative management can reduce the risk for major postoperative complications and can often be accomplished through simple interventions. A detailed review of the patient's pre-illness medications should be performed and assessed for potential drug interactions. It is also important to take note of preexisting cardiac medication, particularly beta-blockers as withdrawal of these medications has been tied to adverse cardiac events [17, 18]. Intraoperative maintenance of normothermia is important as the elderly have impaired thermoregulation [19], and hypothermia is a risk factor for cardiac events [20] and wound complications [21].

Elderly patients are also at increased risk for early postoperative delirium that leads to increased morbidity, prolonged hospital stays, and delayed recovery of functional status [15]. Early recognition is important to allow for appropriate intervention. A vigilant search for common inciting factors such as sepsis, electrolyte disorders, or adverse medications should be undertaken. It is also important to note that inadequate analgesia can exacerbate delirium and lead to increased cardiopulmonary complications [15]. Judicious use of analgesic approach can lead to enhanced recovery and decreased morbidity [22] and should be an integral part of the perioperative plan.

Diagnostic Investigation

As noted above, biliary diseases are the most common cause of surgical pathology in the elderly population [23]. However, unlike young patients with biliary disease, the clinical presentation is often more subtle. Failure to identify and treat surgical conditions can lead to increased mortality even in patients that are admitted to the hospital for observation [24]. There are several physiologic reasons that are responsible for the diagnostic challenge that elderly patients present.

The function of the immune system deteriorates with increasing age [25] which results in an impaired tissue response seen with intra-abdominal inflammatory diseases [24, 26]. This leads to an impaired ability to appropriately respond to an infectious process and also a diminished perception of pain [25]. Together, these changes are felt to account for delays in clinical presentation. Prescribed medications and comorbid conditions can also alter the physical examination findings. Nonsteroidal anti-inflammatory medications can blunt the febrile response, while steroids can alter the leukocyte count and immune response. Patients that present with a "normal" blood pressure with a history of hypertension may actually have ongoing occult hypoperfusion. Additionally, beta-blockers may block the tachycardic response normally seen with serious intra-abdominal pathology. The above pitfalls should be taken into account when evaluating geriatric patients with suspected biliary disease as they can present with frank gallbladder perforation, gangrene, emphysematous cholecystitis, or ascending cholangitis with minimal symptoms [27]. One should have a low threshold for ordering ancillary lab work and imaging investigations to assist with the evaluation and to promptly arrive at the correct diagnosis.

Laboratory Testing

The most common laboratory tests ordered in the evaluation of biliary disease are complete blood count (CBC), electrolytes, aminotransferases, alkaline phosphatase, bilirubin, prothrombin time, and partial thromboplastin time. Each of these can provide clinically useful information but should not be relied upon exclusively for a diagnosis.

Often the most scrutinized value is the white blood cell (WBC) count. It can be helpful when elevated, but in contrast to younger patients, the WBC count can be normal in 30–40 % of older patients with acute gallbladder pathology [25]. The hemoglobin and hematocrit should also be carefully examined as microcytic anemia can be due to an unrelated occult malignancy. Elderly patients often have electrolyte abnormalities, such as hypokalemia, that will need to be corrected prior to anesthesia. This is especially true when the patient is on antihypertensive medications such as diuretics, beta-blockers, ACE inhibitors or angiotensin receptor blockers, and digitalis as these are all known to cause electrolyte abnormalities.

The liver function panel may also be helpful in establishing a diagnosis prior to diagnostic imaging. Aminotransferase elevations are indicative of hepatocyte injury. There may be modest elevations (<500 IU/L) seen with acute/chronic cholecystitis, but the absence of elevation should not exclude this diagnosis as a significant proportion of elderly patients can have normal liver function tests when presenting with acute cholangitis [25]. Markedly elevated aminotransferase levels (>500 IU/L) may be seen with either acute biliary duct obstruction due to choledocholithiasis or biliary pancreatitis.

Markers of cholestasis include serum bilirubin and alkaline phosphatase. Measuring fractionated bilirubin is helpful because it allows discrimination of the predominant source of bilirubin elevation (i.e., conjugated vs. unconjugated). Normally, the total bilirubin is predominantly unconjugated and less than 1.2 mg/dL. Elevations in the conjugated form of bilirubin are indicative of biliary obstruction, particularly when combined with an elevation in alkaline phosphatase. Total bilirubin level is also predictive of benign versus malignant obstruction depending on the serum level [28] and can assist with selecting the appropriate diagnostic workup. Isolated elevation of the alkaline phosphatase level should also not be ignored as it can be elevated with partial biliary duct obstruction.

It is important to also take note of the coagulation panel in elderly patients presenting with suspected extrahepatic biliary disease. Common duct obstruction can cause elevation in the PT/INR due to malabsorption of vitamin K. This fat-soluble vitamin requires bile to aid in its digestion and absorption. Malnutrition is also common in the elderly and can lead to coagulation derangements [29]. Marked elevation in these parameters may be indicative of severe hepatocellular dysfunction or chronic long-standing disease with progression to liver failure.

Noninvasive Imaging

Plain Radiographs

Often one of the earliest tests ordered during the initial evaluation of acute abdominal pain is an upright chest X-ray and abdominal series. Though these are often ordered by the emergency department prior to surgical consultation, they should always be reviewed if available. In Western societies, cholesterol is the main component present in gallstones (>75 %) with the remainder being composed of calcium bilirubinate [30]. The calcified stones can be visualized on plain radiographs [31]. Though the sensitivity for stones is clearly not acceptable for diagnosis, there are other signs of pathology that should be sought after. The presence of pneumobilia

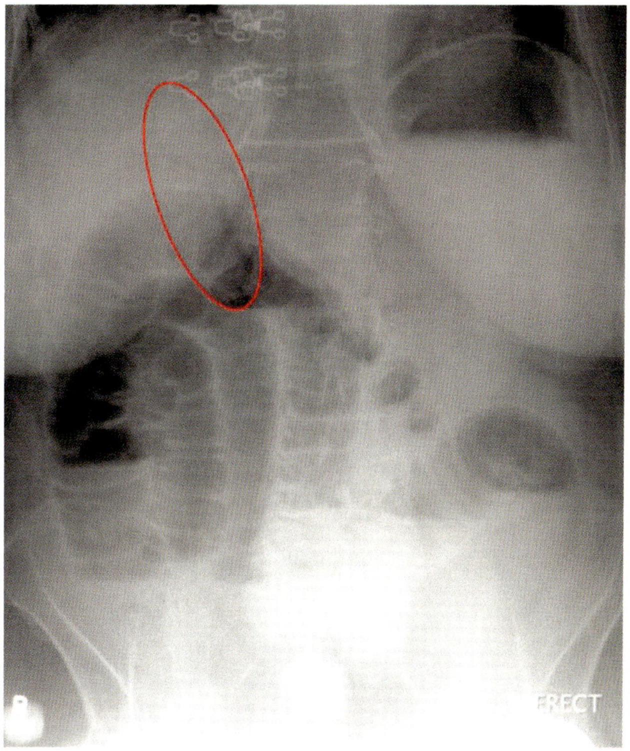

Fig. 12.1 Plain abdominal radiograph of a patient with gallstone ileus. Note the presence of pneumobilia depicted in the *circled area*. Gallstones may not be present due to lack of calcium composition

in a patient that has not been instrumented is pathognomonic for a biliary-enteric fistula. The combination of pneumobilia with clinical signs of a small bowel obstruction (see Fig. 12.1) on plain films, in a patient without any prior abdominal surgery, is virtually diagnostic for gallstone ileus. Lastly, although a rare entity (0.06–0.8 %), calcification in the gallbladder wall ("porcelain gallbladder") may also be diagnosed on plain radiography [32].

Ultrasound

Ultrasound has become the initial diagnostic test of choice in patients with suspected biliary disease. The test can be rapidly performed at the patient's bedside and does not require the use of radiation. Ultrasound is highly accurate for identifying stones that are ≥5 mm in size (>96 %) [31]. In order to diagnose gallstones, there must be demonstration of echogenicity, production of posterior acoustic shadowing, and mobility of the calculi (see Fig. 12.2). False-negative studies may be seen when the examination is performed by an inexperienced sonographer, there is a large amount of bowel gas, or the stones are small (<3 mm) or pigmented [31, 33, 34]. Examining the gallbladder with the patient in multiple different positions can reduce the rate of false-negative exams.

Ultrasonography is also helpful in establishing the diagnosis of acute and chronic cholecystitis. In the setting

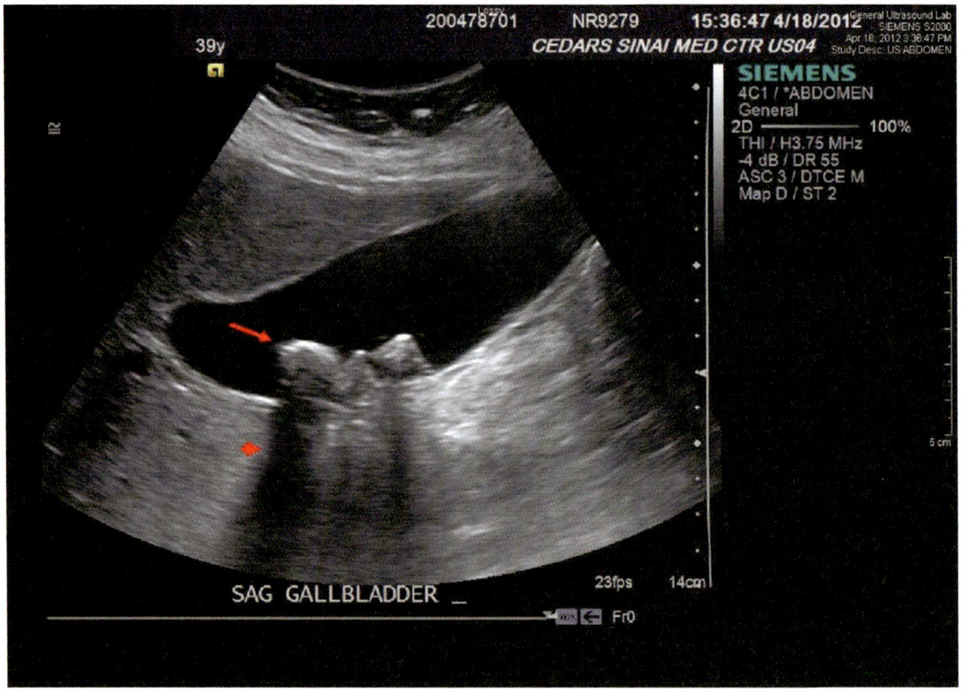

Fig. 12.2 Abdominal ultrasound documenting cholelithiasis. Note the hyperechoic stones (*arrow*) and posterior acoustic shadowing (*arrowhead*)

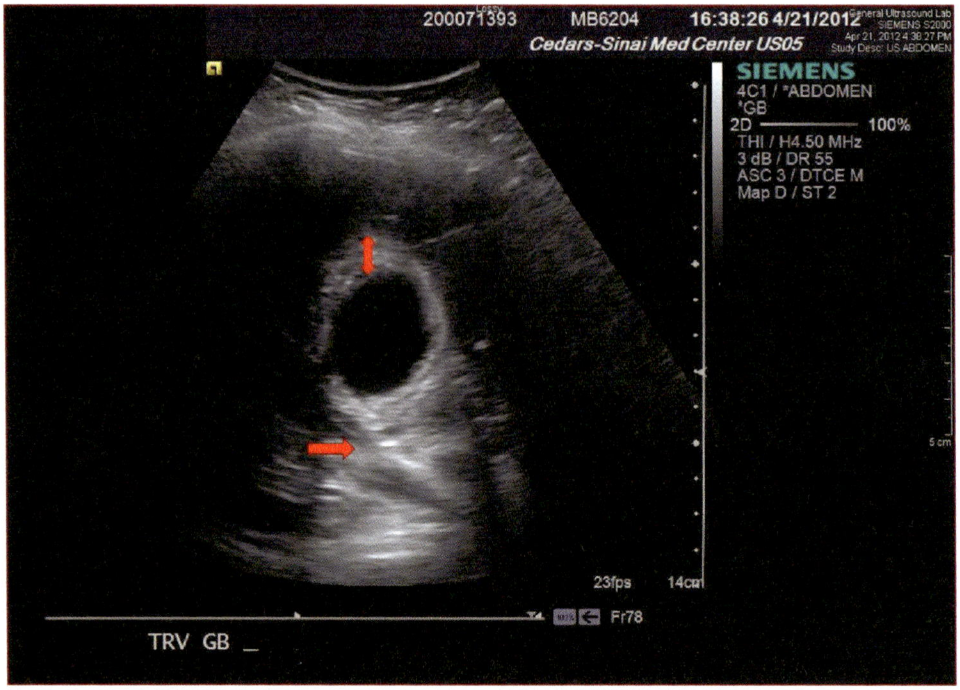

Fig. 12.3 Ultrasound depicting the findings of acute cholecystitis. Note the presence of gallbladder wall thickening (*double arrowhead*) and pericholecystic fluid (*single arrow*)

of acute cholecystitis, the most reliable finding is a sonographic Murphy's sign which is tenderness over the gallbladder with transducer pressure. This finding is 87 % specific for the diagnosis of acute cholecystitis and has a positive predictive value of 92 % when stones are also visualized [35]. The Murphy's sign may not be elicited in patients that are immunosuppressed, obtunded, and recently medicated or have denervated gallbladders (i.e., diabetics or gangrenous cholecystitis) [31]. Other findings that are indicative of acute cholecystitis include gallbladder wall thickening (>3 mm), which is present in 50 % of cases, as well as the presence of pericholecystic fluid (see Fig. 12.3) [31, 35]. It should be noted, however, that these findings alone are nonspecific and may occur with adjacent right

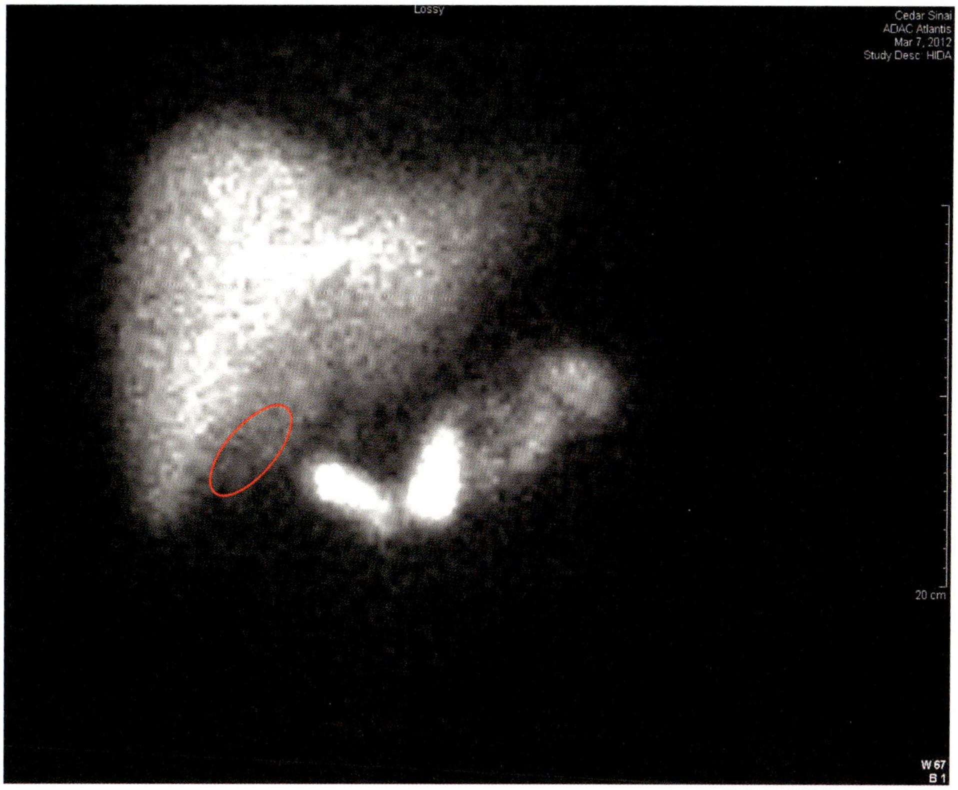

Fig. 12.4 Example of a positive HIDA scan. Note the absence of radioactivity in the area of the gallbladder fossa (*highlighted oval*)

upper quadrant pathology. The ultrasonographic diagnosis of chronic cholecystitis can also be suggested by nonspecific gallbladder wall thickening due to fibrosis with resultant contraction and near obliteration of the gallbladder lumen producing the "double-arc" sign [36].

Ultrasound examination of the right upper quadrant is also the initial imaging study of choice to evaluate for choledocholithiasis. It allows for quick assessment of the extrahepatic and intrahepatic bile duct size and continuity. The extrahepatic common bile duct is routinely measured at the level of the right hepatic artery and should not exceed 6 mm in diameter, while the upper limit for normal diameter of the intrahepatic bile ducts is 2 mm [34]. With adequate sonographer experience, the level of biliary obstruction can be identified in 92 % of patients, and overall sensitivity for choledocholithiasis can reach 75 % [34]. It is important to emphasize that choledocholithiasis can also be present in the absence of biliary ductal dilation in 25–33 % of cases [37]. When this occurs or when stones are less than 5 mm in diameter and overshadowed by bowel gas, the sensitivity of ultrasound is considerably lower. Endoscopic ultrasonography is more sensitive than transabdominal ultrasound for detecting choledocholithiasis (96 %) and should be considered in select cases of presumptive biliary obstruction (i.e., suspected malignancy) due to its more invasive nature [38].

Biliary Scintigraphy (HIDA)

Biliary scintigraphy involves the intravenous administration of radiolabeled technetium iminodiacetic acid which is taken up by the hepatic parenchyma and excreted into the bile with eventual uptake in the gallbladder. The use of hepatobiliary iminodiacetic acid (HIDA) has largely declined into a second-line test for calculous biliary disease due to its increased expense, amount of time needed to complete the study, and the use of ionizing radiation. HIDA is diagnostic for acute cholecystitis when there is non-visualization of the gallbladder 60 min after administration of the technetium (see Fig. 12.4). This test can be carried out in a delayed fashion for up to 4 h; non-visualization during this extended time frame is considered consistent with chronic cholecystitis [39]. Scintigraphy has excellent diagnostic sensitivity (>95 %), particularly in nonhospitalized patients that are much less likely to have false-positive imaging studies [39]. False-positive studies may be seen in up to 30–40 % of patients that are hospitalized for a reason other than abdominal pain, which is a common scenario in the elderly population [40]. Reasons for false-positive exams include prolonged fasting, cholestasis secondary to hepatic disease, or prolonged parenteral nutrition [31]. HIDA can also play a role in diagnosing postoperative biliary complications such as a cystic duct stump leak or biliary motility disorders. However, due to

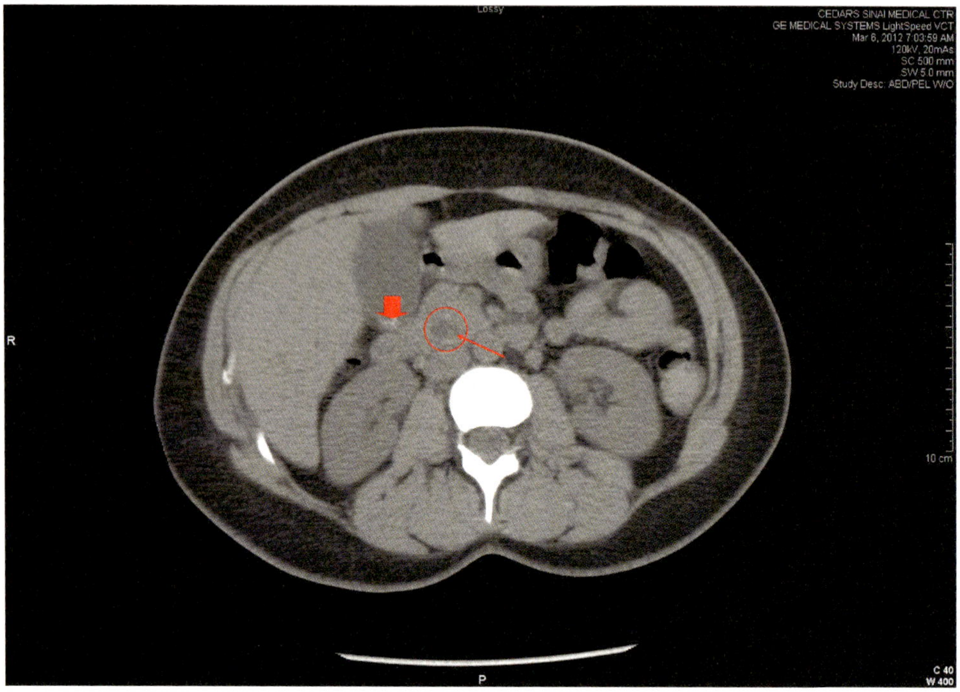

Fig. 12.5 CAT scan of the abdomen showing a stone (*thin arrow*) in a dilated common bile duct (*circled*) along with cholelithiasis (*thick arrow*)

the previously mentioned limitations, differences in cost, and radiation exposure, ultrasonography should be considered as the initial diagnostic imaging test to diagnose cholelithiasis.

Computerized Tomography

Computerized tomography (CT) has variable sensitivity in detecting gallstones secondary to the variable amount of calcification present and thus is also a second-line imaging study for biliary calculi. Calculi that are predominantly composed of cholesterol will be more difficult to identify due to their similar radiographic density as the surrounding bile. CT has similar sensitivity as compared to ultrasonography in identifying choledocholithiasis (75–80 %) (see Fig. 12.5) [31, 38] and can give information regarding ductal anatomy. CT imaging is most useful in demonstrating gallbladder size, wall thickness, and surrounding inflammatory changes associated with acute cholecystitis making it highly specific (99 %) for this particular diagnosis (see Fig. 12.6) [41]. In the setting of suspected malignancy of the head of pancreas or choledochus, CT is the diagnostic image of choice because it allows assessment of not only the gallbladder but adjacent organs such as the liver and the porta hepatis, identification of lymphadenopathy, or pancreaticoduodenal pathology [42]. In the elderly patient with preexisting renal disease, diabetes, or certain medications (i.e., ACE inhibitors, NSAIDs, or metformin), caution should be taken with administering IV contrast as this can precipitate acute kidney injury or exacerbate chronic kidney disease. The nephrotoxicity of the contrast can be reduced with administering intravenous fluid to correct hypovolemia, sodium bicarbonate, and/or Mucomyst. Isoosmolar contrast should also be infused for the dynamic phase of scan [43].

Magnetic Resonance Imaging and Cholangiopancreatography (MRI/MRCP)

MRI, though not frequently used as an initial imaging test, has excellent ability to identify gallstones due to the sharp contrast in signal intensity between bile and stones on T2-weighted images [44]. The resolution with MRCP allows stones as small as 2 mm in diameter to be identified in both the gallbladder and common bile duct (see Fig. 12.7). The sensitivity (81–100 %) and specificity (85–99 %) of MRCP for choledocholithiasis are equivalent to that for endoscopic retrograde cholangiopancreatography (ERCP) but without the inherent risk associated with invasive procedures [45]. However, MRCP is less sensitive for diagnosing microlithiasis, pneumobilia, or calculi in the peri-ampullary region [46]. MRI can also be useful in those with malignant disease as it images the gallbladder wall, liver parenchyma, and biliary tree with high resolution. Unfortunately, elderly patients with dementia or claustrophobia do not tolerate MRI scanning due to the tight confines of the imaging magnet. Also those with a pacemaker or defibrillator device may also not be candidates for MRI, though certain devices have not malfunctioned after imaging [47].

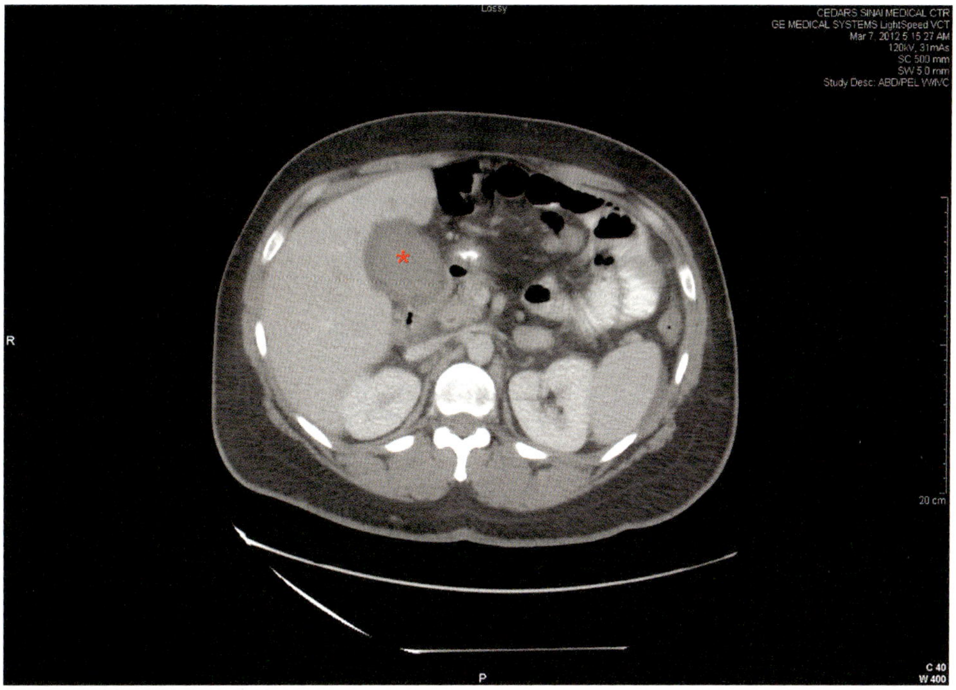

Fig. 12.6 CAT scan of the abdomen showing evidence of acute cholecystitis. Notice distention of the gallbladder (*asterisk*) with surrounding pericholecystic fluid

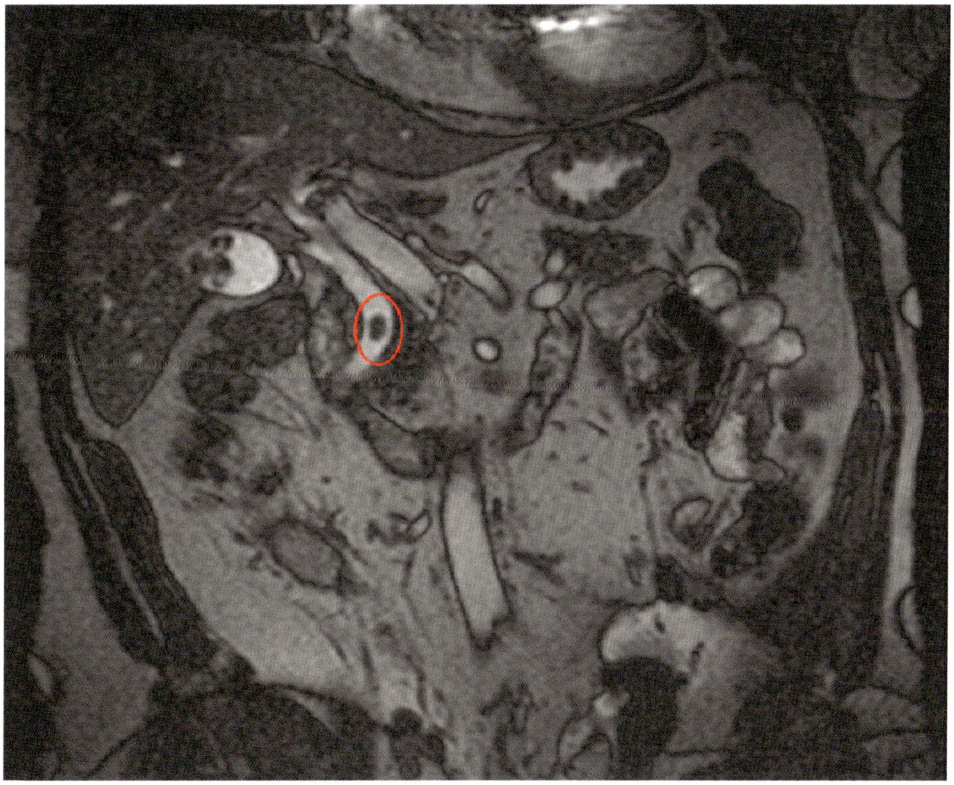

Fig. 12.7 T2-weighted MRCP showing a large stone in the common bile duct (*highlighted oval*)

Invasive Imaging

Endoscopic Retrograde Cholangiopancreatography (ERCP)

Advances in endoscopic techniques and training during the past three decades have made ERCP widely available. It is the gold standard for the diagnosis of the majority of bile duct pathology. However, due to its invasive nature and improvements in the aforementioned noninvasive imaging techniques, ERCP has evolved into more of a planned therapeutic procedure rather than the preferred imaging study for the purpose of obtaining a diagnosis. But those patients

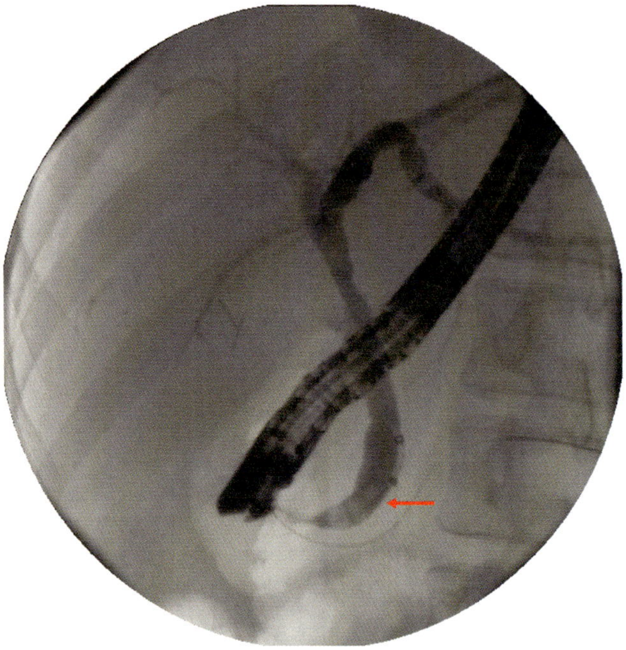

Fig. 12.8 An ERCP demonstrating a dilated common bile duct with multiple stones (*arrow*)

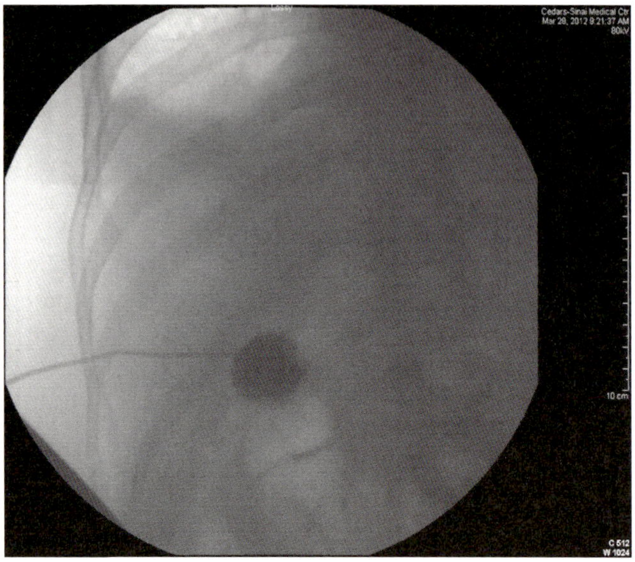

Fig. 12.9 PTC done under fluoroscopy for acute cholecystitis

presenting with symptomatic choledocholithiasis (i.e., Charcot's triad or Reynolds' pentad) or with documented common duct stones on imaging studies are clearly potential candidates for ERCP (see Fig. 12.8). Predicting which asymptomatic patients will ultimately require ERCP is more difficult, but advanced age (>55), hyperbilirubinemia (>1.8 mg/dL), and common bile duct dilation have all been shown to increase the probability of a therapeutic ERCP [48]. The success rate of ERCP for accessing the common bile duct is near 98 % in all patients [49]. A complicating factor in older patients is the presence of a duodenal diverticulum which is found in 20 % of autopsies and on 5–10 % of upper gastrointestinal series. When the diverticulum is juxtapapillary, the endoscopist will frequently have difficulty with safely cannulating the ampulla. Thus, the success rate of ERCP for diagnostic and/or therapeutic purposes in the elder is less than 98 %. Transduodenal imaging of the biliary tree is associated with a number of well-described complications, with the most common being acute pancreatitis. The incidence of post-procedure pancreatitis ranges between 5 and 10 %. Despite the possibility of post-ERCP complications, elderly patients appear to tolerate the procedure as well as their younger counterparts [50].

Percutaneous Transhepatic Cholangiography

Percutaneous transhepatic cholangiography (PTC) involves the passage of a needle into the liver parenchyma under fluoroscopic or ultrasound guidance to access the intrahepatic biliary radicles for diagnostic and/or therapeutic purposes (Fig. 12.9). This technique was initially introduced in 1979 and remains a valuable option for treating biliary pathology when ERCP is either unavailable or unsuccessful, particularly in the critically ill population [51, 52]. PTC can be used to successful treat acute cholecystitis (cholecystostomy tube), cholangitis, choledocholithiasis, or surgically related biliary complications with a high success rate. It should be noted that PTC carries a greater complication risk than ERCP because the catheter traverses the hepatic parenchyma to access the biliary tree; there is a known risk for hemorrhage, septic shock from bacterial translocation, or bile peritonitis.

Benign Calculous Diseases

Acute Calculous Cholecystitis

Clinical Presentation and Diagnosis

The pathophysiology of acute cholecystitis is initiated when a calculus obstructs the cystic duct. Initially, the patient will experience epigastric pain which will localize to the right upper quadrant when the inflammatory process involves the parietal peritoneum. Patients will frequently experience nausea and vomiting. There may be pain referred to the back and right shoulder. The majority of patients will recall prior episodes of similar pain that were consistent with biliary colic. Acute cholecystitis is the initial presentation of gallstone disease in 15–20 % of patients [53]. In addition to the findings on physical examination, there may also be signs of systemic inflammation including fever, tachycardia, and leukocytosis. Laboratory studies that may be abnormal include elevation of C-reactive protein, mild elevation of serum bilirubin, and transaminases (<500 IU/L). If the serum bilirubin is greater than 2 mg/dL, particularly the conjugated form, or serum transaminases are >500 IU/L, choledocholithiasis should be suspected as the incidence of concomitant common bile duct calculi in the elderly is quite high (10–20 %) [49]. It is important to emphasize, however, that the typical presentation in the elderly patient is often the exception rather than the rule as a significant percentage will have no fever, abdominal pain, nausea/vomiting, and normal laboratory findings [25, 54, 55]. In some cases, the only presenting symptom of acute cholecystitis will be a change in mental status or poor oral intake [55, 56]

When the diagnosis of acute cholecystitis is suspected, abdominal ultrasonography is the initial imaging test of choice. A sonographic Murphy's sign combined with the presence of stones, gallbladder wall thickening, and pericholecystic fluid confirms the diagnosis. In cases where the diagnosis is less clear, or when there are no stones visualized, a HIDA scan may be useful. The findings on CT scan of acute cholecystitis as previously described should also be reviewed for possible additional pathology.

Treatment of Acute Calculous Cholecystitis

Ongoing cystic duct obstruction causes inflammation and can lead to bacterial infection in the bile as well as ischemia of the gallbladder wall. Initial supportive measures such as bowel rest (NPO) to reduce stimulation of the gallbladder, intravenous fluid hydration, and analgesics are appropriate. The Infectious Diseases Society of America guidelines recommend empiric antimicrobial therapy in cases of clinically suspected infection [57]. Selection of an antimicrobial(s) should provide coverage of Enterobacteriaceae species. Appropriate antibiotic choices for uncomplicated cholecystitis include second- and third-generation cephalosporins or a combination of fluoroquinolones with metronidazole [57]. For patients who present with severe sepsis or those that are considered high risk (i.e., elderly, diabetics, or immunocompromised), broad-spectrum antibiotics such as piperacillin/tazobactam or aminoglycosides should be considered [57].

Laparoscopic cholecystectomy is the operative intervention of choice due to the low morbidity compared to open surgery [58, 59]. The techniques of laparoscopic cholecystectomy are beyond the scope of this chapter and can be found elsewhere [60]. Elderly patients frequently present with complicated acute cholecystitis (i.e., gangrene, perforation, or emphysematous cholecystitis) all of which are more likely to require emergent surgical intervention with subsequently increased morbidity and mortality [6, 25]. The traditional management of initial nonoperative with supportive measures and antibiotics during the acute inflammatory period followed by delayed surgical cholecystectomy 6 weeks later may still be appropriate for patients with comorbidities associated with increased perioperative risk. However, the recurrence rate of acute cholecystitis can be as high as 30 % over a 3-month waiting period [61, 62].

Two recent systematic reviews of the literature compared outcomes for early laparoscopic cholecystectomy (within 24–72 h) compared to delayed operation (6–12 weeks after initial presentation) [63, 64]. Both meta-analyses found that there were no significant differences in conversion rates to open procedures, incidence of common bile duct injuries, or postoperative complications. Early laparoscopic cholecystectomy is also associated with a shorter hospital length of stay and lower total hospital cost [63]. It should be noted that in one of the meta-analysis, the incidence of bile leaks was higher in the early cholecystectomy group (3 % vs. 0 %) [63]. Also, due to the small number of total patients in these pooled randomized trials (451), the incidence of common duct injury could easily be over or underrepresented in either group due to the low overall incidence of this complication (0.4–0.6 %) [65]. Despite these limitations, the consensus of both meta-analyses is that early laparoscopic cholecystectomy is considered the preferred management for patients with acute cholecystitis. Unfortunately, these reviews did not evaluate outcomes in the elder.

Even with these evidence-based recommendations, elderly patients have been shown to be more likely to be managed differently than younger patients. Previous studies have documented that up to 30 % of elderly patients do not have any surgical intervention for acute gallstone disease during the index hospitalization [66, 67]. This was initially perceived to be due to increased comorbidities or those presenting with acute complicated disease [5, 67]. Recently, in a single institution review, Bergman and colleagues showed that this may not be the reason [6]. They concluded that increasing age was independently associated with a lower likelihood of surgical intervention after adjusting for severity of biliary disease as well as preexisting medical comorbidities. This finding should give surgeons pause as prolonged delay in cholecystectomy increases the subsequent need for emergent surgical intervention [66, 68] with mortality rates as high as 6–15 % [49]. This contrasts with appropriately selected elderly patients that have electively scheduled cholecystectomy and outcomes that are similar to younger patients [13]. Thus, the patient's age alone should not exclude early cholecystectomy if there are no or minimal comorbidities.

Some elderly patients with acute cholecystitis will present with severe sepsis and septic shock or have comorbidities that preclude consideration of early cholecystectomy. These patients need to be admitted to the intensive care unit (ICU) for supportive care in addition to broad-spectrum antibiotics. Obtaining source control in these patients obviously presents a clinical challenge. Two less invasive procedures, percutaneous cholecystostomy (PC) and ERCP, should be considered in these patients once underlying physiologic derangements have been corrected.

PC can either be done with the aid of either ultrasound or CT guidance. The use of ultrasound allows for the procedure to be performed at the bedside which avoids the need for transportation of critically ill patients to the CT scanner. After initial aspiration, a pigtail drainage catheter can be left in place for drainage. Cultures of the bile should be sent to tailor empiric antibiotic therapy, particularly if the elderly patient has come from a nursing facility or has received recent antibiotic exposure as this is associated with a higher incidence of resistant organisms. PC has excellent efficacy and results in the resolution of sepsis in up to 87 % of critically ill patients, with acceptable 30-day mortality rates [69]. This temporizing measure can allow optimization of the patient's organ failure. The drainage catheter should be left in place for 6 weeks to allow for establishment of a fibrous tract prior to removal. In certain patients that are a prohibitive surgical risk due to their underlying medical problems, conservative management with PC cholangiography. All stones can be extracted prior to catheter removal [55, 70].

ERCP with selective cannulation of the cystic duct and stent placement is another treatment modality that may be particularly useful in those critically ill patients that are unable to undergo PC particularly in the setting of coagulopathy or uncontrolled ascites [71]. In experienced hands, this procedure is technically successful in over 90 % of cases with a reported clinical efficacy of 80–90 % [71].

PC should only be used as a treatment modality in those patients that are too critically ill or medically a prohibitive risk for general anesthesia. The procedure is associated with increased hospital lengths of stay and up to a 25 % rate of readmission for biliary related complications. A detailed Cochrane review comparing PC versus cholecystectomy as treatment for severe acute cholecystitis found no evidence to support the use of PC over surgical intervention [72]. A recent large retrospective single institution review reached similar conclusions even when accounting for patients that underwent conversion to open cholecystectomy [52]. Those patients that were treated surgically had shorter lengths of stay, as well as a lower complication rate and number of readmissions compared with those that underwent PC as treatment for acute cholecystitis. Only those patients that presented with comorbidities and medical risk for surgery as defined by the Charlson comorbidity index appeared to benefit from PC over surgical intervention for acute cholecystitis [52].

Chronic Calculous Cholecystitis

Clinical Presentation and Diagnosis

Biliary colic (symptomatic calculous disease) is the most common complication from gallstones. This scenario is typical in the elderly due to the alterations in pain perception and immune response to inflammation that have been described

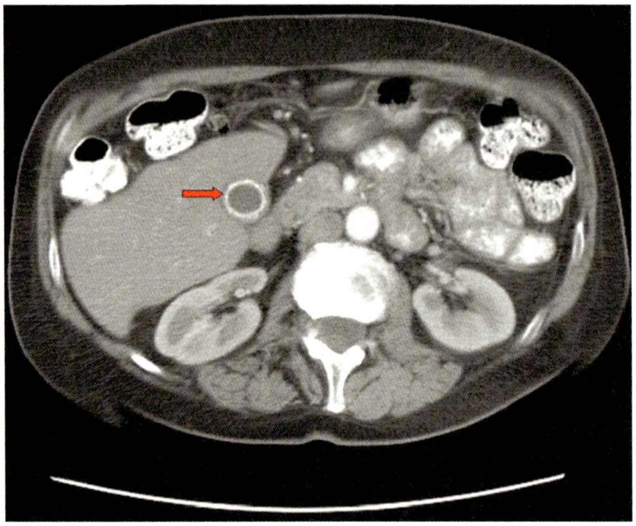

Fig. 12.10 CAT scan of the abdomen showing complete calcification of the gallbladder wall (*arrow*) consistent with a "porcelain" gallbladder

(see section "Diagnostic investigation"). The patient often will present with symptoms similar to those of acute cholecystitis without systemic signs of inflammation. Typically, the pain is located in the epigastrium/right upper quadrant and is dull and of less intensity compared to the pain which occurs with acute cholecystitis. Patients will be afebrile with normal laboratory studies. The metabolic panel should also be checked, particularly in the elderly patient as they often are on medications that can cause fluid and electrolyte derangement. Ultrasound examination should be obtained to confirm the presence of stones. Occasionally, the "double-arc" sign which is pathognomonic for a contracted gallbladder with calculi will be seen on ultrasonography [31]. Rarely, chronic cholecystitis may be associated with mural calcification of the gallbladder. This may involve a portion of the wall or the entire gallbladder otherwise known as a "porcelain" gallbladder (Fig. 12.10). The significance of this finding has been controversial due to the potential association with an underlying carcinoma particularly in older patients [73–75]. This finding on ultrasound should lead one to consider additional imaging such as CT or MRI [76].

Treatment of Chronic Calculous Cholecystitis

The initial treatment for biliary colic should be directed at relieving pain with the judicious use of narcotics. Intravenous fluids should be begun for dehydration. The patient should be seen by an anesthesiologist to determine the patient's ASA score. Reasonable risk patients should be scheduled for elective cholecystectomy as soon as convenient since the recurrence rate for a subsequent episode of biliary colic or acute cholecystitis is 40 % over the next 2 years [77]. Delaying surgery because of age and waiting for an episode of recurrence of disease in the elderly is hazardous as they often present in a delayed fashion and with a higher incidence of complicated calculous disease that may require urgent/emergent cholecystectomy that is associated higher morbidity and mortality [6, 25, 49, 77].

Though the incidence of porcelain gallbladder remains low (0.2 %), there is a small risk for malignancy, particularly in those over 50 years of age (incidence of 0.08 %/year of symptoms) [77]. The management of the porcelain gallbladder has undergone considerable change over the past several decades. Early reports suggested a high association between a calcified gallbladder and carcinoma (up to 60 %) [78] which led to the recommendation for cholecystectomy once the diagnosis was made. Recently, several large clinical series have questioned the significance of the calcification of the gallbladder wall after finding a much lower incidence of malignancy (0–5 %) [74, 75, 78]. The reasons for this dramatic shift are felt to be due to the recent advances and increased usage of abdominal CT imaging which has allowed earlier diagnosis compared to earlier studies which relied on abdominal radiographs for the diagnosis [78].

The overwhelming majority of older patients diagnosed with a porcelain gallbladder also have symptomatic disease which would make them surgical candidates unless their operative risk was found to be prohibitive [74, 75, 78]. The asymptomatic patient with an incidental finding of a porcelain gallbladder represents a clinical impasse on whether to proceed with cholecystectomy or nonoperative management. The risk of surgical intervention, particularly in the patient with comorbidities, should be balanced against the low potential risk of gallbladder carcinoma and discussed with the patient in order to establish a course of action. Laparoscopic cholecystectomy has been found to be technically feasible in patients with a porcelain gallbladder and should be the initial procedure of choice. If carcinoma is confirmed once the gallbladder is resected, the procedure should be converted to an open resection of the liver bed and lymphadenectomy [78, 79].

Choledocholithiasis

Clinical Presentation and Diagnosis

The majority of choledocholithiasis originate from the gallbladder and are associated with a myriad of clinical symptoms. The incidence of symptomatic common bile duct stones is higher in the elderly population (range 15–20 %) compared to younger patients [49]. Up to a third of common duct calculi will spontaneously pass into the duodenum [80], while large stones may lead to common duct obstruction resulting in either gallstone pancreatitis or cholangitis.

Right upper quadrant pains with abnormal liver function tests are present in over 75 % of patients [81]. The laboratory studies usually reveal a cholestatic (elevated serum bilirubin) pattern and transaminases typically higher than 500 IU/L along with elevation of alkaline phosphatase or serum gamma-glutamyltransferase (90 % of cases) [82]. Leukocytosis may also be present in the acute phase, and coagulation parameters should also be evaluated. It should be noted that approximately 10 % of patients will be asymptomatic when the diagnosis is made incidentally on imaging studies obtained for a reason other than biliary symptoms [81, 83]. In the elderly, malaise, altered mental status, or acute deconditioning may be the only presenting symptoms [56].

As noted above, the initial imaging study to evaluate for common bile duct calculi is abdominal ultrasonography. If the ultrasound is normal but clinical and laboratory testings are consistent with choledocholithiasis, then MRCP should be considered as this has higher sensitivity than sonography. ERCP should generally be reserved for therapeutic purposes due to its invasive risks and technical complications.

Treatment of Choledocholithiasis

Once the diagnosis of choledocholithiasis is made, there are a variety of treatment options available, and these should be tailored based upon local expertise and resource availability. Initial treatment should be directed at alleviating pain, fluid resuscitation, and correction of any electrolyte or coagulation disorders that may be present. Complete removal of common duct calculi should be the objective regardless of the intervention chosen because up to 50 % of patients will have recurrence of symptoms if left untreated and 25 % of these recurrent cases will result in potentially serious complications (i.e., biliary pancreatitis or cholangitis) [82].

Endoscopic therapy with ERCP or percutaneous intervention (PTC) are both acceptable methods of ductal clearance according to the Society for Surgery of the Alimentary Tract (SAGES) and British Society of Gastroenterology guidelines [48, 84] and should be chosen based upon local availability and expertise. As elderly patients are often on anticoagulants or antiplatelet medications, these should be withheld in anticipation of therapeutic intervention. Antibiotics should be given periprocedurally and should again be directed primarily against the Enterobacteriaceae family. ERCP with balloon dilation of the sphincter has an excellent clinical success rate and appears to be safe even in the elderly population with known comorbidities [49, 85].

Once the calculi have been removed from the common bile duct, elderly patients should be offered cholecystectomy if they are acceptable surgical candidates because of the potential for recurrent choledocholithiasis or acute cholecystitis. In a 2-year prospective study, Lee et al. found that age and the presence of comorbid conditions were risk factors for recurrent choledocholithiasis [86]. Additionally, these patients were felt to be at higher surgical risk at the time of the second episode than if they had initially had an early

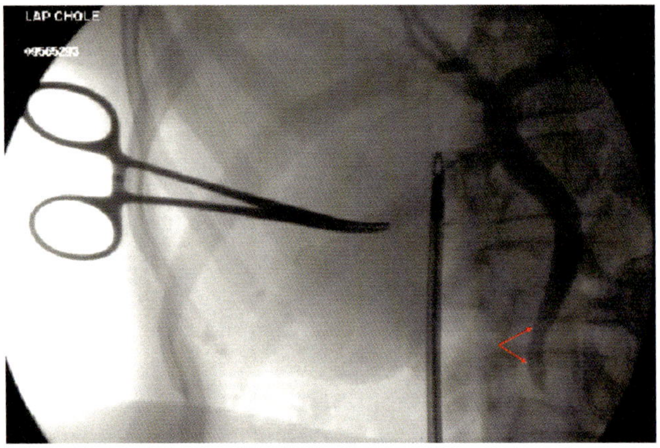

Fig. 12.11 An intraoperative cholangiogram demonstrating two filling defects consistent with common bile duct stones (*arrows*)

cholecystectomy. Similar findings were seen in a large systematic review done by the Cochrane group which found a decreased recurrence rate and increased survival advantage even in patients deemed "high risk" for early cholecystectomy as opposed to a nonoperative approach [87].

The timing of cholecystectomy after ERCP and sphincterotomy has also been investigated. In a prospective, randomized trial comparing early laparoscopic cholecystectomy (within 72 h) versus delayed cholecystectomy (6–8 weeks after ERCP), there were no differences in operative time or rate of conversion to open procedures, while 36 % of patients in the delayed group developed recurrent biliary symptoms [88]. The authors concluded that early cholecystectomy prevented future symptoms related to common duct stones without an increase in morbidity in those undergoing early operation. Patients that undergo ERCP with sphincterotomy and ductal clearance are still at risk for residual choledocholithiasis. Clinical studies assessing this risk have found it to be as high as 13 % [89, 90]. Therefore, the authors recommend routine use of intraoperative cholangiography in patients that had a preoperative ERCP with ductal clearance to reduce the chance of a retained common duct stone going undetected (Fig. 12.11). For those surgeons with advanced laparoscopic skills and institutions that have the instrumentation and imaging capability, single-stage procedures to treat choledocholithiasis (laparoscopic cholecystectomy with intraoperative cholangiogram followed by laparoscopic common bile duct exploration) have gained popularity. This leads to decreased hospital lengths of stay and total charges without an increase in associated morbidity or mortality [91–93]. This management strategy has also been validated in elderly and high-risk patients [94]. The benefits of one-stage treatment of choledocholithiasis have only been observed in uncomplicated cases (i.e., no cirrhosis, cholangitis, or biliary sepsis) [91] and with experienced laparoscopic surgeons [95].

Cholangitis

Clinical Presentation and Diagnosis

Cholangitis can follow a wide spectrum of disease in the elderly patient, from a mild infection to fulminant septic shock with multiple organ dysfunction. Early recognition of which form of disease is present is imperative to achieve good clinical outcomes. Obstructive choledocholithiasis is the most common etiology of cholangitis but may also occur in the presence of benign or malignant biliary strictures. Stasis of bile leads to bacterial overgrowth from the duodenum with *Escherichia coli* being the most common offending organism followed by other members of the family Enterobacteriaceae. Increased pressure in the intrahepatic bile radicles leads to translocation of bacteria into the hepatic veins and systemic bloodstream with resultant toxemia [82]. The classic clinical picture of Charcot's triad (fever, right upper quadrant pain, and jaundice) is present in 70 % of patients [82]. The addition of altered mental status changes and hypotension to Charcot's triad are known as Reynold's pentad and are indicative suppurative cholangitis. In addition to clinical exam findings, laboratory studies often reveal leukocytosis with elevated liver transaminases and cholestasis. Thrombocytopenia, metabolic acidosis, and elevation of creatinine are diagnostic of more severe cholangitis [96]. Coagulation studies should also be assessed in preparation for ductal decompression as biliary obstruction with superimposed sepsis can lead to DIC. Diagnostic imaging is frequently done with ultrasonography that typically reveals dilation of the biliary ducts.

Treatment of Cholangitis

Initial therapy should be to establish intravenous access and begin fluid resuscitation followed by early administration of broad-spectrum antibiotics. Appropriate initial antibiotics include third-generation cephalosporins, fluoroquinolones combined with metronidazole, or beta-lactamase inhibitor combinations (i.e., piperacillin/tazobactam) [57]. Blood cultures should be collected but should not delay initiation of antibiotic therapy. Since most patients present with mild to moderate cholangitis (nonsuppurative), this will lead to clinical improvement within the next 24 h [48]. Even with initial improvement, elderly patients should be closely monitored for decompensation since age (>50 years) has been shown to be a predictor of poor outcomes [97]. Once sepsis has resolved, the duct is decompressed, and the patient is medically optimized, laparoscopic cholecystectomy should be offered to the patient.

Patients that present with florid sepsis and organ dysfunction should be aggressively resuscitated in the intensive care unit with the aid of invasive monitoring. Hemodynamic support with vasopressors may be required in cases of septic shock, and optimization of physiologic parameters should be undertaken to allow for source control through biliary decompression with the least invasive means available. Endoscopic decompression with ERCP has become the initial procedure of choice for most patients, including the elderly [82]. The aim of the procedure is to relieve biliary pressure through minimal manipulation to prevent exacerbation of endotoxemia. Sphincterotomy aids with extraction of the calculi, and then biliary stent placement maintains decompression of the common bile duct. Should ERCP be technically difficult and unsuccessful, PTC is the next option. Even with successful decompression, there is still a mortality rate of 5–10 % [98]. In situations where ERCP/PTC is unsuccessful or unavailable, drainage can be accomplished surgically with open common bile duct exploration and T-tube placement. The mortality for this intervention is much higher than the preferred less invasive techniques (16–40 %) [81]. After successful biliary decompression and stabilization of the patient, antibiotic therapy should be continued for 14 days and the patient evaluated for cholecystectomy once medically optimized.

Biliary Pancreatitis

Clinical Presentation and Diagnosis

A common bile duct stone will frequently impact at the ampulla and obstruct both the bile duct and the pancreatic duct. This results in stasis in both ducts with intraductal activation of enzymes and pancreatic glandular damage which results in a generalized inflammatory response that leads to subsequent symptoms. Risk factors for the development of gallstone pancreatitis include advanced age (>60) and female gender [99]. Most cases of biliary pancreatitis are moderate and will resolve with appropriate supportive care. However, more severe episodes of pancreatic inflammation can lead to sepsis and multiple organ dysfunction with mortality rates that exceed 20 % [100] and require a multidisciplinary approach including critical care support.

Symptoms of gallstone pancreatitis include sharp epigastric pain with radiation to the back that can be confused with acute aortic dissection or myocardial ischemia in the elderly. Nausea and vomiting are common. Signs of systemic inflammation response syndrome (SIRS) such as tachycardia and fever may also be present. In severe acute pancreatitis, patients can also have hypotension and altered mental status. Helpful laboratory investigations include CBC, serum chemistry with a serum calcium level, liver function tests, and serum amylase and lipase. Leukocytosis is often secondary to inflammatory response, and the hematocrit is often elevated from hemoconcentration as a result of third space fluid sequestration. Serum chemistry can also depict signs of impaired tissue perfusion if the serum bicarbonate is low or renal parameters are indicative of acute renal impairment. In cases of biliary pancreatitis, transaminases may be higher than 500 IU/L in the acute phase with a moderate elevation of serum bilirubin. Typically, both the serum amylase and lipase will be elevated, but the hyperamylasemia resolves earlier in the time course of pancreatitis than does the lipase.

Ultrasound examination should be the first imaging study obtained. This test can be done in unstable patients at the patient's bedside. The identification of cholecystolithiasis or sludge in the gallbladder supports the diagnosis. Dilation of the biliary tree may also be noted on the exam. In patients that are clinically stable or that improve with resuscitation, CT imaging can be helpful in predicting the severity of pancreatitis [101]. In the critically ill patient with moderate to severe pancreatitis, the study should be performed without contrast to avoid exposing a hypovolemic elderly patient to a potentially nephrotoxic contrast material. Scans with IV contrast can be obtained at a later time when the patient is clinically stable to delineate areas of potential pancreatic necrosis.

Treatment of Biliary Pancreatitis

Initial therapy is directed at alleviating pain with judicious use of narcotics and nasogastric decompression for those patients presenting with symptoms of ileus. Generous fluid resuscitation should also be undertaken due to the amount of fluid sequestration that can occur in the retroperitoneum. There should be a low threshold to admit elderly patients to the ICU even in moderate cases due to their limited physiologic reserve. Many different scoring systems for determining the severity of pancreatitis have been developed [102–105], but the Ranson score has been shown to have the highest predictive accuracy [102]. A Ranson score of 3 or more is indicative of severe disease, and well-established evidence-based guidelines have been developed for treatment [106, 107]. There are three areas of current debate regarding the optimal therapy of gallstone pancreatitis. The first area of controversy in the treatment of severe pancreatitis is the use of prophylactic antibiotics. Recently several systematic reviews examining the utility of antibiotic prophylaxis in severe acute pancreatitis have been undertaken and have failed to demonstrate any benefit on mortality or the risk of developing infected pancreatic necrosis [108–110]. Due to problems with emerging bacterial resistance, the authors recommend against the routine use of antibiotic administration in sterile cases of severe pancreatitis. In instances when superimposed cholangitis is suspected with biliary pancreatitis, appropriate antibiotic therapy is warranted.

Another controversy involves the use of early (within 24–48 h) ERCP with sphincterotomy. In the past, literature supported early ERCP in patients with biliary pancreatitis that present with severe disease and moderate disease that did not exhibit clinical improvement or experience persistent pain [82]. A recent meta-analysis reexamined this topic utilizing seven prospective randomized trials (ERCP vs. conservative treatment) in patients that presented only with severe biliary pancreatitis without evidence of cholangitis [84]. The authors found that there was no significant benefit or difference in outcome in those patients that underwent early ERCP even when stratifying for disease severity. Therefore, early ductal decompression with ERCP should not be performed routinely as it provides no benefit to the patient.

The final area of discussion involves the timing of cholecystectomy after an episode of biliary pancreatitis. As mentioned in section "Choledocholithiasis", the natural history of biliary pancreatitis is recurrence (up to a third of all patients) if the gallbladder is not removed [111]. Each recurrent episode places the patient at risk of life-threatening pancreatitis or cholangitis. Recently, the group from Harbor-UCLA investigated the feasibility of early cholecystectomy (within 48 h of admission) in patients presenting with moderate biliary pancreatitis (Ranson <3) and found no apparent increase in perioperative complications and a decreased hospital length of stay compared to those that had cholecystectomy delayed until after resolution of all abdominal pain or improved enzymatic parameters [112]. Other studies have found similar findings with the consensus being that laparoscopic cholecystectomy should be performed during the same admission for biliary pancreatitis in patients who are an acceptable surgical risk [111, 113, 114]. Despite the overwhelming evidence favoring cholecystectomy for biliary pancreatitis, a recent appraisal of this approach in elderly patients concluded that over 40 % of patients admitted with a diagnosis of gallstone pancreatitis in a large Medicare sample were not treated surgically and were associated with a high rate of recurrent acute pancreatitis (33 %) [115]. This study demonstrates the practice variations that exist in caring for elderly patients for this disease. For patients that are at a prohibitive surgical risk due to comorbid illnesses, ERCP with sphincterotomy does provide some protection against recurrent episodes of biliary pancreatitis and should be offered to patients that are considered to not be surgical candidates [114, 116].

Gallstone Ileus

Clinical Presentation and Diagnosis

Gallstone ileus is classically a disease of the elderly and is an uncommon cause of bowel obstruction despite its deceptive name. The typical patient for some form of dementia such that the individual has a limited ability to communicate with their caregivers. The onset of symptoms is often subtle but may be preceded by biliary colic or chronic subacute cholecystitis in approximately 50 % of patients [117]. The patient typically experiences nausea and vomiting associated with colicky abdominal pain. These symptoms may be fleeting due to transient episodes of obstruction where the stone intermittently lodges and dislodges in a narrow area of the intestinal tract. This is characteristically known as the "tumbling" phenomenon [118]. The origin of the stones causing the obstruction is secondary to the development of a cholecystoenteric fistula which most commonly is to the duodenum. Less commonly, the stomach or transverse colon is involved. Typically the obstructing calculus is larger than 2.5 cm in diameter which will lodge in the terminal ileum or less commonly at the duodenal-jejunal junction, the duodenal bulb, pyloric region, or colon [81]. The classic radiological findings of pneumobilia, ectopic gallstone, and small bowel obstruction observed on plain films of the abdomen (Rigler's triad) are only seen in approximately 50 % of patients but when present confirm the diagnosis (Fig. 12.1) [119]. CT scan is much more reliable in identifying the diagnosis (93 % sensitivity) when obtained [120]. Only 70 % of cases are diagnosed preoperatively with the remainder being diagnosed at the time of operation [117].

Treatment of Gallstone Ileus

As patients that present with this condition are often elderly and debilitated, initial therapy should be directed at fluid resuscitation for dehydration and the correction of any electrolyte abnormalities in preparation for laparotomy. The optimal surgical procedure for this condition continues to be contested. The easiest technical approach involves relief of the obstruction with enterolithotomy proximal to the obstructing stone for removal and examination of the intestine and gallbladder to ensure multiple stones are not present. The cholecystoenteric fistula is left in situ. Controversy exists about the need to resect the fistula and gallbladder in patients with an acute small bowel obstruction. As this condition is relatively rare, no large randomized studies are available to compare the superiority of one procedure over another [119]. Releasing the bowel obstruction is generally associated with less perioperative morbidity and mortality but may subject the patient to a risk for a recurrence of gallstone ileus (5–17 %) or other complications of cholelithiasis (5–10 %) [119]. Autopsy findings of patients that have undergone enterolithotomy alone have demonstrated that the fistula can close spontaneously in the absence of cholelithiasis [121]. Since no level I data exists regarding the treatment of this condition, surgical therapy should be tailored individually based upon the patient's global condition as wells as intraoperative findings.

Benign Acalculous Diseases

Acute Acalculous Cholecystitis

Clinical Presentation and Diagnosis

Acalculous cholecystitis represents 5–10 % of acute gallbladder pathology in adults [81]. Predisposing risk factors include advanced age, presence of comorbidities, and critical illness. The etiology is multifactorial but thought to be related to biliary stasis [122] and systemic hypoperfusion leading to mucosal ischemia with bacterial overgrowth. Despite increased awareness of this disease entity, mortality rates continue to be as high as 30 % [122].

A high index of suspicion is necessary to diagnose acute acalculous cholecystitis due to the patient's often debilitated state and inability to communicate pain. The presence of sepsis and leukocytosis is frequently associated with nonspecific elevation of AST, ALT, Alk Phos, and bilirubin in many critically ill patients which may make the diagnosis difficult. Abdominal ultrasound is the most useful imaging test with gallbladder wall thickening being the most common diagnostic finding. The sensitivity of ultrasound for diagnosis can vary widely from 29 to 92 % [123] due to false-positive exams that can occur with ascites or other inflammatory conditions. HIDA scan can also be used to confirm the diagnosis in patients with a high suspicion when the ultrasound is equivocal. The sensitivity for HIDA scintigraphy ranges from 67 to 100 % [123]. However, this test typically requires that the patient be transported from the ICU to radiology when portable imaging equipment is not available for a study at the patient's bedside.

Treatment of Acalculous Cholecystitis

Once the diagnosis has been made or clinical suspicion is high enough, percutaneous cholecystostomy is the treatment of choice in critically ill patients. Patients are frequently receiving empiric antibiotics when the diagnosis is confirmed. Cholecystostomy can either be performed at the patient's bedside under ultrasonography or under fluoroscopy with either procedure being clinically effective for resolution of sepsis [69]. Surgical intervention is reserved only for those patients that do not respond to drainage. The cholecystostomy tube can be left in place for 4–6 weeks to allow a tract to establish while the patient convalesces. A repeat cholangiogram can then be performed (Fig. 12.12) to document a patent cystic duct prior to removing the drainage catheter.

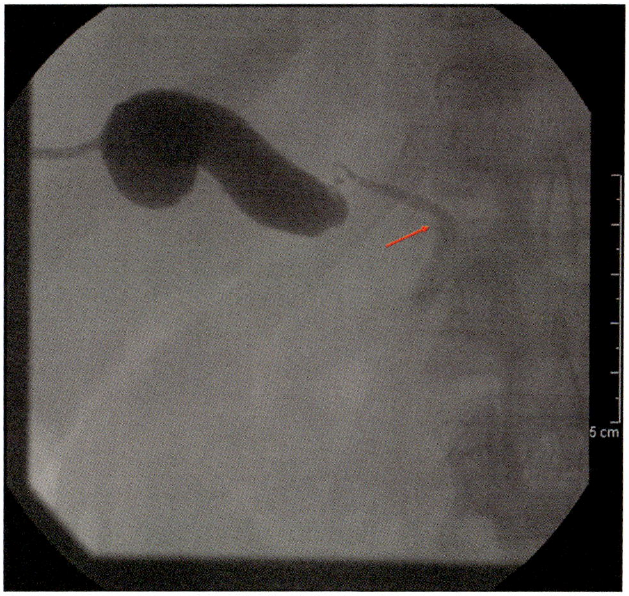

Fig. 12.12 PTC cholangiogram done after convalescence from critical illness secondary to acalculous cholecystitis. Notice the patency of the cystic duct with passage of contrast into the common bile duct (*arrow*)

Motility Disorders of the Biliary Tree

Clinical Presentation and Diagnosis

Motility disorders of the biliary tree include biliary dyskinesia as well as sphincter of Oddi dysfunction. The hallmark of both disorders is a constellation of classic biliary-type symptoms: epigastric or right upper quadrant pain that is episodic and severe enough to interrupt the patient's daily life as defined by the Rome committee [124].

In biliary dyskinesia, laboratory investigations and sonographic imaging are normal. The diagnosis is confirmed by performing a provocative HIDA scan with cholecystokinin infusion. This allows the calculation of an ejection fraction with the normal emptying of the gallbladder being greater than 50 % of the technetium. Abnormal emptying is defined as less than 50 % in response to cholecystokinin [125]. It should be noted that certain medications that are common in elderly patients (i.e., calcium channel blockers and opiates) could also cause impaired gallbladder contraction and emptying and cause an abnormal scintigraphy scan (false-positive) [125].

Sphincter of Oddi dysfunction can present as either recurrent attacks of abdominal pain that mimic biliary colic, recurrent idiopathic pancreatitis, or postcholecystectomy pain. The most classic form of sphincter of Oddi dysfunction is a triad of biliary colic, abnormal liver function tests, and documentation of a dilated common bile duct on imaging without evidence of gallstones [126]. The diagnostic workup [127] should consist of endoscopy with ultrasonography as this may document stones that are not seen on an abdominal ultrasonogram or other imaging modalities. If this is normal, then ERCP should be done to rule out microlithiasis and to perform sphincter manometry. Elevated basal sphincter pressures or paradoxical spasm noted with cholecystokinin infusion are suggestive of the diagnosis.

Treatment of Biliary Motility Disorders

Biliary dyskinesia is treated by laparoscopic cholecystectomy in acceptable risk patients. Pathologic examination will occasionally reveal cholelithiasis that was missed by sonography. Symptom relief after cholecystectomy is seen in between 70 and 90 % of patients [128, 129]. Patients that have typical biliary symptoms, and abnormal HIDA scan, or occult calculi are most likely to have resolution of symptoms [125].

Sphincter of Oddi dysfunction is treated by endoscopic sphincterotomy of both the biliary and pancreatic ducts [130] although a trial of medical management may be undertaken first with calcium channel blockers or anticholinergics [127, 131]. For patients that have an inaccessible papilla or a recurrence of symptoms after sphincterotomy, open transduodenal sphincterotomy is an option [132]. The efficacy of sphincterotomy varies widely from 20 to 91 %. The best predictor of resolution of pain with sphincterotomy is an elevated basal pressure on manometry of the common bile duct [126, 127].

Neoplasms of the Gallbladder

Gallbladder Polyps

Clinical Presentation and Diagnosis

Polyps of the gallbladder are observed in about 5 % of patients that undergo an abdominal ultrasound [133] with most patients being asymptomatic (77 %) [134] and imaged for another reason. The majority of these documented polyps are pseudopolyps with the majority being cholesterol polyps or adenomyomatosis (85 %) followed by inflammatory polyps (10 %) with the remainder being true polyps that are predominantly either adenomas or adenocarcinomas [135].

True polyps are the only form of polyps with malignant potential. Polyp size, vascularity, rate of growth, presence of cholelithiasis, as well as age have been linked to malignant potential [135]. The most commonly cited size that is associated with a risk for malignancy is 10 mm. Using this size, Koga analyzed polyps found in cholecystectomy specimens and observed that 88 % of malignant polyps were greater than 10 mm in size [136]. Recently this size criterion has been challenged due to malignancy being found in polyps of smaller size. A recent Mayo clinic study showed that polyps under 10 mm carried a 7.4 % chance of malignancy and that a size greater than 6 mm was a significant risk factor for malignancy [137]. Using a size of 6 mm resulted in 100 % negative predictive value.

As previously mentioned, age is also a risk factor for polyp malignancy. Two separate studies have concluded that age over 50 years was a risk factor for a polyp being malignant [138, 139]. Based upon the patient's age and size of polyp, the patient can be risk stratified into low or high risk for neoplasm. Endoscopic ultrasound may provide assistance in intermediate cases based upon clinical scoring features of the polyp [140–142].

Treatment of Gallbladder Polyps

Patients that are symptomatic (i.e., biliary colic) without another identifiable etiology for the pain should be offered laparoscopic cholecystectomy [135]. Polyps which are greater than 10 mm in size without symptoms should also be treated with laparoscopic cholecystectomy unless the polyp is greater than 1.8 cm in size [135]. Two different series have shown that polyps above this size are often associated with an invasive cancer and should be treated with an open cholecystectomy and partial liver resection with possible lymphadenectomy if necessary [86, 116, 143]. For asymptomatic lesions that are less than 10 mm, watchful waiting along with serial abdominal ultrasound examinations has been proven to be a safe treatment strategy [134, 144]. Though there are not any well-established guidelines regarding the interval of screening, most experts favor imaging every 6–12 months [144, 145]. Lesions that are of intermediate size (6–10 mm) represent a treatment challenge given the recent evidence that neoplastic growth may occur at polyp sizes in this range. In these cases, endoscopic ultrasonography may be helpful to determine which lesions are suspicious enough to warrant cholecystectomy [135].

Gallbladder Carcinoma

Clinical Presentation and Diagnosis

Although uncommon, gallbladder carcinoma is the most common cancer of the biliary tree with the overwhelming majority of cases being adenocarcinoma (80 %) [146]. The incidence in the United States is 1.2/100,000 with a higher incidence in other countries. Risk factors include advanced age (>65 years), female gender, obesity, and a history of biliary disease (cholelithiasis in particular) [147].

Unfortunately most cases are asymptomatic or have nonspecific complaints leading to delayed presentation with advanced disease (50 %) [148]. Other patients may present with typical biliary symptoms and have undergone cholecystectomy with incidental discovery of cancer on final pathology report (10 %) or have undergone abdominal imaging for another indication revealing gallbladder findings that are concerning for malignancy (i.e., large polyps or a mass with liver involvement) [146].

In the patients where gallbladder cancer is suspected on ultrasound imaging, a CT of the abdomen should be obtained to assess for tumor invasion into the liver or other organ as well as lymph node involvement [148]. Findings on CT that preclude curative resection include invasion of the common hepatic artery or portal vein, lymph node involvement outside the hepatic hilum, or obvious evidence of metastasis [146]. As most patients are often elderly with comorbidities, a reasonable assessment of functional liver reserve should be done to ensure that a large liver resection would not lead to acute fulminant hepatic failure.

Treatment of Gallbladder Carcinoma

When the diagnosis is known or suspected preoperatively, the plan should be to perform an open cholecystectomy with wedge resection of the adjacent liver and a portal lymphadenectomy [149]. Diagnostic laparoscopy may be considered prior to laparotomy as this can identify peritoneal disease or non-contiginous hepatic involvement not seen on preoperative imaging which would preclude curative resection in almost 50 % of patients [150]. Once the specimen is excised, the cystic duct margin should also be sent for frozen section. If there are malignant cells in the margin, excision of the common bile duct with creation of a hepaticojejunostomy [148]. Margins of the liver wedge resection should also be assessed for evidence of tumor, and if present, the resection should be extended until clear margins are obtained [149]. Some tumors require formal anatomic liver resection, but this is usually known preoperatively.

More commonly, patients that have undergone cholecystectomy for presumed benign disease will have the tumor identified on the final pathology report. Tumors that are found to be in situ or only invade the lamina propria (T1a) are considered cured with a 5-year survival rate of greater than 90 % [146]. All other tumors with more extensive invasion should undergo reoperation with wedge resection of the liver, lymphadenectomy, and possible common bile duct excision [149]. All previous laparoscopic port sites should also be excised [146]. Once the tumor extends into the peri-muscular connective tissue of the gallbladder or there is lymph node involvement, the 5-year survival decreases dramatically even with attempts at curative resection as adjuvant chemotherapy remains ineffective [149]. This should be kept in mind when considering extensive resections in the elderly patient. For patients that present with unresectable disease and biliary obstruction, endoscopic or percutaneous interventions with biliary stenting are often successful at providing palliation [49, 149].

References

1. Sanson TG, O'Keefe KP. Evaluation of abdominal pain in the elderly. Emerg Med Clin North Am. 1996;14(3):615–27.
2. Friedman GD, Kannel WB, Dawber TR. The epidemiology of gallbladder disease: observations in the Framingham study. J Chronic Dis. 1966;19(3):273–92.
3. Lirussi F, Nassuato G, Passera D, et al. Gallstone disease in an elderly population: the silea study. Eur J Gastroenterol Hepatol. 1999;11(5):485–91.
4. Ratner J, Lisbona A, Rosenbloom M, Palayew M, Szabolcsi S, Tupaz T. The prevalence of gallstone disease in very old institutionalized persons. JAMA. 1991;265(7):902–3.
5. Urbach DR, Stukel TA. Rate of elective cholecystectomy and the incidence of severe gallstone disease. CMAJ. 2005;172(8):1015–9. doi:10.1503/cmaj.1041363.
6. Bergman S, Sourial N, Vedel I, et al. Gallstone disease in the elderly: are older patients managed differently? Surg Endosc. 2011;25(1):55–61. doi:10.1007/s00464-010-1128-5.
7. Esteller A. Physiology of bile secretion. World J Gastroenterol. 2008;14(37):5641–9.
8. Shaffer EA. The effect of vagotomy on gallbladder function and bile composition in man. Ann Surg. 1982;195(4):413–8.
9. Banfield WJ. Physiology of the gallbladder. Gastroenterology. 1975;69(3):770–7.
10. Shah B, Agrawal R, Goldwasser B, Farah K. Biliary diseases in the elderly. Prac Gastroenterol. 2008;32(9):14–26.
11. Walsh RM. Innovations in treating the elderly who have biliary and pancreatic disease. Clin Geriatr Med. 2006;22(3):545–58. doi:10.1016/j.cger.2006.04.007.
12. Kahng KU, Roslyn JJ. Surgical issues for the elderly patient with hepatobiliary disease. Surg Clin North Am. 1994;74(2):345–73.
13. Glenn F. Surgical management of acute cholecystitis in patients 65 years of age and older. Ann Surg. 1981;193(1):56–9.
14. Eagle KA, Brundage BH, Chaitman BR, et al. Guidelines for perioperative cardiovascular evaluation for noncardiac surgery. report of the American college of Cardiology/American heart association task force on practice guidelines. committee on perioperative cardiovascular evaluation for noncardiac surgery. Circulation. 1996;93(6):1278–317.
15. Jin F, Chung F. Minimizing perioperative adverse events in the elderly. Br J Anaesth. 2001;87(4):608–24.
16. Goldman L, Caldera DL, Nussbaum SR, et al. Multifactorial index of cardiac risk in noncardiac surgical procedures. N Engl J Med. 1977;297(16):845–50. doi:10.1056/NEJM197710202971601.
17. Devereaux PJ, Goldman L, Cook DJ, Gilbert K, Leslie K, Guyatt GH. Perioperative cardiac events in patients undergoing noncardiac surgery: a review of the magnitude of the problem, the pathophysiology of the events and methods to estimate and communicate risk. CMAJ. 2005;173(6):627–34. doi:10.1503/cmaj.050011.
18. American College of Cardiology Foundation/American Heart Association Task Force on Practice Guidelines, American Society of Echocardiography, American Society of Nuclear Cardiology, et al. 2009 ACCF/AHA focused update on perioperative beta blockade. J Am Coll Cardiol. 2009;54(22):2102–28. doi:10.1016/j.jacc.2009.07.004.
19. Vaughan MS, Vaughan RW, Cork RC. Postoperative hypothermia in adults: relationship of age, anesthesia, and shivering to rewarming. Anesth Analg. 1981;60(10):746–51.
20. Frank SM, Higgins MS, Breslow MJ, et al. The catecholamine, cortisol, and hemodynamic responses to mild perioperative hypothermia. A randomized clinical trial. Anesthesiology. 1995;82(1):83–93.
21. Haley RW, Culver DH, Morgan WM, White JW, Emori TG, Hooton TM. Identifying patients at high risk of surgical wound infection. A simple multivariate index of patient susceptibility and wound contamination. Am J Epidemiol. 1985;121(2):206–15.
22. Ballantyne JC, Carr DB, de Ferranti S. The comparative effects of postoperative analgesic therapies on pulmonary outcome: Cumulative meta-analyses of randomized, controlled trials. Anesth Analg. 1998;86(3):598–612.
23. Rosenthal RA, Andersen DK. Surgery in the elderly: observations on the pathophysiology and treatment of cholelithiasis. Exp Gerontol. 1993;28(4–5):459–72.
24. Brewer BJ, Golden GT, Hitch DC, Rudolf LE, Wangensteen SL. Abdominal pain. an analysis of 1,000 consecutive cases in a

university hospital emergency room. Am J Surg. 1976; 131(2):219–23.
25. Martinez JP, Mattu A. Abdominal pain in the elderly. Emerg Med Clin North Am. 2006;24(2):371–88, vii. doi:10.1016/j.emc.2006.01.010.
26. Cooper GS, Shlaes DM, Salata RA. Intraabdominal infection: differences in presentation and outcome between younger patients and the elderly. Clin Infect Dis. 1994;19(1):146–8.
27. Bedirli A, Sakrak O, Sozuer EM, Kerek M, Guler I. Factors effecting the complications in the natural history of acute cholecystitis. Hepatogastroenterology. 2001;48(41):1275–8.
28. Garcea G, Ngu W, Neal CP, Dennison AR, Berry DP. Bilirubin levels predict malignancy in patients with obstructive jaundice. HPB (Oxford). 2011;13(6):426–30. doi:10.1111/j.1477-2574.2011.00312.x; 10.1111/j.1477-2574.2011.00312.x.
29. Potter J, Klipstein K, Reilly JJ, Roberts M. The nutritional status and clinical course of acute admissions to a geriatric unit. Age Ageing. 1995;24(2):131–6.
30. Stewart L, Griffiss JM, Way LW. Spectrum of gallstone disease in the veterans population. Am J Surg. 2005;190(5):746–51. doi:10.1016/j.amjsurg.2005.07.014.
31. Gore RM, Thakrar KH, Newmark GM, Mehta UK, Berlin JW. Gallbladder imaging. Gastroenterol Clin North Am. 2010;39(2):265–87, ix. doi:10.1016/j.gtc.2010.02.009.
32. Liang HP, Cheung WK, Su FH, Chu FY. Porcelain gallbladder. J Am Geriatr Soc. 2008;56(5):960–1. doi:10.1111/j.1532-5415.2008.01664.x.
33. Laing FC. Diagnostic evaluation of patients with suspected acute cholecystitis. Radiol Clin North Am. 1983;21(3):477–93.
34. Laing F. The gallbladder and bile ducts. In: Rumack C, Wilson S, Charboneau J, editors. Diagnostic ultrasound, vol. 1. 1st ed. St. Louis: Mosby-Yearbook; 1998. p. 175–223.
35. Spence SC, Teichgraeber D, Chandrasekhar C. Emergent right upper quadrant sonography. J Ultrasound Med. 2009;28(4): 479–96.
36. Rybicki FJ. The WES, sign. Radiology. 2000;214(3):881–2.
37. Millat B, Decker G, Fingerhut A. Imaging of cholelithiasis: what does the surgeon need? Abdom Imaging. 2001;26(1):3–6.
38. Sugiyama M, Atomi Y. Endoscopic ultrasonography for diagnosing choledocholithiasis: a prospective comparative study with ultrasonography and computed tomography. Gastrointest Endosc. 1997;45(2):143–6.
39. Lin EC, Kuni CC. Radionuclide imaging of hepatic and biliary disease. Semin Liver Dis. 2001;21(2):179–94. doi:10.1055/s-2001-15495.
40. Carroll BA. Preferred imaging techniques for the diagnosis of cholecystitis and cholelithiasis. Ann Surg. 1989;210(1):1–12.
41. Stoker J, van Randen A, Lameris W, Boermeester MA. Imaging patients with acute abdominal pain. Radiology. 2009;253(1): 31–46. doi:10.1148/radiol.2531090302.
42. Furlan A, Ferris JV, Hosseinzadeh K, Borhani AA. Gallbladder carcinoma update: multimodality imaging evaluation, staging, and treatment options. AJR Am J Roentgenol. 2008;191(5): 1440–7. doi:10.2214/AJR.07.3599.
43. Schweiger MJ, Chambers CE, Davidson CJ, et al. Prevention of contrast induced nephropathy: recommendations for the high risk patient undergoing cardiovascular procedures. Catheter Cardiovasc Interv. 2007;69(1):135–40. doi:10.1002/ccd.20964.
44. Tsai HM, Lin XZ, Chen CY, Lin PW, Lin JC. MRI of gallstones with different compositions. AJR Am J Roentgenol. 2004;182(6):1513–9.
45. Hekimoglu K, Ustundag Y, Dusak A, et al. MRCP vs. ERCP in the evaluation of biliary pathologies: review of current literature. J Dig Dis. 2008;9(3):162–9.
46. Irie H, Honda H, Kuroiwa T, et al. Pitfalls in MR cholangiopancreatographic interpretation. Radiographics. 2001;21(1):23–37.
47. Nazarian S, Hansford R, Roguin A, et al. A prospective evaluation of a protocol for magnetic resonance imaging of patients with implanted cardiac devices. Ann Intern Med. 2011;155(7):415–24. doi:10.1059/0003-4819-155-7-201110040-00004.
48. Williams EJ, Green J, Beckingham I, et al. Guidelines on the management of common bile duct stones (CBDS). Gut. 2008;57(7):1004–21. doi:10.1136/gut.2007.121657.
49. Siegel JH, Kasmin FE. Biliary tract diseases in the elderly: management and outcomes. Gut. 1997;41(4):433–5.
50. Sugiyama M, Atomi Y. Endoscopic sphincterotomy for bile duct stones in patients 90 years of age and older. Gastrointest Endosc. 2000;52(2):187–91. doi:10.1067/mge.2000.107285.
51. Elyaderani MK, McDowell DE, Gabriele OF. A preliminary report of percutaneous cholecystostomy under ultrasonography and fluoroscopy guidance. J Clin Gastroenterol. 1983;5(3):277–81.
52. Abi-Haidar Y, Sanchez V, Williams S, Itani K. Revisiting percutaneous cholecystostomy for acute cholecystitis based on a 10-year experience. Arch Surg. 2012;147(5):416–22.
53. Vogt DP. Gallbladder disease: an update on diagnosis and treatment. Cleve Clin J Med. 2002;69(12):977–84.
54. Morrow DJ, Thompson J, Wilson SE. Acute cholecystitis in the elderly: a surgical emergency. Arch Surg. 1978;113(10):1149–52.
55. Strasberg SM. Clinical practice. acute calculous cholecystitis. N Engl J Med. 2008;358(26):2804–11.
56. Cobden I, Lendrum R, Venables CW, James OF. Gallstones presenting as mental and physical debility in the elderly. Lancet. 1984;1(8385):1062–4.
57. Solomkin JS, Mazuski JE, Bradley JS, et al. Diagnosis and management of complicated intra-abdominal infection in adults and children: guidelines by the surgical infection society and the infectious diseases society of America. Surg Infect (Larchmt). 2010;11(1):79–109. doi:10.1089/sur.2009.9930.
58. Keus F, de Jong JA, Gooszen HG, van Laarhoven CJ. Laparoscopic versus open cholecystectomy for patients with symptomatic cholecystolithiasis. Cochrane Database Syst Rev. 2006;(4):CD006231. doi:10.1002/14651858.CD006231.
59. Yamashita Y, Takada T, Kawarada Y, et al. Surgical treatment of patients with acute cholecystitis: Tokyo guidelines. J Hepatobiliary Pancreat Surg. 2007;14(1):91–7. doi:10.1007/s00534-006-1161-x.
60. Overby D, Apelgren K, Bregman K. Guidelines for the clinical application of laparoscopic biliary tract surgery. Society of American Gastrointestinal and Endoscopic Surgeons (SAGES) Web site. http://www.sages.org/publication/id/06/. Published November 2002. Updated 2010. Accessed 22 June 2012.
61. Gurusamy KS, Samraj K. Early versus delayed laparoscopic cholecystectomy for acute cholecystitis. Cochrane Database Syst Rev. 2006;(4):CD005440. doi:10.1002/14651858.CD005440.pub2.
62. Ransohoff DF, Gracie WA. Treatment of gallstones. Ann Intern Med. 1993;119(7 Pt 1):606–19.
63. Gurusamy K, Samraj K, Gluud C, Wilson E, Davidson BR. Meta-analysis of randomized controlled trials on the safety and effectiveness of early versus delayed laparoscopic cholecystectomy for acute cholecystitis. Br J Surg. 2010;97(2):141–50. doi:10.1002/bjs.6870.
64. Siddiqui T, MacDonald A, Chong PS, Jenkins JT. Early versus delayed laparoscopic cholecystectomy for acute cholecystitis: a meta-analysis of randomized clinical trials. Am J Surg. 2008;195(1):40–7. doi:10.1016/j.amjsurg.2007.03.004.
65. Flum DR, Cheadle A, Prela C, Dellinger EP, Chan L. Bile duct injury during cholecystectomy and survival in medicare beneficiaries. JAMA. 2003;290(16):2168–73. doi:10.1001/jama.290.16.2168.
66. Arthur JD, Edwards PR, Chagla LS. Management of gallstone disease in the elderly. Ann R Coll Surg Engl. 2003;85(2):91–6. doi:10.1308/003588403321219849.

67. Chareton B, Letoquart JP, Lucas A, et al. Cholelithiasis in patients over 75 years of age. apropos of 147 cases. J Chir (Paris). 1991;128(10):399–402.
68. Hickman MS, Schwesinger WH, Page CP. Acute cholecystitis in the diabetic. A case–control study of outcome. Arch Surg. 1988; 123(4):409–11.
69. Chok KS, Chu FS, Cheung TT, et al. Results of percutaneous transhepatic cholecystostomy for high surgical risk patients with acute cholecystitis. ANZ J Surg. 2010;80(4):280–3. doi:10.1111/j.1445-2197.2009.05105.x.
70. Van Steenbergen W, Ponette E, Marchal G, et al. Percutaneous transhepatic cholecystostomy for acute complicated cholecystitis in elderly patients. Am J Gastroenterol. 1990;85(10):1363–9.
71. Itoi T, Sofuni A, Itokawa F, et al. Endoscopic transpapillary gallbladder drainage in patients with acute cholecystitis in whom percutaneous transhepatic approach is contraindicated or anatomically impossible (with video). Gastrointest Endosc. 2008;68(3): 455–60. doi:10.1016/j.gie.2008.02.052.
72. Winbladh A, Gullstrand P, Svanvik J, Sandstrom P. Systematic review of cholecystostomy as a treatment option in acute cholecystitis. HPB (Oxford). 2009;11(3):183–93. doi:10.1111/j.1477-2574.2009.00052.x.
73. Polk Jr HC. Carcinoma and the calcified gall bladder. Gastroenterology. 1966;50(4):582–5.
74. Stephen AE, Berger DL. Carcinoma in the porcelain gallbladder: a relationship revisited. Surgery. 2001;129(6):699–703. doi:10.1067/msy.2001.113888.
75. Towfigh S, McFadden DW, Cortina GR, et al. Porcelain gallbladder is not associated with gallbladder carcinoma. Am Surg. 2001;67(1):7–10.
76. Levy AD, Murakata LA, Rohrmann Jr CA. Gallbladder carcinoma: radiologic-pathologic correlation. Radiographics. 2001;21(2):295–314; questionnaire, 549–55.
77. Thistle JL, Cleary PA, Lachin JM, Tyor MP, Hersh T. The natural history of cholelithiasis: the National Cooperative Gallstone Study. Ann Intern Med. 1984;101(2):171–5.
78. Khan ZS, Livingston EH, Huerta S. Reassessing the need for prophylactic surgery in patients with porcelain gallbladder: case series and systematic review of the literature. Arch Surg. 2011;146(10):1143–7. doi:10.1001/archsurg.2011.257.
79. Kim JH, Kim WH, Yoo BM, Kim JH, Kim MW. Should we perform surgical management in all patients with suspected porcelain gallbladder? Hepatogastroenterology. 2009;56(93):943–5.
80. Elmi F, Silverman WB. Long-term biliary endoscopic sphincterotomy restenosis: Incidence, endoscopic management, and complications of retreatment. Dig Dis Sci. 2010;55(7):2102–7. doi:10.1007/s10620-009-0957-3.
81. Dooley J, Lok A, Burrough A, Heathcote E, editors. Sherlock's diseases of the liver and biliary system. 12th ed. Chichester/Hoboken: Blackwell Publishing; 2011.
82. Attasaranya S, Fogel EL, Lehman GA. Choledocholithiasis, ascending cholangitis, and gallstone pancreatitis. Med Clin North Am. 2008;92(4):925–60, x. doi:10.1016/j.mcna.2008.03.001.
83. Tazuma S. Gallstone disease: epidemiology, pathogenesis, and classification of biliary stones (common bile duct and intrahepatic). Best Pract Res Clin Gastroenterol. 2006;20(6):1075–83. doi:10.1016/j.bpg.2006.05.009.
84. Petrov MS, Savides TJ. Systematic review of endoscopic ultrasonography versus endoscopic retrograde cholangiopancreatography for suspected choledocholithiasis. Br J Surg. 2009;96(9): 967–74. doi:10.1002/bjs.6667.
85. Benson ME, Byrne S, Brust DJ, et al. EUS and ERCP complication rates are not increased in elderly patients. Dig Dis Sci. 2010;55(11):3278–83. doi:10.1007/s10620-010-1152-2.
86. Lee KF, Wong J, Li JC, Lai PB. Polypoid lesions of the gallbladder. Am J Surg. 2004;188(2):186–90. doi:10.1016/j.amjsurg.2003.11.043.
87. McAlister VC, Davenport E, Renouf E. Cholecystectomy deferral in patients with endoscopic sphincterotomy. Cochrane Database Syst Rev. 2007;(4):CD006233. doi:10.1002/14651858.CD006233.pub2.
88. Reinders JS, Goud A, Timmer R, et al. Early laparoscopic cholecystectomy improves outcomes after endoscopic sphincterotomy for choledochocystolithiasis. Gastroenterology. 2010;138(7): 2315–20. doi:10.1053/j.gastro.2010.02.052.
89. Edye M, Dalvi A, Canin-Endres J, Baskin-Bey E, Salky B. Intraoperative cholangiography is still indicated after preoperative endoscopic cholangiography for gallstone disease. Surg Endosc. 2002;16(5):799–802. doi:10.1007/s00464-001-8244-1.
90. Pierce RA, Jonnalagadda S, Spitler JA, et al. Incidence of residual choledocholithiasis detected by intraoperative cholangiography at the time of laparoscopic cholecystectomy in patients having undergone preoperative ERCP. Surg Endosc. 2008;22(11): 2365–72. doi:10.1007/s00464-008-9785-3.
91. Kharbutli B, Velanovich V. Management of preoperatively suspected choledocholithiasis: a decision analysis. J Gastrointest Surg. 2008;12(11):1973–80. doi:10.1007/s11605-008-0624-6.
92. Schroeppel TJ, Lambert PJ, Mathiason MA, Kothari SN. An economic analysis of hospital charges for choledocholithiasis by different treatment strategies. Am Surg. 2007;73(5):472–7.
93. Rogers SJ, Cello JP, Horn JK, et al. Prospective randomized trial of LC+LCBDE vs. ERCP/S+LC for common bile duct stone disease. Arch Surg. 2010;145(1):28–33.
94. Noble H, Tranter S, Chesworth T, Norton S, Thompson M. A randomized, clinical trial to compare endoscopic sphincterotomy and subsequent laparoscopic cholecystectomy with primary laparoscopic bile duct exploration during cholecystectomy in higher risk patients with choledocholithiasis. J Laparoendosc Adv Surg Tech A. 2009;19(6):713–20. doi:10.1089/lap.2008.0428.
95. O'Neill CJ, Gillies DM, Gani JS. Choledocholithiasis: overdiagnosed endoscopically and undertreated laparoscopically. ANZ J Surg. 2008;78(6):487–91. doi:10.1111/j.1445-2197.2008.04540.x.
96. Wada K, Takada T, Kawarada Y, et al. Diagnostic criteria and severity assessment of acute cholangitis: Tokyo guidelines. J Hepatobiliary Pancreat Surg. 2007;14(1):52–8. doi:10.1007/s00534-006-1156-7.
97. Gigot JF, Leese T, Dereme T, Coutinho J, Castaing D, Bismuth H. Acute cholangitis. multivariate analysis of risk factors. Ann Surg. 1989;209(4):435–8.
98. Leung JW, Chung SC, Sung JJ, Banez VP, Li AK. Urgent endoscopic drainage for acute suppurative cholangitis. Lancet. 1989;1(8650):1307–9.
99. Whitcomb DC. Clinical practice. acute pancreatitis. N Engl J Med. 2006;354(20):2142–50.
100. Talukdar R, Vege SS. Recent developments in acute pancreatitis. Clin Gastroenterol Hepatol. 2009;7(11 Suppl):S3–9. doi:10.1016/j.cgh.2009.07.037.
101. Koo BC, Chinogureyi A, Shaw AS. Imaging acute pancreatitis. Br J Radiol. 2010;83(986):104–12. doi:10.1259/bjr/13359269.
102. Papachristou GI, Muddana V, Yadav D, et al. Comparison of BISAP, Ranson's, APACHE-II, and CTSI scores in predicting organ failure, complications, and mortality in acute pancreatitis. Am J Gastroenterol. 2010;105(2):435–41. doi:10.1038/ajg.2009.622. quiz 442.
103. Ranson JH, Rifkind KM, Turner JW. Prognostic signs and nonoperative peritoneal lavage in acute pancreatitis. Surg Gynecol Obstet. 1976;143(2):209–19.
104. Wilson C, Heath DI, Imrie CW. Prediction of outcome in acute pancreatitis: a comparative study of APACHE II, clinical assessment and multiple factor scoring systems. Br J Surg. 1990;77(11): 1260–4.
105. Bradley 3rd EL. A clinically based classification system for acute pancreatitis. summary of the international symposium on acute

pancreatitis, Atlanta, GA, September 11 through 13, 1992. Arch Surg. 1993;128(5):586–90.
106. Pezzilli R, Zerbi A, Di Carlo V, Bassi C, Delle Fave GF. Working Group of the Italian Association for the Study of the Pancreas on Acute Pancreatitis. Practical guidelines for acute pancreatitis. Pancreatology. 2010;10(5):523–35. doi:10.1159/000314602.
107. Banks PA, Freeman ML. Practice Parameters Committee of the American College of Gastroenterology. Practice guidelines in acute pancreatitis. Am J Gastroenterol. 2006;101(10):2379–400. doi:10.1111/j.1572-0241.2006.00856.x.
108. Bai Y, Gao J, Zou DW, Li ZS. Prophylactic antibiotics cannot reduce infected pancreatic necrosis and mortality in acute necrotizing pancreatitis: evidence from a meta-analysis of randomized controlled trials. Am J Gastroenterol. 2008;103(1):104–10. doi:10.1111/j.1572-0241.2007.01575.x.
109. Jafri NS, Mahid SS, Idstein SR, Hornung CA, Galandiuk S. Antibiotic prophylaxis is not protective in severe acute pancreatitis: a systematic review and meta-analysis. Am J Surg. 2009;197(6):806–13. doi:10.1016/j.amjsurg.2008.08.016.
110. Wittau M, Mayer B, Scheele J, Henne-Bruns D, Dellinger EP, Isenmann R. Systematic review and meta-analysis of antibiotic prophylaxis in severe acute pancreatitis. Scand J Gastroenterol. 2011;46(3):261–70. doi:10.3109/00365521.2010.531486.
111. Ito K, Ito H, Whang EE. Timing of cholecystectomy for biliary pancreatitis: do the data support current guidelines? J Gastrointest Surg. 2008;12(12):2164–70. doi:10.1007/s11605-008-0603-y.
112. Aboulian A, Chan T, Yaghoubian A, et al. Early cholecystectomy safely decreases hospital stay in patients with mild gallstone pancreatitis: a randomized prospective study. Ann Surg. 2010;251(4):615–9. doi:10.1097/SLA.0b013e3181c38f1f.
113. Hui CK, Lai KC, Yuen MF, et al. The role of cholecystectomy in reducing recurrent gallstone pancreatitis. Endoscopy. 2004;36(3):206–11. doi:10.1055/s-2004-814249.
114. van Geenen EJ, van der Peet DL, Mulder CJ, Cuesta MA, Bruno MJ. Recurrent acute biliary pancreatitis: the protective role of cholecystectomy and endoscopic sphincterotomy. Surg Endosc. 2009;23(5):950–6. doi:10.1007/s00464-009-0339-0.
115. Trust MD, Sheffield KM, Boyd CA, et al. Gallstone pancreatitis in older patients: are we operating enough? Surgery. 2011;150(3):515–25. doi:10.1016/j.surg.2011.07.072.
116. Lee JK, Ryu JK, Park JK, et al. Roles of endoscopic sphincterotomy and cholecystectomy in acute biliary pancreatitis. Hepatogastroenterology. 2008;55(88):1981–5.
117. Clavien PA, Richon J, Burgan S, Rohner A. Gallstone ileus. Br J Surg. 1990;77(7):737–42.
118. Ayantunde AA, Agrawal A. Gallstone ileus: diagnosis and management. World J Surg. 2007;31(6):1292–7. doi:10.1007/s00268-007-9011-9.
119. Ravikumar R, Williams JG. The operative management of gallstone ileus. Ann R Coll Surg Engl. 2010;92(4):279–81. doi:10.1308/003588410X12664192076377.
120. Yu CY, Lin CC, Shyu RY, et al. Value of CT in the diagnosis and management of gallstone ileus. World J Gastroenterol. 2005;11(14):2142–7.
121. Reisner RM, Cohen JR. Gallstone ileus: a review of 1001 reported cases. Am Surg. 1994;60(6):441–6.
122. Barie PS, Eachempati SR. Acute acalculous cholecystitis. Gastroenterol Clin North Am. 2010;39(2):343–57, x. doi:10.1016/j.gtc.2010.02.012.
123. Huffman JL, Schenker S. Acute acalculous cholecystitis: a review. Clin Gastroenterol Hepatol. 2010;8(1):15–22. doi:10.1016/j.cgh.2009.08.034.
124. Drossman DA, Dumitrascu DL. Rome III: new standard for functional gastrointestinal disorders. J Gastrointestin Liver Dis. 2006; 15(3):237–41.
125. Mahid SS, Jafri NS, Brangers BC, Minor KS, Hornung CA, Galandiuk S. Meta-analysis of cholecystectomy in symptomatic patients with positive hepatobiliary iminodiacetic acid scan results without gallstones. Arch Surg. 2009;144(2):180–7. doi:10.1001/archsurg.2008.543.
126. Baillie J. Sphincter of oddi dysfunction. Curr Gastroenterol Rep. 2010;12(2):130–4. doi:10.1007/s11894-010-0096-1.
127. Canlas KR, Branch MS. Role of endoscopic retrograde cholangiopancreatography in acute pancreatitis. World J Gastroenterol. 2007;13(47):6314–20.
128. Sabbaghian MS, Rich BS, Rothberger GD, et al. Evaluation of surgical outcomes and gallbladder characteristics in patients with biliary dyskinesia. J Gastrointest Surg. 2008;12(8):1324–30. doi:10.1007/s11605-008-0546-3.
129. Skipper K, Sligh S, Dunn E, Schwartz A. Laparoscopic cholecystectomy for an abnormal hepato-iminodiacetic acid scan: a worthwhile procedure. Am Surg. 2000;66(1):30–2.
130. Geenen JE, Hogan WJ, Dodds WJ, Toouli J, Venu RP. The efficacy of endoscopic sphincterotomy after cholecystectomy in patients with sphincter-of-oddi dysfunction. N Engl J Med. 1989;320(2):82–7. doi:10.1056/NEJM198901123200203.
131. Behar J, Corazziari E, Guelrud M, Hogan W, Sherman S, Toouli J. Functional gallbladder and sphincter of oddi disorders. Gastroenterology. 2006;130(5):1498–509. doi:10.1053/j.gastro.2005.11.063.
132. Morgan KA, Romagnuolo J, Adams DB. Transduodenal sphincteroplasty in the management of sphincter of oddi dysfunction and pancreas divisum in the modern era. J Am Coll Surg. 2008;206(5):908–14. doi:10.1016/j.jamcollsurg.2007.12.032; discussion 914–7.
133. Ash-Miles J, Roach H, Virjee J, Callaway M. More than just stones: a pictorial review of common and less common gallbladder pathologies. Curr Probl Diagn Radiol. 2008;37(5):189–202. doi:10.1067/j.cpradiol.2007.12.001.
134. Ito H, Hann LE, D'Angelica M, et al. Polypoid lesions of the gallbladder: diagnosis and followup. J Am Coll Surg. 2009;208(4):570–5. doi:10.1016/j.jamcollsurg.2009.01.011.
135. Gallahan WC, Conway JD. Diagnosis and management of gallbladder polyps. Gastroenterol Clin North Am. 2010;39(2):359–67, x. doi:10.1016/j.gtc.2010.02.001.
136. Koga A, Watanabe K, Fukuyama T, Takiguchi S, Nakayama F. Diagnosis and operative indications for polypoid lesions of the gallbladder. Arch Surg. 1988;123(1):26–9.
137. Zielinski MD, Atwell TD, Davis PW, Kendrick ML, Que FG. Comparison of surgically resected polypoid lesions of the gallbladder to their pre-operative ultrasound characteristics. J Gastrointest Surg. 2009;13(1):19–25. doi:10.1007/s11605-008-0725-2.
138. Kwon W, Jang JY, Lee SE, Hwang DW, Kim SW. Clinicopathologic features of polypoid lesions of the gallbladder and risk factors of gallbladder cancer. J Korean Med Sci. 2009;24(3):481–7. doi:10.3346/jkms.2009.24.3.481.
139. Yang HL, Sun YG, Wang Z. Polypoid lesions of the gallbladder: diagnosis and indications for surgery. Br J Surg. 1992; 79(3):227–9.
140. Choi WB, Lee SK, Kim MH, et al. A new strategy to predict the neoplastic polyps of the gallbladder based on a scoring system using EUS. Gastrointest Endosc. 2000;52(3):372–9. doi:10.1067/mge.2000.108041.
141. Mishra G, Conway JD. Endoscopic ultrasound in the evaluation of radiologic abnormalities of the liver and biliary tree. Curr Gastroenterol Rep. 2009;11(2):150–4.
142. Sugiyama M, Atomi Y, Yamato T. Endoscopic ultrasonography for differential diagnosis of polypoid gall bladder lesions: analysis in surgical and follow up series. Gut. 2000;46(2):250–4.

143. Kubota K, Bandai Y, Noie T, Ishizaki Y, Teruya M, Makuuchi M. How should polypoid lesions of the gallbladder be treated in the era of laparoscopic cholecystectomy? Surgery. 1995;117(5):481–7.
144. Colecchia A, Larocca A, Scaioli E, et al. Natural history of small gallbladder polyps is benign: evidence from a clinical and pathogenetic study. Am J Gastroenterol. 2009;104(3):624–9. doi:10.1038/ajg.2008.99.
145. Park JY, Hong SP, Kim YJ, et al. Long-term follow up of gallbladder polyps. J Gastroenterol Hepatol. 2009;24(2):219–22. doi:10.1111/j.1440-1746.2008.05689.x.
146. Sicklick JK, Choti MA. Controversies in the surgical management of cholangiocarcinoma and gallbladder cancer. Semin Oncol. 2005;32(6 Suppl 9):S112–7. doi:10.1053/j.seminoncol.2005.04.018.
147. Eslick GD. Epidemiology of gallbladder cancer. Gastroenterol Clin North Am. 2010;39(2):307–30, ix. doi:10.1016/j.gtc.2010.02.011.
148. Mastoraki A, Papanikolaou IS, Konstandiadou I, Sakorafas G, Safioleas M. Facing the challenge of treating gallbladder carcinoma. review of the literature. Hepatogastroenterology. 2010;57(98):215–9.
149. Jayaraman S, Jarnagin WR. Management of gallbladder cancer. Gastroenterol Clin North Am. 2010;39(2):331–42, x. doi:10.1016/j.gtc.2010.02.006.
150. Weber SM, DeMatteo RP, Fong Y, Blumgart LH, Jarnagin WR. Staging laparoscopy in patients with extrahepatic biliary carcinoma. analysis of 100 patients. Ann Surg. 2002;235(3):392–9.

Diverticulitis

13

Frederick Moore and Chasen A. Croft

Anatomy of the Colon

The colon is a continuous tube extending from the ileocecal valve to the rectum. It is composed of four segments: the ascending colon, transverse colon, descending colon, and sigmoid colon. The first section, the ascending colon, extends along the retroperitoneum for approximately 20 cm from the ileocecal valve upwards towards the transverse colon. The anterior and lateral segments of the ascending colon are completely intraperitoneal whereas the posterior segment is completely retroperitoneal. The transverse colon extends from two fixed positions, the hepatic and splenic flexures. It measures about 45 cm in length. As the transverse colon is completely invested in peritoneum, it is completely mobile. Superiorly, the transverse colon is attached to the greater curvature of the stomach by the gastrocolic ligament which leads to the greater omentum. Posteriorly, it is connected to the retroperitoneum by the transverse mesocolon. The descending colon extends caudally from the splenic flexure towards the sigmoid colon, a distance of approximately 25 cm. Like the ascending colon, the descending colon is fixed within the retroperitoneum. The descending colon is relatively thin walled and transitions to the thicker, mobile sigmoid colon at the pelvic brim. In contrast to other segments of the colon, the sigmoid colon has a small diameter with a thick wall which varies in length from 15 to 50 cm (average 40 cm). It is covered by the peritoneum and, like the transverse colon, is very mobile. The sigmoid colon forms a characteristic S shape as it descends into the pelvis where it transitions into the rectum.

The colon receives arterial blood flow via two main arterial trunks, the superior mesenteric artery (SMA) and the inferior mesenteric artery (IMA). The SMA and IMA are direct branches off of the aorta, with the SMA supplying blood flow to the third and fourth portions of the duodenum, jejunum, and ileum. The ileocolic artery, the terminal branch of the SMA, supplies the terminal ileum, cecum, and appendix. The right colic artery usually arises directly from the SMA and supplies the ascending colon and the hepatic flexure; however, it is absent in up to 20 % of the population. The middle colic artery is a proximal branch of the SMA and divides into the right and left branches, which supply the majority of the transverse colon. The IMA originates proximal to the aortic bifurcation. The first branch, the left colic artery, supplies the distal transverse colon, the splenic flexure, and the descending colon. However, the area of the splenic flexure has inconsistent collateral circulation and is vulnerable to ischemia during even brief periods of hypotension. This is commonly referred to as a "watershed" area. The sigmoid colon is supplied via an arcade, formed from two to six sigmoid branches which collateralize with the left colic artery. This arcade proceeds proximally and connects the SMA and IMA, forming a continuous marginal artery arcade. An additional collateral flow is formed from the arc of Riolan or meandering mesenteric artery. This is a collateral artery that directly connects the SMA to the IMA, forming a vital collateral circulation should one of these arteries become occluded.

The venous and lymphatic drainage of the colon mirrors the arterial supply. The drainage from the ascending and majority of the transverse colon is into the superior mesenteric vein (SMV). The SMV then joins the splenic vein to form the proximal portal vein. The inferior mesenteric vein collects venous blood from the distal transverse colon, descending colon, and sigmoid colon which ends at the distal splenic vein, just before the SMV and splenic vein form the portal vein. The lymphatics follow a similar pattern, draining into the para-aortic lymph basin, which in turn drains into the cisterna chyli.

F. Moore, MD, FACS (✉)
Department of Surgery, University of Florida,
1600 SW Archer Road, Gainesville, FL 32608, USA
e-mail: frederick.moore@surgery.ufl.edu

C.A. Croft, MD
Department of Surgery, Shands at the University of Florida,
1600 SW Archer Road, M-602, 100108, Gainesville, FL 32610, USA
e-mail: chasen.croft@surgery.ufl.edu

J.A. Yelon, F.A. Luchette (eds.), *Geriatric Trauma and Critical Care*,
DOI 10.1007/978-1-4614-8501-8_13, © Springer Science+Business Media New York 2014

Effects of Aging on Colon Motility and Function

The primary function of the colon is to provide a site for bacteria-induced fermentation, storage of waste, and maintenance of water balance. Like all organs of the body, the colon is subject to the effects of aging. However, the exact effects are poorly understood. With the gastrointestinal tract, there is a continuously regulated balance of intestinal epithelial proliferation and apoptosis. Alterations in this balance have been proven to be a causative factor in the development of colorectal cancer [1]. Sipos et al. reported that, on average, 4–5 days are required for colonic mucosa renewal [2]. While it seems intuitive that as the colon ages the rate of colon mucosal regeneration slows, this, in fact, seems to not be the case. Recent data suggests that the rate of colon epithelial proliferation may increase with age, while the rate of apoptosis decreases [3]. This corroborates with the "two-hit" hypothesis of carcinogenesis proposed by Knudson [4].

A frequent problem in the aging population is a slow-transit constipation. Studies of transit times in the aged show either a slower rate of passage through the colon amongst the elderly or no differences with aging [5–7]. As the transit time increases, the transluminal pressure within the colon similarly increases. Stewart et al. studied nearly 3,200 patients aged 65 and older, 26 % of women and 16 % of men reported recurrent constipation, finding a significant increase in reported constipation with increasing age [8]. Of the 13 factors identified as significantly contributing to constipation, the most important were age, sex, total number of medications consumed, pain in the abdomen, and the presence of hemorrhoids. In addition to select demographic factors contributing to slow-transit constipation, immunocytochemistry studies have demonstrated decreased levels of interstitial cells of Cajal, the gastrointestinal pacemakers [9].

Epidemiology and Pathology of Diverticular Disease

Colonic diverticula are herniations of the colonic mucosa and submucosa through defects in the muscular layer resulting in the formation of pulsion or pseudodiverticula. Pseudodiverticula emerge through the muscularis propria along the antimesenteric tenia at points of penetration by the vasa recta, which supply the mucosa and submucosa, creating weak areas within the muscular layer. Although the terminology used to describe the conditions associated with *diverticular disease* are often used interchangeably, the meanings are quite different. Diverticulosis is simply the presence of colonic diverticula, without associated inflammation. Symptomatic diverticular disease is diverticulosis associated with pain or alterations in bowel habits in the absence of radiologic evidence of diverticular inflammation. In contrast, diverticulitis refers to inflammation of one or more diverticula. This term is actually a misnomer, as the disease is actually a perforation of a diverticulum with resultant extraluminal extravasation of feces. The term *peridiverticulitis* has been proposed to more accurately describe the infectious process.

Diverticular disease is a common disease that affects 20 % of men and women older than 40 years of age, 50 % of those older than 60, and more than 60 % of those over the age of 80. In the United States, diverticular disease accounts for greater than 300,000 hospitalizations yearly, with estimated direct health-care costs in excess of $2.4 billion annually [10–13]. One quarter of all patients will develop complicated diverticular disease, defined as diverticulitis associated with phlegmon, abscess, fistula, free perforation, or stricture. The disease is known as the *disease of the industrial revolution*, since there are no reports or pathologic specimens documenting evidence of diverticular disease prior to this period [14]. During the end of the nineteenth century, the process of roller-milling wheat was introduced in Europe and the United States, a technique that removes two-thirds of the fiber content of wheat. Coincident with the implementation of this new technique, diverticulosis was observed in the first decade of the twentieth century. It was initially regarded as a pathologic curiosity. It is now known that a diet low in fiber is a contributing factor in the development of diverticular disease [14, 15]. In a study of nearly 48,000 US men, a low-fiber diet increased the risk of symptomatic diverticular disease by two- to threefold over a 4-year period [16]. In addition to low dietary fiber, alterations in colonic intraluminal pressures have been shown in patients with diverticular disease. Although resting intraluminal pressures between diverticular disease patients and controls do not differ significantly, higher pressures have been demonstrated in segments of colon with diverticula [17]. In addition, later studies indicate increased colonic motility, as assessed by the number and amplitude of bowel wall contractions, in the sigmoid colon of patients with diverticular disease [18–20]. Therefore, both a low-fiber diet and colonic dysmotility have been implicated in the pathogenesis of diverticular disease.

Another cardinal feature of diverticular disease is abnormalities of the muscularis propria. Whiteway et al. demonstrated that the colonic muscle cells in diverticular disease specimens are normal compared to controls; however, the elastin content of the taeniae coli increases by 200 % [21]. The elastin may be responsible for the shortening or "contracture" of the taeniae, which in turn leads to the concertina-like corrugation of the circular muscle [21]. This abnormality can be seen on barium enema radiographs, a pathognomonic sign. Other studies have demonstrated an alteration in the collagen deposition of the aging colon. Thomson et al. showed that as the colon ages, the collagen fibrils of the left colon increase in size and become more tightly packed than those of the right colon [22]. They further showed that these changes are accentuated in diverticular disease patients. Furthermore, the ratio of type I collagen to type III collagen appears to be altered. In diseased segments of the colon, there is decreased mature type I collagen and increased type III collagen, with a resulting lower collagen ratio I/III indicative of scarring [23].

Treatment of Diverticular Disease

Uncomplicated (Simple) Diverticulitis

The treatment of diverticular disease can be divided into two simple categories: medical management and surgical therapy. The decision of which algorithm to follow is determined by the acuity of disease (complicated vs. uncomplicated), patient comorbidities, and patient compliance. Uncomplicated diverticulitis, defined as acute diverticulitis without associated abscess, fistula, obstruction, or free perforation, can be diagnosed on the basis of clinical criteria alone. Most patients will present with left lower quadrant pain, fever, and leukocytosis. Other associated findings may include nausea and vomiting, constipation or diarrhea, dysuria, and urinary frequency. If the clinical picture is unclear, further diagnostic studies should be performed. The two most commonly performed radiologic studies used to aide in the diagnosis of diverticular disease are water-soluble contrast enema and computed tomography scan; however, ultrasonography and magnetic resonance imaging have also been used. Due to the risks of extravasation of barium from the perforation in a patient with acute diverticulitis, barium enema should be avoided in the acute setting. The American College of Radiology currently recommends computed tomography (CT) as the preferred imaging modality in patients with clinically suspected acute diverticulitis [24, 25]. Once the diagnosis of uncomplicated diverticulitis is made, it is should be treated with bowel rest, analgesics, and antibiotics; although, some authors now suggest the use of clear liquids is acceptable [26]. Conservative management has been shown to induce resolution of acute, uncomplicated diverticulitis in 70–100 % of patients [26–29].

The selection of antibiotic for medical management of acute, uncomplicated diverticulitis should cover the spectrum of bacteria commonly found in the colonic flora. This includes gram-negative rods and anaerobes [30]. The most commonly isolated aerobic gram-negative species is *Escherichia coli* and the predominant anaerobe is *Bacteroides fragilis*, present in up to 94 % of patients with intra-abdominal infections [30, 31]. Combination therapy (such as clindamycin and gentamicin) or monotherapy (such as cefoxitin) has been shown to be equally effective in the treatment of uncomplicated diverticulitis [29]. In select patients, particularly those with

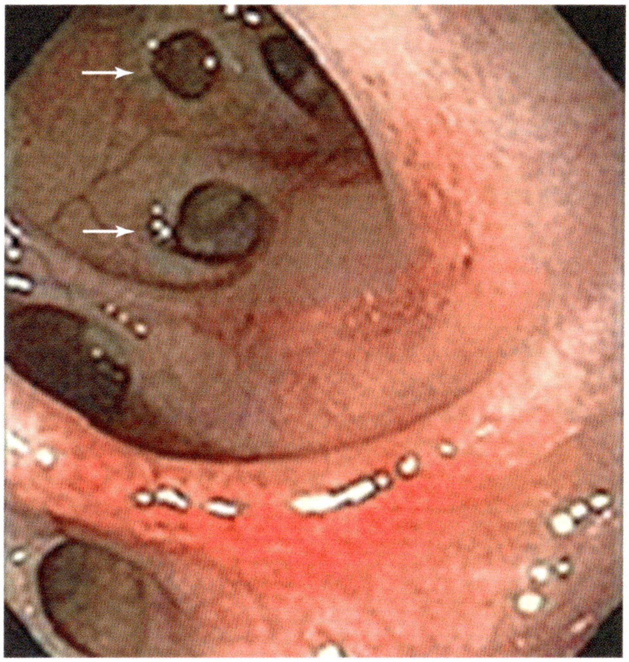

Fig. 13.1 Colonoscopy showing multiple diverticula (*white arrows*) without evidence of diverticulitis

only minimal tenderness and who are otherwise healthy, ambulatory treatment with oral broad-spectrum antibiotics (trimethoprim-sulfamethoxazole, double-strength twice daily, plus metronidazole, 500 mg every 6 h for 10 days to 2 weeks) may be utilized. However, this outpatient regimen should not be offered to immunocompromised patients, including those receiving chronic steroids, as their clinical exam cannot be reliably followed and overwhelming sepsis can ensue with alarming rapidity. Following successful nonoperative treatment of uncomplicated diverticulitis, patients should be placed on a high-fiber diet (30–40 g of soluble fiber per day) once the acute inflammation has resolved.

After recovery of an initial episode of diverticulitis, patients should be evaluated with a complete colonic examination. Appropriate studies include a combination of flexible sigmoidoscopy and single-contrast or double-contrast barium enema or complete colonoscopy [26]. The preferred test is a colonoscopic examination, which can directly visualize the colonic mucosa and evaluate for underlying sigmoid cancer, a condition that may be missed with barium enema alone (Fig. 13.1). More than 75 % of patients respond to conservative management and a recurrence rate of 20–25 % can be expected, mostly within the first 5 years after an initial attack [32–34].

Complicated Diverticulitis

In contrast to uncomplicated diverticulitis, patients with acute, complicated diverticulitis typically present with

Fig. 13.2 Western Trauma Association Complicated Diverticulitis Score (Adapted from Western Trauma Association Critical Decisions on Trauma: Management of Complicated Diverticulitis [45])

Western Trauma Association Complicated Diverticulitis Score	
Grade IA	• Phlegmon with no abscess
Grade IB	• Phlegmon with abscess <4 cm
Grade II	• Phlegmon with abscess >4 cm
Grade III	• Purulent peritonitis
Grade IV	• Feculent Peritonitis

localized or generalized peritonitis, fever, and leukocytosis. The diagnosis should be confirmed radiographically, with either computed tomography or magnetic resonance imaging. In 1978, Hinchey et al. published the first classification system to standardize the nomenclature describing the breadth of perforated diverticular disease [35]. This classification has been used since the 1970s, before the advent of computed tomography. It describes four stages of perforated disease. Stage I disease includes pericolic abscess or phlegmon. Stage II disease is a walled-off pelvic, intra-abdominal, or retroperitoneal abscess. Stage III disease describes generalized purulent peritonitis and stage IV disease is generalized feculent peritonitis. Since the advent of this classification system, few modifications have been introduced. The Western Trauma Association (WTA) consensus has modified this system to reflect contemporary management of complicated diverticular disease (Fig. 13.2).

The optimal treatment of patients with complicated diverticulitis has undergone significant changes with the evolution of surgical techniques and nonoperative therapies. As late as the 1990s, the standard treatment for complicated diverticulitis was surgical resection and colostomy often performed in a multistage procedure, a technique described in the 1920s [36]. A paradigm shift has occurred mostly as the result of advances in antibiotics, interventional radiology, and critical care medicine.

Patients with WTA grade IA (phlegmon with no abscess (Fig. 13.3)) and grade IB (phlegmon with abscess <4 cm) should be treated with hospitalization, bowel rest, and intravenous antibiotics. Those who respond with resolution of pain, fever, and leukocytosis should be started on an oral diet and converted to oral antibiotics. Antibiotics should be continued for 14 days, from the initiation of intravenous antibiotics. Patients should undergo colonoscopy and be placed on a high-fiber diet following resolution of the acute inflammatory process. Those who fail conservative management should undergo definitive resection, described later in this chapter.

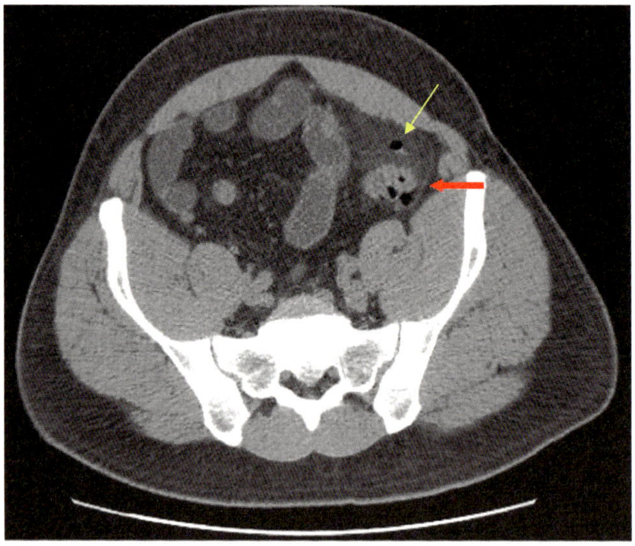

Fig. 13.3 Western Trauma Association Grade IA Complicated Diverticulitis. Computed tomography shows sigmoid diverticulitis (*red arrow*) with pericolonic phlegmon and small focus of extraluminal air (*yellow arrow*)

Patients with WTA grade II disease (phlegmon with abscess >4 cm), or those with abscesses not responding to conservative therapy, should undergo CT-guided percutaneous drainage (PCD) [26, 37]. Seventy to ninety-three percent of patients amenable to CT-guided PCD can be successfully

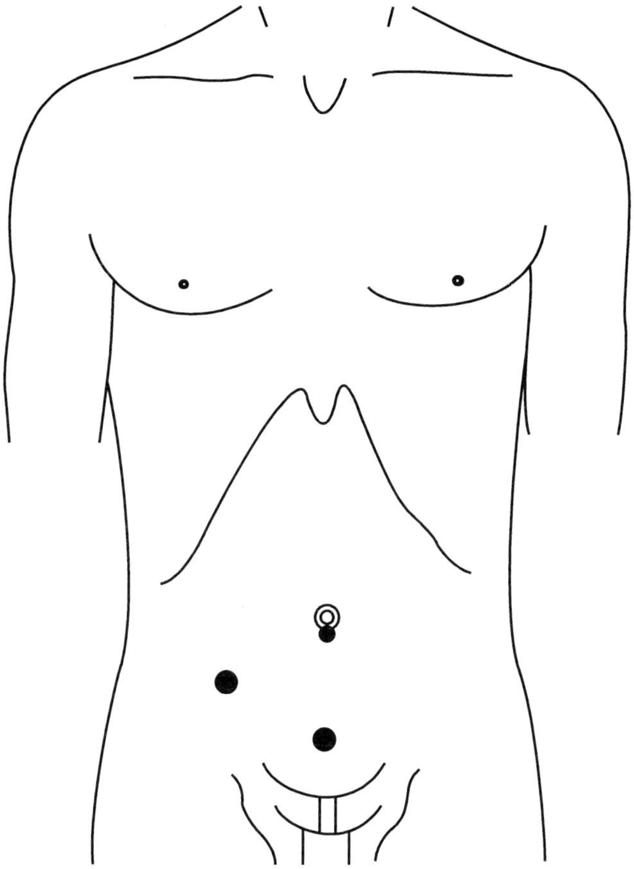

Fig. 13.4 Trocar placement for laparoscopic lavage. A 12 mm trocar is inserted at the umbilicus, and two 5 mm trocars are placed in the right lower quadrant and suprapubic positions

managed with this approach [38]. The preferred approach is transabdominal, either anterior or lateral. Other approaches include transgluteal, transperitoneal, transvaginal, or transanal. The potential advantage to performing CT-guided PCD is that it may avoid the need for urgent operation, allowing defervescence with resolution of inflammation prior to a definitive operation. These admitted patients should be treated with intravenous antibiotics and close clinical observations for evidence of treatment failure. The reported failure rates for CT-guided PCD range from 15 to 30 %. Complications, including bleeding, perforation of a hollow viscus, and fistula formation, occur in up to 5 % of patients. Although some authors suggest CT-guided PCD may avoid the need for definitive resection altogether, the American Society of Colon and Rectal Surgeons does not endorse this concept currently.

In patients whom CT-guided PCD is not feasible, laparoscopic lavage and drainage may be pursued. Once pneumoperitoneum is established, a 12 mm umbilical trocar is placed. Two 5 mm operating trocars are then placed in the right lower quadrant and suprapubic positions to assist with manipulation and lavage (Fig. 13.4). The patient should be positioned in Trendelenburg with a left tilt, with the surgeon and assistant on the patient's right side. The abdomen should be thoroughly inspected and all omental, small bowel, pelvic structures, and abdominal wall attachments should be mobilized away from the inflamed sigmoid colon. However, vigorous manipulation of the diseased segment of colon should be avoided. If there is no evidence of free perforation of the colon, the four quadrants of the abdomen are lavaged until the effluent is clear. A closed-suction drain can be placed in the pelvis and brought out through the right lower quadrant trocar site. Multiple studies have reported the use of laparoscopic lavage in patients with Hinchey II–IV diverticulitis with low complication rates (<8 %) and without the need to convert to an open procedure [39–41]. Successful laparoscopic lavage may control sepsis and allow patients to be bridged for an elective one-stage operation. Of note, in a study of laparoscopic lavage for the management of perforated diverticulitis, only 2 of 88 patients who underwent successful lavage required reoperation for diverticular disease at a median follow-up of 36 months [42]. Similar studies have questioned the need for definitive colon resection following successful laparoscopic lavage. However, trials to date have been limited by low numbers of subjects, and, at this time, definitive operation is the recommended treatment following laparoscopic lavage.

Diverticulitis Associated with Free Perforation

Free perforation associated with acute diverticulitis is classified as WTA grade III (purulent/Hinchey III) or grade IV (feculent/Hinchey IV) peritonitis. Patients who present with florid sepsis, hypotension, and significant metabolic derangements represent a surgical emergency that requires rapid resuscitation, broad-spectrum antibiotics, and prompt operative therapy. Depending on the hemodynamic stability, a truncated or "damage control" laparotomy may be performed. In the unstable patient, a limited resection of the inflamed colon and temporary abdominal closure should be performed. The patient is then returned to the intensive care unit for further resuscitation. Once the physiologic abnormalities are corrected, the patient is returned to the operating room for peritoneal lavage, sigmoid colectomy, and end-colostomy formation.

In patients who present with perforation, but whom are otherwise hemodynamically stable, a definitive resection may be undertaken. Ureteral stents can be used selectively in those patients with abscesses or excessive inflammation in the pelvis, which may aide in the identification of the ureters. The sigmoid colon is then mobilized, extending proximally to an area of the non-inflamed descending colon. The distal dissection should extend to the upper rectum. It should be noted that it is not necessary to resect all diverticula. The current *standard of care* therapy is the Hartmann's procedure, whereby the diseased colon is resected and a temporary end colostomy is performed. This procedure requires a second operation for reversal of the colostomy. However, there is currently much debate as whether to perform a primary resection with anastomosis (PRA) or a Hartmann's procedure (HP). Lidor et al. demonstrated that of more than 53,000 elderly patients studied, patients that underwent emergency surgery for complicated diverticulitis were older (76.8 vs. 73.9 years of age), had increase in-hospital mortality, had a greater rate of intestinal diversion, and had higher 30-day readmission rates [43]. Primary resection and anastomosis of the affected colon segment has been used in an attempt to minimize the morbidity and mortality associated with the reversal of Hartmann's procedure, which has a documented rate of morbidity as high as 50 %. Therefore, the choice of operation should be influenced by factors such as patient age, comorbidities, degree of contamination, and mode of presentation. In a meta-analysis of 15 studies comparing PRA to HP, PRA was shown to have reduced morbidity and mortality, even when used in an emergency setting [44]. However, all studies were limited by significant patient selection bias, where patients with less comorbidity underwent PRA. Currently PRA should be reserved for patients with more favorable comorbid criteria, a lesser degree of contamination, and no preoperative hemodynamic instability.

Summary

Diverticular disease is commonly seen in the elderly population. Thorough history and physical examination combined with computer tomography will diagnose and grade nearly all patients. Treatment algorithms (see Fig. 13.5) will be based upon the patient's preexisting medical conditions, physiologic status, and grade of diverticulitis. Newer concepts including laparoscopic lavage and single-stage operations are gaining acceptance as more data becomes available.

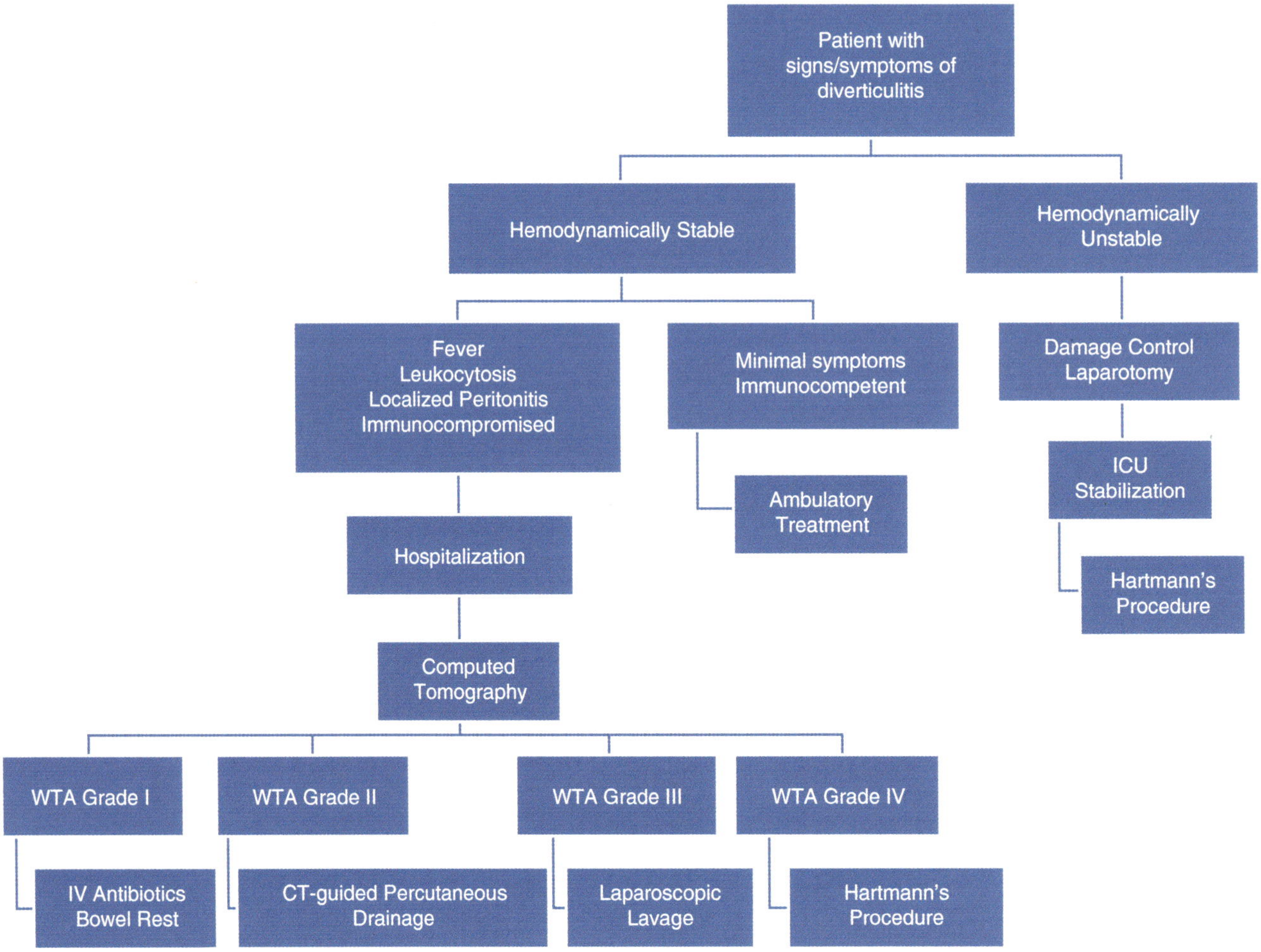

Fig. 13.5 Diverticulitis management algorithm. *Abbreviations*: *WTA* Western Trauma Association, *CT* Computed Tomography

References

1. Fearon ER, Vogelstein B. A genetic model for colorectal tumorigenesis. Cell. 1990;61(5):759–67.
2. Sipos F, et al. Growth in epithelial cell proliferation and apoptosis correlates specifically to the inflammation activity of inflammatory bowel diseases: ulcerative colitis shows specific p53- and EGFR expression alterations. Dis Colon Rectum. 2005;48(4):775–86.
3. Xiao Z-Q, et al. Aging is associated with increased proliferation and decreased apoptosis in the colonic mucosa. Mech Ageing Dev. 2001;122(15):1849–64.
4. Knudson Jr AG. Mutation and cancer: statistical study of retinoblastoma. Proc Natl Acad Sci U S A. 1971;68(4):820–3.
5. Metcalf AM, et al. Simplified assessment of segmental colonic transit. Gastroenterology. 1987;92(1):40–7.
6. Becker U, Elsborg L. A new method for the determination of gastrointestinal transit times. Scand J Gastroenterol. 1979;14(3):355–9.
7. Madsen JL. Effects of gender, age, and body mass index on gastrointestinal transit times. Dig Dis Sci. 1992;37(10):1548–53.
8. Stewart RB, et al. Correlates of constipation in an ambulatory elderly population. Am J Gastroenterol. 1992;87(7):859–64.
9. Lyford GL, et al. Pan-colonic decrease in interstitial cells of Cajal in patients with slow transit constipation. Gut. 2002;51(4):496–501.
10. Kozak LJ, DeFrances CJ, Hall MJ. National hospital discharge survey: 2004 annual summary with detailed diagnosis and procedure data. Vital Health Stat 13. 2004;2006(162):1–209.
11. Sandler RS, et al. The burden of selected digestive diseases in the United States. Gastroenterology. 2002;122(5):1500–11.
12. Almy TP, Howell DA. Medical progress. Diverticular disease of the colon. N Engl J Med. 1980;302(6):324–31.
13. Parks TG. Natural history of diverticular disease of the colon. Clin Gastroenterol. 1975;4(1):53–69.
14. Painter NS, Burkitt DP. Diverticular disease of the colon, a 20th century problem. Clin Gastroenterol. 1975;4(1):3–21.
15. Painter NS. Diverticular disease of the colon. The first of the Western diseases shown to be due to a deficiency of dietary fibre. S Afr Med J. 1982;61(26):1016–20.
16. Aldoori WH, et al. A prospective study of diet and the risk of symptomatic diverticular disease in men. Am J Clin Nutr. 1994;60(5): 757–64.
17. Painter NS, et al. Segmentation and the localization of intraluminal pressures in the human colon, with special reference to the pathogenesis of colonic diverticula. Gastroenterology. 1965;49:169–77.
18. Commane DM, et al. Diet, ageing and genetic factors in the pathogenesis of diverticular disease. World J Gastroenterol. 2009;15(20): 2479–88.
19. Trotman IF, Misiewicz JJ. Sigmoid motility in diverticular disease and the irritable bowel syndrome. Gut. 1988;29(2):218–22.
20. Bassotti G, et al. Twenty-four hour recordings of colonic motility in patients with diverticular disease: evidence for abnormal motility and propulsive activity. Dis Colon Rectum. 2001;44(12): 1814–20.
21. Whiteway J, Morson BC. Elastosis in diverticular disease of the sigmoid colon. Gut. 1985;26(3):258–66.
22. Thomson HJ, et al. Submucosal collagen changes in the normal colon and in diverticular disease. Int J Colorectal Dis. 1987;2(4): 208–13.
23. Stumpf M, et al. Increased distribution of collagen type III and reduced expression of matrix metalloproteinase 1 in patients with diverticular disease. Int J Colorectal Dis. 2001;16(5):271–5.
24. Balfe DM, et al. Evaluation of left lower quadrant pain. American College of Radiology. ACR Appropriateness Criteria. Radiology. 2000;215 Suppl:167–71.
25. Hammond NA, Nikolaidis P, Miller FH. Left lower-quadrant pain: guidelines from the American College of Radiology appropriateness criteria. Am Fam Physician. 2010;82(7):766–70.
26. Wong WD, et al. Practice parameters for the treatment of sigmoid diverticulitis – supporting documentation. The Standards Task Force. The American Society of Colon and Rectal Surgeons. Dis Colon Rectum. 2000;43(3):290–7.
27. Thompson WG, Patel DG. Clinical picture of diverticular disease of the colon. Clin Gastroenterol. 1986;15(4):903–16.
28. Cheskin LJ, Bohlman M, Schuster MM. Diverticular disease in the elderly. Gastroenterol Clin North Am. 1990;19(2):391–403.
29. Kellum JM, et al. Randomized, prospective comparison of cefoxitin and gentamicin-clindamycin in the treatment of acute colonic diverticulitis. Clin Ther. 1992;14(3):376–84.
30. Brook I, Frazier EH. Aerobic and anaerobic microbiology in intra-abdominal infections associated with diverticulitis. J Med Microbiol. 2000;49(9):827–30.
31. Nichols RL. Management of intra-abdominal sepsis. Am J Med. 1986;80(6B):204–9.
32. Larson DM, Masters SS, Spiro HM. Medical and surgical therapy in diverticular disease: a comparative study. Gastroenterology. 1976;71(5):734–7.
33. Makela J, et al. Natural history of diverticular disease: when to operate? Dis Colon Rectum. 1998;41(12):1523–8.
34. Parks TG. Natural history of diverticular disease of the colon. A review of 521 cases. Br Med J. 1969;4(5684):639–42.
35. Hinchey EJ, Schaal PG, Richards GK. Treatment of perforated diverticular disease of the colon. Adv Surg. 1978;12:85–109.
36. Judd ES, Pollock LW. Diverticulitis of the colon. Ann Surg. 1924;80(3):425–38.
37. Soumian S, et al. Management of Hinchey II diverticulitis. World J Gastroenterol. 2008;14(47):7163–9.
38. Kaiser AM, et al. The management of complicated diverticulitis and the role of computed tomography. Am J Gastroenterol. 2005;100(4):910–7.
39. Bretagnol F, et al. Emergency laparoscopic management of perforated sigmoid diverticulitis: a promising alternative to more radical procedures. J Am Coll Surg. 2008;206(4):654–7.
40. Franklin Jr ME, et al. Long-term experience with the laparoscopic approach to perforated diverticulitis plus generalized peritonitis. World J Surg. 2008;32(7):1507–11.
41. Alamili M, Gogenur I, Rosenberg J. Acute complicated diverticulitis managed by laparoscopic lavage. Dis Colon Rectum. 2009;52(7):1345–9.
42. Myers E, et al. Laparoscopic peritoneal lavage for generalized peritonitis due to perforated diverticulitis. Br J Surg. 2008;95(1):97–101.
43. Lidor AO, et al. Elective surgery for diverticulitis is associated with high risk of intestinal diversion and hospital readmission in older adults. J Gastrointest Surg. 2010;14(12):1867–73; discussion 1873–4.
44. Constantinides VA, et al. Primary resection with anastomosis vs. Hartmann's procedure in nonelective surgery for acute colonic diverticulitis: a systematic review. Dis Colon Rectum. 2006; 49(7):966–81.
45. Moore FA, et al. Western Trauma Association/Critical Decisions in Trauma: Management of Complicated Diverticulitis. J Trauma 2012;73:1363–9.

Intestinal Obstruction

14

Andrew H. Stephen, Charles A. Adams Jr., and William G. Cioffi

Introduction

Intestinal obstruction in the elderly is a very challenging entity to manage since it requires timely clinical judgment and the margin for error is narrow. The timing of operative intervention is particularly difficult since the risk to benefit ratio varies widely during the course of the disease process. As our population ages, the burden of this disease on our healthcare system is growing, and the management of intestinal obstruction becomes more complex as patient's age and comorbidities increase. In the elderly intestinal obstruction is a far more frequent cause of abdominal pain than it is in younger patients where nonobstructive etiologies predominate. Also, the elderly are much more likely to present with more diverse causes of obstruction such as gallstone ileus, obturator hernia, bezoars, cecal and sigmoid volvulus, and neoplasms than are younger patients. In addition to these unusual causes of obstruction, the more common etiologies such as postoperative adhesions, ventral and inguinal hernias, and inflammatory bowel disease also affect the geriatric population adding to the complexity of clinical decision making in this group.

Intestinal obstruction is a "surgical disease." This fact is borne out by recent investigations showing decreased mortality and costs, with shorter lengths of stay when patients with obstruction are admitted to a surgical service even though the management typically is nonoperative. In fact, only a small percentage of patients with obstruction require immediate or urgent operation after their initial presentation [1, 2]. However it remains of paramount importance to identify those patients that do require immediate operation as well as those patients who have been initially managed nonoperatively but have progressed to the need for exploration. If the latter is missed, intestinal perforation, bowel ischemia, peritonitis, and loss of significant amounts of bowel occur, all of which greatly increase the mortality of intestinal obstruction in this group. In the elderly, the signs of clinical deterioration are often harder to delineate due to these patients having a greater burden of confounding comorbidities and more frequent alterations of mental status than younger patients. It is precisely these comorbidities coupled with a generalized decrease in physiologic reserve though that make timely management decisions regarding operative intervention even more critical in the elderly. While there is an inherent tendency to have concern over whether an elderly patient can tolerate abdominal exploration, there should also be significant concern over whether such a patient can withstand continued pain, fluid losses, electrolyte derangements, or worse yet peritonitis and ischemic intestine from a delay in operative intervention.

Etiologies

More than 20 % of emergency abdominal surgery is performed for intestinal obstruction and of these small bowel obstructions outweigh colonic obstructions by a 3 a 1 margin [3]. Across all ages, adhesions and hernias remain the two most common causes of small bowel obstruction and this has remained remarkably constant over time since a review from well over 100 years ago to a more recent review document that these are the two dominant etiologies of bowel obstruction [3]. In a geriatric patient, the three most common sources of intestinal obstruction are postoperative adhesions with the

A.H. Stephen, MD
Division of Trauma and Surgical Critical Care, Warren Alpert Medical School at Brown University, Rhode Island Hospital, 593 Eddy Street, Providence, RI 02903, USA
e-mail: andrew_stephen@brown.edu, astephen@lifespan.org

C.A. Adams Jr., MD, FACS
Department of Surgery, Alpert Medical School of Brown University, Rhode Island Hospital, 593 Eddy Street, APC 453, Providence, RI 02903, USA
e-mail: cadams1@lifespan.org

W.G. Cioffi, MD (✉)
Department of Surgery, Rhode Island Hospital, 593 Eddy Street, APC 431, Providence, RI 02903, USA
e-mail: wcioffi@lifespan.org

J.A. Yelon, F.A. Luchette (eds.), *Geriatric Trauma and Critical Care*,
DOI 10.1007/978-1-4614-8501-8_14, © Springer Science+Business Media New York 2014

highest prevalence seen following colorectal and pelvic operations, incarcerated or strangulated hernias, and neoplasms. Bowel obstruction in the elderly is a very serious condition since it must be remembered that greater than half the deaths in obstructed patients occur after the age of 65. In accordance with an aging population, the peak age of patients undergoing operation for intestinal obstructions has risen to the seventh decade [4]. In light of the fact that over 30 % of our population will be over the age of 65 by the year 2030, it is very likely that an even larger percentage of patients requiring admission and intervention for intestinal obstruction will be of advanced age.

Other causes of small intestinal obstruction in the elderly that are less common but must be considered include small bowel tumors, both primary and secondary from metastatic melanoma or direct invasion from colon cancers, Crohn's disease, volvulus, intussusception, internal hernia, bezoar formation, strictures, and gallstone ileus. While primary small bowel tumors only make up approximately 5 % of all gastrointestinal neoplasms, intestinal obstruction is the most frequent presenting sign of a host of neoplastic processes including small bowel lymphomas, stromal tumors, carcinoid tumors, adenocarcinomas, and metastases [5]. Gallstone ileus resulting from cholecystoenteric fistula and subsequent stone impaction in the terminal ileum is a particularly interesting etiology that almost exclusively presents in the elderly population and accounts for 1–4 % of mechanical intestinal obstructions [6]. Patients that suffer from gallstone ileus also tend to be debilitated and have significant comorbidities and diagnosis can be challenging. Small bowel obstruction in the elderly patient with no prior history of surgery and no hernias should raise the possibility of gallstone ileus or malignant obstruction, but the finding of air in the biliary tree is pathognomonic of gallstone ileus.

Colonic obstructions are significantly more prevalent in elderly patients rather than younger patients. In developing nations, where the dietary intake of crude fiber is very high, colonic volvulus and specifically sigmoid volvulus is a major etiology of large bowel obstructions. Many years ago this was also true in the United States but now colonic tumors are by far the most common etiology of large bowel obstruction followed by inflammation from repeated episodes of diverticulitis, ischemic stricture, and incarcerated hernias. The sigmoid colon is the most frequent location of obstructing colon cancers, and in general the likelihood of a cancer-causing obstruction increases as its location moves distally. Other important causes of large bowel obstruction include the functional, nonmechanical etiologies that are generally pertinent only to those of advanced age with significant debilitation, namely, colonic pseudo-obstruction, also known as Ogilvie's syndrome. The approach to treatment of colonic dysfunction is very different from that of mechanical causes of obstruction and will be discussed later in detail. Lastly, in the elderly population constipation and stool impaction are not trivial causes of colonic obstruction and must be considered in the differential diagnosis.

Presentation

Patients with intestinal obstruction pose significant diagnostic challenges due to the varied nature of how the patient presents. In order to create a systematic approach to the patient with suspected obstruction, all signs and symptoms of obstruction should be considered separately. The most specific symptom of bowel obstruction is a prolonged period without bowel function, namely, a complete cessation of the production of flatus or stool. Every effort should be made when obtaining a history of present illness to determine from the patient or family members when the last signs of bowel function occurred and also to gather an estimate of how often the patient's bowel function normally occurs as in the elderly this can be quite variable. Additional commonly reported symptoms include abdominal pain that is colicky in nature but that can progress to more diffuse, severe, and constant pain, which is typically accompanied by nausea and emesis. Depending on the location of the obstruction, the emesis can range from minimal, as with proximal obstructions, to voluminous as seen with distal pathology. In the case of gastric volvulus, there can be severe retching but almost little or no production of vomitus. More distal obstructions tend to produce large emesis since in addition to whatever food or fluid has been consumed, the proximal gastrointestinal tract makes several liters of secretions when the summation of gastric, biliary, duodenal, and pancreatic secretions are considered and contribute to the amount of emesis. Feculent emesis due to long-standing pooling and bacterial overgrowth of intestinal contents proximal to an obstruction is not an unusual finding. Cheadle's review on "The importance of early diagnosis of small bowel obstruction" found abdominal pain and vomiting to be the most commonly noted symptoms in 92 and 82 % of patients, respectively, in a review of 3,000 patients presenting with bowel obstruction [7]. There are also several less-specific symptoms frequently reported that are likely related to dehydration and lack of nutritional intake associated with obstruction including fatigue, general malaise, and weakness.

Abdominal tenderness and distention are the two most commonly noted and classical physical findings of intestinal obstruction. In multiple investigations and reviews, it is unclear which of these two findings is more commonly present, but regardless they are each seen in greater than half of patients with obstruction [7]. Distention though tends to be less noticeable in more proximal obstructions such as gastric volvulus, gastric outlet obstruction, duodenal obstruction, and jejunal obstruction, while more distal obstructions such as small bowel obstruction due to adhesions or hernias involving the ileum, cecal volvulus, colonic masses, and colonic pseudo-obstruction can lead to marked and impressive distention due to large volumes of air and fluid that can accumulate in the gastrointestinal tract. Abdominal tenderness implies irritation of the peritoneal surfaces and in the initial stages is usually due to the apposition of a dilated viscus against the peritoneum.

While it is difficult to quantify, it is important to evaluate the degree of the presenting symptoms and signs to aid in determining what surgical process is occurring. Patients with partial obstructions often report a decrease in their stool production or frequency or that they have recently developed intermittent loose stools and do not report total and prolonged obstipation as is more commonly reported by patients with complete obstructions. Patients with partial obstructions tend to present with relapsing and remitting degrees of tolerance of oral intake or that they have altered their diet to take mainly liquids as they feel this does not lead to as much abdominal pain as taking solid food. Conversely patients with strangulated intestinal obstruction with resulting ischemic bowel that requires urgent surgical intervention tend to present with greater degrees of abdominal tenderness and even peritonitis. While all patients should be assessed carefully, it is true that peritoneal signs such as abdominal guarding and rebound tenderness have been shown to be present in less than 50 % of patients with small bowel obstruction and are also of limited sensitivity and specificity in detecting strangulation [8, 9]. While nonspecific, the general appearance of patients harboring ischemic intestine from obstruction is often ominous and patients can appear in significant distress and discomfort, as well as appear diaphoretic.

Unfortunately there is no set of symptoms, signs, or any criteria that can be utilized to determine the presence of nonviable bowel due to obstruction, but presenting vital signs may yield important clues. Tachycardia can be due to dehydration and hypovolemia related to obstruction, pain, or marked inflammation and cytokine release from ischemic intestine. Fever can also be an ominous vital sign derangement, but much like tachycardia it has been shown in multiple reviews to have no significant correlation to the presence of nonviable intestine. As mentioned above, the entire presentation of the patient with suspected intestinal obstruction including symptoms and signs needs to be assimilated to establish a differential diagnosis that includes intestinal obstruction and to determine the degree of surgical urgency of an obstruction. This is reflected in Stewardson's 1978 hallmark review of the records of 238 patients with small bowel obstruction; the 4 "classical" findings of leukocytosis, tachycardia, fever, and localized tenderness were examined, and when none were present patients could be safely managed nonoperatively initially without significant morbidity or mortality [10].

Workup and Evaluation

The primary and initial goal in the evaluation of elderly patients with suspected intestinal obstructions is to determine whether there is a complete mechanical bowel obstruction, a strangulated or closed-loop obstruction, or ischemic intestine requiring immediate operation. Unfortunately retrospective analyses of elderly patients with operative findings of strangulated and compromised intestine from obstruction have shown that classic clinical signs and symptoms mentioned above such as peritonitis and abnormal vital signs are only present in the minority of patients [11]. Thus, maintaining a high degree of suspicion on initial presentation and continued vigilance if an initial period of nonoperative management is chosen is of paramount importance. This is aptly described in one review of small bowel obstruction: "identification of those at risk for bowel ischemia and bowel death is an art as much as it is a science" [12]. The reasons why the elderly may "hide" compromised bowel are unclear but likely are related to a diminished immune-inflammatory response, a blunted nociceptive response, or the presence of delirium and or dementia.

All patients should undergo a thorough history and physical examination. It is particularly important to ask patients and family about comorbidities, past surgical history, colonoscopic and endoscopic history, and whether there have ever been similar prior episodes or admissions for intestinal obstruction. Physical examination should be done in a comprehensive fashion with particular focus on the patient's general appearance and abdomen. Cope's Early Diagnosis of the Acute Abdomen advocates that "one should always take the time to watch the patient quietly for several minutes" to gauge if there is an abdominal emergency [13]. The abdominal exam should be done systematically starting with inspection, followed by auscultation and palpation. Distention and tympany tend to be more profound with more distal obstructions as mentioned above, while auscultation can be revealing if there are hypoactive or high-pitched bowel sounds, but little data has shown support for auscultation as a means of reliable diagnosis. Palpation is performed to evaluate for tenderness, rebound tenderness, and guarding; and a thorough exam for abdominal wall or groin hernias should be undertaken. Lastly a rectal examination must be done to evaluate for impacted stool, gross blood, and rectal masses.

A complete blood count and metabolic panel should be obtained in order to augment the history and physical examination findings that have been elicited. Leukocytosis with bandemia may be indicative of compromised intestine; however this too has been shown to be nonspecific. Significant fluid losses and dehydration can occur from emesis, bowel edema, and intraluminal fluid accumulation, as well as from decreased oral intake. Dehydration may also lead to hemoconcentration with marked elevation in hematocrit, and in severe cases, renal failure and azotemia may ensue. The classically described hypokalemic, hypochloremic alkalosis that results from loss of gastric hydrogen ions, potassium, and chloride compounded by renal tubular mechanisms excreting hydrogen ions in the urine in order to retain sodium is more often seen with proximal obstructions. Distal obstructions tend to have an unpredictable electrolyte profile and patients can present with marked hypernatremia or hyponatremia depending on what compensatory mechanism has predominated. Elevations in serum amylase are commonly seen in bowel obstructions; however striking elevations should increase the index of suspicion for ischemic bowel and or perforation. Due to the variation and nonspecificity of laboratory data, management decisions, especially the need for operative intervention, should never be solely based on laboratory data.

Radiologic evaluation should start with a plain chest film (CXR), preferably upright, in order to evaluate for free intraperitoneal air and the need for prompt exploration. Supine and upright abdominal films assess for dilated loops of bowel, "step laddering" indicating fluid collecting in the dependent portions of intestinal loops, and most importantly for the presence of air in the descending colon and rectum. Air in the distal colon signifies that complete obstruction, and thus immediate operative intervention, is unlikely. Overall, the sensitivity and specificity of plain x-rays for diagnosing obstruction is between 50 and 80 % [14]. CT scan with oral and intravenous contrast can also be done in the initial evaluation, but plain films should be obtained first to look for signs such as free intraperitoneal air that prove that further workup is unnecessary. CT scans have a sensitivity and specificity for diagnosis of complete obstruction of greater than 90 % in recent meta-analysis with the key findings including proximal dilated intestine, a transition point, and fecalized intestinal contents [15]. CT scan evaluation for ischemic intestine is not quite as reliable, and sensitivity and specificity have been shown to be roughly 80 and 90 %, respectively, with the key findings of ischemia being reduced intestinal wall enhancement and mesenteric attenuation << [16, 17]. Other findings on CT scan include air in the biliary tree from a cholecystoenteric fistula or portal venous gas, the latter of which portends a dismal prognosis. These two entities are easily differentiated by remembering that air in the biliary tree tends to remain centralized in the liver while porto-venous gas typically moves to the periphery.

Other worthwhile diagnostic studies are follow-up plain films in the patient that has undergone CT scan evaluation with oral contrast to assess progression of the contrast. The presence of such contrast in the colon within 24 h of administration has been shown to be 97 % sensitive and 96 % specific for resolution of adhesion-related obstruction in meta-analysis [18]. Interestingly, diatrizoate meglumine (Gastrografin®), but not barium contrast agents, has been speculated to promote bowel motility, and there is limited data that it may shorten hospital stay in patients with adhesion-related obstruction [18]. Ultrasound and MRI both have significant limitations that render them unhelpful in the workup of intestinal obstruction. Ultrasound reliability is affected markedly by bowel gas and is very much operator dependent while MRI is expensive, time consuming, and it is considerably unwise to position an elderly patient with potential obstruction in the supine position for a prolonged period due to risk of vomiting, aspiration, and death.

Patients that present in extremis due to presumed abdominal emergency, with signs of peritonitis, or with clearly incarcerated or strangulated hernia do not require any radiologic evaluation, and in fact operative therapy and fluid resuscitation should not be delayed for imaging. Also, as previously noted, elderly patients may not present with obvious symptoms or findings on physical exam and tend to mask serious abdominal emergencies such as intestinal ischemia due to various comorbidities, alterations in mental status including delirium from electrolyte derangement and dehydration, and dementia and other cognitive disturbances common with aging; thus a very high index of suspicion must be maintained when dealing with this patient population.

Treatment and Intervention

Patients with signs and symptoms of intestinal strangulation, intestinal ischemia, and closed-loop obstruction should be promptly brought to the operating room for abdominal exploration once intravenous access and fluid resuscitation have been started in the emergency room. Patients who are more likely to have success with nonoperative management include those with postoperative obstruction, obstruction due to inflammatory bowel disease such as Crohn's, partial obstruction due to adhesions from prior operations, and carcinomatosis. One of the more difficult clinical decisions is the management of the elderly patient with signs of obstruction but with no history of prior operation and no signs of incarcerated or strangulated hernia on examination. It must be remembered that there is a significant probability of neoplastic disease in these patients; thus abdominal exploration is likely warranted even in the absence of significant physical exam, laboratory, and radiographic evidence indicating that exploration is warranted.

After the initial workup and evaluation has been completed and decision to trial a period of a nonoperative approach has been made, the elderly patient with intestinal obstruction needs a multifaceted approach to their care. All patients with intestinal obstruction tend to be significantly hypovolemic, and this is especially true of the elderly who tend to be chronically hypovolemic due to diuretic therapy, decreased thirst mechanisms, and loss of lean muscle mass, thus prompt resuscitation with isotonic intravenous fluid is warranted. Either lactated Ringer's solution or normal saline can be utilized, and the choice of fluid should be made based on their initial electrolyte profile, but either is effective in restoring the circulating volume to euvolemia. Whether the patient is to undergo urgent laparotomy or nonoperative management, starting a fluid resuscitation should not be delayed in the emergency room as there can be a tendency to overlook this when there are many tasks occurring simultaneously in getting a patient prepared for the operating room. With these same concerns for volume depletion, a Foley catheter should be placed and urine output monitored on an hourly basis to guide the fluid resuscitation. While one may wish to consider patient comfort and avoid urethral catheterization, it is not possible to adequately monitor urine output and resuscitation by relying on a sick elderly patient to save all urine in a collection chamber, nor will they urinate often enough to make hourly monitoring possible. In retrospective analysis, patients with intestinal obstruction and acute renal failure have been shown to have increased mortality and requirement for bowel resection thus the risks of bladder catheterization are outweighed by the information it yields [1].

A nasogastric tube (NGT) of fairly large caliber should also be placed at this time to decompress the stomach to lessen the risk of aspiration of vomitus and to reduce the continued air contributing to the intestine distention proximal to the obstruction. Smaller-caliber NGTs are prone to clogging from fecalized contents and can lead to emesis and aspiration. Special attention should be paid to insertion technique and confirmation of proper location as NGT placement is a procedure shown in literature review to have significant potential for error with rates of 1.9–89.5 % reported [19]. Good NGT insertion technique is especially important in the elderly population since these patients are more likely to have aspiration during the procedure. The passage of the NGT should always occur in the upright position with an assistant present, and auscultation should be done while the tube is being flushed with air to assess its position. This alone is inadequate for confirmation of placement and CXR should be performed as this is the most reliable means for assessing placement. Recently, emerging evidence supports the use of bedside ultrasound being an even more prompt and reliable method of identifying correct NGT placement [20]. The NGT should then be placed to medium continuous suction, 80–100 mmHg, and its patency maintained by gentle, occasional flushing with a catheter-tipped syringe. Most NGTs in use today are Salem sumps, and as such, a continuous aspiration of room air through the sump port should be observed if the tube is correctly located in the gastric lumen. Lack of air sumping or the backup of bilious gastric fluid in the air port signifies that the tube is incorrectly positioned which may place the patient at risk for aspiration and subsequent death despite the presence of the NGT.

Not only should all patients with intestinal obstruction be evaluated early by a surgeon, these patients should always be admitted to the surgical service as outcomes of mortality, time to operation, length of hospital stay, and cost have been shown to be reduced in multiple series that have compared surgical service to medical service admission for patients with obstruction. Serial examinations and continued vigilance then become the key tenets to determine whether the patient is improving and regaining bowel function or worsening and in need of operative exploration. Trending white blood cell counts and other laboratory information remain an unreliable basis for decision making regarding exploration. Vital sign monitoring also has significant limitation for accurately predicting whether a patient has developed ischemic or strangulated bowel as the elderly often are unable to mount a tachycardia to a developing inflammatory process due to the frequent presence of cardiovascular comorbidities or use of adrenergic blocking agents; thus serial abdominal exams by a skilled examiner are mandatory. In a large retrospective analysis of patients with intestinal obstruction, greater than 50 % of patients over the age of 75 were shown to have a significant medical comorbidity with cardiovascular disease the most common [21]. Age has also been shown to confer markedly increased risk for the presence of strangulated, nonviable intestine and mortality from obstruction further supporting the need for a truly vigilant approach with frequent examination of elderly patients. Each examination should include the patient's subjective report of symptoms, vital signs, physical exam findings, and any new laboratory data should be compiled to consider the overall progress of the patient. Second opinions should also be obtained from more senior surgeons, especially in teaching institutions, due to the complexity of clinical decision making in the obstructed elderly patient.

A question that frequently arises is "how long can we wait or observe this obstruction?" This is difficult to answer, and while prior edicts mention to "never let the sun rise or set on a small bowel obstruction," there are a number of conditions such as postoperative obstruction and partial obstruction from adhesions that can be present that can be managed nonoperatively for several days as long as peritonitis or other concerning signs do not develop. There is limited data of successful nonoperative management of up to or greater than 5 days duration, and when the obstruction occurs in the early postoperative period, this interval of nonoperative management can likely be extended to 7–14 days with success [16].

Patients that require operation for peritonitis, concern for strangulated or ischemic intestine, or failure to progress with nonoperative management may require bowel resection, repair of hernias, and even damage control approaches due to patient instability. The technical details of the operative management of these patients is beyond the scope of this chapter as the breadth of disease processes that cause obstruction require a vast array of different surgical approaches. Diagnostic and therapeutic success has even been shown with a laparoscopic approach to small intestinal obstruction in a few small series but this is likely a function of the laparoscopic skill set of the operator [22, 23]. The theoretical benefits of laparoscopic approaches must be weighed against the likelihood of prolonged operative times and inadequate exploration.

Special Considerations and Conclusion

One final aspect of management that deserves mention is whether narcotic pain medication should be administered or withheld from the elderly patient with intestinal obstruction. While some feel it may obscure the examination and lead to delay in recognition of the patient with ischemic or strangulated intestine, there is some limited randomized data that early use of morphine for patients with abdominal pain does not lead to delays in treatment. In Cope's *Early Diagnosis of the Acute Abdomen*, the author goes as far as to describe the withholding of narcotic pain medication as a "cruel practice [that] is to be condemned" [13]. The liberal use of narcotic medications should be offset with vigilant serial abdominal exams, preferably by the same examiner in order to detect subtle changes in the exam or worsening of the clinical scenario.

In summary, elderly patients with intestinal obstruction present very unique challenges. The breadth of etiologies of obstruction is far greater in the elderly population, and unusual processes such as gallstone ileus, colonic volvulus, and colonic pseudo-obstruction must be considered among many other more common causes such as hernia, adhesions, and neoplasms. Also, the more limited physiologic reserve of the elderly patient coupled with their greater burden of comorbidities needs to make the provider practice an even more vigilant approach to diagnosis, management, and resuscitation and if necessary to provide the most timely surgical intervention possible to avoid the discovery of ischemic or nonviable intestine.

References

1. Oyasiji T, Angelo S, Kyriakides TC, Helton SW. Small bowel obstruction: outcome and cost implications of admitting service. Am Surg. 2010;76(7):687–91.
2. Schwab DP, Blackhurst DW, Sticca RP. Operative acute small bowel obstruction: admitting service impacts outcome. Am Surg. 2001;67(11):1034–8.
3. Drozdz W, Budzynski P. Change in mechanical bowel obstruction demographic and etiological patterns during the past century: observations from one health care institution. Arch Surg. 2012; 147(2):175–80.
4. Markogiannakis H, Messaris E, Dardamanis D, Pararas N, Tzertzemelis D, Giannopoulos P, Larentzakis A, Lagoudianakis E, Manouras A, Bramis I. Acute mechanical bowel obstruction: clinical presentation, etiology, management and outcome. World J Gastroenterol. 2007;13(3):432–7.
5. Catena F, Ansaloni L, Gazzotti F, Gagliardi S, Di Saverio S, De Cataldis A, Taffurelli M. Small bowel tumours in emergency surgery: specificity of clinical presentation. ANZ J Surg. 2005; 75(11):997–9.
6. Ayantunde AA, Agrawal A. Gallstone ileus: diagnosis and management. World J Surg. 2007;31(6):1292–7.
7. Cheadle WG, Garr EE, Richardson JD. The importance of early diagnosis of small bowel obstruction. Am Surg. 1988;54:565–9.
8. Sarr M, Bulkley G, Zuidema G. Preoperative recognition of intestinal strangulation obstruction: prospective evaluation of diagnostic capability. Am J Surg. 1983;145:176.
9. Eskelinen M, Ikonen J, Lipponen P. Contributions of history taking, physical examination, and computer assistance to diagnosis of acute small bowel obstruction: a prospective study of 1333 patients with acute abdominal pain. Scan J Gastroenterol. 1994;29:715.
10. Stewardson RH, Bombeck CT, Nyhus LM. Critical operative management of small bowel obstruction. Ann Surg. 1978;187(2):189–93.
11. Zadeh BJ, Davis JM, Canizaro PC. Small bowel obstruction in the elderly. Am Surg. 1985;51(8):470–3.
12. Trevino C. Small bowel obstruction: the art of management. AACN Adv Crit Care. 2010;21(2):187–94.
13. Silen W. Cope's early diagnosis of the acute abdomen. 18th ed. New York: Oxford Press; 1991.
14. Suri S, Gupta S, Sudhakar PJ, Venkataramu NK, Sood B, Wig JD. Comparative evaluation of plain films, ultrasound and CT in the diagnosis of intestinal obstruction. Acta Radiol. 1999;40(4): 422–8.
15. Mallo RD, Salem L, Lalani T, Flum DR. Computed tomography diagnosis of ischemia and complete obstruction in small bowel obstruction: a systematic review. J Gastrointest Surg. 2005;9(5): 690–4.
16. Diaz JJ, Bokhari F, Mowery NT, et al. Guidelines for management of small bowel obstruction. J Trauma. 2008;64:1651–64.
17. Maglinte DD, Heitkamp DE, Howard TJ, Kelvin FM, Lappas JC. Current concepts in imaging of small bowel obstruction. Radiol Clin North Am. 2003;41:263–83.
18. Abbas SM, Bissett IP, Parry BR. Meta-analysis of oral water-soluble contrast agent in the management of adhesive small bowel obstruction. Br J Surg. 2007;94:404–11.
19. Ellett ML. What is known about methods of correctly placing gastric tubes in adults and children. Gastroenterol Nurs. 2004;27(6): 253–9.
20. Nguyen L, Lewiss RE, Drew J, Saul T. A novel approach to confirming nasogastric tube placement in the ED. Am J Emerg Med. 2012;30(8):1662.e5–7.
21. Fevang BT, Fevang J, Stangeland L, Soreide O, Svanes K, Viste A. Complications and death after surgical treatment of small bowel obstruction: a 35-year institutional experience. Ann Surg. 2000; 231(4):529–37.
22. Schuster KM, Davis KA, Rosenbaum SH. Emergency and urgent surgery. Med Clin North Am. 2009;93:1131–48.
23. Szomstein S, Lo Menzo E, Simpfendorfer C, Zundel N, Rosenthal RJ. Laparoscopic lysis of adhesions. World J Surg. 2006;30: 535–40.

15 Intestinal Hemorrhage in the Elderly

Todd W. Costantini, Leslie M. Kobayashi, and Raul Coimbra

Introduction

Intestinal hemorrhage is a common clinical problem with an overall incidence of approximately 100 cases per 100,000 of the general population [1]. Hospitalization for GI bleeding is a frequent occurrence in the United States. The incidence of hospitalization for upper GI bleeding is 60.6/100,000 and greater compared to the incidence of hospitalization of 35.7/100,000 for lower GI bleeding. However over the past decade, the incidence of hospitalizations for upper GI bleeding have been decreasing, while admissions for lower GI bleeding have remained relatively stable [2]. Mortality from intestinal hemorrhage is approximately 3 %, which has decreased slightly over the past decade. Mortality due to upper GI bleeding tends to be higher than mortality for lower GI bleeding.

Rates of both upper and lower GI hemorrhage increase significantly with aging. The incidence of hospitalization in patients older than 75 years for upper GI bleeding and lower GI bleeding is 425.2/100,000 and 380.1/100,00, respectively. The mortality rate for GI bleeding also increases with aging but remains low overall with the rate being just over 3 % in patients aged 65–84 and 5.2 % in patients over age 85 years [3]. Pre-hospitalization functional status impacts outcomes in elderly patients admitted to the hospital for intestinal bleeding and may influence treatment strategies in patients who have functional impairments affecting normal activities of daily living. A study by Inouye et al. found that measures of physical and cognitive function are strong predictors of 90-day and 2-year mortality in patients 70 years or older [4]. In addition, among geriatric patients who present with GI bleeding and do not undergo definitive therapy with either angiography or surgery, only a quarter will experience a recurrent bleeding event within the following 4 years [5, 6]. Therefore, weighing the risks and benefits of aggressive treatment of elderly patients admitted for an initial bleed must take into account comorbid conditions and functional status considering the overall low mortality rate and recurrence rate.

Causes of Gastrointestinal Bleeding

The combination of advancing age, comorbid disease, and polypharmacy places the elderly patient at increased risk for developing intestinal bleeding. Patients over 65 years of age commonly are prescribed numerous medications which may compromise mucosal integrity and predispose the mucosa to bleeding, particularly in patients requiring therapeutic anticoagulation [7]. The widespread use of aspirin for the primary prevention of coronary events has caused an increase in major gastrointestinal bleeding episodes [8]. Elderly patients are also frequently treated with anticoagulant and antiplatelet medications for several conditions including stroke, atrial fibrillation, and prevention of vascular stent thrombosis [9]. Hemorrhage is a major concern in patients who are prescribed with these medications, with an incidence of 13.1 episodes of major hemorrhage per 100 patient years during the first year of anticoagulation in the population older than 80 years. This compares to an incidence of major hemorrhage of 4.7 per 100 patient years in individuals younger than 80 [10]. The differential diagnosis of GI bleeding is broad and requires an organized approach to ensure prompt localization of the bleeding source (Table 15.1).

Upper Gastrointestinal Bleeding

Upper GI bleeding is characterized as bleeding proximal to the ligament of Treitz including the stomach, duodenum, and esophagus. Patients with upper GI bleeding may present with symptoms such as hematemesis (vomiting of fresh,

T.W. Costantini, MD • L.M. Kobayashi, MD
R. Coimbra, MD, PhD, FACS (✉)
Division of Trauma, Surgical Critical Care, and Burns, Department of Surgery, University of California San Diego Health Sciences, 200 West Arbor Drive, #8896, San Diego, CA 92103, USA
e-mail: tcostantini@ucsd.edu; lkobayashi@ucsd.edu; rcoimbra@ucsd.edu

J.A. Yelon, F.A. Luchette (eds.), *Geriatric Trauma and Critical Care*,
DOI 10.1007/978-1-4614-8501-8_15, © Springer Science+Business Media New York 2014

Table 15.1 Common causes of gastrointestinal bleeding in the elderly

Upper GI bleeding
Peptic ulcer disease
Gastritis
Esophageal/gastric varices
Mallory-Weiss tear
Boerhaave's syndrome
Malignancy
Lower GI bleeding
Diverticulosis
Angiodysplasia
Malignancy
Inflammatory bowel disease
Colitis (ischemic or infectious)
Hemorrhoids
Anal fissure
Solitary rectal ulcer

bright red blood, coffee ground emesis) or melena (passage of black or tarry stools). It may also be occult and present with hemoccult positive stools or as a microcytic anemia. Symptoms of upper GI bleeding may include lightheadedness, orthostatic hypotension, and syncope related to blood loss and hypovolemia. Bleeding from the foregut is estimated to be five times more common that lower GI bleeding [11]. The mortality rate for hemorrhage from the upper GI tract has also been shown to increase with aging [6].

The most common sources of hemorrhage in the elderly are peptic ulcer disease and gastropathy which together account for between 55 and 80 % of patients presenting to the emergency department [12]. Esophagitis and esophageal/gastric varices account for the remaining sources of bleeding. Less common etiologies of hemorrhage include esophageal tears due to Boerhaave's syndrome or Mallory-Weiss syndrome, duodenal diverticula, Dieulafoy's lesion, angiodysplasia, hemobilia, aortoenteric fistulae, and neoplasms. History should focus on prior diagnosis of peptic ulcer disease, treatment for *Helicobacter Pylori*, smoking, alcohol use, previous abdominal surgeries, and steroid use. Liver disease is another key risk factor and may suggest variceal bleeding. Elderly critically ill patients are at increased risk for development of stress gastritis with mechanical ventilation, traumatic brain injury, major burn wound, or trauma injury all being known risk factors. Confounding factors include the use of anticoagulants, antiplatelet agents, and recent use of nonsteroidal anti-inflammatory drugs (NSAIDS).

Lower Gastrointestinal Bleeding

Intestinal bleeding from a source distal to the ligament of Treitz is considered to be a lower GI bleed. While lower GI bleeding is less common than upper GI bleeding in the general population, the incidence of lower GI hemorrhage is higher in the elderly. It is important to remember that one of the most common sources of blood per rectum is actually the upper GI tract, and therefore, upper GI bleeding should always be considered first and investigated as the source. Nearly 80 % of patients presenting with a lower GI hemorrhage will stop bleeding without intervention, however, the recurrence rate can be as high as 25 % [13].

The most common cause of lower GI bleeding is diverticulosis of the colon which is usually characterized by abrupt onset of painless hematochezia. Angiodysplasia is also a common cause of painless bleeding from the anus, especially in the elderly. It accounts for up to 30 % of lower GI bleeding in patients over the age of 65 years. A less common source is a colonic neoplasm where ulceration of the mucosal surface by the tumor results in bleeding. Bleeding from colonic neoplasms is often more subtle than diverticular bleeding and may lead to slow blood loss over a prolonged period of time. Less common etiologies include infectious colitis, mesenteric ischemia, and inflammatory bowel disease [14].

Obtaining a detailed history of the events related to the bleeding episode is crucial and should include the color and quantity of blood passed. Patients should be queried regarding any previous history of colon malignancy, diverticulosis, and personal or family history of inflammatory bowel disease. Anorectal bleeding should also be considered and may be characterized by bright red bleeding from hemorrhoids, a solitary rectal ulcer, or anal fissures.

Obscure Gastrointestinal Bleeding

Rarely, the source of hemorrhage is not identified by either colonoscopy or esophagogastroduodenoscopy (EGD) and is then referred to as obscure GI bleeding. In these situations, the etiology of the bleeding may be from a small bowel source or may originate from a source in the upper GI tract or colon that was not visualized during prior diagnostic attempts. While obscure GI bleeding is less common than a defined upper or lower GI source, this cause of bleeding is often challenging to diagnose and treat and may lead to ongoing blood loss with prolonged hospital stays.

Diagnosis

Endoscopy

Endoscopy, including EGD and colonoscopy, is the diagnostic test of choice and may also allow for therapeutic intervention. EGD is safe and effective in the elderly population and has been reported to allow for a diagnosis in over 90 % of patients [7]. Colonoscopy and EGD generally require conscious sedation to ensure patient comfort and to allow for the technical completion of the study. Sedation is generally well tolerated in the elderly patient. A randomized controlled trial of geriatric patients comparing the use of midazolam versus saline for sedation during EGD found that treatment with midazolam increased the probability that patients would successfully tolerate the exam with no significant increase in the number of hypotensive episodes [15]. However, this study did find a significantly higher incidence of desaturation in geriatric patients sedated with midazolam, which is in agreement with previous studies [16]. Elderly patients may also be at increased risk of aspiration during upper endoscopy procedures and tolerate such events poorly due to underlying lack of physiologic reserve. Lastly, patients older than 80 years have been shown to have a greater risk of colon perforation during colonoscopy [17].

Angiography

Angiography is another useful modality in the diagnosis of GI bleeding. Angiography allows for localization of the bleeding source when the rate is as low as 0.5 ml/min. Diagnostic angiography is safe and well tolerated with risks including puncture site complications such as bleeding, hematoma, and pseudoaneurysm. There is also risk of acute kidney injury associated with the administration of iodinated intravenous contrast [18]. In addition to its diagnostic capabilities, angiography also possesses the added benefit of potential therapeutic intervention. Catheter-based interventions including vasopressin injection and angioembolization will be discussed later in this chapter.

Nuclear Medicine

Nuclear scintigraphy can be used to identify the source of intestinal bleeding and involves Tc-99m-labeled red blood cells or technetium-99m (Tc-99m) sulfur colloid. Radiolabeled red blood cells maintain their activity for longer periods of time compared to injection of Tc-99m sulfur colloid, allowing for serial imaging, and may give better results when used to diagnose lower GI bleeding. Nuclear scintigraphy is safe, noninvasive, and an accurate method of localizing the source of GI bleeding [19]. The benefits of this imaging technique for detecting GI bleeding include its sensitivity for very slow bleeding, with the ability to detect bleeding rates as low as 0.1 ml/min and its noninvasiveness [20].

Computed Tomographic Scanning

Contrast-enhanced multidetector-row helical computed tomography (MDCT) scanning is a newer technology

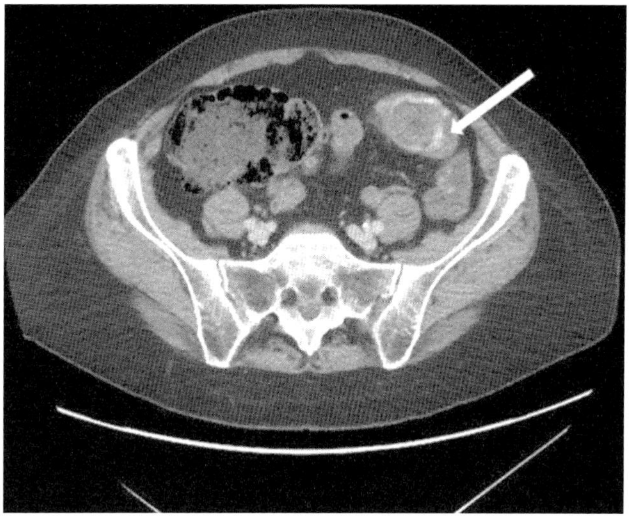

Fig. 15.1 Lower GI bleeding diagnosed by contrast-enhanced computed tomographic (CT) scan. The *arrow* indicates area of active arterial extravasation seen in the descending colon

which can be used to identify the area of intestinal blood loss. This technique of CT scan allows images to be obtained during the arterial phase of contrast administration which allows identification of contrast extravasation into the bowel lumen (Fig. 15.1). Areas concerning on the arterial phase can be further investigated using delayed images to assess for residual contrast, or pooling of contrast, which further supports the presence of active arterial bleeding. As with angiography, MDCT appears to be most effective in detecting active or symptomatic bleeding, however unlike angiography, MDCT has been reported to detect bleeding rates as low as 0.4 ml/min, similar to those for nuclear scintigraphy [6]. It also has the advantage of being noninvasive, widely available, avoids the risks associated with arterial puncture required for conventional angiography, and has the added benefit of identifying extraluminal pathology or causes of hemorrhage. However, MDCT is associated with complications related to the use of intravenous contrast administration and radiation exposure [19]. Using MDCT to diagnose the source of bleeding may be an efficient method to facilitate directed interventions via either endoscopy or angiography [21].

CT Enterography

As the technology of CT scanning improves the sensitivity of imaging with the advent of multidetector imaging systems with 64 channels has improved image resolution and introduced more applications for the use of CT scans in the diagnosis of GI bleeding. CT enterography utilizes orally delivered, neutral contrast material which improves the visualization of pathology within the lumen of the intestine. The protocols require the oral administration of contrast in several doses at 20-min intervals in order to distend the lumen of the intestine. With the neutral background provided by the enterally delivered contrast material, active hemorrhage can be visualized and localized more easily than traditional CT scanning protocols. The large volume of oral contrast required to perform CT enterography does place elderly patients at risk of aspiration. CT enteroclysis is another option which delivers contrast enterally at a continuous rate via a nasojejunal tube which is placed under fluoroscopic guidance, potentially decreasing the risk of vomiting, reflux, and aspiration [22].

Magnetic Resonance Imaging

The use of Magnetic Resonance Imaging (MRI) to diagnosis the cause of GI bleeding continues to evolve, however, it is currently considered to be experimental for localizing the source. However, its use in the evaluation of obscure GI bleeding has shown a diagnostic yield of only 40 % with improved localization of pathology in the distal small bowel compared to the proximal small bowel [23]. MRI enterography has a low-diagnostic yield for identifying intraluminal small bowel bleeding sources causing occult GI bleed, however, this imaging has been shown to identify extraintestinal pathology which may aid in the diagnosis of the cause of hemorrhage [24]. Further studies are needed to define the role of MRI in the diagnosis of occult GI bleeding; however, it may be an adjunctive diagnostic test to consider in patients with bleeding sources not localized by other, more traditional imaging techniques.

Capsule Endoscopy

Improvements in technology have allowed for the more widespread use of capsule endoscopy to aid in the diagnosis of obscure GI bleeding. The capsule, which is the size of a large pill, is swallowed and advances the length of the GI tract through peristalsis. Capsule endoscopy is especially useful in identifying the etiology of small bowel blood loss with imaging completed to the cecum in nearly 75 % of cases [25]. This technology is purely diagnostic with a yield near 50 % but unfortunately does not allow for intervention [26–28]. Clinical studies evaluating the effectiveness of capsule endoscopy for obscure GI bleeding have shown a diagnostic yield between 30 and 68 % with angiodysplasia the most common diagnosis [29–31]. The test is well tolerated and safe, with retained capsule representing the most significant risk associated with this procedure [32, 33].

Management

Initial Evaluation

As with any acute illness associated with blood loss, the initial assessment of GI bleeding should include evaluation of the airway, breathing, and circulation. The patient should be evaluated in the appropriate level of care with frequent monitoring of vital signs. With significant hemorrhage, patients should have two large bore IV's placed for transfusion of blood or IV fluids as needed. The primary treatment goals in patients presenting with a major intestinal bleed include adequate resuscitation, localization and/or diagnosis of the cause of hemorrhage, and control of the bleeding source with endoscopy, angiography, or surgery. A nasogastric tube may be placed and saline lavage performed to give some insight as to whether the bleeding is originating from an upper GI source. A Foley catheter should be placed to monitor urine output and assess the response to fluid resuscitation. If the index of suspicion is high for an upper GI source of bleeding, high dose proton pump inhibitor infusion therapy should be initiated.

Aspiration Risk in Elderly

Elderly patients who are hospitalized with GI bleeding have been shown to experience complications early in their hospital course, frequently within 96 h of admission [34]. Among the most frequent complications are pneumonia and aspiration [12]. Therefore, airway protection and pulmonary toilet are of significant importance during the resuscitation and hospitalization of patients presenting with GI bleeding.

All patients should be administered supplemental oxygen and the head of bed should remain elevated at all times. Supplemental oxygen by nasal cannula is an important adjunct at the time of endoscopy as it has been shown to prevent hypoxemia, oxygen desaturation, and cardiac arrhythmias [35]. Consideration should be given to early, prophylactic intubation in order to secure the airway and limit the risk of aspiration. This is especially true in patients undergoing endoscopy who will be receiving conscious sedation. Elderly patients generally require lower doses of sedative medications during endoscopic procedures compared to their younger counterparts [36]. However, older patients may experience an unexpected respiratory arrest that may necessitate emergent endotracheal intubation further increasing the risk of aspiration. Paradoxic reactions to conscious sedation which may result in altered mental status are also more frequent in the elderly making endoscopic interventions difficult [6]. Current guidelines from the American Society for Gastrointestinal Endoscopy recommend heightened attention to the dose and effects of standard sedatives used during endoscopic procedures on the elderly and emphasize the importance of lower initial doses of sedatives with more gradual titration [37].

Fluid Resuscitation

Normal saline and lactated ringers are the most common resuscitation fluids used in the treatment of hypovolemic shock. Studies comparing the use of normal saline and lactated ringers in patients with acute hemorrhage show equivalent outcomes [17, 38]. There is a theoretical risk of hyperkalemia with the use of lactated ringers which may be exacerbated in patients with acute kidney injury or chronic renal insufficiency seen in many elderly patients. Resuscitation with colloids has theoretical benefits over crystalloid resuscitation due to its ability to restore intravascular volume more efficiently due to the higher oncotic pressure resulting in decreased losses into the extravascular space. This may be beneficial in elderly patients as colloid resuscitation may allow for lower total infusion volume required to restore intravascular volume. Unfortunately, several studies have compared crystalloid versus colloid resuscitation showing no statistical benefit with colloid resuscitation [39, 40]. A large randomized controlled trial compared 3,497 patients who received 4 % albumin to 3,500 patients receiving normal saline [15]. This study found no significant difference in mortality, need for renal replacement therapy, or hospital length of stay suggesting no benefit in the use of colloid resuscitation compared to crystalloid resuscitation.

Recent research from the trauma population suggests that early transfusion of blood products may be beneficial in patients with acute hemorrhage. Not only does early transfusion of packed red blood cells (PRBCs) appear to be superior to crystalloid resuscitation in patients with hemorrhage, but the transfusion of other blood components may be beneficial as well. Studies suggest that transfusion of fresh frozen plasma (FFP) and platelets in addition to PRBCs may decrease mortality [13]. The optimal transfusion strategy appears to be a 1:1 ratio of FFP to PRBCs [19]. Studies also suggest that increasing the ratio of platelets to PRBCs may be beneficial as well [41].

Medications

Elderly patients who are diagnosed with GI bleeding should be queried regarding their current medication regimen with particular focus on antiplatelet and anticoagulant medications. Laboratory studies including complete blood count, PT/INR, and PTT should be measured to diagnose any derangements in the clotting cascade. Classical measures of coagulopathy may not address all coagulation abnormalities and thus may fail to correctly diagnose coagulopathy. The classical measures fail to measure platelet dysfunction due to medications or fibrinolysis. Limitations of these traditional laboratory measures of coagulopathy have led to increased interest in the use of alternative measures of coagulation, clot strength, and fibrinolysis. Thromboelastography (TEG) and thromboelastometry (TEM) are an established method for measuring the viscoelastic properties of blood for hemostasis testing [3, 14, 23]. TEG and TEM have the benefit of providing detailed information on clot formation and clot strength and provide results more rapidly than conventional measures of coagulation.

Treatment with fresh frozen plasma is a common method used to reverse anticoagulation in patients taking Coumadin. FFP is effective; however, it takes time to transfuse and may require the infusion of large volumes of fluid in order to correct the INR. In elderly patients who are actively bleeding, strategies need to be considered that more rapidly correct the coagulopathy and prevent large volume infusions that may be problematic in patients with comorbid disease such as congestive heart failure. Pharmacologic agents such as factor VIIa and prothrombin complex should be considered as they result in rapid correction of the clotting abnormality and require minimal volume infusion.

Recombinant factor VIIa has traditionally been used as a treatment for uncontrolled bleeding in patients with hemophilia. It has been used to treat GI bleeding in patients with liver disease and in the treatment of trauma-induced coagulopathy [22, 24]. Randomized controlled trials have failed to show improvements in mortality in cirrhotic patients with acute upper intestinal hemorrhage compared with placebo [42, 43]. There are case reports which suggest that recombinant factor VIIa may be a useful strategy in elderly patients with GI hemorrhage who are poor candidates for aggressive intervention, however, further randomized controlled trials will be need to define its role in treating acute bleeding from the GI tract the elderly [44]. There are concerns regarding increased thromboembolic complications, particularly those affecting the arterial circulation, associated with the use of Factor VIIa. Therefore, while the use of Factor VIIa may be a useful strategy to quickly reverse coagulopathy in patients, its risks and benefits must be weighed carefully.

Several studies have compared the use of prothrombin complex to FFP and vitamin K for reversal of coagulopathy following injury or in anticipation of an invasive procedure. These studies have concluded that prothrombin complex corrected the INR more quickly and effectively than the combination of FFP and vitamin K. Coagulation was normalized 30 min after administration of prothrombin complex. Treatment with prothrombin complex is generally safe; however, the reversal of coagulopathy is not as durable as that achieved with vitamin K. Further studies are needed to better define the role of prothrombin complex in the treatment of elderly patients with GI bleeding, but it should be part of the armamentarium in the treatment of the exsanguinating patient.

Patients on antiplatelet medications such as clopidogrel (Plavix), and to a lesser degree aspirin, experience alterations in the platelet function that may cause coagulopathy which contributes to ongoing bleeding. Point of care testing is available to determine the degree of platelet inhibition caused by clopidogrel, which can vary significantly among patients [34]. Treatment with platelet transfusion can be considered in bleeding patients with pharmacologically induced platelet inhibition despite normal platelet counts.

While Coumadin therapy prolongs the INR, which allows for a quantification of the clotting abnormality, newer antithrombotic medications may not cause any changes in basic laboratory measures even when therapeutically anticoagulated. Medications such as dabigatran (Pradaxa) and other new direct thrombin inhibitors have effects that cannot be measured by conventional clinical laboratory assays, and TEG and TEM are required to detect their effects. Currently, the therapeutic effect of these agents cannot be reversed with conventional interventions such as FFP, platelet infusion, or recombinant factor VIIa making management of patients difficult. Dabigatran can only be removed by hemodialysis which is difficult to perform in patients with ongoing hemorrhage [35].

Endoscopy

Endoscopy is the primary diagnostic and treatment modality for both upper and bleeding from the proximal and distal intestine. Endoscopy is generally a safe and well tolerated procedure; however, mortality rates are higher for EGD when performed for hemorrhage [45]. Once the bleeding source is diagnosed, therapeutic maneuvers can be immediately implemented including placement of hemoclips, thermocoagulation, argon beam coagulation, injection of epinephrine, or placement of bands around varices. Certain endoscopic findings are associated with increased risk of rebleeding including active pulsatile bleeding or the presence of a visible vessel within the base of a duodenal ulcer. Timing of upper GI endoscopy for non-variceal bleeding has been studied, and evidence suggests that EGD should be performed in an urgent though not emergent fashion. Multiple studies demonstrate that endoscopy within the first 24 h of admission is safe and more urgent endoscopy within the first 6 h of admission offers no additional benefit [37, 46].

Complication rates associated with colonoscopy are generally less than 3 % and it has a high-diagnostic utility in identifying the source of a lower GI bleed. However, there is no consensus on the optimal timing for colonoscopic examination. Recent studies suggest that early intervention may offer a benefit. Colonoscopy performed within the first 24 h of admission has been shown to provide a definitive diagnosis in up to 96 % of patients [47]. Adequate visualization during colonoscopy requires bowel preparation which has been shown to be safe and effective during acute GI bleeding [45, 48]. Similar to upper endoscopy, colonoscopy allows the opportunity to treat the source of bleeding using mechanical clipping, electrical coagulation, or injection of epinephrine. Even if bleeding cannot be treated endoscopically, the bleeding site can be localized and marked to facilitate other intervention. Clips left at the time of endoscopy may help localize the bleeding site during angiographic intervention. Localizing the site of bleeding with ink tattooing at the time of colonoscopy can also facilitate the surgeon in identifying the portion of colon for resection if there is recurrent bleeding.

While colonoscopy is a safe procedure, elderly patients are at increased risk of complications. A systematic review of adverse events in elderly patients undergoing colonoscopy found that octogenarians have a high risk of complications with 29 cardiovascular and pulmonary complications per 1,000 scopes compared to 19 cardiovascular and pulmonary complication per 1,000 scopes in patients 65–80 years [49].

Angiography

Once bleeding is localized using digital subtraction angiography, treatment can be performed using transcatheter arterial embolization. Arterial embolization is highly effective with bleeding controlled in 80–90 % of patients [50, 51]. Recurrent hemorrhage after angiographic embolization is infrequent; the rate of rebleeding is higher with angiodysplasia and arteriovenous malformation. Recurrent bleeding episodes can be evaluated with repeat angiography and further embolization if needed. Risks of arterial embolization include bowel ischemia which may result in ulceration, necrosis, or perforation. Bowel ischemia is a rare event after embolization with an incidence less than 5 % in most series [49, 52]. Contrast-induced nephropathy causing acute kidney injury (AKI) is also a concern after diagnostic and therapeutic angiography with rates ranging between 2 and 25 % [53]. Risk factors for contrast-induced AKI include diabetes mellitus, congestive heart failure, and dehydration prior to the procedure which is a frequent occurrence among patients with acute hemorrhage [54]. Interventions to reduce contrast-induced nephropathy have been investigated and include administration of acetylcysteine and bicarbonate fluid hydration. Acetylcysteine has been shown to provide minimal protection from acute kidney injury after contrast administration in multiple randomized control trials [55–57]. Bolus infusion of sodium bicarbonate in addition to standard hydration may decrease contrast-induced nephropathy compared to standard hydration alone [28, 58]. Clearly, aggressive fluid rehydration should be performed prior to angiographic intervention and the delivery of contrast in order to limit the risk of contrast-induced AKI.

Catheter directed infusion therapy may be used to treat bleeding in locations where arterial embolization is not ideal. Vasopressin causes arterial vasoconstriction and thus reduced perfusion at the site of bleeding which may provide more beneficial conditions to allow clot formation. While catheter directed vasopressin infusion is effective in controlling bleeding, rebleeding rates reach 50 % [59, 60]. Vasopressin is often not an ideal treatment in the elderly as it is generally discouraged in patients with severe coronary artery disease or cardiac arrhythmias and may also cause bowel ischemia.

Surgery

Attempts to stop hemorrhage from an upper GI source using endoscopy or angiography may be unsuccessful, or the rate of bleeding leads to hemodynamic instability that requires operative intervention. Emergent surgery for upper GI bleeding has a high rate of morbidity and mortality, especially in the elderly [56]. If bleeding is suspected from a gastric source, an anterior gastrotomy can be performed with identification and ligation of the bleeding source. Rarely, in cases of unlocalized hemorrhage, gastric devascularization can be performed. In this procedure, the blood supply to the stomach is ligated with the exception of the short gastric vessels.

Bleeding from the duodenum is most commonly due to a posterior ulcer in the first portion of the duodenum. Surgical treatment options for these lesions include an anterior gastroduodenostomy with oversewing of the bleeding vessel alone versus oversewing the bleeding vessel with a definitive antiacid operation. Simple oversewing of the bleeding ulcer is recommended in hemodynamically unstable patients or those with multiple medical comorbidities.

If non-surgical means fail to control bleeding from the lower GI tract, surgery may be needed to control the hemorrhage. Criteria for emergent bowel resection for bleeding include the transfusion of 4–6 units of blood in 24 h, ongoing hemodynamic instability, and/or the inability to stop bleeding by endoscopic or angiographic means. Subtotal colectomy may be required if the specific location of bleeding cannot be localized. Mortality rates in patients undergoing subtotal colectomy remain high, ranging from 20 to 35 % [61, 62]. Segmental colon resection is preferred in order to preserve uninvolved colon and is associated with decreased mortality compared to subtotal colectomy. Segmental colon resection requires that the bleeding source has been localized thus ensuring that resection will control the hemorrhage. Despite preoperative angiographic localization of the bleeding source, there is a risk for rebleeding after hemicolectomy that requires repeat operation for completion colectomy [63]. Operative risks are also determined by the preoperative functional status of the patients. A review of a large Medicare database demonstrated that the mortality rate for nursing home patients is 32 % compared with 13 % mortality in non-institutionalized counterparts [55].

Summary

Gastrointestinal hemorrhage is a common problem in the elderly which results in frequent hospitalization and places this population of patients at risk for significant morbidity and mortality. Clinicians must consider the patients comorbid conditions, medication usage, and functional status when diagnosing and treating GI bleeding in the geriatric patient. Special attention should be given for the potential coagulopathy that may exist in the elderly patient taking anticoagulant or antiplatelet medications. The management of GI bleeding often requires a multidisciplinary approach including the emergency room physician, acute care surgeon, endoscopists, and radiologist. While endoscopy remains a mainstay in the management of GI bleeding, the clinician should be familiar with the various diagnostic and treatment modalities available to diagnose and treat upper, lower, and obscure GI bleeding. Treatment algorithms for the diagnosis and treatment of patients with upper and lower GI bleeds are shown in Figs. 15.2 and 15.3.

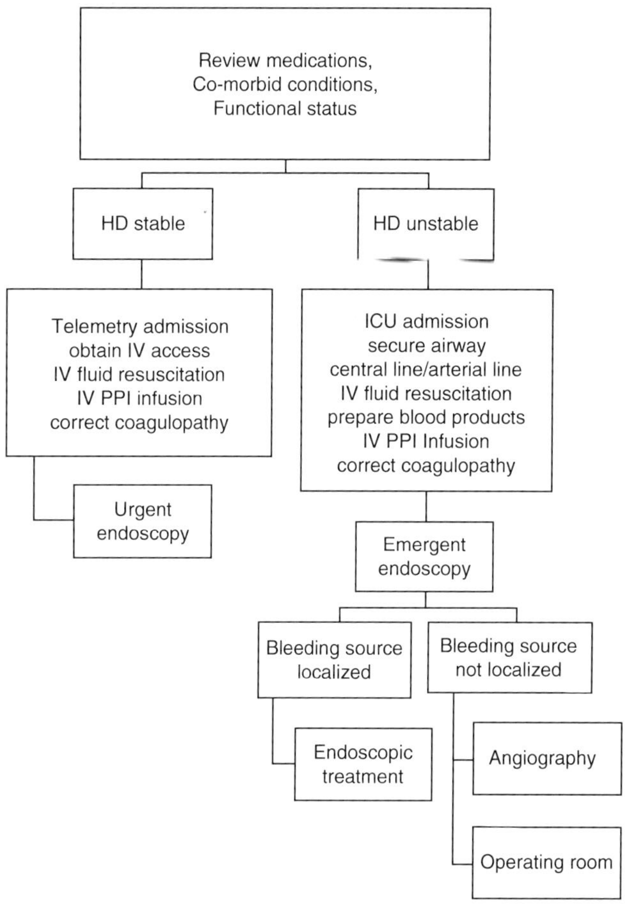

Fig. 15.2 Algorithm for the management of upper GI bleeding

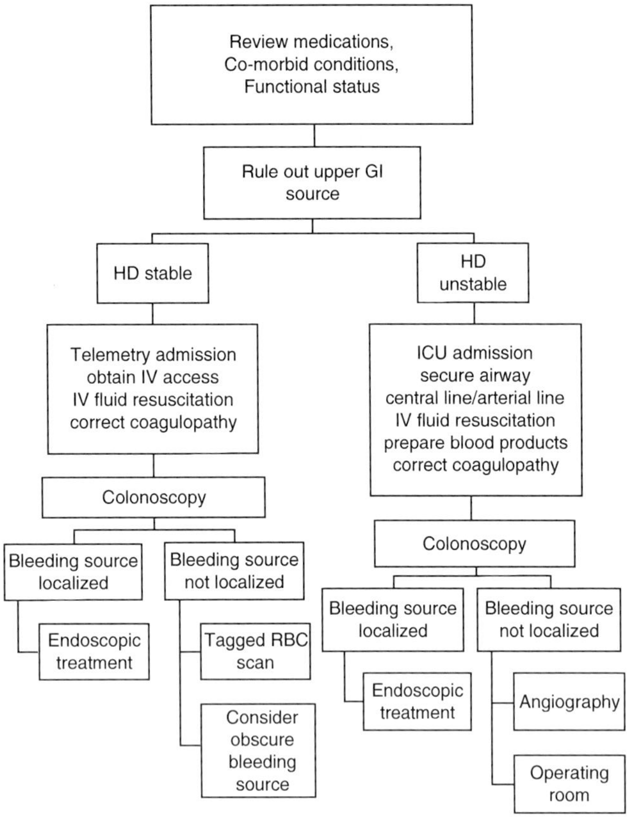

Fig. 15.3 Algorithm for the management of lower GI bleeding

References

1. Fallah MA, Prakash C, Edmundowicz S. Acute gastrointestinal bleeding. Medical Clin North Am. 2000;84(5):1183–208. Epub 2000/10/12.
2. Laine L, Yang H, Chang SC, Datto C. Trends for incidence of hospitalization and death Due to GI complications in the United States from 2001 to 2009. Am J Gastroenterol. 2012;107(8):1190–5. Epub 2012/06/13.
3. El-Tawil AM. Trends on gastrointestinal bleeding and mortality: where are we standing? World J Gastroenterol. 2012;18(11): 1154–8. Epub 2012/04/03.
4. Inouye SK, Peduzzi PN, Robison JT, Hughes JS, Horwitz RI, Concato J. Importance of functional measures in predicting mortality among older hospitalized patients. JAMA. 1998;279(15): 1187–93. Epub 1998/04/29.
5. Longstreth GF. Epidemiology of hospitalization for acute upper gastrointestinal hemorrhage: a population-based study. Am J Gastroenterol. 1995;90(2):206–10.
6. Katschinski B, Logan R, Davies J, Faulkner G, Pearson J, Langman M. Prognostic factors in upper gastrointestinal bleeding. Dig Dis Sci. 1994;39(4):706–12. Epub 1994/04/01.
7. Jafri SM, Monkemuller K, Lukens FJ. Endoscopy in the elderly: a review of the efficacy and safety of colonoscopy, esophagogastroduodenoscopy, and endoscopic retrograde cholangiopancreatography. J Clin Gastroenterol. 2010;44(3):161–6. Epub 2010/01/01.
8. Nikolsky E, Mehran R, Stone GW. Gastrointestinal bleeding in percutaneous coronary intervention and acute coronary syndromes. Am J Cardiol. 2009;104(5 Suppl):22C–9. Epub 2009/08/27.
9. Sinnaeve PR, Brueckmann M, Clemens A, Oldgren J, Eikelboom J, Healey JS. Stroke prevention in elderly patients with atrial fibrillation: challenges for anticoagulation. J Intern Med. 2012;271(1): 15–24. Epub 2011/10/15.
10. Hylek EM, Evans-Molina C, Shea C, Henault LE, Regan S. Major hemorrhage and tolerability of warfarin in the first year of therapy among elderly patients with atrial fibrillation. Circulation. 2007;115(21):2689–96. Epub 2007/05/23.
11. Longstreth GF. Epidemiology and outcome of patients hospitalized with acute lower gastrointestinal hemorrhage: a population-based study. Am J Gastroenterol. 1997;92(3):419–24.
12. Yachimski PS, Friedman LS. Gastrointestinal bleeding in the elderly. Nat Clin Pract Gastroenterol Hepatol. 2008;5(2):80–93. Epub 2008/02/07.
13. McGuire Jr HH. Bleeding colonic diverticula. A reappraisal of natural history and management. Ann Surg. 1994;220(5): 653–6.
14. Sharma R, Gorbien MJ. Angiodysplasia and lower gastrointestinal tract bleeding in elderly patients. Arch Intern Med. 1995;155(8): 807–12. Epub 1995/04/24.
15. Christe C, Janssens JP, Armenian B, Herrmann F, Vogt N. Midazolam sedation for upper gastrointestinal endoscopy in older persons: a randomized, double-blind, placebo-controlled study. J Am Geriatr Soc. 2000;48(11):1398–403. Epub 2000/11/18.
16. Lukens FJ, Loeb DS, Machicao VI, Achem SR, Picco MF. Colonoscopy in octogenarians: a prospective outpatient study. Am J Gastroenterol. 2002;97(7):1722–5. Epub 2002/07/24.
17. Arora G, Mannalithara A, Singh G, Gerson LB, Triadafilopoulos G. Risk of perforation from a colonoscopy in adults: a large population-based study. Gastrointest Endosc. 2009;69(3 Pt 2):654–64. Epub 2009/03/11.
18. Calvin AD, Misra S, Pflueger A. Contrast-induced acute kidney injury and diabetic nephropathy. Nat Rev Nephrol. 2010;6(11): 679–88. Epub 2010/09/30.
19. Zink SI, Ohki SK, Stein B, Zambuto DA, Rosenberg RJ, Choi JJ, et al. Noninvasive evaluation of active lower gastrointestinal bleeding: comparison between contrast-enhanced MDCT and 99mTc-labeled RBC scintigraphy. AJR Am J Roentgenol. 2008;191(4): 1107–14. Epub 2008/09/23.
20. Howarth DM. The role of nuclear medicine in the detection of acute gastrointestinal bleeding. Semin Nucl Med. 2006;36(2):133–46. Epub 2006/03/07.
21. Geffroy Y, Rodallec MH, Boulay-Coletta I, Julles MC, Ridereau-Zins C, Zins M. Multidetector CT angiography in acute gastrointestinal bleeding: why, when, and how. Radiographics. 2011; 31(3):E35–46. Epub 2011/07/02.
22. Filippone A, Cianci R, Milano A, Valeriano S, Di Mizio V, Storto ML. Obscure gastrointestinal bleeding and small bowel pathology: comparison between wireless capsule endoscopy and multidetector-row CT enteroclysis. Abdom Imaging. 2008;33(4):398–406. Epub 2007/07/10.
23. Bocker U, Dinter D, Litterer C, Hummel F, Knebel P, Franke A, et al. Comparison of magnetic resonance imaging and video capsule enteroscopy in diagnosing small-bowel pathology: localization-dependent diagnostic yield. Scand J Gastroenterol. 2010;45(4): 490–500. Epub 2010/02/06.
24. Golder SK, Schreyer AG, Endlicher E, Feuerbach S, Scholmerich J, Kullmann F, et al. Comparison of capsule endoscopy and magnetic resonance (MR) enteroclysis in suspected small bowel disease. Int J Colorect Dis. 2006;21(2):97–104. Epub 2005/04/23.
25. Scaglione G, Russo F, Franco MR, Sarracco P, Pietrini L, Sorrentini I. Age and video capsule endoscopy in obscure gastrointestinal bleeding: a prospective study on hospitalized patients. Dig Dis Sci. 2011;56(4):1188–93. Epub 2010/09/23.
26. Matsumura T, Arai M, Sazuka S, Saito M, Takahashi Y, Maruoka D, et al. Negative capsule endoscopy for obscure gastrointestinal

bleeding is closely associated with the use of low-dose aspirin. Scand J Gastroenterol. 2011;46(5):621–6. Epub 2010/12/30.
27. Katsinelos P, Chatzimavroudis G, Terzoudis S, Patsis I, Fasoulas K, Katsinelos T, et al. Diagnostic yield and clinical impact of capsule endoscopy in obscure gastrointestinal bleeding during routine clinical practice: a single-center experience. Med Princ Pract. 2011;20(1):60–5. Epub 2010/12/17.
28. van Turenhout ST, Jacobs MA, van Weyenberg SJ, Herdes E, Stam F, Mulder CJ, et al. Diagnostic yield of capsule endoscopy in a tertiary hospital in patients with obscure gastrointestinal bleeding. J Gastrointestin Liver Dis. 2010;19(2):141–5. Epub 2010/07/02.
29. Laine L, Sahota A, Shah A. Does capsule endoscopy improve outcomes in obscure gastrointestinal bleeding? Randomized trial versus dedicated small bowel radiography. Gastroenterology. 2010;138(5):1673–80.e1; quiz e11–2. Epub 2010/02/09.
30. Estevez E, Gonzalez-Conde B, Vazquez-Iglesias JL, de Los Angeles Vazquez-Millan M, Pertega S, Alonso PA, et al. Diagnostic yield and clinical outcomes after capsule endoscopy in 100 consecutive patients with obscure gastrointestinal bleeding. Eur J Gastroenterol Hepatol. 2006;18(8):881–8. Epub 2006/07/11.
31. Redondo-Cerezo E, Perez-Vigara G, Perez-Sola A, Gomez-Ruiz CJ, Chicano MV, Sanchez-Manjavacas N, et al. Diagnostic yield and impact of capsule endoscopy on management of patients with gastrointestinal bleeding of obscure origin. Dig Dis Sci. 2007;52(5):1376–81. Epub 2007/03/16.
32. Liao Z, Gao R, Xu C, Li ZS. Indications and detection, completion, and retention rates of small-bowel capsule endoscopy: a systematic review. Gastrointest Endosc. 2010;71(2):280–6. Epub 2010/02/16.
33. Kelley SR, Lohr JM. Retained wireless video enteroscopy capsule: a case report and review of the literature. J Surg Educ. 2009;66(5):296–300. Epub 2009/12/17.
34. Hay JA, Lyubashevsky E, Elashoff J, Maldonado L, Weingarten SR, Ellrodt AG. Upper gastrointestinal hemorrhage clinical–guideline determining the optimal hospital length of stay. Am J Med. 1996;100(3):313–22. Epub 1996/03/01.
35. Bell GD, Bown S, Morden A, Coady T, Logan RF. Prevention of hypoxaemia during upper-gastrointestinal endoscopy by means of oxygen via nasal cannulae. Lancet. 1987;1(8540):1022–4. Epub 1987/05/02.
36. Scholer SG, Schafer DF, Potter JF. The effect of age on the relative potency of midazolam and diazepam for sedation in upper gastrointestinal endoscopy. J Clin Gastroenterol. 1990;12(2):145–7. Epub 1990/04/01.
37. Qureshi WA, Zuckerman MJ, Adler DG, Davila RE, Egan JV, Gan SI, et al. ASGE guideline: modifications in endoscopic practice for the elderly. Gastrointest Endosc. 2006;63(4):566–9. Epub 2006/03/28.
38. Moore FA, McKinley BA, Moore EE, Nathens AB, West M, Shapiro MB, et al. Inflammation and the Host Response to Injury, a large-scale collaborative project: patient-oriented research core–standard operating procedures for clinical care. III. Guidelines for shock resuscitation. J Trauma. 2006;61(1):82–9. Epub 2006/07/13.
39. Alderson P, Bunn F, Lefebvre C, Li WP, Li L, Roberts I, et al. Human albumin solution for resuscitation and volume expansion in critically ill patients. Cochrane Database Syst Rev. 2002;1, CD001208. Epub 2002/03/01.
40. Ament A, Baltussen R, Duru G, Rigaud-Bully C, de Graeve D, Ortqvist A, et al. Cost-effectiveness of pneumococcal vaccination of older people: a study in 5 western European countries. Clin Infect Dis. 2000;31(2):444–50. Epub 2000/09/15.
41. Inaba K, Lustenberger T, Rhee P, Holcomb JB, Blackbourne LH, Shulman I, et al. The impact of platelet transfusion in massively transfused trauma patients. J Am Coll Surg. 2010;211(5):573–9. Epub 2010/09/18.
42. Bosch J, Thabut D, Bendtsen F, D'Amico G, Albillos A, Gonzalez Abraldes J, et al. Recombinant factor VIIa for upper gastrointestinal bleeding in patients with cirrhosis: a randomized, double-blind trial. Gastroenterology. 2004;127(4):1123–30. Epub 2004/10/14.
43. Bosch J, Thabut D, Albillos A, Carbonell N, Spicak J, Massard J, et al. Recombinant factor VIIa for variceal bleeding in patients with advanced cirrhosis: a randomized, controlled trial. Hepatology. 2008;47(5):1604–14. Epub 2008/04/09.
44. Ali ZS, Al-Shaalan H, Jorgensen J. Successful treatment of massive acute lower gastrointestinal bleeding in diverticular disease of colon, with activated recombinant factor VII (NovoSeven). Blood Coagul Fibrinolysis. 2006;17(4):327–9.
45. Gilbert DA, Silverstein FE, Tedesco FJ. National ASGE survey on upper gastrointestinal bleeding: complications of endoscopy. Dig Dis Sci. 1981;26(7 Suppl):55S–9. Epub 1981/07/01.
46. Sarin N, Monga N, Adams PC. Time to endoscopy and outcomes in upper gastrointestinal bleeding. Can J Gastroenterol. 2009;23(7):489–93.
47. Lipof T, Sardella WV, Bartus CM, Johnson KH, Vignati PV, Cohen JL. The efficacy and durability of super-selective embolization in the treatment of lower gastrointestinal bleeding. Dis Colon Rectum. 2008;51(3):301–5. Epub 2008/01/22.
48. Gilbert DA, Silverstein FE, Tedesco FJ, Buenger NK, Persing J. The national ASGE survey on upper gastrointestinal bleeding. III. Endoscopy in upper gastrointestinal bleeding. Gastrointest Endosc. 1981;27(2):94–102. Epub 1981/05/01.
49. Day LW, Kwon A, Inadomi JM, Walter LC, Somsouk M. Adverse events in older patients undergoing colonoscopy: a systematic review and meta-analysis. Gastrointest Endosc. 2011;74(4): 885–96. Epub 2011/09/29.
50. Kuo WT. Transcatheter treatment for lower gastrointestinal hemorrhage. Tech Vasc Interv Radiol. 2004;7(3):143–50.
51. Bandi R, Shetty PC, Sharma RP, Burke TH, Burke MW, Kastan D. Superselective arterial embolization for the treatment of lower gastrointestinal hemorrhage. J Vasc Interv Radiol. 2001;12(12): 1399–405. Epub 2001/12/14.
52. Kuo WT, Lee DE, Saad WE, Patel N, Sahler LG, Waldman DL. Superselective microcoil embolization for the treatment of lower gastrointestinal hemorrhage. J Vasc Interv Radiol. 2003;14(12): 1503–9.
53. Mehran R, Aymong ED, Nikolsky E, Lasic Z, Iakovou I, Fahy M, et al. A simple risk score for prediction of contrast-induced nephropathy after percutaneous coronary intervention: development and initial validation. J Am Coll Cardiol. 2004;44(7):1393–9. Epub 2004/10/07.
54. Day L. The Otago strength and balance exercise programme lowers the risk of death and falls in the older people at 12 months. Evid Based Nurs. 2011;14(3):76–8. Epub 2011/03/26.
55. Finlayson E, Wang L, Landefeld CS, Dudley RA. Major abdominal surgery in nursing home residents: a national study. Ann Surg. 2011;254(6):921–6. Epub 2011/10/25.
56. Clarke MG, Bunting D, Smart NJ, Lowes J, Mitchell SJ. The surgical management of acute upper gastrointestinal bleeding: a 12-year experience. Int J Surg. 2010;8(5):377–80. Epub 2010/06/12.
57. Tepel M, van der Giet M, Schwarzfeld C, Laufer U, Liermann D, Zidek W. Prevention of radiographic-contrast-agent-induced reductions in renal function by acetylcysteine. N Engl J Med. 2000;343(3):180–4. Epub 2000/07/20.
58. Tamura A, Goto Y, Miyamoto K, Naono S, Kawano Y, Kotoku M, et al. Efficacy of single-bolus administration of sodium bicarbonate to prevent contrast-induced nephropathy in patients with mild renal insufficiency undergoing an elective coronary procedure. Am J Cardiol. 2009;104(7):921–5. Epub 2009/09/22.
59. Clark RA, Colley DP, Eggers FM. Acute arterial gastrointestinal hemorrhage: efficacy of transcatheter control. AJR Am J Roentgenol. 1981;136(6):1185–9. Epub 1981/06/01.

60. Gimson AE, Westaby D, Hegarty J, Watson A, Williams R. A randomized trial of vasopressin and vasopressin plus nitroglycerin in the control of acute variceal hemorrhage. Hepatology. 1986;6(3):410–3. Epub 1986/05/01.
61. Gianfrancisco JA, Abcarian H. Pitfalls in the treatment of massive lower gastrointestinal bleeding with "blind" subtotal colectomy. Dis Colon Rectum. 1982;25(5):441–5.
62. Setya V, Singer JA, Minken SL. Subtotal colectomy as a last resort for unrelenting, unlocalized, lower gastrointestinal hemorrhage: experience with 12 cases. Am Surg. 1992;58(5):295–9.
63. Cohn SM, Moller BA, Zieg PM, Milner KA, Angood PB. Angiography for preoperative evaluation in patients with lower gastrointestinal bleeding: are the benefits worth the risks? Arch Surg. 1998;133(1):50–5. Epub 1998/01/23.

16 Acute Abdomen

Ronald M. Jou and David Spain

Acute Abdomen

Abdominal pain is one of the most common chief complaints for patients presenting for emergency medical care, regardless of age [1]. Older patients tend to present to medical attention in a more delayed fashion. For appendicitis and other intra-abdominal infections, the average duration of symptoms prior to presentation is 1–5 days longer in elderly patients compared to younger patients [2, 3].

Perhaps because of the tendency toward later presentation and the presence of comorbidities, older patients tend to have higher acuity of disease compared to younger patients with similar complaints and diagnoses. Forty to sixty percent of geriatric patients with acute abdominal pain require hospital admission, 10–30 % will require an operation or invasive procedure, and ultimately, the mortality rate is 5–8 %. The rates of admission and invasive intervention are roughly twice as high as those for younger patients with similar presentations, and the mortality rate is as much as five- or tenfold higher [4–7]. Accurately determining the diagnosis and the need for an operation in a timely fashion is both important and challenging in this patient population.

History and Physical Exam

A careful and complete history is fundamental to the evaluation of the acute abdomen. Unfortunately, geriatric patients presenting with acute abdominal symptoms often have nonspecific abdominal pain, leading to diagnostic inaccuracy which increases with age [6, 7]. Memory loss, with or without dementia, affects 3–8 % of the elderly population, which can present a significant obstacle to obtaining an accurate history [8, 9]. Furthermore, 25–45 % of elderly patient have significant hearing loss that can impair speech recognition in noisy settings such as the emergency department [10].

The presence of a family member, caretaker, or close friend can be invaluable in providing the history, clarifying the timeline or sequence of events, and to establish the patient's baseline level of function prior to the onset of acute illness.

Open-ended questions often provide a more accurate story than closed-ended questions, which tends to confirm the preconceived notions of the medical team. The time course, location, quality, and radiation of pain should be established, along with any inciting or exacerbating factors such as positioning, movement, or coughing. Changes in the location or intensity of pain are important clues.

Associated symptoms including fevers, chills, nausea, vomiting, or changes in bowel or bladder habits should be elicited. The onset and quality of the vomitus may indicate the level of obstruction, be it distal or proximal. The frequency, consistency, and color of bowel movements may indicate obstruction, inflammation, or bleeding.

The majority of elderly patients have at least one comorbid condition that complicates their acute abdominal pain, and a careful review of cardiac and respiratory symptoms may help to identify important nonsurgical causes of acute abdominal pain such as pneumonia or myocardial infarction [3, 11]. Urinary symptoms should also be elicited, and postmenopausal bleeding is always significant and concerning for malignancy.

Previous operations and their indications should be well documented. Medications should be reviewed, paying particular attention to anticoagulants, antihypertensives, NSAIDs, steroids, antimicrobials, and immunosuppressants. The majority of elderly patients are taking at least one long-term medication, and the addition of a new medication has the potential to cause adverse drug reactions. Many of these

R.M. Jou, MD
Department of Surgery, Stanford Hospital and Clinic, 300 Pasteur Drive, S-067, Stanford, CA 94305, USA
e-mail: ronald.jou@gmail.com, rjou@stanford.edu

D. Spain, MD (✉)
Department of Surgery, Stanford University Medical Center, 300 Pasteur Drive, S-067, Stanford, CA 94305-5655, USA
e-mail: dspain@stanford.edu

J.A. Yelon, F.A. Luchette (eds.), *Geriatric Trauma and Critical Care*,
DOI 10.1007/978-1-4614-8501-8_16, © Springer Science+Business Media New York 2014

reactions are gastrointestinal in nature and can mimic acute intra-abdominal pathology [12, 13]. Age-appropriate cancer screening study results should be reviewed.

Important aspects of the physical exam can be obtained, while the history is taken. The overall appearance of the patient, whether ill-appearing or obvious distressed, is crucial. Observations about the patient's dress, grooming, or hygiene can be proxies for overall care access to medical attention and elder abuse. The patient's habitus and the presence of cachexia are important indicators of nutrition and the ability to withstand a surgical intervention. The quality and rate of the pulse, skin turgor, and capillary refill time can provide important clues about systemic toxicity and overall volume status. The presence of fever is important, as many elderly patients with an acute surgical disease do mount a febrile response [14].

One major contributor to difficulties in diagnosis is the high prevalence of cognitive impairment present in this patient population. Although definitions of cognitive impairment vary, 17–20 % of elderly patients have some impairment in language, visuospatial awareness, or attention that can impair the examiner's ability to elicit physical examination findings [9, 15]. Nonverbal signs of pain or tenderness such as wincing, grimacing, changes in breathing patterns, or tensing of the abdominal wall musculature take on a greater importance for patients who may not be able to communicate directly.

The sclera should be inspected for jaundice, and detection of conjunctival pallor can be a rapid way to screen for profound anemia. The mucous membranes of the face should be inspected for color and moisture. Neck masses and lymphadenopathy are important findings that can be associated with infection or malignancy.

The lung fields should be auscultated carefully to find signs of pneumonia or pleural effusions that sometimes mimic or accompany intra-abdominal pathology. The heart sounds should be auscultated carefully, as pericarditis and heart failure can both be present with abdominal pain. The flanks should be palpated and percussed for costovertebral angle tenderness as a sign of nephrolithiasis or upper urinary tract infection.

The abdomen is best examined from the patient's right side, with the patient in the supine position and arms down at the sides. Having the patient flex both knees may allow for better relaxation of the abdominal wall and less guarding. The abdomen is inspected for distention and any obvious lesions or hernias. The stigmata of liver disease such as jaundice, spider angiomas, and caput medusae should be noted. The auscultation of high-pitched bowel sounds can occasionally be helpful in cases of suspected bowel obstruction.

When examining a tender abdomen, the goal is to elicit sufficient information without causing undue pain or discomfort. Asking the patient to cough prior to palpation may cause localized abdominal tenderness as a sign of peritoneal irritation. All four quadrants should be palpated, beginning in a quadrant away from the site of pain, and starting with gentle palpation and moving to deeper palpation as tolerated by the patient. Exquisite tenderness to percussion or light palpation signifies peritonitis, which does not need to be verified by deeper palpation. Assessing rebound in a patient when localized or generalized peritonitis has already been established is unnecessary, and only serves to distract the patient, thereby decreasing the sensitivity of other aspects of physical examination. Voluntary guarding, involuntary guarding, and "washboard" rigidity signify increasing degrees of visceral and parietal peritonitis. Obvious masses should be noted. Dullness to percussion or a palpable fluid wave signifies ascites that may be associated with liver disease, heart disease, malnutrition, or malignancy.

The digital rectal examination is a fundamental part of the evaluation and should not be omitted. The presence of rectal masses, tenderness, blood, and the presence and quality of stool in the rectal vault are all important clues.

In men, the genitalia and scrotum should be examined for hernias, torsion, and epididymitis. In women, a pelvic examination may be required to evaluate for adnexal masses, tenderness, or signs of a pelvic wall or floor hernia.

The pulse exam including palpation of extremity and abdominal pulsations is important to detect signs of vascular insufficiency and aneurysm related to mesenteric ischemia or abdominal aortic aneurysm disease as causes of acute abdominal pain. Peripheral edema can be a sign of venous occlusion or fluid overload.

Laboratory Analyses

Although laboratory analyses do not differentiate between surgical and nonsurgical causes of abdominal pain in elderly patients [16], routine evaluation should include a complete blood count, serum chemistries, liver function tests, serum amylase and/or lipase, and a urinalysis [16]. In general, most laboratory values in healthy elderly patients fall into the same reference ranges as younger patients [17–19].

The presence of leukocytosis can signify inflammation, infection, or malignancy. Hints to the chronicity and cause of anemia detected in the blood count can be found in the mean corpuscular volume, which may be microcytic in anemia of iron deficiency or chronic disease, or macrocytic in the setting of liver disease or malnutrition. Thrombocytopenia is a sensitive marker of portal hypertension.

Assessment of renal function including serum urea nitrogen (BUN) and serum creatinine is important for elderly patients with abdominal complaints. In addition to the azotemia from any fluid losses during acute illness, these patients may have underlying chronic kidney insufficiency.

Furthermore, many patients with abdominal pain will undergo intravenous iodinated contrast injection for CT scanning, and an assessment of renal function is important to stratify risk for contrast nephropathy.

Measurement of electrolytes is important for patients who have had fluid losses from vomiting or diarrhea. Elderly patients taking diuretics also have a tendency to have electrolyte abnormalities even when healthy [19]. Glucose measurement may detect hypoglycemia from lack of oral intake and compounded by hypoglycemic therapy or hyperglycemia from diabetic ketoacidosis (DKA) or hyperosmolar non-ketotic coma (HONC) as causes of nonsurgical abdominal pain. Liver function tests are useful when liver or biliary disease is suspected. The measurement of serum amylase and/or lipase is mandatory if pancreatitis is a possibility.

Although elderly patients have a high incidence of malignancy, the measurement of serum tumor markers to screen for various cancers in patients with acute abdominal pain is costly, untimely, and unlikely to provide any useful information during the initial evaluation.

Diagnostic Imaging

Ideally, an imaging test is ordered to evaluate the diagnostic hypotheses generated by the history, physical exam, and laboratory analyses. Although advances in imaging technology continue to provide greater resolution, no radiographic test provides perfect diagnostic information for abdominal pain. Instead, the clinician's must deal with probabilities and likelihoods, where the pretest probability of having a particular disease is modified by the likelihood ratio of the chosen imaging test result, which gives the posttest probability of having confirmed that particular diagnosis. Accordingly, the choice of imaging for each case depends on the performance of each imaging test to provide a high (or low) likelihood ratio in that particular situation.

The acute abdominal radiograph series is an inexpensive, widely available, and low-risk test for acute abdominal pain. Generally, this test involves acquiring an upright chest radiograph, an upright abdominal radiograph, and a supine abdominal radiograph. If the patient cannot tolerate standing upright, then a lateral decubitus or supine cross-table radiograph may be substituted. The chest radiograph can evaluate for acute cardiopulmonary disease such as pneumonia but, more importantly, is considered the most sensitive plain radiograph for the detection of pneumoperitoneum, i.e., free air. While plain abdominal radiographs may demonstrate foreign bodies and bowel obstruction as well as evidence of volvulus, bowel ischemia, and stones, they are generally insensitive for diagnosing acute abdominal pathology [20].

Abdominal ultrasound continues to be the test of choice for evaluating right upper quadrant pain [21, 22]. Although this modality is somewhat dependent on operator skill and experience, ultrasound is a sensitive test for evaluating for gallstones and acute cholecystitis. While elderly patients do tend to have larger caliber extrahepatic bile ducts on ultrasound, the vast majority of elderly patients without biliary disease have calibers below 6–7 mm, the generally accepted upper range of normal [23, 24]. Abdominal ultrasound can also demonstrate perinephric fluid collections or hydronephrosis associated with urinary tract pathology. The use of abdominal ultrasonography in the diagnosis of acute appendicitis in adults is controversial, and further study is needed, especially in the elderly population. Ultrasound is very accurate in the diagnosis of abdominal aortic aneurysms [25].

In elderly female patients with pelvic complaints, transvaginal ultrasound is an efficient modality that does not involve contrast injection or ionizing radiation. Although diagnoses such as ectopic pregnancy and pelvic inflammatory disease are not concerns in the elderly population, transvaginal ultrasound is sensitive for the detection of endometrial cancer and adnexal masses, both benign and malignant [26, 27].

Computed tomography (CT) scanning is relatively fast, widely available, and has been shown to be helpful in the diagnosis of a wide variety of diseases in patients with acute abdominal pain [28]. In elderly patients with acute abdominal pain where accurate diagnosis can be challenging, CT has been shown to alter clinical decision making in a significant portion of cases [29]. CT also provides spatial anatomic information that may be useful to surgeons or other interventionalists. CT does require exposure to ionizing radiation and the risk for the induction of malignancy, although this risk is lower for older patients whose postexposure lifetimes are generally shorter. Although non-contrast CT scans do provide some diagnostic information, the utility of CT is greatly augmented by the administration of intravenous radiocontrast during the examination. Kidney injury from contrast administration continues to be an important complication of CT examinations and advanced age has been associated with increased risk, independent of other known risk factors such as renal insufficiency, diabetes mellitus, and cardiovascular disease [30]. Therefore, before intravenous contrast is given, the potential benefit of the examination should be assessed along with the risk of contrast nephropathy and the possible need for incorporation of prevention strategies.

Although magnetic resonance imaging (MRI) has been found to be accurate in the diagnosis of acute appendicitis, diverticulitis, acute cholecystitis, and acute pancreatitis [31], it is not widely available, and utility of MR in acute abdominal pain is limited by lengthy examination times and higher cost compared to CT.

Differential Diagnosis

When caring for a patient with acute abdominal pain, the most important question is whether or not the patient requires an urgent operation. If hemodynamic instability, generalized peritonitis, or clinical deterioration is present, the safest course of action is often to proceed directly to the operating room or surgical intensive care unit under the care of a surgical team. With few exceptions, if a patient presents in extremis with acute abdominal pain, they suffer from one of a few catastrophes: ruptured abdominal aortic aneurysm, severe pancreatitis, bowel infarction, or sepsis from some uncontrolled source of infection such as cholangitis or urosepsis. In this situation, information is often limited, and the task is to determine rapidly the most likely cause and proceed as quickly as possible with stabilization and definitive treatment. In this situation, further efforts to diagnose the patient more accurately or thoroughly in the emergency department serve only to delay the potentially life-saving intervention that is required.

If the patient with acute abdominal pain is hemodynamically stable and peritonitis is absent, then there is time to review all relevant clinical information and develop a differential diagnosis. Here, the location and nature of pain are particularly helpful. In general, the differential for acute abdominal pain in the elderly patient will not differ significantly from that of a younger patient, although certain diagnoses such as ectopic pregnancy are not encountered in elderly patients.

In comparison to generalized peritonitis where late-stage inflammation is usually related to a perforated hollow viscus, the cardinal presentation of localized pain and tenderness provides some information about which viscera is diseased. Furthermore, observational studies of elderly patients presenting with acute abdominal pain have described the most common diagnoses in this cohort [4, 6, 11, 32–34]. Among causes of right upper quadrant pain and tenderness, biliary colic, acute cholecystitis, and cholangitis are most common. Right lower quadrant findings suggest acute appendicitis or an unusual presentation of diverticulitis. Left lower quadrant pain and tenderness would be a more usual presentation of diverticulitis. Epigastric pain and tenderness invoke peptic ulcer disease or pancreatitis. Suprapubic or flank findings suggest a urinary source such as infection or stone disease, which are both quite common in the elderly population [6].

The cardinal presentation of distention, nausea, and vomiting suggests bowel obstruction. When accompanied by colicky pain, small bowel obstruction would be most common, due to incarcerated hernia, adhesions, or malignancy [32, 33]. When distention is more prominent than pain, large bowel obstruction from diverticular disease, malignancy, volvulus, or constipation are most common [32, 33].

Given the higher rates of malignancy for elderly patients and the significant rates of malignancy in elderly patients presenting with abdominal pain cancer should always be considered as a possibility [11, 32, 34].

Important nonsurgical causes of abdominal pain include myocardial infarction, pulmonary embolism, pneumonia, toxic ingestion, and drug or alcohol withdrawal.

Pitfalls

The term "nonspecific abdominal pain" should be used with caution. Especially in the elderly patient, the absence of a diagnosis does not indicate that a life-threatening process does not exist. Important causes of abdominal pain tend to progress with time, and a period of observation is prudent for any elderly patient who presents with acute abdominal pain. The observation period allows for the integration of serial physical examinations and follow-up laboratory or imaging data either to make an accurate diagnosis or to decide that the patient requires an urgent intervention.

References

1. National Hospital Ambulatory Medical Care Survey: 2008 Emergency Department Summary Tables [Internet]. National Center for Health Statistics and U.S. Census Bureau. 2008.
2. Kraemer M, Franke C, Ohmann C, Yang Q. Acute appendicitis in late adulthood: incidence, presentation, and outcome. Results of a prospective multicenter acute abdominal pain study and a review of the literature. Langenbecks Arch Surg. 2000;385(7):470–81. PubMed PMID: 11131250.
3. Cooper GS, Shlaes DM, Salata RA. Intraabdominal infection: differences in presentation and outcome between younger patients and the elderly. Clin Infect Dis. 1994;19(1):146–8. PubMed PMID: 7948517.
4. Marco CA, Schoenfeld CN, Keyl PM, Menkes ED, Doehring MC. Abdominal pain in geriatric emergency patients: variables associated with adverse outcomes. Acad Emerg Med. 1998;5(12):1163–8. PubMed PMID: 9864129.
5. Brewer BJ, Golden GT, Hitch DC, Rudolf LE, Wangensteen SL. Abdominal pain. An analysis of 1,000 consecutive cases in a University Hospital emergency room. Am J Surg. 1976; 131(2):219–23.
6. Lewis LM, Banet GA, Blanda M, Hustey FM, Meldon SW, Gerson LW. Etiology and clinical course of abdominal pain in senior patients: a prospective, multicenter study. J Gerontol A Biol Sci Med Sci. 2005;60(8):1071–6. PubMed PMID: 16127115.
7. de Dombal FT. Acute abdominal pain in the elderly. J Clin Gastroenterol. 1994;19(4):331–5. PubMed PMID: 7876517.
8. Rocca WA, Petersen RC, Knopman DS, Hebert LE, Evans DA, Hall KS, et al. Trends in the incidence and prevalence of Alzheimer's disease, dementia, and cognitive impairment in the United States. Alzheimers Dement. 2011;7(1):80–93. PubMed PMID: 21255746.
9. Graham JE, Rockwood K, Beattie BL, Eastwood R, Gauthier S, Tuokko H, et al. Prevalence and severity of cognitive impairment with and without dementia in an elderly population. Lancet. 1997;349(9068):1793–6. PubMed PMID: 9269213.

10. Li-Korotky HS. Age-related hearing loss: quality of care for quality of life. Gerontologist. 2012;52(2):265–71. PubMed PMID: 22383543.
11. Fenyo G. Acute abdominal disease in the elderly: experience from two series in Stockholm. Am J Surg. 1982;143(6):751–4. PubMed PMID: 7091511.
12. Veehof LJ, Stewart RE, Meyboom-de Jong B, Haaijer-Ruskamp FM. Adverse drug reactions and polypharmacy in the elderly in general practice. Eur J Clin Pharmacol. 1999;55(7):533–6. PubMed PMID: 10501824.
13. Dang C, Aguilera P, Dang A, Salem L. Acute abdominal pain. Four classifications can guide assessment and management. Geriatrics. 2002;57(3):30–2, 5–6, 41–2. PubMed PMID: 11899547.
14. Potts FE, Vukov LF. Utility of fever and leukocytosis in acute surgical abdomens in octogenarians and beyond. J Gerontol A Biol Sci Med Sci. 1999;54(2):M55–8. PubMed PMID: 10051855.
15. DeCarli C. Mild cognitive impairment: prevalence, prognosis, aetiology, and treatment. Lancet Neurol. 2003;2(1):15–21. PubMed PMID: 12849297.
16. Parker JS, Vukov LF, Wollan PC. Abdominal pain in the elderly: use of temperature and laboratory testing to screen for surgical disease. Fam Med. 1996;28(3):193–7. PubMed PMID: 8900552.
17. Coodley EL. Laboratory tests in the elderly. What is abnormal? Postgrad Med. 1989;85(1):333–8.
18. Huber KR, Mostafaie N, Stangl G, Worofka B, Kittl E, Hofmann J, et al. Clinical chemistry reference values for 75-year-old apparently healthy persons. Clin Chem Lab Med. 2006;44(11):1355–60. PubMed PMID: 17087648.
19. Hale WE, Stewart RB, Marks RG. Haematological and biochemical laboratory values in an ambulatory elderly population: an analysis of the effects of age, sex and drugs. Age Ageing. 1983;12(4):275–84. PubMed PMID: 6660137.
20. Ahn SH, Mayo-Smith WW, Murphy BL, Reinert SE, Cronan JJ. Acute nontraumatic abdominal pain in adult patients: abdominal radiography compared with CT evaluation. Radiology. 2002;225(1):159–64. PubMed PMID: 12355000.
21. Carroll BA. Preferred imaging techniques for the diagnosis of cholecystitis and cholelithiasis. Ann Surg. 1989;210(1):1–12. PubMed PMID: 2662921.
22. Walsh PF, Crawford D, Crossling FT, Sutherland GR, Negrette JJ, Shand J. The value of immediate ultrasound in acute abdominal conditions: a critical appraisal. Clin Radiol. 1990;42(1):47–9. PubMed PMID: 2202538.
23. Perret RS, Sloop GD, Borne JA. Common bile duct measurements in an elderly population. J Ultrasound Med. 2000;19(11):727–30, quiz 31. PubMed PMID: 11065260.
24. Horrow MM, Horrow JC, Niakosari A, Kirby CL, Rosenberg HK. Is age associated with size of adult extrahepatic bile duct: sonographic study. Radiology. 2001;221(2):411–4. PubMed PMID: 11687684.
25. Barkin AZ, Rosen CL. Ultrasound detection of abdominal aortic aneurysm. Emerg Med Clin North Am. 2004;22(3):675–82. PubMed PMID: 15301845.
26. Taipale P, Tarjanne H, Heinonen UM. The diagnostic value of transvaginal sonography in the diagnosis of endometrial malignancy in women with peri- and postmenopausal bleeding. Acta Obstet Gynecol Scand. 1994;73(10):819–23. PubMed PMID: 7817736.
27. Fleischer AC, Rogers WH, Rao BK, Kepple DM, Jones HW. Transvaginal color Doppler sonography of ovarian masses with pathological correlation. Ultrasound Obstet Gynecol. 1991;1(4):275–8. PubMed PMID: 12797059.
28. Lameris W, van Randen A, van Es HW, van Heesewijk JP, van Ramshorst B, Bouma WH, et al. Imaging strategies for detection of urgent conditions in patients with acute abdominal pain: diagnostic accuracy study. BMJ. 2009;338:b2431. PubMed PMID: 19561056.
29. Esses D, Birnbaum A, Bijur P, Shah S, Gleyzer A, Gallagher EJ. Ability of CT to alter decision making in elderly patients with acute abdominal pain. Am J Emerg Med. 2004;22(4):270–2. PubMed PMID: 15258866.
30. Goldenberg I, Matetzky S. Nephropathy induced by contrast media: pathogenesis, risk factors and preventive strategies. CMAJ. 2005;172(11):1461–71. PubMed PMID: 15911862.
31. Stoker J. Magnetic resonance imaging and the acute abdomen. Br J Surg. 2008;95(10):1193–4. PubMed PMID: 18763236.
32. Costamagna D, Pipitone Federico NS, Erra S, Tribocco M, Poncina F, Botto G, et al. Acute abdomen in the elderly. A peripheral general hospital experience. G Chir. 2009;30(6–7):315–22. PubMed PMID: 19580715.
33. van Geloven AA, Biesheuvel TH, Luitse JS, Hoitsma HF, Obertop H. Hospital admissions of patients aged over 80 with acute abdominal complaints. Eur J Surg. 2000;166(11):866–71. PubMed PMID: 11097153.
34. Bugliosi TF, Meloy TD, Vukov LF. Acute abdominal pain in the elderly. Ann Emerg Med. 1990;19(12):1383–6. PubMed PMID: 2240749.

Necrotizing Soft Tissue Infections

17

D. Dante Yeh and George Velmahos

> Many were attacked by the erysipelas all over the body when the exciting cause was a trivial accident or a very small wound...Flesh, sinews, and bone fell away in large quantities. The flux which formed was not like pus but a different sort of putrefaction...Fever was sometimes present and sometimes absent... there were many deaths. The course of the disease was the same to whatever part of the body it spread... The most dangerous cases of all such cases were when the pubes and genital organs were attacked. [1]
>
> – Hippocrates (circa 500 B.C.)

Since its first description in antiquity, man has been afflicted by aggressive soft tissue infections arising from seemingly trivial wounds or often without any provocation. Centuries later, Ambroise Pare (1510–1590) reported that "there can happen no greater than a Gangrene, as that which may cause the mortification and death of the part, and oft times the whole body... mortification and death of the part, which it feafth upon, dying little by little" [2]. The first descriptions in English are credited to Leonard Gillespie, Sir Gilbert Blane, and Thomas Trotter (a British naval surgeon and two British naval physicians, respectively) in the late eighteenth century [3, 4]. In the United States, Joseph Jones, a Confederate medical officer in the American Civil War, first published in 1871 a report describing "hospital gangrene" [5, 6]. Jones, authorized by the United States Sanitary Commission, described 2,642 cases with a mortality rate of 46 % [5]. Meleney, reporting on 20 cases in China, is credited with establishing streptococcus as the major etiologic agent in 1924. His description of the deadly disease remains relevant almost a century later:

> The disease is characterized by its alarmingly rapid development....the affect member becomes greatly swollen, hot, red and tender, with symptoms and signs of acute inflammation spreading rapidly both proximally and distally from the original focus... As the part swells, the stiffness, pain and increased weight rend it quite useless. In some cases, the pain of onset is replaced by a numbness, which later develops into a complete anesthesia for the affected portion... blisters and bullae begin to form... sometimes the area of skin necrosis is very small, while the subcutaneous gangrene is very extensive... in other cases, the extent of the subcutaneous necrosis is not recognized until an incision is made... the process continues to advance rapidly until several large areas of skin have become gangrenous, and the intoxication renders the patient dull.... [7]

The term "necrotizing fasciitis" was first coined by Wilson in 1952 and referred to both gas-forming and non-gas-forming infections. In the 1990s, the term "flesh-eating bacteria" was popularized by the media. Various names have been used to describe this deadly disease: hospital gangrene, necrotizing erysipelas, necrotizing myositis, acute necrotizing cellulitis, Streptococcal gangrene, suppurative fasciitis, gas gangrene, Clostridial gangrene, Clostridial cellulitis, Clostridial myositis, malignant ulcer, gangrenous ulcer, Cullen ulcer, putrid ulcer, phagedena ("eating away"), phagedenic ulcer, phagedena gangrenosa, progressive synergistic bacterial gangrene, acute synergistic gangrene, acute dermal gangrene, etc. [4, 8, 9]. The numerous monikers used to describe this cluster of disease in the literature has created much confusion and may contribute to misdiagnosis and delay in treatment. All forms of this disease include necrotic or devitalized tissue which encourages the rapid growth of bacteria and also precludes delivery of antibiotics and host defenses [8]. Because the treatment is the same regardless of location or depth, the all-encompassing term *necrotizing soft tissue infection* (*NSTI*) is now preferred.

Incidence

According to the United States Center for Disease Control and Prevention, the estimated incidence of NSTI in the United States is between 500 and 1,500 cases per year and

D.D. Yeh, MD (✉) • G. Velmahos, MD, PhD
Department of Surgery, Massachusetts General Hospital, 165 Cambridge St. #810, Boston, MA 02114, USA

Division of Trauma Emergency Surgery, and Surgical Critical Care, Massachusetts General Hospital, 165 Cambridge St. #810, Boston, MA 02114 USA
e-mail: dyeh2@partners.org; gvelmahos@partners.org

J.A. Yelon, F.A. Luchette (eds.), *Geriatric Trauma and Critical Care*,
DOI 10.1007/978-1-4614-8501-8_17, © Springer Science+Business Media New York 2014

most cases are community acquired [9, 10]. This disease affects men slightly more than women [11–15]. Although NSTI has been described in all ages, the mean age is between 50 and 60 years in most series [11–13, 16, 17]. Infants and children are rarely affected. The incidence of NSTI increases with increasing age, being three times higher in those over age 65 (0.55 per 100,000) when compared to those under the age of 45 (0.15 per 100,000) [10, 18]. This is likely related to the prevalence of risk factors for NSTI, almost all are more prevalent in the older population.

The hospitalization rate is approximately 1.3 cases/100,000 population with an average cost of $50,000 to $100,000 per case, not including the costs of rehabilitation and indirect costs [19]. The average length of stay for survivors ranges between 13 and 40 days in most reports [13–16, 19–27]. Only about one-half of surviving patients are discharged home [27], the remainder discharged to rehabilitation facilities or nursing homes. Interestingly, when compared with the general population (controlled for age, sex, and geographic area), the long-term survival of NSTI survivors is markedly decreased [28]. Annual deaths due to infectious causes are significantly higher (14 % vs. 2.9 %) when compared with the general population.

Mortality

Despite improvements in diagnostic modalities and advances in critical care, mortality rates have not improved significantly over the past century [5, 20]. Although a wide range of mortality rates (6–76 %) is reported in the literature, modern series mortality rates are about 30 % [8, 13, 16, 20]. Like other infectious processes, early deaths are due to overwhelming septic shock, while late deaths are usually secondary to progressive multiorgan failure [11]. Much has been written about risk factors for mortality, with delay in surgical excision the most commonly cited [11, 25, 29–32]. Advanced age is another strong predictor of mortality [16, 17, 24, 28, 31, 33, 34] with one series reporting a fivefold greater risk of death occurring in patients age > 60 compared with younger patients [19, 33]. Other reported prognosticators of mortality include the presence of hypotension [25], tachycardia [34], hypothermia [34], thrombocytopenia [31], bacteremia [10, 16, 17], acidosis, leukocytosis [34, 35], elevated hematocrit [21], bandemia [25], coagulopathy [17], APACHE II score > 20 [21, 26], SOFA score > 8 [32], heart disease, renal failure (acute and chronic) [34], cirrhosis [36], diabetes mellitus (DM), peripheral vascular disease (PVD), immunosuppression [24], number of comorbid medical diseases, malnutrition, cancer, extent of total body surface area (TBSA) involved [30], and obesity [11, 16, 17, 25]. Ethnic race has not been shown to be associated with mortality [33]. Interestingly, female gender has been reported to be a mortality risk factor, although the mechanism is not clear [33].

Etiology

Risk Factors

Predisposing factors to the development of NSTI vary by series and are influenced by geography and patient population. Some series report intravenous (IV) drug abuse as a strong risk factor [15], whereas in others unintentional trauma and surgical operations are most common [11, 17, 20, 25]. Amongst all comorbid medical conditions, DM is most strongly associated with NSTI, present in up to 50 % of confirmed cases [12, 13, 25, 28, 30, 37]. Importantly, no predisposing risk factor is present (idiopathic) in a high percentage of patients with NSTI, between 15 and 40 % in most reports [11, 13, 15, 17, 20, 22, 25, 27, 35].

Classification

NSTI are typically classified according to microbiologic causative organisms, though the distinction is of questionable clinical relevance as the initial treatment does not differ.

Type 1 (*Polymicrobial*) – this is the most common type, occurring in approximately 75 % of confirmed cases [12, 20, 30, 38]. There are typically between two and four organisms cultured per patient [11, 12, 39] and up to 11 organisms in one series [4]. The milieu contains a combination of anaerobic, aerobic, Gram-positive, and Gram-negative bacteria [11]. These infections tend to occur on the trunk, particularly postoperatively [4]. Immunocompromised patients are especially at risk of developing Type 1 NSTI [38].

Type 2 (*Streptococcus pyogenes alone or in combination*) – in contrast to Type 1 NSTI, Type 2 infections tend to occur in younger, immunocompetent patients such as IV drug abusers and athletes [38]. Monomicrobial infections are more common on the extremities [4].

Type 3 (*marine Vibrios*) – this type of NSTI is characterized by a particularly aggressive and fulminant clinical course caused by *Vibrio* spp. (*V. vulnificus*, *V. parahaemolyticus*, *V. damsela*) [40]. As etiologic agents, *Vibrio* spp. are associated with increased mortality [17, 25]. Cirrhosis (especially from chronic hepatitis B) is a strong risk factor for the development of Type 3 NSTI [38], which commonly involves both lower extremities without any obvious entry sites. This type is almost exclusively acquired in the community after exposure to seawater [36]. Interesting, the GI tract has been reported to be a possible portal of entry, with case reports describing NSTI after ingestion of raw oysters [41].

Microbiology

Although NSTIs are most frequently polymicrobial, certain organisms appear most commonly and an understanding of these "usual suspects" is crucial in directing initial empiric antibiotic therapy. Multiple infecting organisms are the rule and it is believed that these facultative bacteria behave synergistically.

S. pyogenes – is amongst the most commonly isolated organisms in both monomicrobial and polymicrobial infections [12]. Expression of surface proteins M-1 and M-3 are believed to increase streptococcal adhesion to tissues, preventing phagocytosis by neutrophils [42, 43]. Release of streptococcal exotoxins A, B, C, and superantigen contributes to host cytokine release (TNF-α, IL-1, IL-6) and platelet/neutrophil aggregate-mediated microvascular occlusion and may occasionally lead to the deadly toxic shock syndrome [4, 38, 42].

MRSA – in recent years, increasing prevalence of MRSA as a causative organism in NSTI has been reported (29–39 %), rivaling *S. pyogenes* in some series [16, 17, 37, 44]. Interestingly, MRSA NSTI occurs most commonly as a monomicrobial infection [37] in patients without coexisting risk factors [8, 44] and is often characterized by a subacute presentation. Several authors have suggested that this form of NSTI may be less virulent than those caused by other agents [37, 44].

Clostridium spp. – Clostridia are saprophytes found widespread in soil, clothing, and as resident flora of the gastrointestinal tract in humans and animals. While *Clostridium* spp. (especially *C. perfringens*) have been historically closely linked to NSTI (previously known as "gas gangrene"), in the modern era, Clostridium is a very rare causative agent in NSTI (<5 %), found most commonly in cases involving injection drug abuse [17, 23, 45]. Like *S. pyogenes*, the virulence of Clostridia is attributable to the elaboration of exotoxins, alpha-toxin, and theta-toxin in this case [38]. In addition to local tissue effects (myonecrosis and microvascular thrombosis), alpha-toxin also depresses cardiac contractility and activates cytokine expression [5]. These systemic effects may explain the higher mortality rates encountered with Clostridial infection [21].

Zygomycete – this ubiquitous fungus is responsible for a rare but devastating form of NSTI known as *mucormycosis*, seen predominantly in diabetics, especially in the presence of uncontrolled hyperglycemia and ketoacidosis [5]. Infection usually begins with minor trauma followed by rapid spread to periorbital structures, the maxillary sinus, hard palate, and the cranial vault. This form of NSTI is rare and highly lethal.

Others – dozens of other organisms have been reported to be associated with NSTI in varying degrees of frequency (Table 17.1). Aerobic agents include *E. coli*, *Enterobacter*, *Klebsiella*, *Haemophilus influenza*, and *Pseudomonas*; common anaerobes include *Bacteroides*, *Peptostreptococcus*, *Prevotella*, and *Fusobacterium*. Atypical pathogens (seen mainly in immunosuppressed patients) include *Mycobacterium kansasii*, *M. chelonae*, and *M. smegmatis*.

Table 17.1 Organisms identified in necrotizing fasciitis

Gram-positive aerobic bacteria	*Bacillus* sp.
	Coagulase-negative staphylococci
	Enterococci
	Group A, β-hemolytic streptococcus
	Group B streptococcus
	Staphylococcus aureus
Gram-negative aerobic bacteria	*Acinetobacter* spp.
	Citrobacter spp.
	Enterobacter spp.
	Escherichia coli
	Haemophilus influenza
	Klebsiella spp.
	Pasteurella multocida
	Proteus spp.
	Pseudomonas aeruginosa
	Serratia spp.
Anaerobic bacteria	*Bacteroides* spp.
	Clostridium spp.
	Fusobacterium spp.
	Peptostreptococcus spp.
	Prevotella spp.
Marine *Vibrio* spp.	*Vibrio alginolyticus*
	Vibrio damsela
	Vibrio parahaemolyticus
	Vibrio vulnificus
Atypical	*Mycobacterium kansasii*
	M. chelonae
	M. smegmatis
Fungi	*Aspergillus* spp.
	Candida spp.
	Rhizopus

Location

NSTI can affect any part of the body. For simplicity, the body regions most commonly affected are usually categorized in order of decreasing incidence: extremities, perineum and buttocks, trunk, and head and neck. The body region affected varies according to the study patient population, for example, IV drug abusers are disproportionately affected in the extremities at the sites of injection [15–17, 20], while Fournier's gangrene is seen most commonly in diabetics [20, 33]. Fournier's gangrene, named after French dermatologist Jean Alfred Fournier described a series of five male patients in 1883, is the eponymous name used to describe NSTI of the perineum (Figs. 17.1 and 17.2). This form of NSTI affects men ten times more

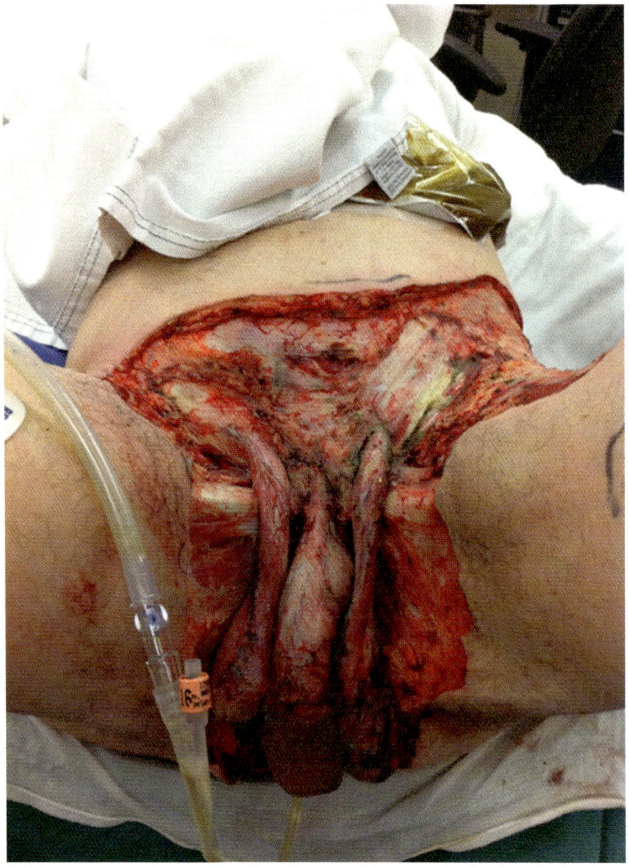

Fig. 17.1 Fournier's gangrene after radical debridement. Author's collection

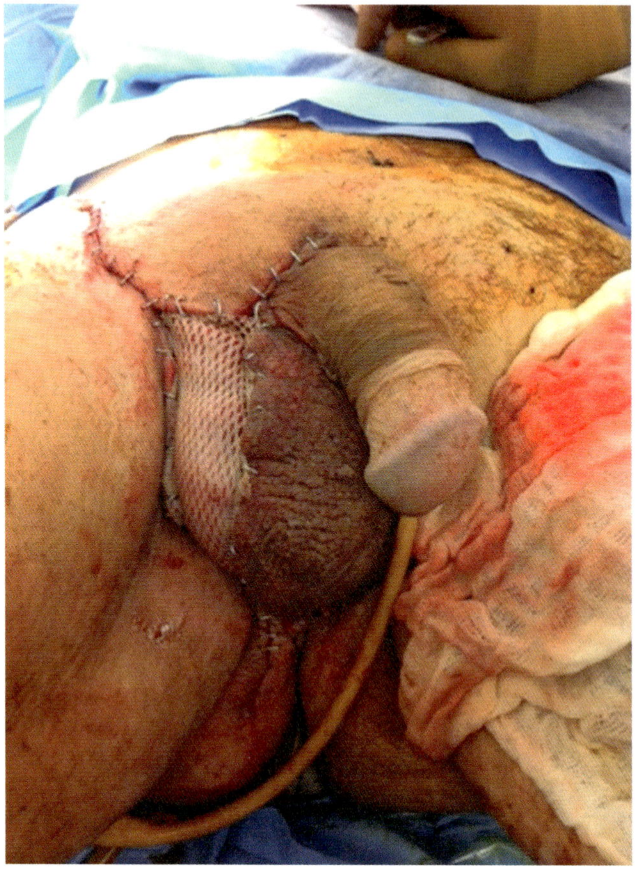

Fig. 17.2 Fournier's gangrene after partial wound closure and skin grafting. Author's collection

commonly than women. NSTI of the head and neck is most commonly preceded by a dental infection [46, 47].

NSTI can occur following insect bites and muscle strains. Non-recreational drug use needle injection-related NSTI has been reported after tattooing [18], acupuncture [30, 48], and insulin administration [30] (Figs. 17.3 and 17.4). Case reports of postsurgical NSTI have been reported for appendectomy, inguinal hernia, various gynecologic operations, orthopedic fixation, dental procedures, transanal procedures, urologic procedures (including circumcision), angiographic interventions, and laparoscopic procedures [6, 49, 50]. As a general rule, infections adjacent to mucous membranes (oral cavity, rectum, vagina) are caused by the normal resident flora of those mucous membranes, while infections in distant areas are usually caused by resident skin flora [51].

Diagnosis

The distinction between NSTI and non-necrotizing infections is of prime importance, the latter being treated with antibiotics alone. The main differential diagnosis includes simple cellulitis, erysipelas, abscess, Clostridial and non-Clostridial myonecrosis, toxic epidermal necrolysis (TEN), staphylococcal scalded skin syndrome, and rarely, cutaneous anthrax (Table 17.2).

Clinical Exam

The physical exam findings in NSTI have been known since the first description by Hippocrates: soft tissue edema (71–83.7 %) [11, 17, 25], erythema (52–85.6 %) [11, 13, 17, 25], and skin blebs and bullae (13.3–44.9 %) [11, 13, 15, 17, 23, 25]. Crepitus and skin necrosis, highly specific signs, are present in less than a third of patients [5, 33]. The symptom most characteristic of NSTI is severe pain (often out of proportion to exam) (54.7–86.6 %) [11, 16, 17, 23, 25]. Absence of pain and numbness may result, however, from destruction of cutaneous nerves. Systemic symptoms such as fever (32.5–60 %) and hypotension are variably present [11, 13, 17, 23, 25, 30]. No single physical finding is universally present. Reliance upon the physical exam for diagnosis may result in delayed recognition and treatment [12, 43]. In fact, NSTI is the admitting diagnosis in only a minority of confirmed cases [8, 23].

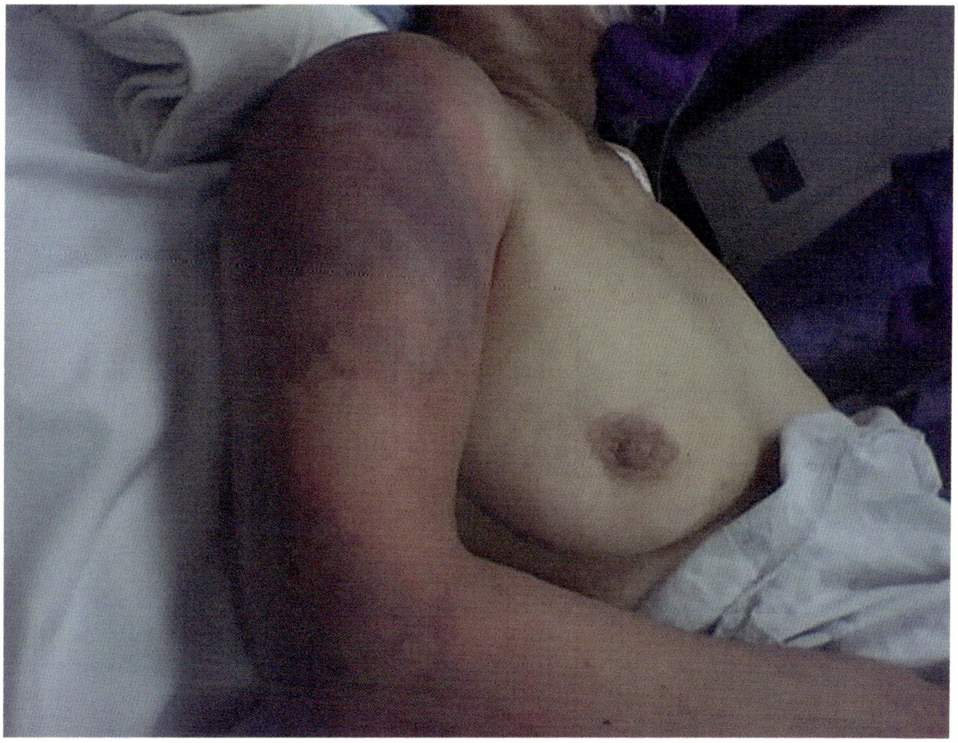

Fig. 17.3 Preoperative appearance of upper extremity NSTI. Author's collection

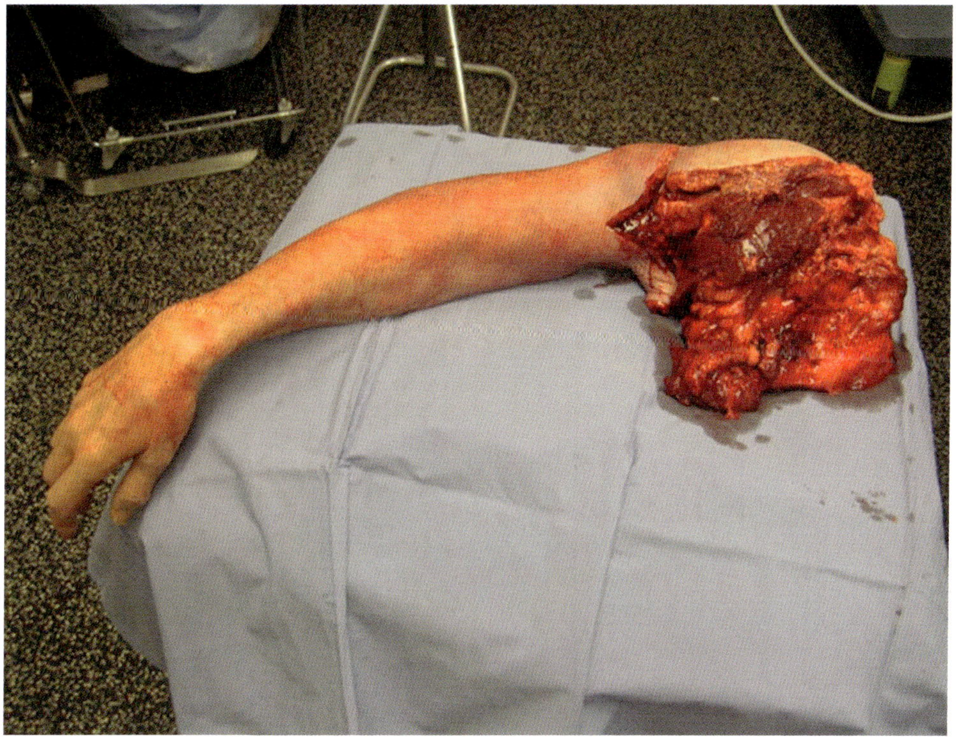

Fig. 17.4 Life-saving upper extremity amputation required for NSTI. Author's collection

Radiology

Plain Films

Plain films were once considered essential in the diagnostic work-up of NSTI. In recent series, however, soft tissue gas evident on X-rays is present in only about 30 % of cases of confirmed NSTI [11, 15, 30]. This is likely due to the presence of non-gas forming pathogenic bacteria and variable stages of disease upon presentation. While the presence of subcutaneous emphysema is very specific and can confirm the diagnosis when clinically suspected, the absence of subcutaneous gas is not sufficiently sensitive to rule out the

Table 17.2 Differential diagnosis of NSTI

Abscess
Anthrax (cutaneous)
Cellulitis
Erysipelas
Lymphedema
Myonecrosis (Clostridial and non-Clostridial)
Myxedema
Noninfectious fasciitis
Phlegmasia cerulea dolens
Staphylococcal scalded skin syndrome
Toxic epidermal necrolysis (TEN)

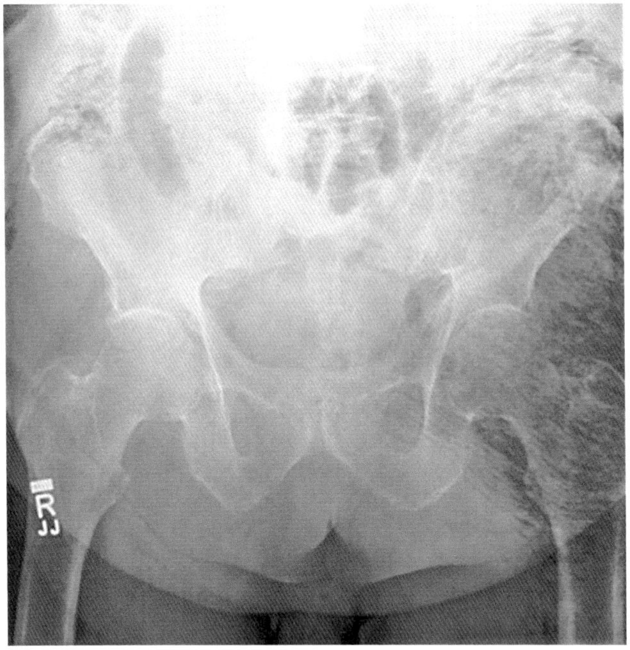

Fig. 17.5 Subcutaneous emphysema evident on plain films. Author's collection

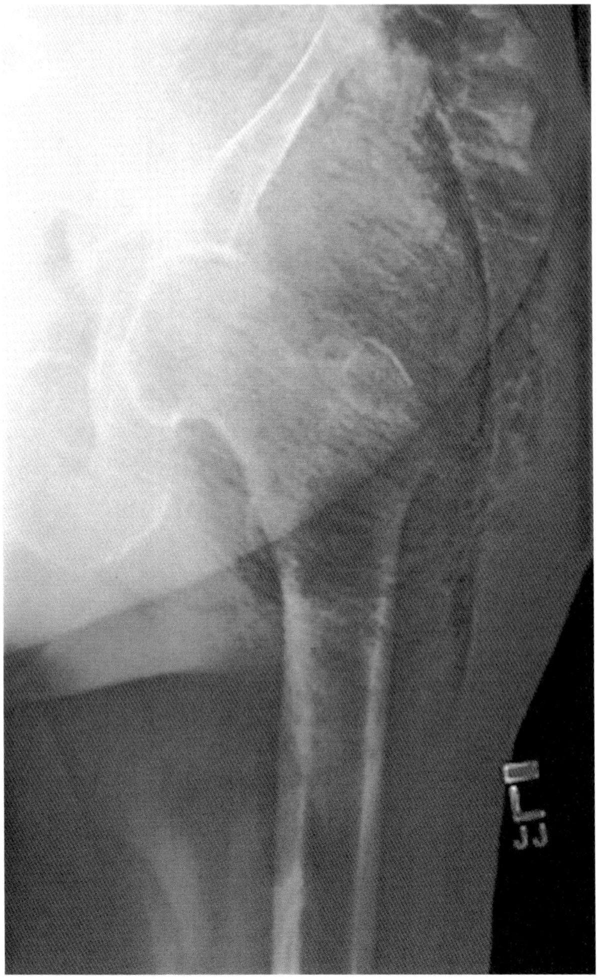

Fig. 17.6 Subcutaneous emphysema evident on plain films. Author's collection

diagnosis of NSTI (Figs. 17.5 and 17.6). Awaiting the results of plain films should not delay surgical consultation or intervention.

Ultrasound

The use of ultrasonography (US) in the diagnosis of NSTI has been described in several single institution studies. Findings characteristic of NSTI include "a diffuse thickening of the subcutaneous tissue, accompanied by a layer of fluid accumulation more than 4 mm in depth along the deep fascial layer when compared with the contralateral position on the corresponding normal limb" [52]. Preliminary work in cadavers suggests that ultrasound is accurate in the detection of subcutaneous air [53].

Using operative and histological findings as the reference standard, Yen et al. report a sensitivity of 88.2 %, specificity of 93.3 %, positive predictive value (PPV) of 83.3 %, negative predictive value of 95.4 %, and an accuracy of 91.9 % [52]. Limitations of this modality include the dependence on operative experience and availability. Until larger, multicenter studies confirm these preliminary results, routine use of US for the diagnosis of NSTI cannot be recommended.

Computed Tomography (CT)

The literature on the use of CT to aid in the diagnosis of NSTI is conflicting; earlier studies reporting inaccuracy are limited by older CT technology and small sample sizes. Newer generation scanners (16-slice and above) have increased sensitivity in detecting pathological changes associated with NSTI: asymmetrical and diffuse areas of soft tissue inflammation and ischemia, muscle necrosis, gas across tissue planes, and fluid collections (Fig. 17.7). Using these four CT criteria, Zacharias et al. report a sensitivity of 100 %, specificity 81 %, PPV 76 %, and NPV 100 % [14]. Thus, the utility of CT seems to be greatest in ruling out

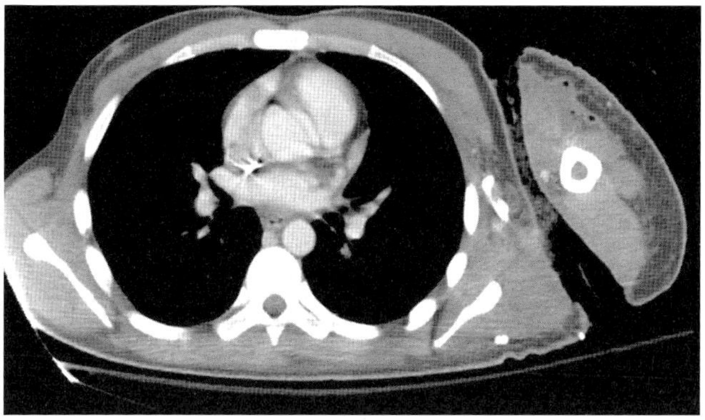

Fig. 17.7 NSTI computed tomography appearance. Author's collection

NSTI in clinically equivocal cases, thus avoiding unnecessary operative explorations (Figs. 17.8, 17.9, and 17.10).

Magnetic Resonance Imaging (MRI)

Without question, MRI is more sensitive than plain films, US, or CT in the detection of acute inflammation. In general, NSTI manifests as high signal intensity on T2-weighted images and as low-signal intensity on T1-weighted images [54]. Absence of Gd-DTPA contrast enhancement is strongly suggestive of tissue necrosis [55]. There are two main drawbacks of MRI. Firstly, this modality may be too sensitive. Falsely positive MRI scans may result in unnecessary surgical explorations for cellulitis. Secondly, MRI may not be immediately available in all institutions. Reliance on this modality for diagnosis may cause therapeutic delay. Routine application cannot be recommended.

Laboratory

No single laboratory value has sufficient accuracy to assist in the diagnosis of NSTI. Bacteremia is present in <30 % [12, 17, 25] and leukocytosis is nonspecific. In cases with equivocal physical exam and radiologic findings, a constellation of laboratory values may help distinguish the diagnosis of NSTI from cellulitis. Wong et al. have described a Laboratory Risk Indicator for Necrotizing Fasciitis (LRINEC) score to stratify patients into low-, moderate-, or high-risk categories using commonly ordered laboratory tests: C-reactive protein, WBC, hemoglobin, sodium, creatinine, and glucose [56]. According to the authors, at a cut-off LRINEC score of ≥ 6, their model has a PPV of 92 % and NPV of 96 %. While these results are impressive, one must apply the LRINEC with caution, as the LRINEC score may be less accurate in patients with multiple medical comorbidities and/or a blunted inflammatory response, both of which are present in the geriatric population.

A second group, Wall et al., have proposed a simple laboratory model based on two values: WBC > 15.4 and serum sodium < 135 [15]. These authors report that their model can distinguish NSTI from non-NSTI with a NPV of 99 %. Again, one must proceed with caution in the evaluation of the elderly patient as this model has not been validated in this population.

Surgical Exploration

It cannot be overemphasized that wide surgical debridement is the only effective therapy for NSTI and that time is of the utmost essence. Delay in surgical therapy has been repeatedly demonstrated to be associated with increased mortality and increased number of required debridements [29]. Even with severe hemodynamic and metabolic derangement, surgical exploration and debridement must proceed; physiologic resuscitation and correction is futile in the continued presence of infected, necrotic tissue. Because of the difficulty in establishing the diagnosis non-invasively, several authors have described bedside tests, including aspiration with Gram-stain [57], frozen section biopsy [58], and "the finger test." The "finger test" is performed by making a small incision (2 cm) through the skin down to the fascia and bluntly probing the wound with a finger. A positive test (indicating NSTI) results if one can dissect the subcutaneous tissue off the fascia with minimal resistance [22]. Because of the possibility of sample bias and the potential delay in diagnosis and therapy, these lesser diagnostic operations are not recommended; in most instances the morbidity associated with delayed treatment of NSTI outweighs the morbidity of an exploratory incision in superficial skin and soft tissue infection.

The surgical approach at the first debridement should resemble a "search-and-destroy" mission. All frankly necrotic and infected tissue should be excised irrespective of anatomic or functional boundaries (Fig. 17.11). As this disease pays no respect to anatomic planes, neither should the treating surgeon hesitate to remove tissue when the patient's life is at stake. At operation, affected tissue is easily recognized by lack of bleeding and lack of normal resistance to blunt dissection. In elderly patients, however, ease of tissue separation alone may not be a reliable indicator of infection.

A clinical caveat: finger dissection should be utilized with care in injection drug abusers as broken needle tips may reside in the subcutaneous tissues (Fig. 17.12). Necrotic fascia is noted to be discolored (grayish) and sometimes surrounded by a thin, foul-smelling "dishwater" liquid distinct from the garden variety creamy thick pus encountered in simple abscesses. Intraoperative aerobic and anaerobic cultures should be taken to aid in future targeted antibiotic therapy; these cultures should be taken from subcutaneous tissues, not from the skin surface or blister fluid. Tissue biopsies should be taken from the interface between necrotic and

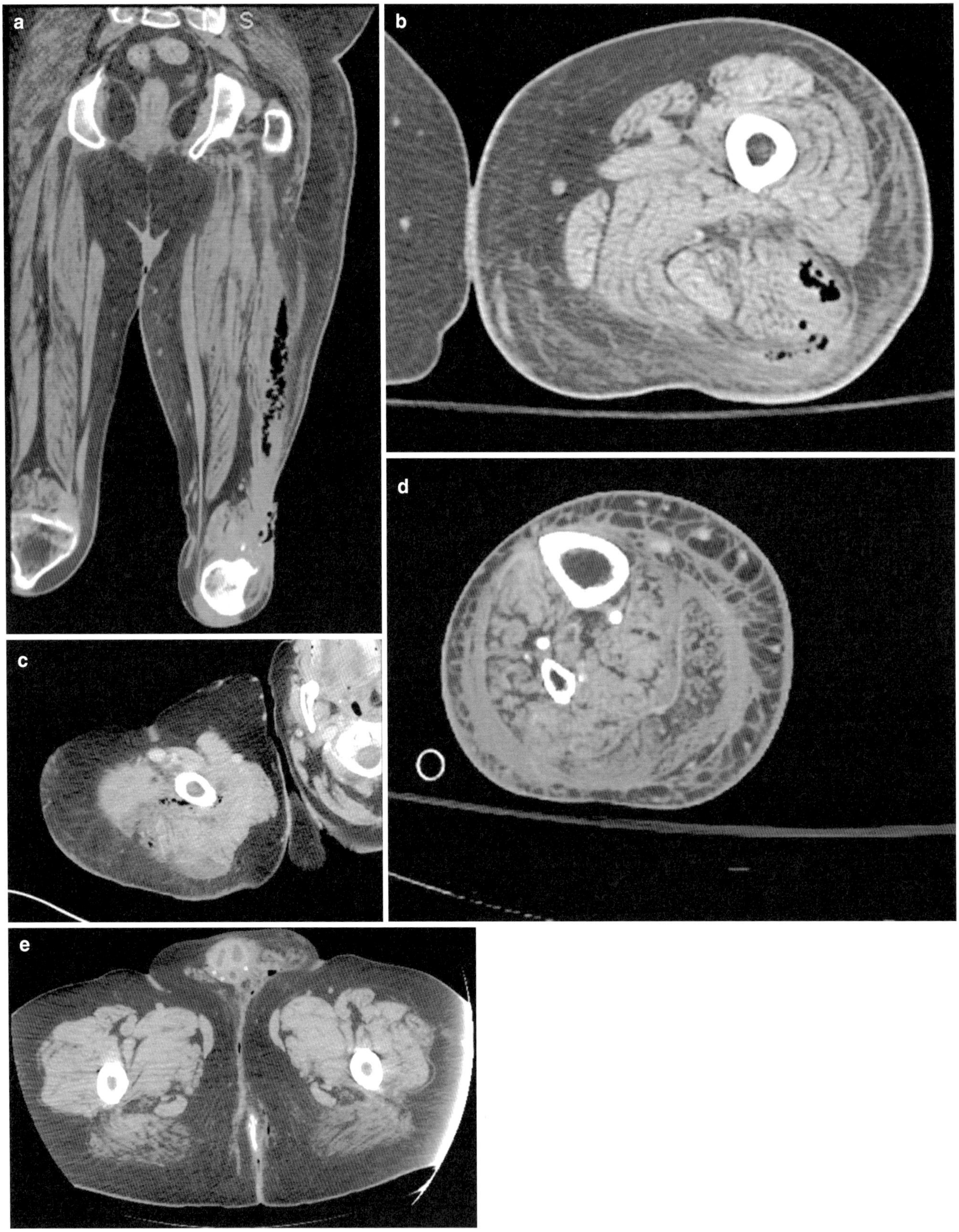

Fig. 17.8 (**a**–**e**) Confirmed NSTI

alive tissue for optimal diagnostic yield [38]. Skin should be debrided until brisk capillary dermal bleeding without epidermal discoloration is encountered. Large skin flaps may impede wound drainage and it may be prudent to excise skin with extensive underlining to facilitate wound care. Muscle and fascia should be debrided to healthy tissue with normal contractile function (in response to electrocautery).

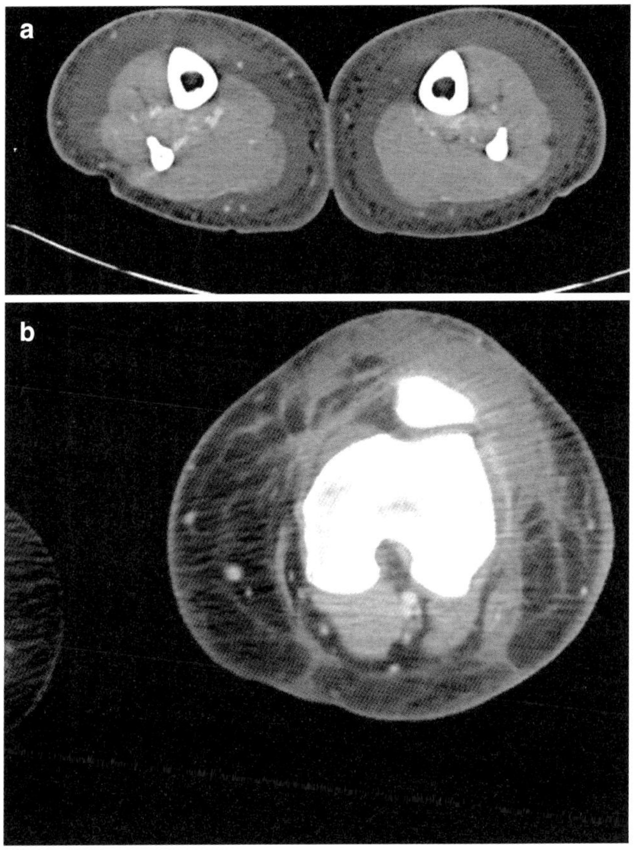

Fig. 17.9 (a, b) Cellulitis – no NSTI

Attempts to preserve marginal tissue are ill-advised as residual infection only serves as a nidus for further spread. Much like with a wildfire, the goal is to dig a trench beyond the advancing front (in unburned forest) to halt the progression. A scheduled second-look operation is highly recommended, although the appropriate timing is unknown. Common intervals are between 12 and 48 h; however, this may be influenced by changes in clinical condition. Frequently, additional debridement is required and multiple operations are the rule. The average number of debridements required has been reported to be between 2.3 and 5.6 [11, 13, 15, 17, 21, 23–25]. Wound closure at the initial operation is strongly discouraged. Adjunctive use of 5 % mafenide acetate solution has been reported to decrease the number of debridements required and increase success of subsequent wound closure [59].

Reported amputation rates range between 11.7 and 26.3 % [10, 11, 13, 21, 23, 25, 31] and risk factors for amputation include PVD, DM [11], and age over 65 years [21]. Even without amputation, 30 % of survivors are left with functional disability at discharge [16].

For perineal NSTI, two pearls are offered. Firstly, the necessity of a temporary diverting colostomy is not usually apparent in the first few days and delaying this additional procedure is recommended as many patients will not ultimately require fecal diversion. Additionally, since these infections may spread along the anterior abdominal wall, it is prudent to await the final anterosuperior demarcation before committing to ostomy placement. Secondly, orchiectomy is almost never required even when the entire scrotum has been debrided. Consultation with a urologist is recommended for ultimate testicular disposition, however, in the acute setting, the viable testes may be wrapped in petroleum gauze.

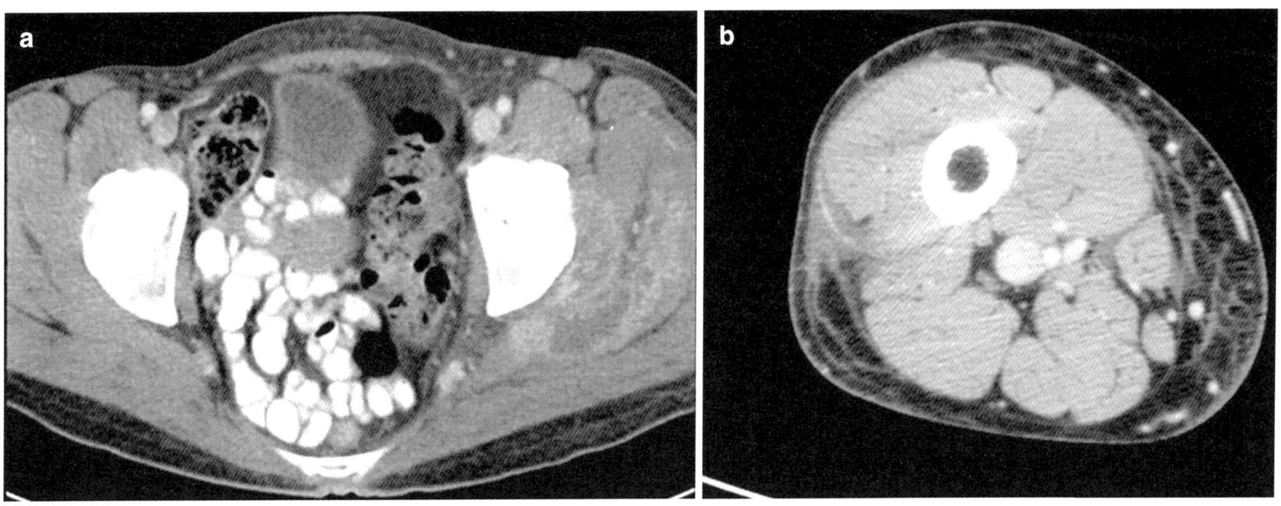

Fig. 17.10 (a, b) Abscess – no NSTI

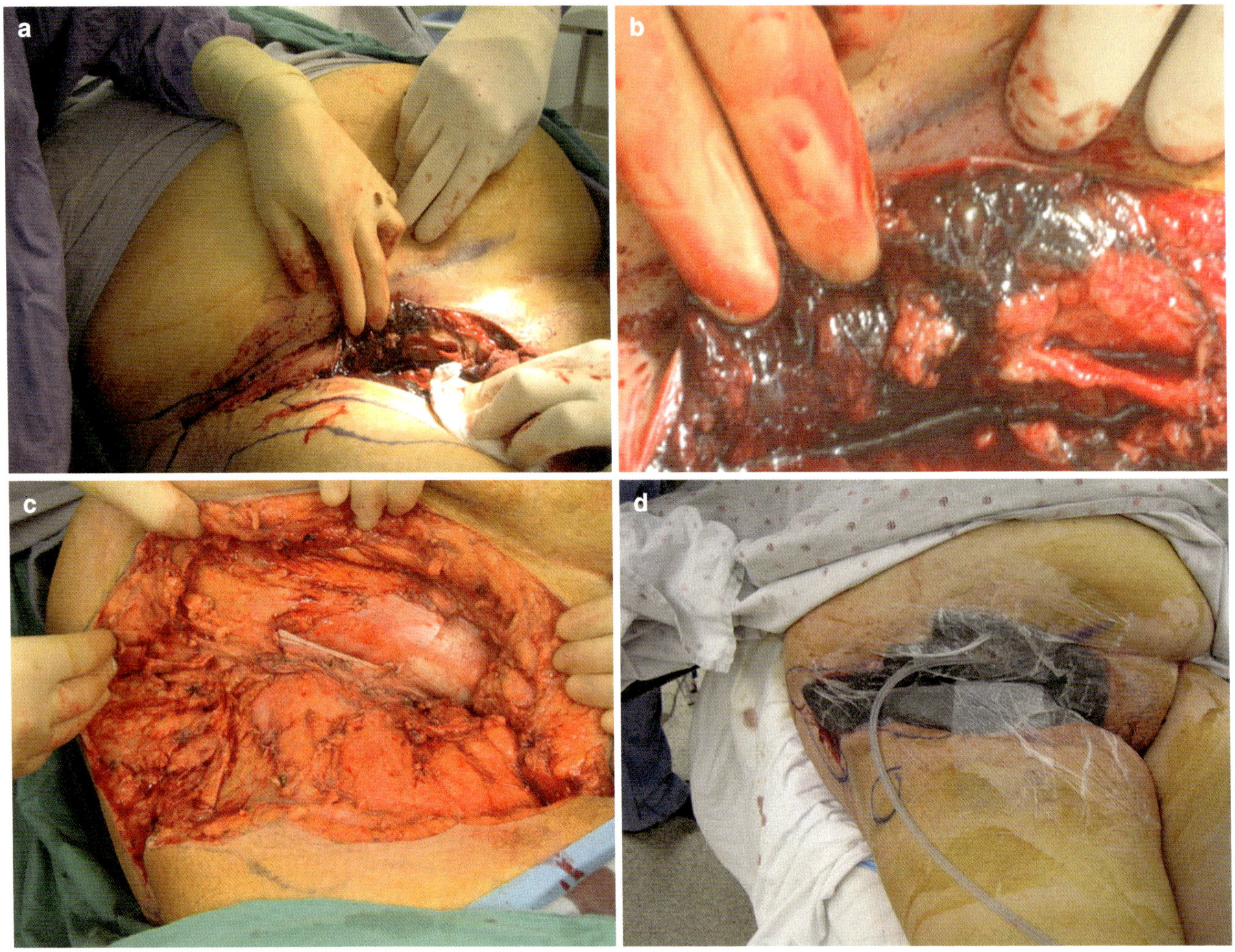

Fig. 17.11 NSTI intraoperative appearance. (**a**) Necrotic muscle and fat is evident; (**b**) necrotic muscle and fat is evident; (**c**) wound debrided to healthy, viable tissue; (**d**) VAC dressing on open wound. Author's collection

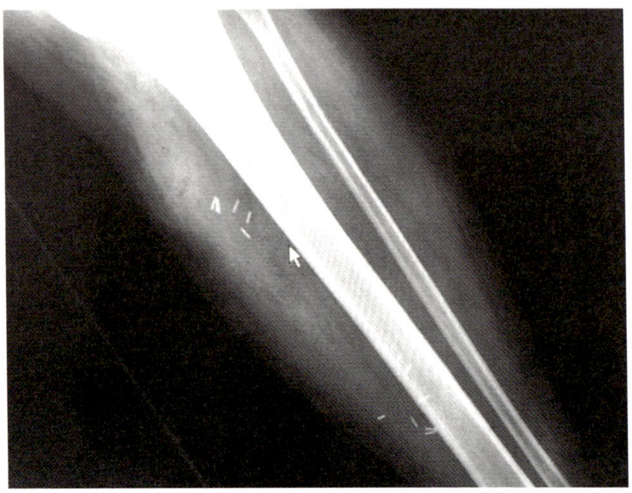

Fig. 17.12 Broken hypodermic needle tips embedded within the tissue. Author's collection

Once no further debridements are required and the infection cleared, the surgeon must deal with the residual defect. Accumulating experience and evidence supports the use of vacuum-assisted closure dressings to hasten the formation of granulation tissue [38]. If primary closure is not feasible, ultimate closure will often require skin grafting or flap coverage.

Adjunctive Treatments

Antibiotics

Once the diagnosis of NSTI is suspected, broad-spectrum antibiotic therapy should be instituted immediately to mitigate the systemic effects of infection; however, without surgical excision, mortality is almost universal despite appropriate microbial coverage. Antifungal therapy is not routinely given unless the clinician suspects invasive mucormycosis. Although numerous combinations of regimens have been described, none have been demonstrated to be superior to any other. Because of the polymicrobial nature of NSTI, initial empiric therapy must adequately cover Gram-positive, Gram-negative, aerobic, and anaerobic organisms, including MRSA. The addition of a protein synthesis inhibitor (such as clindamycin, erythromycin, or linezolid) is also recommended as it is believed to inhibit exotoxin and M protein production [5, 9, 38, 42]. Clindamycin has several other theoretical advantages: it reduces the synthesis of penicillin-binding protein, has a longer post-antibiotic effect than the β-lactams, suppresses TNF-α synthesis, and facilitates phagocytosis of group A Streptococcus [57]. It is generally agreed upon that antibiotic therapy should continue until no further debridements are required and the patient's clinical condition has improved. Prolonged treatment is not associated with improved outcomes and will only contribute to the selection of resistant microorganisms.

Hyperbaric Oxygen

The use of hyperbaric oxygen (HBO) to inhibit anaerobic infections was first described in the early 1960s [60], and it is believed that increased tissue oxygen tension enhances local defense mechanisms, mitigates reperfusion injury, and moderates the systemic inflammatory response by decreasing proinflammatory cytokine and exotoxin production [38, 60, 61]. Laboratory and animal studies demonstrated that at >1 atm absolute pressure, oxygen enhances bacterial killing (especially *Clostridium*); arrests toxin production [62]; and increases collagen formation, fibroblast growth, and superoxide dismutase production [4]. The recommended HBO treatment protocol for NSTI is 2.0–2.5 atm absolute pressure for 90 min twice daily (3.0 atm thrice daily if *Clostridium* is suspected) until no further debridements are required.

Routine application of this treatment modality is much debated and many studies show conflicting results. Supporters report decreased number of debridements, decreased amputation rate, and decreased mortality [63–65]. However, the literature supporting its use comprises mainly animal studies, case series, and retrospective studies. Most are single center and underpowered and none are randomized. Perhaps the strongest evidence to date supporting the use of HBO is an analysis of the Nationwide Inpatient Sample (NIS), an administrative database, in which propensity scoring derived from multivariate logistic regression of known confounders was used to compare outcomes in patients who received HBO with those who did not. The authors report higher cost of hospitalization and longer length of stay but significantly lower in-hospital mortality rates (4.5 % vs. 9.4 %, $p=0.001$) [66]. Opponents report no difference in outcomes in other studies [67, 68]. Concerns about recommending its use include limited availability and the transport of a critically ill patient to the dive chamber. All agree that HBO therapy or transfer to an HBO-capable center should not delay surgical debridement. Until a well-controlled, adequately powered prospective study is performed, the use of HBO as adjunctive treatment for NSTI will remain controversial.

IVIG

Rarer still (and even more controversial), is the use of intravenous immunoglobulin (IVIG) as adjunctive therapy for NSTI. The biologic rational supporting its use is that the administered immunoglobulin antibodies can neutralize circulating exotoxin and superantigen and reduce plasma concentrations of proinflammatory cytokines, thus mitigating the systemic inflammatory response [5, 42]. Clinical evidence supporting its use is scant [69, 70], and IVIG is not currently FDA approved for the treatment of NSTI.

Conclusion

NSTI is a rare and deadly disease primarily affecting middle- and older-aged individuals. Misdiagnosis leading to delay in treatment is common and a high index of suspicion must be maintained. Pain is the most consistent presenting symptom. The use of laboratory markers and radiologic imaging may assist in ruling in or out the disease. Treatment is expedient surgical excision and should be regarded as a surgical emergency. Amputation rates are high and multiple debridements are the rule. Empiric antibiotic therapy should be broad-spectrum and should include a protein-synthesis inhibitor such as clindamycin. The use of adjuvant therapies such as HBO and IVIG is controversial. Mortality remains between 10 and 30 % and long-term disability is common.

References

1. Descamps V, Aitken J, Lee MG. Hippocrates on necrotising fasciitis. Lancet. 1994;344(8921):556.
2. Pace A, van den Spiegel A. The Workes of that Famous Chururgian Ambrose Parey. In: Clarke J, editor. The Complutense University of Madrid (trans: Johnson T). R. Cotes and Willi Dugard; 2011, pp. 837.
3. Salcido RS. Necrotizing fasciitis: reviewing the causes and treatment strategies. Adv Skin Wound Care. 2007;20(5):288–93, quiz 294–5.

4. Green RJ, Dafoe DC, Raffin TA. Necrotizing fasciitis. Chest. 1996; 110(1):219–29.
5. Phan HH, Cocanour CS. Necrotizing soft tissue infections in the intensive care unit. Crit Care Med. 2010;38(9 Suppl):S460–8.
6. Quirk Jr WF, Sternbach G. Joseph Jones: infection with flesh eating bacteria. J Emerg Med. 1996;14(6):747–53.
7. Meleney F. Hemolytic Streptococcus Gangrene. Arch Surg. 1924; 9:317–64.
8. May AK. Skin and soft tissue infections. Surg Clin North Am. 2009;89(2):403–20, viii.
9. Anaya DA, Dellinger EP. Necrotizing soft-tissue infection: diagnosis and management. Clin Infect Dis. 2007;44(5):705–10.
10. Kaul R, et al. Population-based surveillance for group A streptococcal necrotizing fasciitis: clinical features, prognostic indicators, and microbiologic analysis of seventy-seven cases. Ontario Group A Streptococcal Study. Am J Med. 1997;103(1):18–24.
11. McHenry CR, et al. Determinants of mortality for necrotizing soft-tissue infections. Ann Surg. 1995;221(5):558–63; discussion 563–5.
12. Elliott D, Kufera JA, Myers RA. The microbiology of necrotizing soft tissue infections. Am J Surg. 2000;179(5):361–6.
13. Su YC, et al. Laboratory risk indicator for necrotizing fasciitis score and the outcomes. ANZ J Surg. 2008;78(11):968–72.
14. Zacharias N, et al. Diagnosis of necrotizing soft tissue infections by computed tomography. Arch Surg. 2010;145(5):452–5.
15. Wall DB, et al. A simple model to help distinguish necrotizing fasciitis from nonnecrotizing soft tissue infection. J Am Coll Surg. 2000;191(3):227–31.
16. Kao LS, et al. Local variations in the epidemiology, microbiology, and outcome of necrotizing soft-tissue infections: a multicenter study. Am J Surg. 2011;202(2):139–45.
17. Huang KF, et al. Independent predictors of mortality for necrotizing fasciitis: a retrospective analysis in a single institution. J Trauma. 2011;71(2):467–73; discussion 473.
18. Das DK, Baker MG, Venugopal K. Increasing incidence of necrotizing fasciitis in New Zealand: a nationwide study over the period 1990 to 2006. J Infect. 2011;63(6):429–33.
19. Mulla ZD, Gibbs SG, Aronoff DM. Correlates of length of stay, cost of care, and mortality among patients hospitalized for necrotizing fasciitis. Epidemiol Infect. 2007;135(5):868–76.
20. Singh G, et al. Necrotising infections of soft tissues – a clinical profile. Eur J Surg. 2002;168(6):366–71.
21. Anaya DA, et al. Predictors of mortality and limb loss in necrotizing soft tissue infections. Arch Surg. 2005;140(2):151–7; discussion 158.
22. Childers BJ, et al. Necrotizing fasciitis: a fourteen-year retrospective study of 163 consecutive patients. Am Surg. 2002;68(2): 109–16.
23. Wong CH, et al. Necrotizing fasciitis: clinical presentation, microbiology, and determinants of mortality. J Bone Joint Surg Am. 2003;85-A(8):1454–60.
24. Brandt MM, Corpron CA, Wahl WL. Necrotizing soft tissue infections: a surgical disease. Am Surg. 2000;66(10):967–70; discussion 970–1.
25. Hsiao CT, et al. Predictors of mortality in patients with necrotizing fasciitis. Am J Emerg Med. 2008;26(2):170–5.
26. Yilmazlar T, et al. Necrotizing soft tissue infections: APACHE II score, dissemination, and survival. World J Surg. 2007;31(9): 1858–62.
27. Endorf FW, Supple KG, Gamelli RL. The evolving characteristics and care of necrotizing soft-tissue infections. Burns. 2005;31(3): 269–73.
28. Light TD, et al. Long-term outcomes of patients with necrotizing fasciitis. J Burn Care Res. 2010;31(1):93–9.
29. Kobayashi L, et al. Necrotizing soft tissue infections: delayed surgical treatment is associated with increased number of surgical debridements and morbidity. J Trauma. 2011;71(5):1400–5.
30. Bosshardt TL, Henderson VJ, Organ Jr CH. Necrotizing soft-tissue infections. Arch Surg. 1996;131(8):846–52; discussion 852–4.
31. Liu YM, et al. Microbiology and factors affecting mortality in necrotizing fasciitis. J Microbiol Immunol Infect. 2005;38(6):430–5.
32. Pessa ME, Howard RJ. Necrotizing fasciitis. Surg Gynecol Obstet. 1985;161(4):357–61.
33. Elliott DC, Kufera JA, Myers RA. Necrotizing soft tissue infections. Risk factors for mortality and strategies for management. Ann Surg. 1996;224(5):672–83.
34. Anaya DA, et al. Predicting death in necrotizing soft tissue infections: a clinical score. Surg Infect (Larchmt). 2009;10(6):517–22.
35. Tillou A, et al. Necrotizing soft tissue infections: improved outcomes with modern care. Am Surg. 2004;70(10):841–4.
36. Lee CC, et al. Necrotizing fasciitis in patients with liver cirrhosis: predominance of monomicrobial Gram-negative bacillary infections. Diagn Microbiol Infect Dis. 2008;62(2):219–25.
37. Lee TC, et al. Incidence and clinical characteristics of methicillin-resistant *Staphylococcus aureus* necrotizing fasciitis in a large urban hospital. Am J Surg. 2007;194(6):809–12; discussion 812–3.
38. Sarani B, et al. Necrotizing fasciitis: current concepts and review of the literature. J Am Coll Surg. 2009;208(2):279–88.
39. Voros D, et al. Role of early and extensive surgery in the treatment of severe necrotizing soft tissue infection. Br J Surg. 1993;80(9): 1190–1.
40. Wong CH, Wang YS. The diagnosis of necrotizing fasciitis. Curr Opin Infect Dis. 2005;18(2):101–6.
41. NIH. Highly invasive new bacterium isolated from US east coast waters. JAMA. 1984;251(3):323–5.
42. Cainzos M, Gonzalez-Rodriguez FJ. Necrotizing soft tissue infections. Curr Opin Crit Care. 2007;13(4):433–9.
43. Stone DR, Gorbach SL. Necrotizing fasciitis. The changing spectrum. Dermatol Clin. 1997;15(2):213–20.
44. Miller LG, et al. Necrotizing fasciitis caused by community-associated methicillin-resistant *Staphylococcus aureus* in Los Angeles. N Engl J Med. 2005;352(14):1445–53.
45. Dunbar NM, Harruff RC. Necrotizing fasciitis: manifestations, microbiology and connection with black tar heroin. J Forensic Sci. 2007;52(4):920–3.
46. Tovi F, Fliss DM, Zirkin HJ. Necrotizing soft-tissue infections in the head and neck: a clinicopathological study. Laryngoscope. 1991;101(6 Pt 1):619–25.
47. Maisel RH, Karlen R. Cervical necrotizing fasciitis. Laryngoscope. 1994;104(7):795–8.
48. Hsieh RL, Huang CH, Uen WC. Necrotizing fasciitis after acupuncture in a patient with aplastic anemia. J Altern Complement Med. 2011;17(9):871–4.
49. Eke N. Fournier's gangrene: a review of 1726 cases. Br J Surg. 2000;87(6):718–28.
50. Rea WJ, Wyrick Jr WJ. Necrotizing fasciitis. Ann Surg. 1970; 172(6):957–64.
51. Brook I, Frazier EH. Clinical and microbiological features of necrotizing fasciitis. J Clin Microbiol. 1995;33(9):2382–7.
52. Yen ZS, et al. Ultrasonographic screening of clinically-suspected necrotizing fasciitis. Acad Emerg Med. 2002;9(12):1448–51.
53. Butcher CH, Dooley RW, Levitov AB. Detection of subcutaneous and intramuscular air with sonography: a sensitive and specific modality. J Ultrasound Med. 2011;30(6):791–5.
54. Schmid MR, Kossmann T, Duewell S. Differentiation of necrotizing fasciitis and cellulitis using MR imaging. AJR Am J Roentgenol. 1998;170(3):615–20.
55. Brothers TE, et al. Magnetic resonance imaging differentiates between necrotizing and non-necrotizing fasciitis of the lower extremity. J Am Coll Surg. 1998;187(4):416–21.
56. Wong CH, et al. The LRINEC (Laboratory Risk Indicator for Necrotizing Fasciitis) score: a tool for distinguishing necrotizing

fasciitis from other soft tissue infections. Crit Care Med. 2004;32(7):1535–41.
57. Edlich RF, et al. Modern concepts of the diagnosis and treatment of necrotizing fasciitis. J Emerg Med. 2010;39(2):261–5.
58. Stamenkovic I, Lew PD. Early recognition of potentially fatal necrotizing fasciitis. The use of frozen-section biopsy. N Engl J Med. 1984;310(26):1689–93.
59. Heinle EC, et al. The use of 5% mafenide acetate solution in the postgraft treatment of necrotizing fasciitis. J Burn Care Rehabil. 2001;22(1):35–40.
60. Jallali N, Withey S, Butler PE. Hyperbaric oxygen as adjuvant therapy in the management of necrotizing fasciitis. Am J Surg. 2005;189(4):462–6.
61. Sheridan RL, Shank ES. Hyperbaric oxygen treatment: a brief overview of a controversial topic. J Trauma. 1999;47(2):426–35.
62. Van U. Inhibition of toxin production in *Clostridium perfringens* in vitro by hyperbaric oxygen. Antonie Van Leeuwenhoek. 1965; 31:181–6.
63. Wilkinson D, Doolette D. Hyperbaric oxygen treatment and survival from necrotizing soft tissue infection. Arch Surg. 2004; 139(12):1339–45.
64. Riseman JA, et al. Hyperbaric oxygen therapy for necrotizing fasciitis reduces mortality and the need for debridements. Surgery. 1990;108(5):847–50.
65. Escobar SJ, et al. Adjuvant hyperbaric oxygen therapy (HBO2)for treatment of necrotizing fasciitis reduces mortality and amputation rate. Undersea Hyperb Med. 2005;32(6):437–43.
66. Soh CR, et al. Hyperbaric oxygen therapy in necrotising soft tissue infections: a study of patients in the United States Nationwide Inpatient Sample. Intensive Care Med. 2012;38(7):1143–51.
67. Brown DR, et al. A multicenter review of the treatment of major truncal necrotizing infections with and without hyperbaric oxygen therapy. Am J Surg. 1994;167(5):485–9.
68. Shupak A, et al. Necrotizing fasciitis: an indication for hyperbaric oxygenation therapy? Surgery. 1995;118(5):873–8.
69. Darenberg J, et al. Intravenous immunoglobulin G therapy in streptococcal toxic shock syndrome: a European randomized, double-blind, placebo-controlled trial. Clin Infect Dis. 2003;37(3):333–40.
70. Kaul R, et al. Intravenous immunoglobulin therapy for streptococcal toxic shock syndrome – a comparative observational study. The Canadian Streptococcal Study Group. Clin Infect Dis. 1999; 28(4):800–7.

18 Acute Vascular Insufficiency in the Elderly

Michael J. Sise

Introduction

The incidence of peripheral arterial disease (PAD), coronary artery disease (CAD), and cardiac arrhythmias among the elderly is extremely high and increasing yearly [1–4]. Coupled with the steadily rising life expectancy, the problems of acute limb ischemia and acute mesenteric ischemia are of growing importance to acute care surgeons. More than 25 % of the elderly have clinically significant and active health problems related to PAD, CAD, or atrial fibrillation [3, 5]. Acute vascular insufficiency presents in a variety of settings. Although the emergency department remains the most common location to encounter these patients, the ICU, medial-surgical floors, and the operating room may also be the site of consultation for these emergencies. However, the workup remains straight forward and is based upon a thorough history, an appropriate examination, adjunctive Doppler pressure measurements or CT imaging studies, and, in a few compelling clinical settings, an immediate operation. The time urgency of diagnosis and effective treatment is based upon the "Golden Period" of 6–8 h within which adequate blood flow must be restored if limb-threatening tissue loss or life-threatening bowel necrosis is to be prevented. Decisive action is essential to successful management. Acute limb ischemia is much more common than acute mesenteric ischemia but shares a number of characteristic including etiology, pathophysiology, and the need for immediate diagnosis and treatment [6, 7].

M.J. Sise, MD, FACS
Trauma Service, Scripps Mercy Hospital,
4077 5th Avenue MER-62, San Diego, CA 92103, USA
e-mail: sise.mike@scrippshealth.org

Acute Limb Ischemia

The call from the emergency department, the ICU, the medial-surgical floor, or the operating room for a patient with an ischemic extremity is always the beginning of a challenging clinical problem. Acute, nontraumatic limb ischemia is usually due to either emboli originating in the heart or thrombotic occlusion of preexisting occlusive arterial disease [8]. Although less common, iatrogenic arterial occlusion is a growing problem for the acute care surgeon [9]. Most, if not all of these patients have major comorbidities that complicate their management. Prompt diagnosis and treatment are essential to successful management.

Pathophysiology

Extremity ischemia is the result of either acute arterial occlusion or acute thrombosis of chronic occlusive disease. Infrequently, severe acute venous occlusion results in ischemia secondary to arterial vasoconstriction and venous hypertension (phlegmasia cerulea dolens) [10]. The vascular anatomy of the extremities and the tissue mass perfused give rise to important differences in the presentation of upper and lower extremity acute ischemia.

Both the arms and legs have a single major proximal vessel that traverses the mid-extremity joint and divides into three vessels supplying the distal limb. There are key collaterals that determine the severity of ischemia and acute occlusion. However, the embryologic development of that single proximal vessel is distinctly different in the upper and lower extremity. In the arm, the brachial artery traverses medially in a straight course down the upper arm accompanied by the median nerve without passing through any muscular skeletal structures until it passes under the flexor aponeurosis at the antecubital fossa. In the leg, the superficial femoral artery (SFA) develops in the embryo as an anterior anastomosis between the femoral region and the popliteal artery. The initial embryonic blood supply is via a posterior sciatic artery

J.A. Yelon, F.A. Luchette (eds.), *Geriatric Trauma and Critical Care*,
DOI 10.1007/978-1-4614-8501-8_18, © Springer Science+Business Media New York 2014

which involutes [11]. This explains the spiral anterior to posterior-medial course of the SFA as it passes through the adductor magnus aponeurosis at Hunter's canal. It is accompanied by the small sural nerve.

Collateral flow into the most proximal portion of the extremities is typically adequate to prevent limb-threatening ischemia with inflow occlusion in the arm, but this is not true in the leg. Acute subclavian or axillary artery occlusion usually does not result in limb-threatening arm ischemia because of the abundant collaterals around the shoulder [6]. In contrast, occlusion of the inflow vessels of the leg (external iliac or common femoral arteries) threatens viability of the limb because pelvic collaterals to the upper thigh are not adequate to provide perfusion to the large muscle mass of the leg [10].

The arterial collateral supply in the arm is via the proximal superior contribution of the profunda brachial artery and the distal ulnar and radial collateral branches from the upper forearm. They are usually not sufficient to mitigate the ischemia that results from acute occlusion of the brachial artery. In the leg, which has a larger muscle mass, the collateral flow from the profunda femoral artery proximal to the branches of the distal popliteal artery are not adequate to prevent acute ischemia with sudden SFA occlusion [6].

The chronic and progressive occlusive disease of atherosclerosis in the lower extremities results in the development of collaterals which prevent ischemia at rest in the early stages of the disease [6]. Progressive disease with obliteration of distal vessels will lead to chronic ischemia at rest. Acute thrombosis of extensively atherosclerotic vessels can result in acute limb-threatening ischemia [12]. In patients with previous extremity angioplasty and stent placement or arterial bypass surgery, acute thrombosis may cause limb-threatening ischemia if preexisting collateral flow is insufficient [5, 7].

The most common etiology of acute arterial occlusion is cardiac source embolism. In extremity embolism, the typically lozenge-shaped chronic thrombus that dislodges from the fibrillating left atrium usually lodges in the brachial artery or the proximal femoral vessels of the leg. If the organized thrombus is large enough, it may occlude distal flow beyond the aortic bifurcation as a saddle embolism. If it flows to the upper extremity, it will occlude the subclavian or axillary artery. Less commonly, fresh and less organized thrombus from an acutely ischemic ventricular wall, a ventricular aneurysm with thrombus, or paradoxical embolism of venous thrombus through a patent foramen ovale diffusely distributes itself in multiple levels of the extremity [10, 14, 15] (Table 18.1).

Peripheral arterial aneurysms are an uncommon but important source of distal emboli. At the time of presentation, there is usually evidence of multiple prior episodes of small emboli followed by the current complete thrombosis and acute distal limb ischemia [15]. These aneurysms can be of both atherosclerotic and, less commonly, a congenital origin. Popliteal artery atherosclerotic aneurysms are the most common peripheral aneurysms and are associated with bilateral lesions in 50 % and abdominal aortic aneurysms in 60 % of patients [16]. Congenital popliteal entrapment and thoracic outlet syndrome with arterial compression can lead to aneurysms with embolic and thrombotic complications [17, 18]. Rupture of peripheral aneurysms is rare [16]. If left untreated, these rare congenital aneurysms are associated with a significant risk of limb loss because of chronic small distal emboli, acute thrombosis, and delay in diagnosis [17, 18].

Table 18.1 Sources of arterial emboli by frequency

1.	Organized chronic cardiac thrombus from atrial fibrillation
2.	Subacute thrombus from ischemia endocardium of acute MI
3.	Iatrogenic catheter-induced thrombus
4.	Paradoxical embolism from DVT, multiple PE with patent foramen ovale
5.	Peripheral artery aneurysm – congenital or atherosclerotic origins
6.	Atherosclerotic aortic plaque
7.	Aortic aneurysm

The increasing use of the extremity arteries for diagnostic and therapeutic endovascular techniques had resulted in a rise in iatrogenic acute limb ischemia [9, 19, 20]. Catheterization site arterial occlusion may result from an intimal dissection, accumulation of thrombus along indwelling catheter sheaths with subsequent thrombosis or distal embolism, and intravascular occlusion from misplaced closure devices. Diagnosis of this source of acute ischemia is also frequently delayed. Similarly, the outcome is dependent upon prompt recognition and treatment.

The ischemic pattern with the classic "five P's" of arterial occlusion occurs one level distal to the area of occlusion [5, 12]. If complete, this ischemia results in skeletal muscle and nerve tissue death at approximately 6 h [12]. This has given rise to the concept of a "Golden Period" of 6 h. This is the period of time between the onset of ischemia and the successful restoration of flow to save the limb from permanent loss of muscle and nerve tissue (Table 18.2).

Iatrogenic arterial occlusion is an increasingly common cause of acute limb ischemia [9]. The use of the femoral artery for catheter access for endovascular cardiac and peripheral interventions places a large number of patients at risk for acute ischemia from access site occlusions [19, 20]. Orthopedic surgical procedures in the hip and knee also put the femoral artery and the popliteal artery at risk for acute occlusion [22].

Acute massive venous thrombosis with outflow occlusion can cause acute limb ischemia. This entity is known as phlegmasia cerulea dolens or painful blue edema [23]. The venous obstruction and engorgement with desaturated

Table 18.2 Acute and chronic signs and symptoms of extremity arterial occlusive disease

Acute ischemia
Sudden onset of the "5 P's"
Pain
Pulselessness
Pallor
Paresthesias
Paralysis
Absent or monophasic Doppler tones at the ankle or wrist
Chronic arterial occlusion
Mild
Diminished distal pulses
Mild claudication of legs or exercise-induced muscle pain arm
Relieved by rest
Ankle or wrist pressure index 0.6–0.75
Moderate
Absent distal pulses
Severe exercise-induced extremity pain
Extremity pressure index < 0.6
Severe
Night pain forefoot or numbness of hand
No exercise tolerance
Extremity pressure index < 0.5
Limb threat
Rest pain in the extremity
Nonhealing ulcers on digits, heel, or palm
Dependent rubor
Blanching on elevation
Absent or monophasic distal Doppler tones

blood is associated with significant pain and resulting in arterial vasoconstriction. Left untreated, limb-threatening ischemia results from the accumulation of desaturated venous blood, decreased arterial flow, and compartment syndrome [23].

Clinical Presentation and Diagnosis

Acute limb ischemia presents with sudden onset of pain followed quickly by numbness and weakness. In patients with preexisting occlusive disease, these symptoms may be less distinct [5, 12]. The most common clinical setting of acute limb ischemia includes a history of atrial fibrillation [5, 15]. Preexisting lower extremity occlusive arterial disease is the next most common setting. These acute on chronic limb ischemia patients will have a history of claudication past extremity angioplasty with stent placement or arterial bypass surgery. The third most common clinical setting is a history of either acute or chronic ischemic heart disease with thromboembolism when mural thrombus dislodges form the damaged endocardium [15]. There is rising incidence of catheterization site occlusion in patients undergoing cardiac endovascular procedures [9, 19]. These iatrogenic lesions also occur in the setting of associated cardiac disease.

History and physical examination quickly reveal the most likely source of the acute occlusion in the vast majority of patients. Cardiac source emboli usually occur in the setting of atrial fibrillation or acute myocardial infarction. Less commonly, emboli result from paradoxical embolism of venous thrombus through a patent foramen ovale in patients with lower extremity deep venous thrombosis and multiple pulmonary emboli [14]. The resulting pulmonary hypertension with opening of an incompletely closed foramen ovale allows the next venous embolism to cross from the right atrium through the foramen ovale into the left atrium and out to the systemic circulation. Rarely, emboli from atherosclerotic arterial plaque or a peripheral aneurysm present as acute limb ischemia [8, 15]. These lesions more commonly cause digital ischemia. Thrombosis of a preexisting bypass graft or a stent is an important source of acute ischemia in patients with previous surgical or endovascular management of chronic disease [13]. This group of patients usually has a progression of distal occlusive disease and less commonly, occlusion of a patent graft in the absence of identifiable progression of disease. These patients must undergo detailed catheter arteriography and often are candidates for thrombolytic therapy [13]. Consultation with a vascular surgeon colleague is usually required in this setting.

Most patients with acute limb ischemia from embolism do not have a history of claudication and have normal pulses in the contralateral, non-affected extremity [5, 8, 15]. Saddle embolism to the aortic bifurcation may result in an absence of palpable pulses in both legs [24]. Acute thrombosis of preexisting arterial occlusive disease usually occurs in the setting of preexisting claudication. Physical exam usually reveals diminished pulses in the contralateral extremity and signs of chronic ischemia in the affected extremity. Ankle brachial indices may also reveal contralateral occlusive disease (Table 18.2).

Complete thrombosis of the infrarenal aorta is a rare and usually catastrophic event [25]. Practically all of these patients have significant cardiac disease with poor cardiac output that leads to thrombosis of chronic occlusive disease of the distal aorta and iliac bifurcation. The clinical presentation may include buttock and leg muscle weakness or paraplegia from distal spinal cord and lumbar plexus ischemia. The diagnosis is often delayed because of the baffling constellation of clinical findings despite the fact that physical examination reveals the bilateral absence of pulses from the femoral arteries distally with lower body and leg mottling. The mortality rate in these patients exceeds 50 % [25].

Phlegmasia cerulea dolens presents in the setting of massive lower extremity DVT complicated by arterial vasoconstriction and dehydration [23]. This lower extremity and, rarely, upper extremity syndrome is striking in its appearance with a swollen, blue, and cool to the touch limb [23]. Severe pain is always present. The compelling nature of these findings usually prompts venous duplex studies which confirm the diagnosis.

Doppler assessment of arterial flow in the extremity is an essential adjunctive measure to add to physical examination. Although the experienced examiner can assess flow based on the character of the audible Doppler signals, the best way to use the Doppler device is in conjunction with an extremity systolic blood pressure determination. The manual blood pressure cuff is placed at the wrist or ankle and the probe placed over the distal vessel. The cuff is slowly inflated and the cessation of signals indicates the systolic blood pressure at the level of the cuff. Normal ankle brachial index (ABI) is 1.1 [6]. Less than 0.8 is abnormal. In general claudication begins to be significant at that level of reduced flow. Below an ABI 0.5 or an ankle systolic pressure of 60 Torr, potentially limb-threatening ischemia begins [6] (Table 18.2).

Once the diagnosis of acute limb ischemia due to cardiac source embolism is made, there is an important decision to carefully consider. If the patient with distal limb ischemia has atrial fibrillation, no history of prior claudication or arm exercise intolerance, and an otherwise normal peripheral vascular examination with a normal groin or axillary pulse proximal to the ischemic area, and normal contralateral limb pulses, immediate operative exploration for embolectomy is indicated [8]. Preoperative CT or catheter arteriography is essential in patients who do not have a clearly identifiable cardiac source embolism or an obvious level of arterial occlusion. Acute on chronic occlusion needs to be delineated with detailed arteriography [12]. Although CT angiography may be adequate, catheter arteriography is preferred. In the setting of preexisting chronic occlusive disease, catheter arteriography also allows for endovascular techniques when appropriate [26, 27].

The most important factor to consider in obtaining arteriography is the time it takes and the potential delay to the operating room. Remembering the "Golden Period," there must be a rapid workup if arterial flow is to be successfully restored within 6 h. Therefore, if endovascular therapy is not an option, high-resolution CT angiography may be the best option if catheter arteriography is not immediately available.

Compartment syndrome should be anticipated in patients with acute limb ischemia [28]. All muscle compartments in the extremities are vulnerable to reperfusion intracompartmental hypertension that can lead to muscle necrosis after revascularization [49]. Compartment syndrome results from post-ischemia swelling of muscle in the confined space created by the muscle fascia in the extremities. This swelling increases the tissue pressure within the compartment compressing venous and lymphatic outflow as well as arteriolar inflow [28]. Ultimately the tissue perfusion pressure threshold of 25 mmHg is exceeded and ischemic neurolysis and myonecrosis occurs. It may take hours to occur after restoration of flow and therefore serial examinations are essential to prevent delaying diagnosis and treatment. Compartment pressures should be measured with the Stryker device or by other devices (Fig. 18.1). Compartment syndrome occurs most commonly in the muscle compartments of the calf and is relatively uncommon in nontraumatic arterial occlusion in the upper extremity [28].

Operative Management

The performance of emergency vascular surgery should be limited to those surgeons who are capable and qualified. That does not limit these procedures to those who are board certified in vascular surgery. There are many general surgeons who are very skilled in vascular technique by virtue of their interest and experience. There is a simple test to consider when deciding who should manage vascular emergencies.

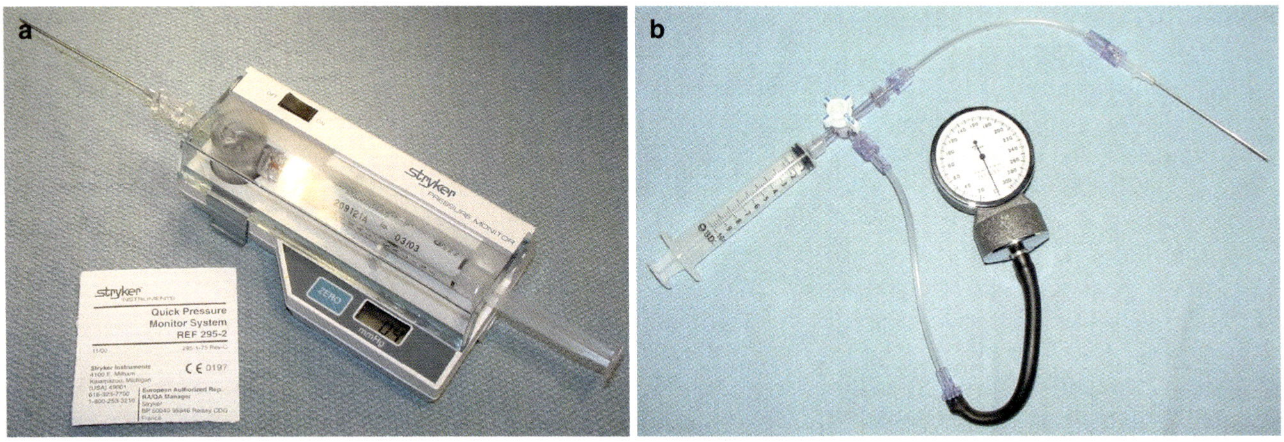

Fig. 18.1 (**a**) Stryker™ pressure monitoring device for muscle compartment pressure measurement. (**b**) Alternative pressure monitoring device for muscle compartment pressure measurement. The syringe and half of the line to the manometer is filled with saline (Reproduced, with permission, from Mattox KL, Moore EE, Fleiciano DV, eds. TRAUMA: New York: McGraw Hill; 2013)

Table 18.3 Checklist for femoral thrombectomy for cardiac source embolism and ischemic leg

1.	Pull up A-grams on PACS, position patient, pads under ankles, time out, (start dextran 40), give antibiotics, choose sutures
2.	Decide on early fasciotomy
3.	Mark landmarks and sketch incision sites on leg
3.	Expose vessels and control with vessel loops
4.	Administer heparin bolus 5,000 units
5.	Choose transverse vs. longitudinal arteriotomy
6.	Fogarty catheter thrombectomy proximal and distal vessels
7.	Flush with heparinized saline
8.	Supplemental dose of 2,500 units of heparin at 50 min
9.	Close artery (PTFE patch if longitudinal arteriotomy)
10.	Pulse, Doppler interrogation, on-table agram as indicated
11.	If distal occlusion, go to distal popliteal via medial upper calf incision – repeat steps 5 and 6
12.	Protamine, hemostasis, close wound, reassess pulses, Doppler if needed
13.	Reassess calf muscle compartments, measure pressures, fasciotomy if needed
14.	Talk to family, referring MD, and dictate

"Would I be comfortable having someone with this surgeon's level of experience caring for a member of my family?" There should be a designated call panel for appropriate vascular surgical backup at all times for an acute care surgery service.

The use of checklists to manage acute surgical emergencies is strongly recommended. These are best prepared in advance and should be printed and posted in the operating room. In my practice, I have created short checklists for each of the most common vascular emergencies. I print three copies just before the operation and give one to the anesthesiologist, one to be posted on the operating room white board, one to hang on an i.v. pole at the head of the table within reading distance of the surgeons. If checklists haven't been created, I recommend writing the important goals of the operation on the white board for all to see and to remind the team of the intended operative plan. Examples of checklists are provided below and I recommend each surgeon create their own version to include their choices for operative management (Tables 18.3 and 18.4).

The patient should be widely prepped and draped with generous inclusion of the entire upper or lower extremity and the shoulder or lower abdomen. One leg should also be prepped and draped from inguinal region to toes to allow for saphenous vein harvest. Adjunctive measures such as bolus intravenous systemic heparinization, the administration of a continuous infusion of low molecular weight Dextran™, and administration of intravenous antibiotics should be considered and utilized where appropriate. Preparation for surgery should also include appropriate management of associated cardiopulmonary disease by your anesthesia colleague.

Table 18.4 Checklist for 4-compartment calf fasciotomy

Calf fasciotomy checklist	
1.	Mark landmarks and incision lines – note head of fibula and mark 2 finger breadths below for exclusion zone for peroneal nerve safety
2.	Skin incisions – full length medial and lateral to create full dermotomy
3.	Incise anterior compartment fascia through lateral incision proximally and distally, avoiding peroneal nerve exclusion zone proximally
4.	Probe under fascia to the tibia to assure in the anterior compartment
5.	Release lateral compartment fascia in similar fashion probing under fascia to confirm in proper space posterior to the intermuscular septum
6.	Posterior compartment release – generous longitudinal medial incision 2 cm behind tibia and avoid the saphenous vein
7.	Deep posterior release under direct vision to locate and avoid posterior tibial artery
8.	Hemostasis on skin, check muscle contraction with electrocautery in all compartments
9.	Place loose moist sponge or Kerlix in wounds – wrap leg loosely
10.	Recheck perfusion at DP, PT, dictate and complete chart work
11.	Reassess wounds for hemorrhage and dressing tension every 4–6 h for the next 24 h – avoid recurrent compression from dressings as muscle compartments swell after release

Surgical exposure requires generous incisions placed to both maximize exposure and provide appropriate options for exploration and reconstruction. In the upper extremity, the axillary artery is exposed by making a transverse infraclavicular incision over the deltopectoral groove. A muscle-splitting incision is carried down through the pectoralis major muscle. The pectoralis minor muscle is divided close to the coracoid process and the axillary artery and vein exposed where they traverse just below the plane of the muscle. There are cords of the brachial plexus, nerves to the pectoral muscles, and large muscular branches of the artery in this area. Proximal and distal exposure of the artery should be carefully obtained avoiding damage to the brachial plexus and the axillary vein. Silastic vessel loops should be double passed proximally and distally and used to gently occlude the vessel. The artery is relatively fragile and pulling too vigorously on the vessel loops may fracture the arterial intima causing a dissection. A transverse arteriotomy is performed and proximal and distal thrombectomy with appropriately sized Fogarty catheters is carried out. A gentle heparinized saline flush (10 units heparin per ml) proximally and distally is performed taking care to not flush air or residual thrombus back up the vertebral arteries or the common carotid artery on the right side which can cause cerebral emboli and stroke.

The brachial artery is best exposed through a longitudinal incision along the medial aspect of the upper arm over the groove between the triceps and biceps muscles. The incision can be extended distally with an "S"-shaped extension across the antecubital fossa from ulnar to radial aspect and onto the forearm to expose the origins of the forearm vessels when the occluding thrombus is located at that level. (See below in Case Presentation 1.)

The location of incisions for acute lower extremity ischemia is determined by the level of the embolic occlusion. If the acute ischemic episode is due to a thrombosis of severe preexisting occlusive disease, a bypass graft, or a stented arterial segment, a vascular surgery colleague should be consulted to appropriately manage this complex problem. Iliac or femoral artery occlusion from an embolism is best approached through a longitudinal incision over the common femoral artery in the groin. The common, superficial, and profunda femoral arteries are controlled with silastic vessel loops. If the common femoral is soft and free of significant atherosclerotic plaque, a transverse arteriotomy is made. If it is not and chronic atherosclerotic changes are present, a longitudinal arteriotomy is the safest approach. Proximal and distal Fogarty catheter thrombectomy is carried out followed by gentle flushing with heparinized saline. The transverse arteriotomy is closed primarily with a running Prolene™ suture. A longitudinal arteriotomy should be closed with a patch angioplasty. Distal flow is assessed by pulse and Doppler examination or, if needed, completion intraoperative arteriogram. If distal thrombus is present and needs to be removed, a medial longitudinal incision along the posterior aspect of the tibia below the knee provides access to the distal popliteal artery. The exposure of the proximal tibial vessels may be required for distal control and should be carefully performed to avoid injury to the popliteal vein and the tibial nerve (Fig. 18.2). A checklist for management of lower extremity acute ischemia due to a cardiac source embolism is helpful for even the most experienced surgeon (Table 18.3).

The treatment of phlegmasia cerulea dolens is based on prompt anticoagulation and catheter-directed thrombolytic therapy [23]. Pain management and hydration are also important. An inferior vena cava filter should be placed at the initiation of thrombolysis because of the risk of pulmonary embolism [30]. Open thrombectomy of the common femoral and iliac vein is very infrequently required [30]. At the time of opening the common femoral vein, careful use of a large Fogarty catheter in the iliac vein retrieves distal thrombus. Wrapping the leg firmly with a sterile elastic bandage will milk out proximal thrombus. Retrograde Fogarty catheter passage down the veins of the leg risks significant damage to the valves and worsens the risk of recurrent thrombosis.

Fasciotomy

Failure to perform an adequate fasciotomy when indicated after revascularization of an acutely ischemic limb is the

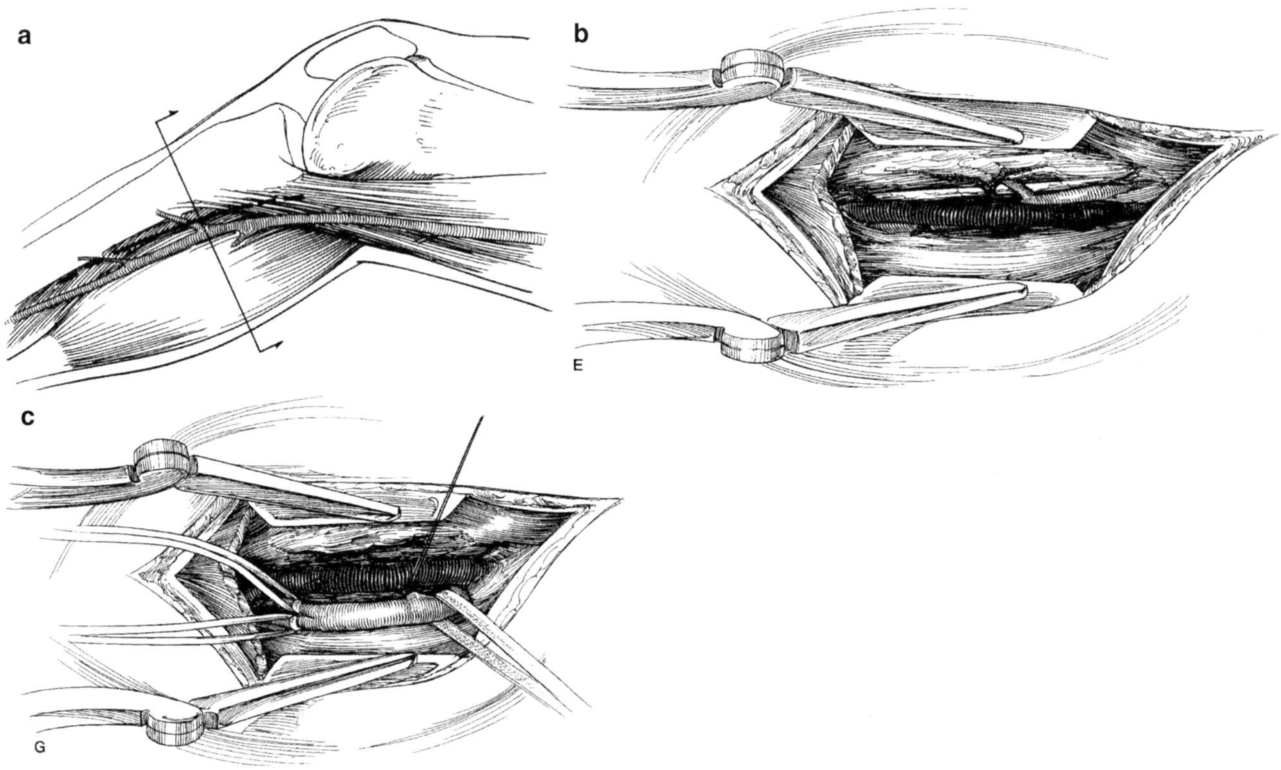

Fig. 18.2 (**a**) Incision for exposure vessels in the upper calf. (**b**) Dissection to expose distal popliteal artery. (**c**) Dissection to expose origins of tibial vessels (Reproduced, with permission, from Rutherford RB, ed. Atlas of Vascular Surgery: Basic Techniques and Exposures. Phoadelphia: WB Saunders; 1993. © Elsevier)

most common cause of preventable limb loss [28, 29]. Calf compartment syndrome is common and forearm compartment syndrome is relatively rare in nontraumatic acute limb ischemia [28]. Calf fasciotomy, particularly in the setting of prolonged ischemia, must always be considered prior to completion of the operation. Intraoperative compartment pressure measurements may provide decision-making data [28, 29]. However, if normal pressures are initially obtained, eventual reperfusion edema and subsequent swelling may occur with delayed compartment syndrome. Serial post-operative compartment pressure measurements may be required. There are four compartments in the calf that need to be released. These include the anterior and lateral compartments on the anterolateral aspect of the calf and the deep and superficial posterior compartments (Fig. 18.3). The best approach for release is two long incisions: one on the lateral side and one on the medial side of the calf [31] (Fig. 18.4). Although isolated anterior compartment syndrome occurs in some settings, four compartment release is usually required. A checklist for fasciotomy is strongly recommended and an example is included in Table 18.4.

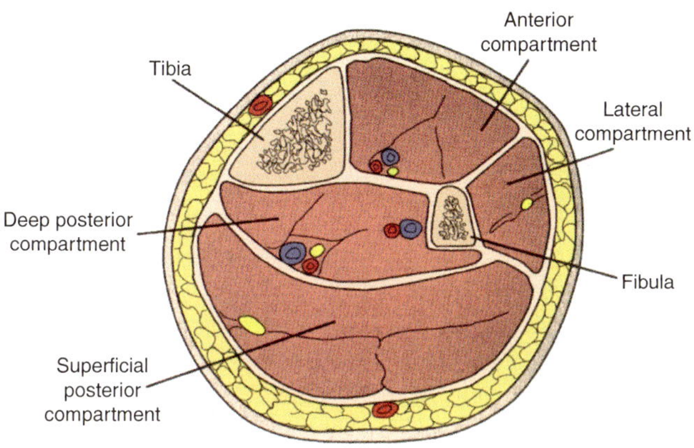

Fig. 18.3 Calf muscle compartments (Reproduced, with permission, from Frykberg ER: Compartment Syndrome, in Current Surgical Therapy, Cameron JD (ed) 5th edition, /WB Saunders, Philadelphia, 1995. © Elsevier)

The lateral calf incision should be generous. Start proximally no higher than 3–4 cm below the fibular head in order to avoid the superficial branch of the peroneal nerve. The incision should be taken distally to within 3–4 cm of the lateral malleolus. The fascia of both the anterior and the lateral compartments need to be incised longitudinally through the full length of the skin incision. Take care not to carry the incision beyond the limits of the skin incision proximally to avoid injuring the peroneal nerve. Make certain that the anterior compartment is fully released by palpating the tibia anteriorly under the fascia. Misplacing the incision lateral to the interosseous membrane will fail to decompress the anterior compartment with devastating consequences.

The medial incision should be made 1–2 cm posterior to the posterior edge of the tibia avoiding laceration of the greater saphenous vein. The fascia over the gastrocnemius should be fully incised proximally and distally. The gastrocnemius and soleus muscles are retracted posteriorly in the distal calf to expose the deep posterior fascia. This layer needs to be incised under direct vision to avoid lacerating the posterior tibial artery.

Once all four compartments are adequately released and adequate hemostasis is obtained, a loose dressing is applied. Care should be taken to avoid tight dressings which can recreate the compartment syndrome when muscle swelling occurs. Subsequent wound closure is performed in 2–3 days

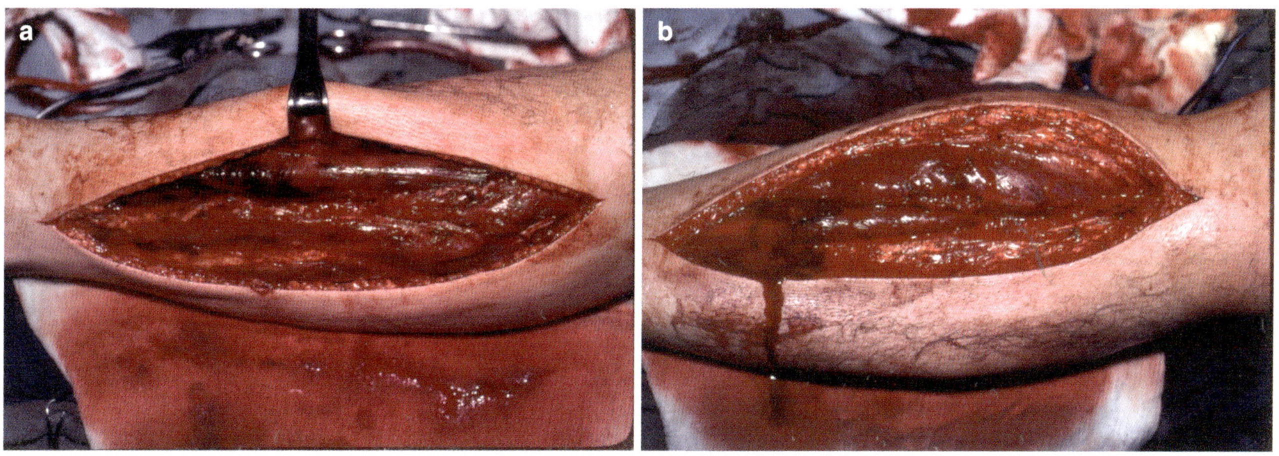

Fig. 18.4 (**a**) Lateral incision for release anterior and lateral muscle compartments. (**b**) Medial incision for posterior and deep posterior compartments

or when edema has sufficiently resolved. Split thickness skin graft may be required for closure.

Postoperative Considerations

Serial examinations after successful restoration of flow are essential to detect reocclusion or compartment syndrome and promptly treat these limb-threatening complications. These patients usually have significant comorbidities, and postoperative care should include a period of monitoring in the intensive care unit or a specialized telemetry unit. The nursing staff needs to have training and experience in monitoring the vascular status of extremities. Any evidence of recurrent ischemia, operative site hemorrhage, or compartment syndrome should prompt an immediate return to the operating room. In patients with cardiac source embolism, systemic anticoagulation should be started at 12 h or so after operation. The risk of recurrent embolism outweighs the risk of operative site bleeding. Continuous heparin infusion without a bolus is recommended instead of weight-based subcutaneous fractionated heparin. In the early postoperative period it is best to preserve the ability to reverse the intravenous infusion of heparin with protamine if needed because of bleeding complications. Once the patient is stable, the subcutaneous fractionated heparin every 12 h and oral warfarin can be administered. Lifelong anticoagulation is the standard of care in patients with a cardiac source embolism.

Acute Mesenteric Ischemia

Acute mesenteric ischemia is a potentially lethal process which requires prompt recognition and treatment for successful management. The mortality rate remains more than 50 % and there is little room for either delay or errors in management [32, 33]. Symptoms vary from the insidious onset of vague generalized abdominal pain to the sudden onset of severe and constant pain. There are four common causes: acute cardiac source embolism to the superior mesenteric artery, acute thrombosis of previous partial occlusion from an atherosclerotic lesion, splanchnic vasoconstriction leading to low flow and regional ischemia known also as nonocclusive mesenteric ischemia, and mesenteric venous thrombosis (Table 18.5). Each of these causes is a secondary phenomenon which results from other major diseases and occurs in a high-risk setting [34, 35] (Table 18.6).

Table 18.5 Etiology of mesenteric ischemia

50 %	Arterial embolism
20 %	Arterial thrombosis
20 %	Small vessel occlusion
10 %	Venous thrombosis

Table 18.6 Risk factors for mesenteric ischemia

Arterial embolism or thrombosis
Cardiac disease:
Atrial fibrillation
Recent myocardial infarction
Congestive heart failure
Digitalis therapy
Previous arterial emboli
Hypercoagulable state
Hypovolemia, shock
Venous thrombosis
Portal hypertension
Intra-abdominal inflammation
Trauma or major bowel surgery
Prothrombotic state
Chronic renal failure

Pathophysiology

The arterial blood supply of the gut is divided into four areas defined by the arteries that supply them. Collaterals connect the perfusion of each area (Table 18.7) [36, 37, 39]. In the absence of preexisting occlusive disease and compensatory enlargement of collateral vessels, these connections are not sufficient to provide adequate flow if the superior mesenteric artery is acutely occluded. In chronic mesenteric occlusive disease from atherosclerosis, patients may have total gut perfusion via a single remaining mesenteric artery or the bilateral hypogastric arteries via collateral flow to the other vessels [38]. However, many of these patients have intestinal angina when eating large meals. The venous drainage of the gut is via the portal venous system. Gastric drainage is via the splenic vein. The small bowel and the proximal colon up to the splenic flexure drain via the superior mesenteric vein. The descending colon drains via the inferior mesenteric vein. Collateral venous vessels are also present and connect each major area.

Cardiac source emboli have a predilection to enter the orifice of the relatively large superior mesenteric artery and then typically lodge distal to the origin of proximal jejunal branches and the middle colic artery [38]. This gives rise to a pattern of small intestine and colon ischemia with sparing of the proximal jejunum and perfusion of the transverse colon and distal colon. Celiac artery emboli are less common as are emboli to the inferior mesenteric artery and hypogastric artery emboli rarely cause ischemia due to a variety of pelvic collateral arteries [38].

The clinical manifestations of mesenteric ischemia are the result of insufficient blood flow to meet the metabolic demands of the bowel [36, 37]. The onset of acute ischemia leads to initial hyperperistalsis with gut emptying and vomiting and diarrhea. This is accompanied by intense ischemic pain from gut wall ischemia. This visceral pain is vague

Table 18.7 Gut regions, their blood supply, and collateral connections

Region	Blood supply	Collateral connections
Foregut Distal esophagus through the ampulla of Vater in the duodenum	Celiac artery	Pancreaticoduodenal arteries and arc of Buhler distally
Midgut Ampulla of Vater region of the duodenum to splenic flexure of the colon	Superior mesenteric artery	Pancreaticoduodenal arteries and arc of Buhler proximally Marginal artery of Drummond and arc of Riolan distally
Hindgut Splenic flexure of the colon to distal sigmoid colon	Inferior mesenteric artery	Marginal artery of Drummond and arc of Riolan proximally Superior hemorrhoidal to middle hemorrhoidal arteries distally
Cloacal derivatives	Branches of the bilateral hypogastric arteries	Middle hemorrhoidal to superior hemorrhoidal arteries proximally

and projected across the area of the superficial abdominal wall depending upon the area of visceral innervation [36, 37]. Foregut structures generate pain in the epigastrium, midgut in the periumbilical regions, hindgut in the infraumbilical region, and cloacal derivatives (rectum and genitourinary organs) in the suprapubic region of the abdomen [39]. Visceral ischemic pain is intense and constant and does not increase with palpation nor is it associated with abdominal wall rigidity. This gives rise to the pathognomonic "pain out of proportion to physical findings" attributed to acute mesenteric ischemia [36, 37]. The initial vomiting and diarrhea frequently diverts the examining physicians attention to consider other diagnoses [36, 37]. Ultimately, when ischemia leads to necrosis, inflammation of the gut surface leads to abdominal tenderness and associated physical findings of peritonitis. At the point of intestinal infarction, a systemic inflammatory response is initiated with an extremely high associated mortality rate [36, 37]. Elderly patients with this diagnosis typically have cardiopulmonary and other comorbidities which further limit their ability to recover.

Clinical Presentation and Diagnosis

Acute intestinal ischemia from sudden embolic occlusion of the superior mesenteric artery causes the classical findings outlined above. Acute on chronic occlusion of a preexisting atherosclerotic lesion may lead to a more insidious onset of pain because of preexisting collateral flow which mitigates the severity of the resulting ischemia [7, 36, 37]. There may be a history of intestinal angina (postprandial pain), fear of food, and weight loss. The least common etiology, mesenteric venous thrombosis, causes an insidious onset of initially vague symptoms which worsen progressively over time [40, 41]. Nonocclusive acute mesenteric ischemia from vasoconstriction occurs in the setting of critical illness with reduced cardiac output and is associated with vague symptoms or undetectable symptoms in the intubated patient on a critical care unit.

Table 18.8 Common symptoms and findings in patients with chronic mesenteric arterial occlusive disease

1. Postprandial pain	100 %
2. Weight loss	85 %
3. Abdominal bruit	70 %
4. Nausea, vomiting	60 %

Atrial fibrillation is the most common etiology of embolism [7, 36, 37]. Patients usually report sudden onset of pain associated with nausea, vomiting, and diarrhea. Mild abdominal distension and hypoactive bowel sounds without abdominal tenderness are the most common initial findings. In patients with acute worsening of chronic mesenteric ischemia, there is frequently a history of postprandial pain and weight loss occurs in close to 90 % of patients (Table 18.8). Mesenteric venous thrombosis usually is associated with congenital or acquired hypercoagulability and a variety of comorbidities (Table 18.6) [40, 41].

The laboratory studies of patients with acute mesenteric ischemia are initially normal except for an often profound leukocytosis [7, 36]. The white blood cell count is often in excess of 20,000. This finding is an important early indicator and, when present, should prompt the inclusion of acute intestinal ischemia in the differential diagnosis. Metabolic acidosis is a late finding and usually indicates intestinal infarction. Hyperamylasemia and elevated serum lipase may also be seen early in the course of mesenteric ischemia [32, 33, 36, 42].

The best hope for an early diagnosis of acute mesenteric ischemia in patients at risk is a promptly performed CT scan of the abdomen with intravenous contrast [43, 44] (See below Case Presentation 9). This exam definitively rules in the presence of mesenteric arterial and venous occlusion or rules it out and indicates the presence of one of the other etiologies of these clinical findings. Early discovery with CT scanning allows timely diagnosis before significant bowel compromise occurs [33, 38, 43, 44]. End-stage intestinal necrosis causes severe shock and an overwhelming inflammatory response with an attendant high mortality rate [45, 46]. The outcome of acute mesenteric ischemia has not significantly improved in the last four decades because of the high incidence of both intestinal infarction at the time of diagnosis and the common associated significant comorbidities [32, 33, 36, 47, 48]. The only hope to improve outcome remains prompt recognition, early diagnosis, and successful management prior to bowel necrosis [32, 33, 36].

Management of Mesenteric Ischemia

The overarching principles of management of acute mesenteric ischemia are summarized in Fig. 18.5. The decision for an immediate open surgical approach versus an endovascular approach is based upon the duration and severity of bowel ischemic, the nature of the occlusive lesion, and the ready availability and the capability of the emergency center's interventional radiology or vascular surgical intervention program [32, 33, 36, 49]. Patients with suspected bowel infarction or impending infarction need to go directly to the operating room for open surgical therapy [33, 49]. Embolic occlusion usually is due to organized cardiac thrombus which is not amenable to thrombolytic therapy. Prompt operation with superior mesenteric artery embolectomy combined with inspection of the bowel for necrosis is appropriate.

Chronic occlusive disease may be managed with endovascular techniques with stenting the mesenteric arterial lesion [36, 37, 50–53]. Thrombolytic therapy has limited application in acute mesenteric ischemia [36, 37, 52, 53]. None of these endovascular techniques should be attempted unless there is an active preexisting program with adequate

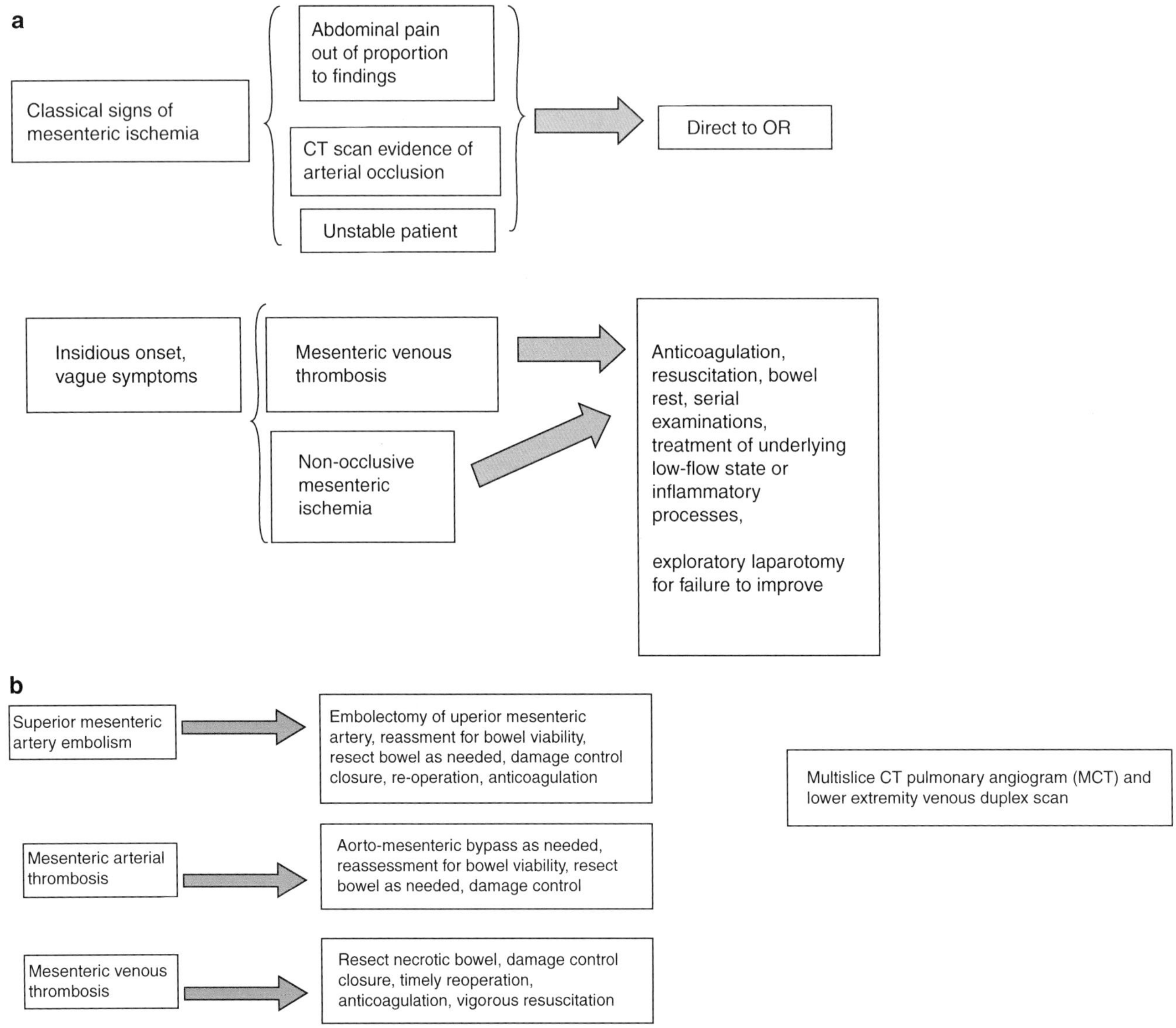

Fig. 18.5 (**a**) Decision making in the management of mesenteric ischemia. (**b**) Intraoperative management of mesenteric ischemia

personnel, equipment, and timely staffing at the emergency center. The risk of bowel necrosis and subsequent peritonitis requires prompt abdominal exploration to assess bowel viability even when arterial flow has been restored by endovascular techniques. Laparoscopy does not have a role in the management of mesenteric ischemia [36, 37, 49].

The celiac and mesenteric artery origins from the aorta are closely associated with the renal artery origins in the upper abdomen. The celiac axis lies just below the aortic hiatus of the diaphragm. The proximal portions of the celiac and superior mesenteric arteries are each covered by a closely applied plexus of lymphatic and neurologic tissue. These vessels are relatively thin walled and must be handled with care. The portal vein and major mesenteric veins are also thin walled and easily torn during exposure.

Intraoperative assessment of intestinal blood flow requires inspection of the entire intestinal tract by running the bowel, assessing color, peristaltic activity, and palpating the mesenteric arcade arteries. The main trunk of the superior mesenteric artery is located by upward retraction of the transverse colon, downward retraction of the small bowel, and palpation of the root of the mesentery along the inferior margin of the body of the pancreas. The celiac artery and its branches are palpated through the lesser sac just below the left lobe of the liver. The inferior mesenteric is palpated along left anterolateral area of the infrarenal aorta at the base of the left colon mesentery. Assessment of the mesenteric border for Doppler signals aids in the assessment of areas of questionable perfusion. Angiography with Fluorescein and an ultraviolet lamp can be helpful in assessing the return of perfusion [54].

The pattern and appearance of ischemic bowel is essential in determining the cause of mesenteric ischemia if it is first encountered in the operating room [32, 36, 37]. Embolism to the superior mesenteric artery most often lodges in the main vessel distal to the origin of the proximal jejunal branches and the middle colic artery. There is proximal sparing of the jejunum and the transverse colon with ischemia of the remaining small bowel and ascending colon. Superior mesenteric artery occlusion secondary to thrombosis of the origin leads to ischemia throughout its distribution from the duodenum to the splenic flexure of the colon. If the celiac artery and the inferior mesenteric artery are also occluded, more proximal and distal areas of ischemia are encountered. Acute thrombosis of both vessels leads to total intestinal ischemia from the distal esophagus to the rectum in a few catastrophic cases.

A transverse incision in the main trunk of the superior mesenteric artery at the mesenteric root below the pancreas is used to remove emboli [37, 55]. This visceral artery is a relatively fragile artery and requires careful handling to avoid tears and dissections. Fogarty embolectomy catheters should also be used gently proximally and distally to avoid arterial injury. Careful flushing with heparinized saline (10 units of heparin per ml) proximally and distally should be performed. Do not flush forcibly proximally in order to avoid dislodging thrombus into the aorta and causing distal embolism. Closure of the arteriotomy must be done with either running monofilament suture or interrupted sutures. Placing proximal and distal vascular clamps and gently retracting the artery towards the arteriotomy site minimizes tension during the closure. Once flow has been reestablished, placing warm laparotomy packs and waiting 10–15 min to reassess is helpful to relieve spasm. Injection of papaverine hydrochloride into the superior mesenteric artery (2 ml of a 30 mg/ml solution) may also reduce vasospasm and improve flow. Damage control closure and re-inspection in 24–36 h is prudent unless there is prompt complete restoration of normal intestinal blood flow without questionable areas of bowel at the initial operation [36, 37].

Proximal mesenteric arterial thrombosis and acute ischemia requires experience and skill in advanced vascular surgical technique [36, 37, 50]. It is best to involve an experienced vascular surgeon colleague to assist if you are not comfortable and capable to perform the necessary aorto-mesenteric bypass. There are a variety of bypasses described. Although seemingly easier to perform, retrograde iliac artery to mesenteric artery bypass is often more difficult than antegrade supraceliac aorto-mesenteric bypass and may have inferior results [56–58]. The iliac arteries are often involved with atherosclerotic occlusive disease in this setting. The donor vessel is difficult to sew into and the bypass is difficult to complete without kinking. This bypass also places synthetic graft in proximity to the duodenum with the risk of eventual erosion and graft infection.

The best choice for restoring flow in acute mesenteric ischemia from proximal mesenteric arterial thrombosis is antegrade aorto mesenteric bypass from the supraceliac aorta [56]. This requires exposure of the retrocrural aorta by mobilizing the left lobe of the liver and opening the lesser omentum. The left hepatic lobe is retracted medially and, with the stomach retracted caudally, the crura of the diaphragm divided longitudinally over the aorta to expose the area for the proximal end-to-side anastomosis. The tunnel for the graft to the superior mesenteric artery at the root of the mesentery is relatively easily made along the left anterior margin of the aorta with gentle blunt dissection behind the pancreas. It is also possible to dissect directly down the superior mesenteric artery behind the pancreas if the stenotic lesion is limited to the ostium. The celiac artery may also be exposed at its bifurcation into the splenic and common hepatic branches for performing a second bypass limb if needed. The patient is systemically heparinized (5,000 unit heparin bolus IV) and proximal and distal totally occluding aortic clamps are placed. Partial occluding clamps may damage the aorta or cause distal emboli. The distal anastomoses are performed end to side with careful flushing and, if indicated, balloon catheter thrombectomy. The bowel is inspected for viability once flow has been reestablished (see description above).

The management of the bowel after restoration of arterial blood flow in acute on chronic occlusive lesions should also include damage control techniques [2, 35–37, 59]. Obviously necrotic bowel should be resected by stapling and dividing at healthy margins and anastomosis of bowel segments deferred until reoperation at 24–36 h to make certain further necrosis and failure of the anastomosis does not occur. Temporary abdominal wall closure followed by prompt transfer to the intensive care unit for further postoperative critical care management should happen expeditiously. Early anticoagulation with intravenous heparin should be added despite the risk of operative site hemorrhage in order to prevent re-thrombosis of mesenteric vessels.

Mesenteric venous thrombosis leading to bowel necrosis is insidious in its onset and much more difficult to manage than arterial mesenteric ischemia [40, 41]. By the time intestinal infarction occurs from venous engorgement and impeded arterial flow, there are few options that will relieve venous congestion. Mesenteric and portal venous thrombectomy is dangerous and not effective. Systemic anticoagulation coupled with resection of necrotic bowel, damage control closure, and aggressive resuscitative measures are all essential for optimal management. Multiple reoperations to reassess bowel for viability are often required. Patients who survive extensive bowel resection for mesenteric venous thrombosis are often left with short gut syndrome [60].

Summary

Successful management of acute limb ischemia and acute mesenteric ischemia requires prompt recognition and timely treatment. There is a period of approximately 6 h of acute ischemia after which permanent nerve and muscle damage in the extremity and bowel necrosis in the abdomen occurs and the threat of limb loss increases as does the risk of an overwhelming intra-abdominal catastrophe. CT scan or catheter arteriography should be promptly obtained only when necessary but should not delay operative management. Carefully chosen incision sites and proper vascular technique are required. Fasciotomy should be considered in the setting of prolonged extremity ischemia or when compartment pressures are high. Damage control laparotomy is a mainstay of successful management of acute mesenteric ischemia. There is a role for the use of checklists to help organize your efforts in the care of these critically ill patients.

Illustrative Case Presentations

Case 1

History: 87-year-old male retired physician with atrial fibrillation on warfarin has sudden onset of pain and paralysis at the right forearm 3½ h earlier. Presents to the emergency department. Past history of hypertension, hyperlipidemia, CABG 12 years ago, open prostatectomy 5 years ago. Other meds include beta blocker, statin, and antihypertensive. No prior events similar to this. Lives a very active life style – hunting, fishing, and volunteering at his church.

Exam: BP 140/70, HR 70 and irregular, resp. 18, temp. 37C, absent pulses, paralysis and paresthesia right forearm, and palpable right axillary pulse but no pulse at antecubital fossa. Normal pulses left arm and both legs. EKG: atrial fibrillation, no other findings. Chest x-ray normal. CBC and chemistry panel normal. INR is 1.5.

Decision Making: Patient has history and physical examination strongly suggesting brachial artery embolism with limb-threatening arm ischemia. Peripheral pulse examination otherwise normal. It is now approaching 4 h since the onset of symptoms. Imaging studies are not necessary with this straight forward presentation and may waste time. This patient needs to go promptly to the operating room for expeditious thrombectomy. However, if the distribution of ischemia is not clear or if proximal pulses are absent, CT angiogram of the upper extremity would be appropriate and can be rapidly performed. Preoperative preparation should include administration of an i.v. bolus of 5,000 units of heparin as soon as possible.

Operative Management: Sterile prep and drape right arm and axilla. Draw an S-shaped course for the incision forming the distal brachial artery course across the antecubital fossa with a marking pen. Begin with a longitudinal incision over the distal brachial artery above the antecubital fossa (Fig. 18.6). A transverse incision is made in the distal brachial artery. Local Fogarty catheter thrombectomy is performed proximally and distally into all vessels with adequate flushing of all embolic material. Heparinized saline (10u heparin per ml) is flushed taking care to limit infusion volume proximally to avoid air and debris flushing into origin of vertebral artery with the risk of stroke. Arteriotomy should be closed with a running 5-0 or 6-0 Prolene suture.

Distal pulses and Doppler flow assessed and found to be normal and wound closed primarily.

Postoperative Plan: Serial right arm pulse examinations, neurologic examinations, and assessment muscle compartments in addition to inspection of wound site for presence hematoma. Plan to begin continuous heparin infusion without a bolus at 8–12 h. Begin warfarin at postoperative day 2 if operative site stable. Consult cardiology and patient's primary physician and discuss concerns that patient be kept in therapeutic range with anticoagulant therapy.

Outcome: Fully recovered without neurologic deficit and with normal upper extremity blood flow.

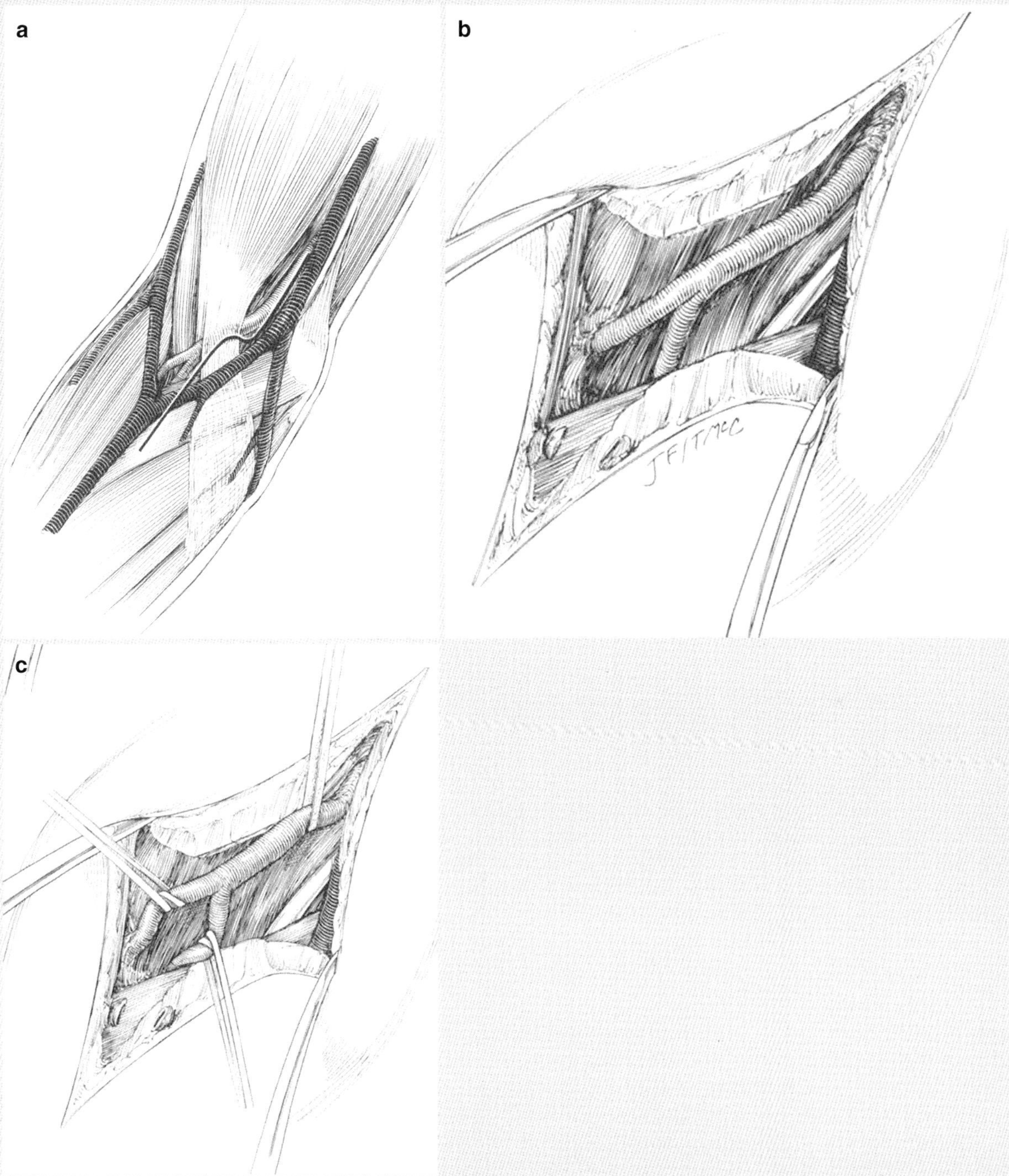

Fig. 18.6 (**a**) Course of incision to expose distal brachial artery. (**b**) Divided flexor aponeurosis and brachial bifurcation. (**c**) Vessel loop control of brachial, ulnar, and radial arteries (Reproduced, with permission, from Rutherford RB, ed. Atlas of Vascular Surgery: Basic Techniques and Exposures. Phoadelphia: WB Saunders; 1993. © Elsevier)

Case 2

History: 74-year-old male on the ICU post-op resection of diverticular abscess with septic shock and cold right leg with faint Doppler tones. Patient sedated with mechanical ventilation, weaning off pressors. Had workup for claudication with arteriogram 8 months ago. Told to quit smoking, take cilostazol, and walk regularly. Arteriogram from 8 months ago on PACS reveals superficial femoral artery occlusion with traceable collateral flow to the proximal popliteal artery (Fig. 18.7).

Exam: BP 100/70, HR 110 on SIMV mode ventilation, temp. 38C, absent pulses, cool somewhat mottled legs bilateral. Absent pulses below the femoral level bilaterally. Brisk Doppler flow on the left, diminished flow on the right. Ankle brachial index 0.5 on the right and 0.08 on the left.

Decision Making: Patient has history and physical examination strongly suggesting chronic preexisting occlusive disease at the right leg with vasoconstriction of collateral flow due to critical illness and vasoconstricting drug therapy. This is near limb-threatening ischemia and needs to be promptly addresses with medial management before tissue loss occurs.

Management: Optimize fluid resuscitation and cardiac output. Actively wean from pressor agents as soon as possible. Keep feet well-padded and avoid pressure lesions. Perform serial examinations with Doppler pressures.

Outcome: Slow but steady recovery without tissue loss. After discharge, claudication stable.

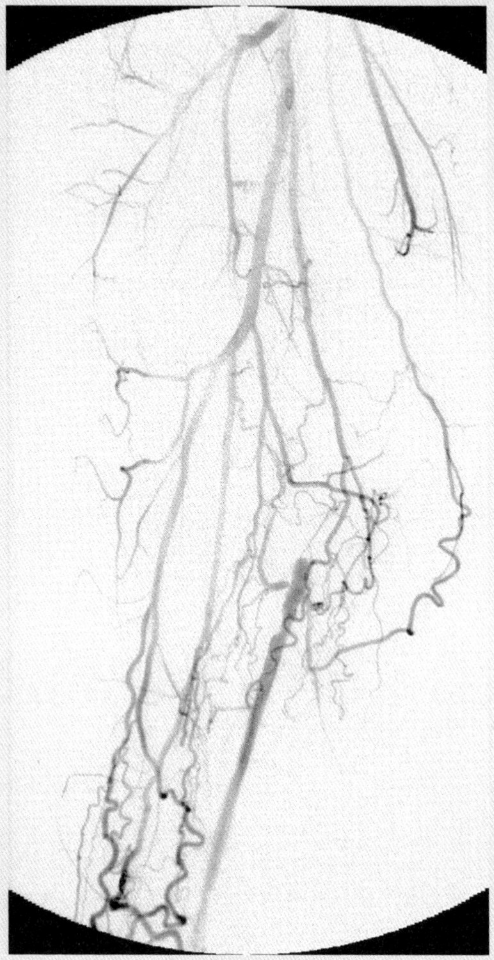

Fig. 18.7 Arteriogram from 8 months earlier with collateral flow to popliteal artery from profunda femoral artery branches

Case 3

History: 67-year-old woman on warfarin for recurrent DVT now has sudden onset 4 h ago of severe pain and marked weakness in both legs. The INR is 2.5.

Exam: BP 120/70, HR 100 and regular, resp. 28, temp. 37C, O_2 Saturation 92 % on mask O_2. Absent pulses, paralysis, pallor, and paresthesia in both legs.

Decision Making: Is this aortic dissection, massive cardiac source arterial embolism, or thrombosis of the aortoiliac segment, or is there some other cause? Patient has history of DVT and now apparent acute limb ischemia. Recurrent DVT can cause pulmonary hypertension which opens a previously physiologically sealed but anatomically patent foramen ovale (present in 15 % of adults) leading to a right-to-left atrial shunt and access to the systemic circulation for the next venous thromboembolic episode. Paradoxical embolism must be ruled out with CT angiogram of the aorta and of the pulmonary vasculature. CT scan reveals presence of both saddle pulmonary embolism and aortoiliac embolism (Fig. 18.8).

Operative Management: Patient at risk for both fatal pulmonary embolism and limb-threatening ischemia. Immediate operative thrombectomy through bilateral common femoral artery exposures is required. After restoring flow, compartment pressure needs to be measured in both calves to assess for compartment syndrome. Immediately after completion of the operation, an inferior vena cava filter should be placed. Intravenous heparin administration should be prompt.

Postoperative Plan: Serial examinations and, if indicated, repeat calf compartment pressures should be performed. The patient will need lifelong anticoagulant therapy. If not already completed, a thorough workup for underlying hypercoagulation syndrome also needs to be done.

Outcome: Successful thrombectomy. Discharge on warfarin and bridging enoxaparin 1 mg/kg q12 hours. Long-term follow-up for postphlebitic syndrome legs and disciplined use of support stocking and elevation extremities.

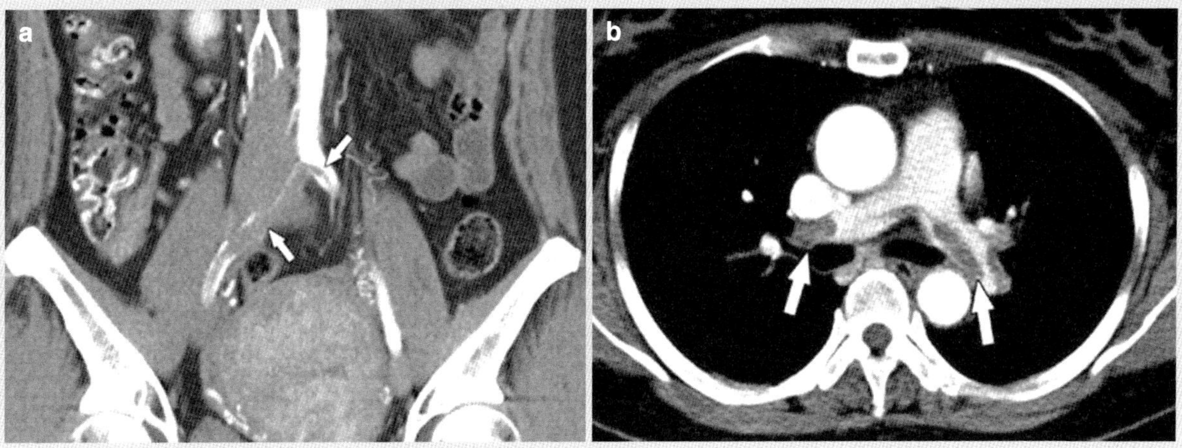

Fig. 18.8 (**a**) CT angiogram reveals a saddle embolism at the aortic bifurcation. (**b**) CT angiogram of the chest reveals large bilateral pulmonary emboli

Case 4

History: 67-year-old female retired teacher who presents to the emergency department with 2-day history of severe left calf claudication at less than a block. History of hypertension, hyperlipidemia, and smoking. Past CABG for three vessel coronary artery disease. She had two to three block bilateral calf claudication prior to this event. At rest she had no symptoms.

Exam: BP 150/80, HR 60 and regular. Absent pulses below femoral level left leg and decreased capillary fill left foot. Ankle brachial index 0.48.

Decision Making: This is a sudden acceleration of symptoms which suggests acute on chronic occlusive disease. The ankle brachial index suggests significant occlusive disease but not limb threatening.

Management: Arteriography will be needed to delineate arterial anatomy and plan therapy. It may be possible to perform an endovascular intervention to relieve this acute event.

Outcome: Successful angioplasty and resolution of left calf claudication (Fig. 18.9). Patient discharge on clopidogrel, cilostazol, and nicotine patches with counseling on smoking cessation. Exercise program initiated and patient followed regularly to assess progress.

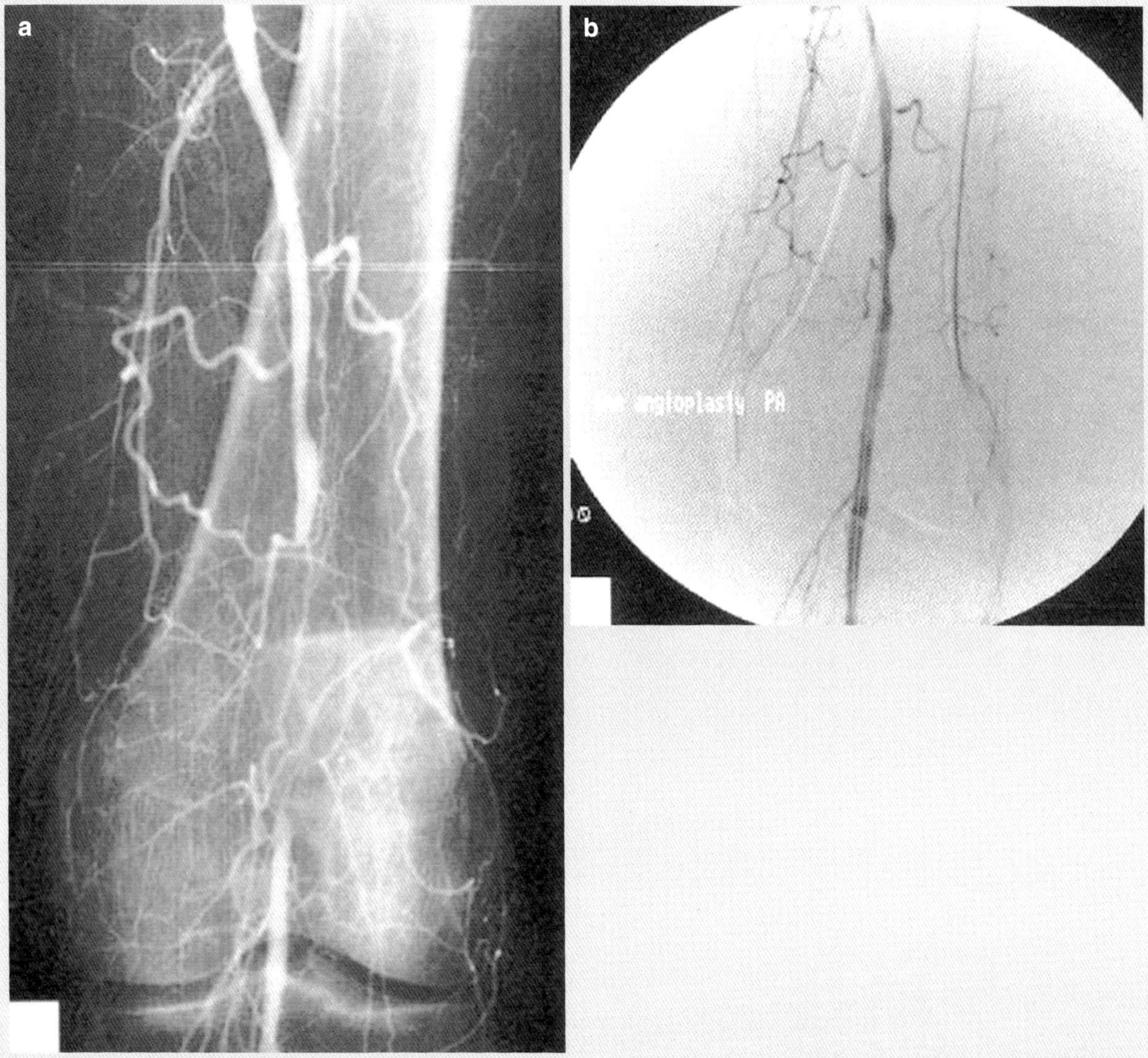

Fig. 18.9 (**a**) Catheter angiogram reveals proximal short segment popliteal occlusion. (**b**) Short segment angioplasty and stent placement

Case 5

History: 72-year-old man on warfarin for atrial fibrillation presents to emergency department with 4 days of right leg pain and paralysis. Wheel chair-bound for 5 years from right hemisphere stroke and left hemiparesis. History of coronary artery disease, congestive heart failure, and diabetes. The patient has an advance directive indicating no CPR.

Exam: BP 110/70, HR 100 and irregular. Paralysis, pallor, absent pulses throughout right leg, and absent Doppler signals at popliteal and pedal level. Firm, tender muscle compartments right calf, and paresthesia both legs. CPK over 50,000 IU/L, and myoglobin present in urine. CT angiogram reveals complete occlusion left external iliac, common femoral, superficial femoral, and popliteal arteries with few collaterals. The patient is not communicative and is disoriented.

Decision Making: This is advanced ischemia of many days duration and is not compatible with limb salvage. Left untreated, this patient will die of the systemic efforts of massive muscle necrosis. The only treatment option would be a high above-knee amputation. However, with his advanced cardiac disease, hemiparesis, and limited life expectancy, discussion of goals of therapy with the patient and his family is essential. Comfort care may well be the most appropriate treatment.

Management: You meet at length with the family reviewing the patient's course to this point and the trajectory of his decline explaining that this would have happened sooner or later given the severe nature of his health problems. You query them regarding the patient's wishes and they state that he did not want care that wouldn't lead to his recovery. You counsel them that the prognosis is extremely poor no matter what medial or surgical choices are pursued and that it is best to begin comfort care.

Outcome: Patient chooses comfort care and is transferred to hospice dying with family in attendance 3 days later.

Case 6

History: You are called to the recovery room by an orthopedic surgery colleague who has completed a redo right hip replacement in a 75-year-old woman with degenerative joint disease 2½ h ago. Her right leg is now cool, painful, paralyzed, and pulseless. The patient has a history of hypertension, hyperlipidemia, and breast cancer. There is no history of calf claudication.

Exam: BP 145/80, HR 75 and regular. Absent pulses at the femoral level and below right leg and blanched-appearing foot. Pulses are present and normal throughout the left leg. There are no Doppler tones at the femoral level and below in the right leg.

Decision Making: This is an apparent total occlusion of the femoral artery caused by the operative procedure. It is now well into the 6-h "Golden Period" and flow needs to be reestablished ASAP in order to prevent nerve and muscle tissue loss and possible limb loss. The proximity of the acetabulum to the femoral vessels places them at risk for intraoperative trauma. CT or catheter arteriography is not necessary and time consuming. The absence of a history of calf claudication and the presence of normal pulses in the contralateral leg suggest that the vessels were patent with significant chronic occlusive disease prior to this event. Immediate return to the operating room for exploration of the femoral artery and fasciotomy are called for.

Management: The patient is given an intravenous bolus of 5,000 units of heparin and promptly returned to the operating room. The patient is prepped from the umbilicus to toes on the right and mid-thigh on the left. The femoral vessels are exposed through a longitudinal incision, and the common femoral artery is found to be thrombosed with a through-and-through penetration from one of the sharp-ended acetabulum retractors (Fig. 18.10). A longitudinal artery is performed and there is a moderate-sized posterior atherosclerotic plaque with extensive disruption and thrombosis. Fogarty catheter thrombectomy yields a moderate amount of thrombus from the superficial and profunda femoral arteries. A PTFE interposition graft is placed from proximal common femoral artery to the bifurcation (Fig. 18.11). Intraoperative Doppler and pulse examination reveals flow throughout the right leg. Four compartment fasciotomy of the calf is performed through generous medial and lateral incisions.

Outcome: The patient recovers after closure of calf fasciotomy wounds with a skin graft over the lateral incision and primary closure of the medial incision at 72 h. You compliment your colleague's prompt recognition of this complication to the patient and her family and follow closely throughout her hospital stay. She is satisfied with her care and continues to be followed by you and your colleague as an outpatient.

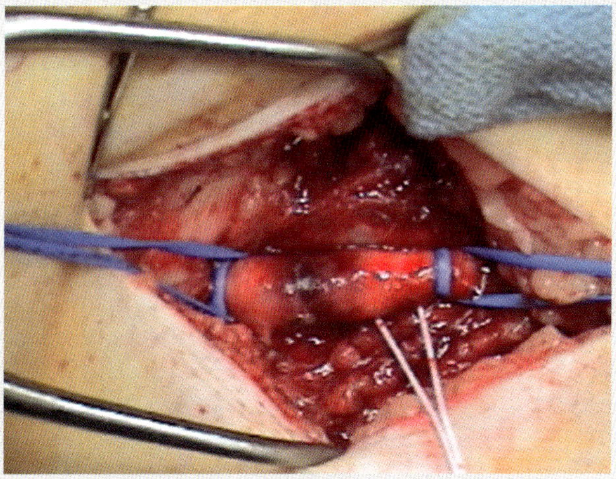

Fig. 18.10 Common femoral artery with perforation and thrombosis from a sharp-ended retractor used in the acetabulum during hip replacement (Left is proximal, right is distal)

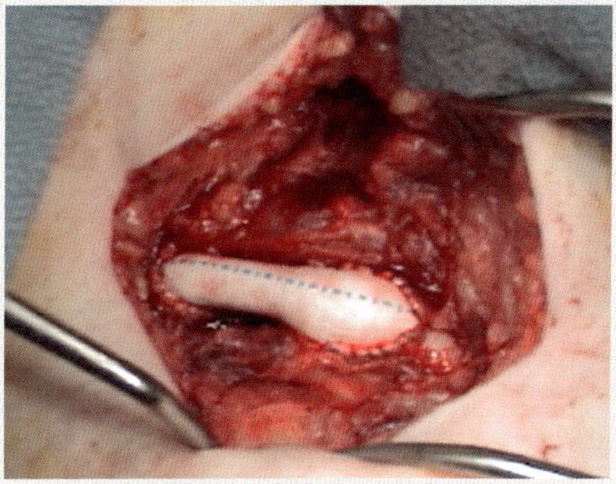

Fig. 18.11 PTFE interposition graft from common femoral (*left*) to the bifurcation at the origins of the superficial femoral and profunda femoral arteries (*right*)

Case 7

History: You are called by a cardiologist colleague to evaluate a 66-year-old man who underwent a coronary angioplasty via a right femoral access site for a STEMI 2 h ago. His right leg is now cool, painful, paralyzed, and pulseless. The patient has a history of smoking, hypertension, hyperlipidemia, and non-insulin-dependent type II diabetes. There is also a history of bilateral calf claudication. The patient has been given Plavix and is on an eptifibatide drip.

Exam: BP 140/70, HR 60 and regular. Absent pulses at the femoral level and below right leg and blanched-appearing foot. Pulses are present at the left femoral artery but absent at the popliteal and pedal level in the left leg. There are no Doppler tones at the femoral level and below in the right leg. There are Doppler tones present throughout the left leg and the left ankle brachial index is 0.65.

Decision Making: This is an apparent total occlusion of the femoral artery caused by the interventional cardiology procedure. It occurred in the setting of preexisting arterial occlusive disease. It is unclear what the site of occlusion is – at the site of catheter entry or more proximal in the iliac artery. A clear delineation of arterial anatomy is essential to successful management. The patient needs an immediate catheter aortoiliac and runoff arteriogram. Also, endovascular management is a possibility at the time of arteriography. Operative management, if required, must occur promptly after arteriography to avoid limb-threatening ischemia.

Management: The patient is given an immediate intravenous bolus of 5,000 units of heparin and undergoes arteriography at 3 h status postcoronary stent placement. There is an occluded proximal right external iliac artery which appears to have a dissection plane. A wire crosses the occlusion and a covered stent is placed. Distally, there is a patent common femoral artery and a profunda femoral artery. The superficial femoral artery is occluded but collaterals from the profunda femoral artery promptly fill the proximal popliteal artery. There is no distal thrombotic material seen and you conclude this is due to the powerful antiplatelet agents the patient is receiving as part of the STEMI protocol. After the completion of the arteriogram and covered stent placement, the patient has no pain in the right leg and has a normal right leg neurologic examination. The right ankle brachial index is 0.75.

Outcome: The patient is discharged home in 2 days, quits smoking, and is placed on a walking program. His walking tolerance improves.

Case 8

History: 65-year-old male in the emergency department with painful severely swollen left leg with deep bluish discoloration. First noted rapid onset left leg swelling 3 days ago and noted rapid worsening last 12 h. Four weeks earlier he was riding a horse and had left leg pinned between horse and a gate post with a large resulting thigh and calf hematoma. Patient has a history of hypertension, hyperlipidemia, and smoking.

Exam: BP 130/80, HR 90, and resp. 25. Markedly swollen left leg with bluish discoloration. Foot cool, no palpable pedal pulses, and markedly diminished arterial Doppler flow signals at foot. Duplex can reveal extensive popliteal, femoral, and iliac venous thrombosis.

Decision Making: Patient has history and physical examination consistent with massive venous thrombosis, marked entrapment of venous blood, pain, and arterial vasoconstriction – all the elements of phlegmasia cerulea dolens. This uncommon syndrome is the result of untreated lower extremity DVT with extension into the iliac vein. The patient needs immediate anticoagulation, pain management, hydration, and limb elevation. There is also a role for direct intravenous thrombolytic therapy. Failure to respond to thrombolysis in the first 8–12 h should prompt venous thrombectomy at the common femoral vein in the groin. Left untreated, the rate of limb loss and eventual death for the systemic effects of tissue necrosis. Both thrombolytic therapy and operative thrombectomy should be accompanied by inferior vena cava filter placement because of the high risk of pulmonary embolism.

Management: Immediate bolus i.v. administration of 10,000 units of heparin, infusion of 2 l of normal saline, intravenous pain management with a PCA pump, and elevation of left leg are accomplished, and admission to the ICU is accomplished. Within 90 min, the patient has placement of an IVC filter on internal jugular vein site and the initiation of thrombolysis via both a popliteal vein access site and a common femoral site.

Outcome: The patient immediately has relief of pain and the deep bluish discoloration steadily decreases over the first day. Pulses are palpable at the ankle by 2 h. It takes 3 days of thrombolysis to clear all but a persistent area of thrombus in the below-knee popliteal vein. Workup for thrombophilia fails to identify an underlying cause. The patient begins enoxaparin 1 mg/kg q 12 hours and warfarin at the end of the thrombolytic therapy. Lifelong warfarin is planned and the filter is left in place. On discharge, the patient begins wearing a below-knee support stocking with instructions to use it daily and keep renewing the prescription to keep appropriate compression.

Case 9

History: 73-year-old male first seen in the emergency department with severe abdominal pain of sudden onset first noted 6 h ago. CT scan reveals an abrupt cut off of flow in the main trunk of the superior mesenteric artery (Fig. 18.12). Patient has a history of hypertension, hyperlipidemia, and smoking. Patient denies chest pain, past history of myocardial infarction, and has no history of cardiac arrhythmias.

Exam: BP 140/80, HR 95 and irregular, resp. 25. Abdomen mildly distended and diffusely tender to palpation without signs of peritoneal irritation. Peripheral pulses in the extremities are normal. EKG reveals atrial fibrillation.

Decision Making: Patient has history, physical examination findings, and CT scan consistent with cardiac source embolism to the superior mesenteric artery. The time since onset of symptoms and physical examination findings are worrisome for impending bowel infarction. The patient should go directly to the operating room for thrombectomy of the superior mesenteric artery and evaluation of the bowel for viability.

Management: Immediate bolus i.v. administration of 5,000 units of heparin and transfer to the operating room for expeditious exploratory laparotomy. Superior mesenteric thrombectomy needs to be performed through a transverse incision. The anesthesiologist needs to be prepared to deal with the systemic effects of an introduction of the products of prolonged ischemia from the bowel when it is reperfused. The bowel should be inspected after 15 min application of warm packs. Necrotic areas should undergo damage control resection without anastomosis. Damage control closure should be performed and a hepa rin drip stated. Reoperation at 24–36 h will be needed to reassess bowel viability. The patient will require lifelong warfarin.

Outcome: The patient has a brief period of hemodynamic instability after reperfusion of the gut. There are a few questionable areas of bowel perfusion. At 30 h the bowel has all reperfused and no resection is required. The abdomen is closed. The patient has evidence of a non-STEMI myocardial infarction by cardiac enzyme determination after the first operation but remains hemodynamically stable. A cardiac catheterization is performed and a stent placed in the right coronary artery distribution. The patient is discharged to a rehabilitation facility on warfarin at 2 weeks.

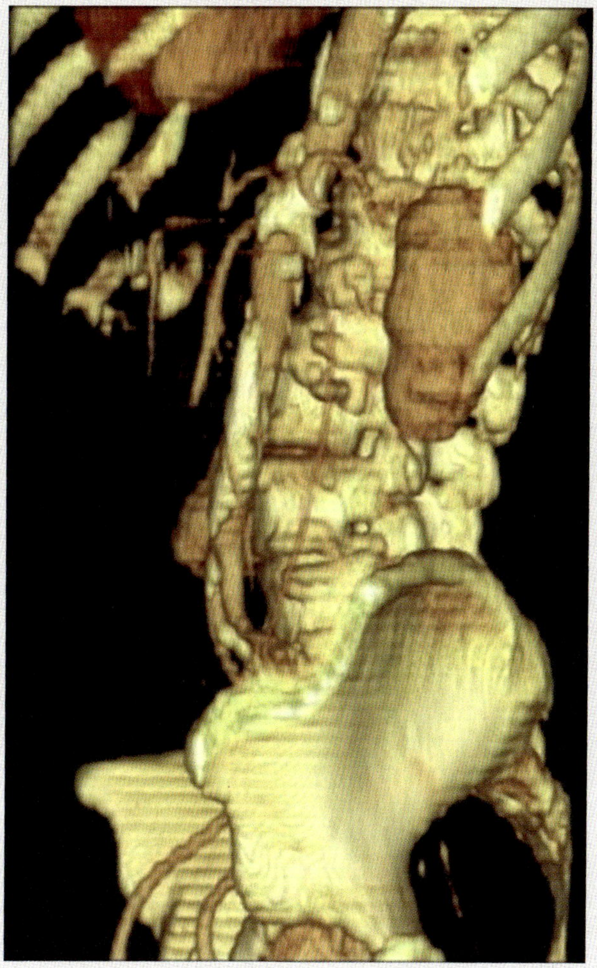

Fig. 18.12 CT angiogram VTR view of abdomen revealing occluded superior mesenteric artery

Case 10

History: 67-year-old female in the emergency department with vague abdominal pain and nausea and vomiting for the third time in 3 weeks. She suffered from a bout of apparent viral gastroenteritis approximately 1 month ago. Patient has been healthy in the past. Family history is positive for a brother who died from pulmonary embolism following a femur fracture. WBC 25,000; CT scan reveals a partial occlusion of the superior mesenteric and portal vein with thrombus.

Exam: Vital signs are normal. Abdominal exam is unremarkable.

Decision Making: This patient has mesenteric venous thrombosis. The paucity of abdominal exam findings and leukocytosis with the CT scan findings are typical of this diagnosis. The prodrome of an inflammatory bowel condition like viral gastroenteritis is also common. The positive family history for venous thromboembolic disease suggests an inherited hypercoagulability. Factor V Leiden is the most likely inherited disease associated with these complications. The late onset is suggestive of the heterozygote state for this patient rather than the homozygote pattern of early thrombotic complications.

Management: This patient needs hospital admission, immediate systemic anticoagulation, hydration, and bowel rest. Serial abdominal examinations are essential to detect intestinal complications related to venous congestion and infarction. The patient should be given an intravenous bolus of 5,000 units of heparin and a continuous heparin infusion. A generous infusion of normal saline should be started and a urinary catheter placed to monitor output. Pain should promptly decrease with anticoagulation and hydration. Continued pain is worrisome for bowel inflammation and impeding infarction. For the first 72 h, the patient should receive nothing by mouth. Serial abdominal examinations are required to make certain that bowel inflammation is not progressing. Any hemodynamic instability or signs of peritoneal irritation would indicate bowel infarction and should prompt immediate exploratory laparotomy. However, with appropriate anticoagulation and bowel rest, intestinal infarction is unlikely in patients who have the diagnosis made in a timely fashion. A workup for hypercoagulability should be performed on this hospitalization and the patient should be placed on lifelong warfarin prior to discharge.

Outcome: The patient resumes oral intake with a clear liquid diet at 72 h and is counseled to eat frequent small meals for the next 6–8 weeks. Workup reveals that she is heterozygous for Factor V Leiden. She recovers and continues warfarin. Her surviving siblings are tested and one is also heterozygous for Factor V Leiden. That sister is referred to a hematologist for counseling and treatment.

Case 11

History: 71-year-old male with severe pneumonia on the ventilator in the medial ICU for 5 days. Patient also has significant coronary artery disease and has required intravenous pressors during septic episodes. The patient has abdominal distension and underwent a CT scan with contrast which shows patent mesenteric arteries but an ischemic pattern in the small bowel.

Exam: BP 90/50, HR 95, resp. 18 (ventilator). Abdomen mildly distended and mildly tender to palpation without signs of peritoneal irritation. Peripheral pulses in the extremities are reduced but brisk Doppler tones present with patient on intravenous dopamine drip. WBC is 22,000, the serum amylase is elevated, and arterial blood gases reveal a mild metabolic alkalosis and marginal oxygenation.

Decision Making: Patient has history, physical examination findings, and CT scan consistent with low cardiac output, visceral vasoconstriction, and "nonocclusive" mesenteric ischemia. The examination and laboratory results suggest low visceral blood flow and the risk of infarction. The optimization of cardiac function and improved visceral perfusion is the best option to prevent the devastating complication of bowel infarction. This patient needs aggressive critical care management. Progression to bowel infarction in a patient with severe pneumonia and compromised cardiac function is almost always lethal.

Management: The medial critical care team boluses intravenous fluids, weans pressors, and begins a heparin infusion at your suggestion. You follow closely for signs of worsening.

Outcome: The patient steadily improves and is weaned, undergoes percutaneous tracheostomy, and eventual weaning form mechanical support. He is transferred to a rehabilitation facility 2 weeks later.

Case 12

History: 83-year-old female first seen in the emergency department with severe diffuse abdominal pain of gradual onset 8 h ago. She has an 18-month history of postprandial pain and has lost 25 lb of weight. She also had hypertension, hyperlipidemia, past myocardial infarction, and smokes a pack of cigarettes every 2 days. She also has claudication in both calves at two blocks. WBC is 27,000 and CT scan reveals severe aorto-mesenteric calcification with occlusion of the celiac artery and a long severe stenosis of the proximal superior mesenteric artery. There is diffuse distal aorta and iliac artery atherosclerotic plaque and tandem stenoses.

Exam: The patient is a very thin woman with little body fat. BP 140/80, HR 95, and resp. 25. Abdomen mildly distended and diffusely tender to palpation without signs of peritoneal irritation. Peripheral pulses in the extremities are diminished but Doppler tones are present. EKG reveals atrial fibrillation.

Decision Making: Patient has history, physical examination findings, and CT scan consistent with acute on chronic mesenteric ischemia. Her history of postprandial pain and weight loss is typical of this disease which is progressive and carries a high mortality because of the associated cardiac disease. She is at a significant risk of intestinal infarction and needs prompt restoration of adequate flow. This presentation does not yet indicate the risk but probably not the presence of infarction, and catheter arteriography allows for delineate of arterial anatomy and possible endovascular therapy. Open therapy with mesenteric artery bypass will be required if endovascular therapy is not possible. Exploratory laparotomy may also be required with successful endovascular therapy if there is a suspicion of bowel infarction.

Management: Immediate bolus i.v. administration of 5,000 units of heparin and transfer to the interventional radiology suite for arteriography. Superior mesenteric artery stenosis is successfully relieved with a stent and there is evidence of flow to all major areas. The patient is admitted to the surgical intensive care unit. Three hours later, she is febrile and abdominal pain and tenderness has increased. Exploratory laparotomy is performed because of the suspicion of bowel infarction. A 20 cm segment of distal ileum and the cecum is found to be infarcted and is resected with stapled ends of bowel left and a damage control closure is performed. The patient is returned to the operating room at 28 h and bowel anastomosis performed with closure of the abdomen.

Outcome: Patient requires a subsequent 2-week hospitalization. Although the patient has cardiac enzyme elevation and evidence of a non-ST segment change myocardial infarction, she recovers and is discharged on clopidogrel and counseled on smoking cessation.

References

1. Roger VL, Go AS, Lloyd-Jones DM, et al. Heart disease and stroke statistics 2011 update: a report from the American Heart Association. Circulation. 2011;123:e18–209.
2. Hirsch AT, Haskal ZJ, Hertzer NR, et al. ACC/AHA 2005 Practice guidelines for the management of patients with peripheral arterial disease (lower extremity, renal, mesenteric, and abdominal aortic). Circulation. 2006;113:463–654.
3. Go AS, Hylek EM, Phillops KA, et al. Prevalence of diagnosed atrial fibrillation in adults. JAMA. 2001;285:2370–5.
4. Fang J, Shaw KM, Keenan NL. Prevalence of coronary heart disease – United States, 2006–2010. CDC MMWR. 2011;60:1377–411.
5. Eliason JL, Wainess RM, Proctor MC, et al. A national and single institutional experience in the contemporary treatment of acute lower extremity ischemia. Ann Surg. 2003;238:382–90.
6. Creager MA, Loscalzo J. Vascular diseases of the extremities. In: Fauci AS, Braunwald E, Kasper DL, et al., editors. Harrison's principles of internal medicine. 17th ed. New York: McGraw Hill; 2008.
7. Burns BJ, Brandt LJ. Intestinal ischemia. Gastroenterol Clin North Am. 2003;32:1127–43.
8. Dale WA. Differential management of acute peripheral arterial ischemia. J Vasc Surg. 1984;1:269.
9. Giswold ME, Landry GJ, Taylor LM, Moneta GL. Iatrogenic arterial injury is an increasingly important cause of arterial trauma. Am J Surg. 2004;187:590–3.
10. Rooke TW, Wennberg PW. Diagnosis and management of diseases of the peripheral arteries and veins. In: Walsh RA, Simon DI, Hoit BD, et al., editors. Hurst's the heart. 12th ed. New York: McGraw Hill; 2007.
11. Brantley SK, Rigdon EE, Raju S. Persistent sciatic artery: embryology, pathology, and treatment. J Vasc Surg. 1993;18:242–8.
12. Cambria RP, Abbott WM. Acute arterial thrombosis of the lower extremity. Arch Surg. 1984;119:784.
13. Comerota AJ, Malone MD. Simplified approach to thrombolytic therapy of arterial and graft occlusion. In: Yao JST, Pearce WH, editors. Practical vascular surgery. Stamford: Appleton and Lange; 1999. p. 321–34.
14. Travis JA, Fuller SB, Ligush J, et al. Diagnosis and treatment of paradoxical embolus. J Vasc Surg. 2001;34:860.
15. Tawes RL, Harris EJ, Brown WH, et al. Arterial thromboembolism: a 20-year experience. Arch Surg. 1985;120:595.
16. Galland RB. Popliteal aneurysms: from John Hunter to the 21st century. Ann R Coll Surg Engl. 2007;89:466–71.
17. Sinha S, Houghton J, Holt PJ, et al. Popliteal entrapment syndrome. J Vasc Surg. 2012;55:252–62.
18. Sanders RJ, Hammond SL, Rao NM. Diagnosis of thoracic outlet syndrome. J Vasc Surg. 2004;46:601–4.
19. Nehler MR, Lawrence WA, Whitehill TA, Charette SD, et al. Iatrogenic vascular injuries from percutaneous vascular suturing devices. J Vasc Surg. 2001;33:943–7.
20. Natali J, Benhamou AC. Iatrogenic vascular injuries. A review of 125 cases (excluding angiographic injuries). J Cardiovasc Surg. 1979;20:169–76.
21. Mills JL, Porter JM. Basic data related to clinical decision making in acute limb ischemia. Ann Vasc Surg. 1991;5:96–8.
22. Freischlag JA, Sise MJ, Hye R, et al. Vascular complications associated with orthopedic procedures. Surg Gynecol Obstet. 1989;169:147–52.
23. Patel NH, Plorde JJ, Meissner M. Catheter-directed thrombolysis in the treatment of phlegmasia cerulea dolens. Ann Vasc Surg. 1998;12:471–5.
24. Busuttil RW, Keehn G, Milliken J, et al. Aortic saddle embolus. A twenty-year experience. Ann Surg. 1983;197:698–706.
25. Danto LA, Fry WJ, Kraft RO. Acute aortic thrombosis. Arch Surg. 1972;104:569–72.
26. Hynes BG, Margey RJ, Ruggiero N, et al. Endovascular management of acute limb ischemia. Ann Vasc Surg. 2012;26:110–24.
27. Vikram S, Kashyap VS, Gilani R, Bena JF, et al. Endovascular therapy for acute limb ischemia. J Vasc Surg. 2011;53:340–6.
28. Matsen FA. Compartment syndromes. New York: Grune and Stratton; 1980.
29. Whitesides TE, Heckman MM. Acute compartment syndrome: update on diagnosis and treatment. J Am Acad Orthop Surg. 1996;4:209.
30. Hartung O, Benmiloud F, Barthelemy P, et al. Late results of surgical venous thrombectomy with iliocaval stenting. J Vasc Surg. 2008;47:381–7.

31. Mubarak SJ, Owen CA. Double-incision fasciotomy of the the leg for decompression in compartment syndrome. J Bone Joint Surg. 1976;58:549–50.
32. Wyers MC. Acute mesenteric ischemia: diagnostic approach and surgical treatment. Semin Vasc Surg. 2010;23:9–20.
33. Kougias P, Lau D, El Sayed FH, et al. Determinants of mortality and treatment outcome following surgical interventions for acute mesenteric ischemia. J Vasc Surg. 2007;46:467–74.
34. Schoots IG, Koffeman GI, Legemate DA, et al. Systematic review of survival after acute mesenteric ischemia according to disease aetiology. Br J Surg. 2004;91:17–27.
35. Schermerhorn ML, Giles KA, Allen D, Hamdan AD, et al. Mesenteric revascularization: management and outcomes in the United States 1988–2006. J Vasc Surg. 2009;50:341–8.
36. Oldenburg WA, Lau LL, Rodenberg TL, et al. Acute mesenteric ischemia. Arch Intern Med. 2004;164:1054–62.
37. McKinsey JF, Gewertz BL. Acute mesenteric ischemia. Surg Clin North Am. 1997;77:307–18.
38. Moore WS. Visceral ischemic syndromes. In: Moore WS, editor. Vascular and endovascular surgery. 7th ed. New York: Saunders; 2005.
39. Curie DJ. Abdominal pain. Washington, DC: Hemisphere Pub Corp; 1979.
40. Boley SJ, Kaleya RN, Brandt LJ. Mesenteric venous thrombosis. Surg Clin North Am. 1992;72:183–201.
41. Rhee RY, Gloviczki P, Mendonca CT, et al. Mesenteric venous thrombosis: still a lethal disease in the 1990s. J Vasc Surg. 1994;20:688–97.
42. Horton KM, Fishman EK. Multidetector CT angiography in the diagnosis of mesenteric ischemia. Radiol Clin North Am. 2007;45:275–88.
43. Cikrit DF, Harris VJ, Hemmer CG, et al. Comparison of spiral CT scan and arteriography for evaluation of renal and visceral arteries. Ann Vasc Surg. 1996;10:109–16.
44. Ridley N, Green SE. Mesenteric arterial thrombosis diagnosed on CT. Am J Roentgenol. 2001;176:549.
45. Moore EE, Moore FA, Franciose RJ, et al. The postischemic gut serves as a priming bed for circulating neutrophils that provoke multiple organ failure. J Trauma. 1994;37:881–7.
46. Hassoun HT, Kone BC, Mercer DW, et al. Post-injury multiple organ failure: the role of the gut. Shock. 2001;15:1–10.
47. Klempnauer J, Grothues F, Bekras H, et al. Long-term results after surgery for acute mesenteric ischemia. Surgery. 1997;121:239–43.
48. Cho JS, Carr JA, Jacobsen G, et al. Long-term outcome after mesenteric artery reconstruction: a 37-year experience. J Vasc Surg. 2002;35:453–60.
49. Endean ED, Barnes SL, Kwolek CJ, et al. Surgical management of thrombotic acute intestinal ischemia. Ann Surg. 2001;233:801–8.
50. Park WM, Gloviczki P, Cherry KJ, et al. Contemporary management of acute mesenteric ischemia: factors associated with survival. J Vasc Surg. 2002;35:445–52.
51. Hansen KJ, Wilson DB, Craven TE, Pearce JD. Mesenteric artery disease in the elderly. J Vasc Surg. 2004;40:45–52.
52. Kasirajan K, O'Hara PJ, Gray BH, et al. Chronic mesenteric ischemia: open surgery versus percutaneous angioplasty and stenting. J Vasc Surg. 2001;33:63–71.
53. Matsumoto AH, Angle JF, Spinosa DJ, et al. Percutaneous transluminal angioplasty and stenting in the treatment of chronic mesenteric ischemia: results and long-term follow up. J Am Coll Surg. 2002;194:S22–31.
54. Ballard J, Stone W, Hallett J, et al. A critical analysis of adjuvant techniques used to assess bowel viability in acute mesenteric ischemia. Am Surg. 1993;7:309–11.
55. Bjorek M, Acosta S, Lindber F, et al. Revascularization of the superior mesenteric artery after acute thromboembolic occlusion. Br J Surg. 2002;89:923–7.
56. Hermeck J, et al. Role of supraceliac aortic bypass in visceral artery reconstruction. Am J Surg. 1991;162:611–4.
57. Foley MI, Moneta G, Abu-Zamzam AM, et al. Revascularization of the superior mesenteric artery alone for treatment of intestinal ischemia. J Vasc Surg. 2000;32:37–47.
58. Gentile A, Moneta G, Taylor L, et al. Isolated bypass to the superior mesenteric artery for intestinal ischemia. Arch Surg. 1994;129:926–32.
59. Ryer EJ, ManjuKalra M, Oderich GS, et al. Revascularization for acute mesenteric ischemia. J Vasc Surg. 2012;55:1682–9.
60. Thompson JS, Langnas AN, Pinch LW, et al. Surgical approach to short-bowel syndrome. Experience in a population of 160 patients. Ann Surg. 1995;222:600–5.

Thoracic Diseases in the Elderly

19

Matthew V. Benns and J. David Richardson

Introduction

Thoracic diseases in the geriatric patient that require emergency surgery are highly varied and can be quite challenging. They will often present with similar symptom complexes and can easily be confused with medically treated diseases. Unfortunately, many are imminently fatal if prompt diagnosis and management is not initiated. In this chapter, a broad range of thoracic surgical emergencies will be discussed. Specific focus will be given to those etiologies found most commonly in the geriatric population. In most cases, treatment of these conditions does not differ with advancing age.

Respiratory Tract

Airway Obstruction

The causes of acute upper airway obstruction are highly varied and include aspiration of foreign bodies, tumors, strictures, and tracheomalacia. Most conditions other than aspiration will be associated with some chronic symptoms of stridor, cough, or dyspnea. However, they still may present acutely if a chronic lesion progresses past a critical threshold, or respiratory secretions cause a sudden obstruction of an already narrowed lumen. The initial assessment and management in the acute setting does not differ between etiologies and with advanced age [1].

Clinical Presentation and Initial Management

Patients with proximal airway obstruction will generally present with choking, cough, and stridor. More distal obstructions may have few or no associated symptoms, other than wheezing on exam. Immediate airway assessment and control, if necessary, is of paramount importance. The preferred method of airway stabilization when required is endotracheal intubation. However, this may not be possible in the setting of proximal obstruction. Repeated unsuccessful attempts may only cause further edema or bleeding within the airway; thus, clinicians should proceed to a surgical airway without delay when intubation fails [1, 2].

Surgical management of supraglottic acute airway obstruction is usually accomplished via cricothyroidotomy, given the speed with which it can be performed and the limited required supplies. Access to the airway needs to be gained below the level of obstruction; thus, patients with known laryngeal pathology should undergo tracheostomy. If the level of obstruction is unknown when access is required, cricothyroidotomy should be the default point of access. Once the airway is secured, diagnosis of the underlying etiology may proceed. In the case of foreign body aspiration, these can often be extracted or dislodged through the airway incision.

One potential complicating factor that is almost exclusive to older patients is the presence of tracheal calcification. This phenomenon is associated with normal aging and may also occur with long-term warfarin use [3, 4]. It may lead to a distortion of the tracheal anatomy, and the calcified trachea may be difficult to incise. Bony fragments may pierce the cuff of a tracheostomy tube on insertion, and the risk of fracturing or tearing the trachea may be higher. If extreme calcification of the trachea is noted on chest radiographs or computed tomography, consideration for performing a surgical airway in the operating room should be given. The patient may be better served by the improved lighting, broader scope of instruments, and anesthesia support of the operating room environment. Patient condition and emergent operating room availability will obviously dictate the feasibility of this approach.

Diagnosis

After the airway has been assessed and controlled (if necessary), the diagnostic workup for airway obstruction may proceed. Many etiologies will be suggested based on history and

M.V. Benns, MD • J.D. Richardson, MD (✉)
Department of Surgery, University of Louisville,
550 S. Jackson Street, Louisville,
KY 40292, USA
e-mail: m0benn02@louisville.edu; jdrich01@louisville.edu

J.A. Yelon, F.A. Luchette (eds.), *Geriatric Trauma and Critical Care*,
DOI 10.1007/978-1-4614-8501-8_19, © Springer Science+Business Media New York 2014

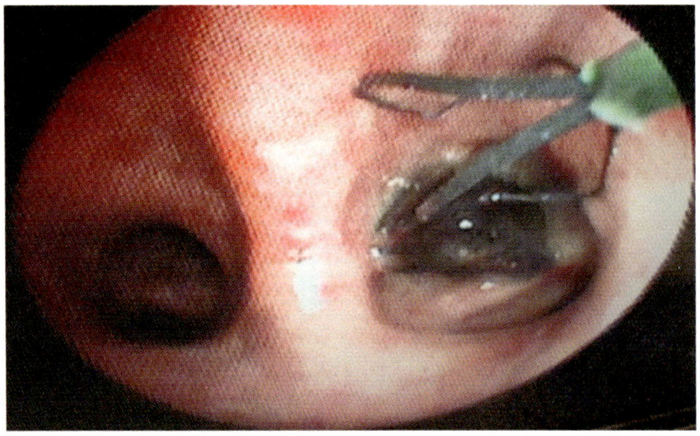

Fig. 19.1 Bronchoscopic removal of aspirated foreign body

physical alone. The gold standard for definitive diagnosis is direct visualization via bronchoscopy, but most patients will undergo some form of radiographic workup first. Plain films of the chest and neck are commonly performed and can be very useful. Positive findings include atelectasis, pneumonia, hyperinflation (in cases of partial obstruction), or aspirated foreign bodies (if radiopaque). Computed tomography is rarely indicated, but may similarly demonstrate the cause or sequelae of obstruction. Patients who have a consistent history, but a negative radiographic workup should still undergo diagnostic bronchoscopy. The complications of a delay in diagnosis include recurrent pneumonia, hemoptysis, pleural effusion, empyema, and bronchial injury.

Aspiration

The aspiration of foreign bodies is the most common cause of acute airway obstruction in the geriatric population. Dental or medical appliances are the most common objects aspirated. Risk factors include dental procedures, conditions leading to depressed mental status, and dysphagia. Advanced age is not an independent risk factor for foreign body aspiration [5, 6].

The treatment of foreign body aspiration is via bronchoscopy, either rigid or flexible. The choice depends on the comfort level of the treating physician in most cases, but flexible bronchoscopy is more commonly utilized. Prior to inserting the bronchoscope, the patient's airway should either be definitively secured or preparations for an emergency airway should be in place.

A variety of bronchoscopic instruments can be used to retrieve foreign bodies including forceps, snares, baskets, and balloon catheters (Fig. 19.1). Magnetic probes are available and can be useful for metallic objects. Occasionally, laser coagulation of surrounding granulation tissue is necessary in order to dislodge the object. If the identity of the foreign body is known and can be duplicated, it is often useful to determine what instrument would be most useful for retrieval extracorporeally. Flexible bronchoscopy should be performed through the mouth to prevent loss of the object within the nasal passages. Once grasped, the scope, retrieval instrument, and foreign body should be removed together [6].

Complications associated with bronchoscopic foreign body removal occur in less than 10 % of patients and include bronchospasm, laryngospasm, pneumonia, pneumothorax, pneumomediastinum, and bleeding. It has an overall success rate of greater than 85 %. Failure of bronchoscopic removal generally requires tracheostomy or thoracotomy for object removal. Surprisingly, location or duration of time in the airway does not seem to predict complications or success [5, 6].

Massive Hemoptysis

Hemoptysis may be a common complaint among geriatric patients presenting to the emergency room, but "massive" hemoptysis will frequently prompt acute care surgery consultation. The amount of blood loss to be considered massive is variable, but generally greater than 600 ml/24 h. The actual amount may not be important, however, as significant oxygenation and ventilation deficiencies can occur with a much smaller volume of blood. Most patients presenting with massive hemoptysis will develop life-threatening respiratory failure before hemodynamically significant blood loss occurs [7]. This is of particular importance to the geriatric population who may already have diminished pulmonary reserve.

Ninety percent of the bleeding in cases of massive hemoptysis originates from the bronchial arteries. Only 5 % of hemoptysis occurs from pulmonary arterial sources and is generally less threatening secondary to the lower pressures. The specific causes of massive hemoptysis are broad, but certain etiologies are more common among the geriatric population. Neoplastic etiologies including both primary and metastatic lesions are the most common. Other causes include infections such as bronchiectasis, tuberculosis, fungal balls, lung abscess, and necrotizing pneumonia. Vascular etiologies are less common, but may still be seen and include AV malformations, thoracic aneurysm, pulmonary embolism/infarction, and mitral stenosis. Medical causes such as Goodpasture syndrome and Behcet's disease are also causes, but are rare among the elderly [7].

Clinical Presentation and Diagnosis

Patients presenting with massive hemoptysis require a prompt assessment that should mirror that of a trauma resuscitation (Fig. 19.2). The airway must be assessed first. Patients with severe bleeding or signs of respiratory failure should be intubated without delay. The largest possible endotracheal tube should be used to facilitate suctioning as well as bronchoscopy. Physical exam may reveal the side of bleeding in some patients. If this is the case, patients should

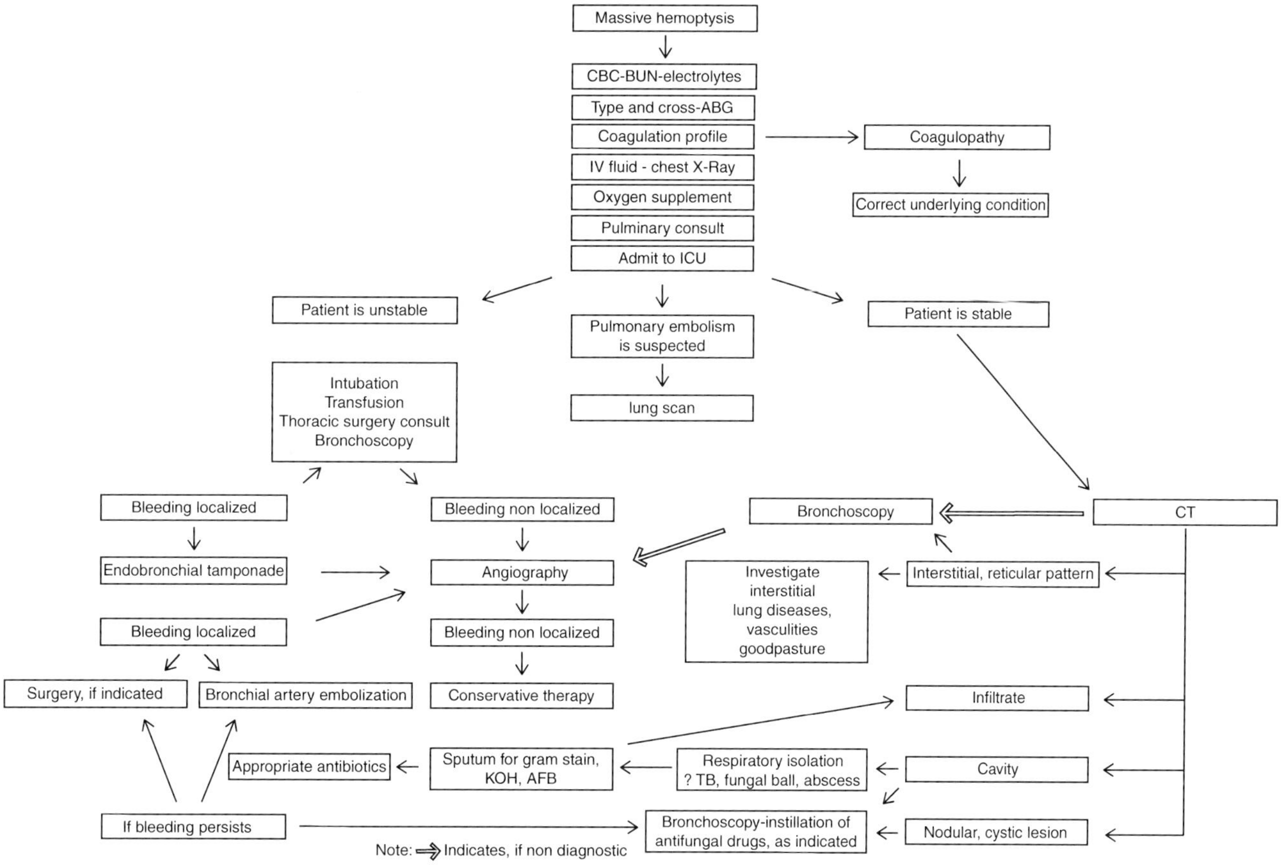

Fig. 19.2 Management of massive hemoptysis [7]

be placed in the lateral decubitus position toward the side of bleeding in order to diminish the risk of aspirating blood into the contralateral lung. Large-bore intravenous access should be in place and fluid resuscitation should commence. Patients with unstable vital signs should be transfused packed red blood cells [7].

The diagnostic evaluation of massive hemoptysis is secondary to the initial stabilization and resuscitation, but can generally proceed in tandem. A sputum examination is recommended for all patients to look for the presence of bacteria. Cultures should be obtained, especially looking for mycobacterium and fungus. Chest x-ray is also a useful initial diagnostic tool. Parenchymal pathologies such as tumors, cavitary lesions, and infiltrates may be readily apparent and help localize the portion of lung responsible for bleeding. It is important to note, however, that greater than 20 % of patients with massive hemoptysis may have a normal chest x-ray. Computed tomography (CT) is also an important tool for evaluation. It may demonstrate small lesions such as tumors or bronchiectasis not readily seen on plain films. When performed with intravenous contrast, it is the preferred method to diagnose thoracic aneurysm or other vascular abnormalities. Caution should be exercised in obtaining CT scans on patients with unstable vital signs or unsecured airways [7, 8].

Bronchoscopy is usually the most effective method for bleeding localization. Both rigid and flexible bronchoscopy can be performed. Rigid bronchoscopy has the benefit of greater suctioning ability and maintenance of airway patency in cases of heavy bleeding, but cannot be used to access peripheral lesions. It also requires general anesthesia in all but the most experienced hands. Flexible bronchoscopy can be performed at the bedside and may easily reach the distal bronchioles, but visualization of heavily bleeding lesions may prove challenging. Occasionally, the installation of dilute epinephrine or other vasoactive agents may reduce bleeding and improve visualization [7, 8].

Therapeutic Options

Therapeutic options for massive hemoptysis are broad and vary depending upon the etiology. Surgical intervention was traditionally the method of choice, but other less invasive options can be effective. In some cases, definitive surgical therapy may be delayed following temporary control of bleeding to allow for preoperative optimization.

Endobronchial methods are commonly first-line therapies, as they can be instituted at the time of bronchoscopic localization. Techniques include the installation of local hemostatic agents, photocoagulation, and endobronchial tamponade using balloon catheters. Endobronchial methods are most often utilized as temporary measures to allow for resuscitation and planning of more definitive intervention, but this depends upon the etiology [7, 8].

Bronchial artery embolization is a highly effective technique with a greater than 90 % success rate at 24 h. Selective angiography is used to identify the bleeding bronchial artery, followed by the instillation of coils or other thrombotic particles. Failure of this technique may occur secondary to non-bronchial collateral circulation [7, 9].

Patients with massive hemoptysis secondary to aspergilloma may be treated with the direct installation of antifungal drugs into the bleeding cavity. This can be accomplished via either percutaneous or transbronchial catheter access. This minimally invasive technique may be particularly useful for patients who are poor surgical candidates. External beam radiation therapy has also been used with success in hemoptysis from fungal balls, but only for those with low rates of bleeding [7].

Surgical intervention includes the full spectrum of pulmonary resection, including pneumonectomy. Patients who have a localized source of bleeding that would be amenable to complete resection and who are otherwise appropriate candidates for surgery should be considered. It is the treatment of choice for patients with malignancies or cavitary diseases in which vascular control alone would not be curative. Surgery is contraindicated in patients with lung carcinoma invading the mediastinum, trachea, heart, great vessels, or parietal pleura. Options must be carefully considered among patients with significant preexisting lung dysfunction, as emergent lobectomy or pneumonectomy will be poorly tolerated with diminished pulmonary reserve [7–9].

Outcome

The mortality rate for patients with massive hemoptysis is difficult to quantify and depends heavily on the underlying etiology. Patients with malignancy or significant bleeding (>1,000 ml/24 h) tend to do worse than those with other presentations. There is no evidence to suggest that age in and of itself is a risk factor for poor outcome [7].

Lung Abscess

Lung abscess is a well-circumscribed collection of pus within the lung that leads to cavity formation and the presence of an air-fluid level on imaging studies. It is most commonly formed by anaerobic bacteria and follows aspiration. Other etiologies include necrotizing pneumonia, septic emboli, and prior cavitation. Patients with a predisposition to aspiration, underlying immunocompromised state, or bronchial obstruction are at increased risk. Advanced age in and of itself is not a risk factor for lung abscess development, but has been associated with poor outcome when present [10–13].

Clinical Presentation and Diagnosis

Lung abscess typically presents with cough, pleuritic chest pain, fevers, weight loss, hemoptysis, or dyspnea. Patients will typically have one or more underlying risk factors by history and usually describe a prolonged course of symptoms prior to presentation. Diagnosis is usually straightforward and can be accomplished with plain chest radiography or computed tomography.

Management

The majority of lung abscess cavities will communicate with the bronchial tree and drain spontaneously; thus, antibiotic therapy alone is the primary treatment (Fig. 19.1). Antibiotics are usually chosen empirically because accurate culture data from within the abscess cannot be obtained noninvasively. There is an increasing incidence of gram-negative pathogens among community-acquired organisms. Current regimens use a β-lactam with a β-lactamase inhibitor or combination therapy with an advanced-generation cephalosporin and clindamycin or metronidazole. Unusual organisms such as gram-positive aerobes are rarely found to be the etiology of lung abscess and are more common in nosocomial cases [10].

Prolonged antibiotic therapy is successful in greater than 85 % of cases. Unfortunately, the geriatric population is at increased risk for conservative treatment failure. Other risk factors for failure include immunocompromised states, large abscess cavities, and unresolved bronchial obstruction. Antibiotic treatment failure requires improved drainage of the abscess. This can usually be accomplished percutaneously with radiographic guidance and represents definitive therapy for the majority of patients. A small minority of patients will require surgery for clearance. Surgical intervention for lung abscess includes varying degrees of pulmonary resection, including complete pneumonectomy in rare cases. Both traditional and minimally invasive techniques can be utilized. As surgery is taking place in an infected field, there is an increased risk of bronchial stump breakdown and bronchopleural fistula. Tissue coverage over the bronchial stump is recommended if possible [10, 12].

Outcome

Despite improvements in antibiotics and supportive care, the mortality of lung abscess remains at 15–20 %. Patients who do survive typically have a prolonged hospital course with significant morbidity. The risk of death is greater with an increasing number of predisposing conditions [10, 12, 13].

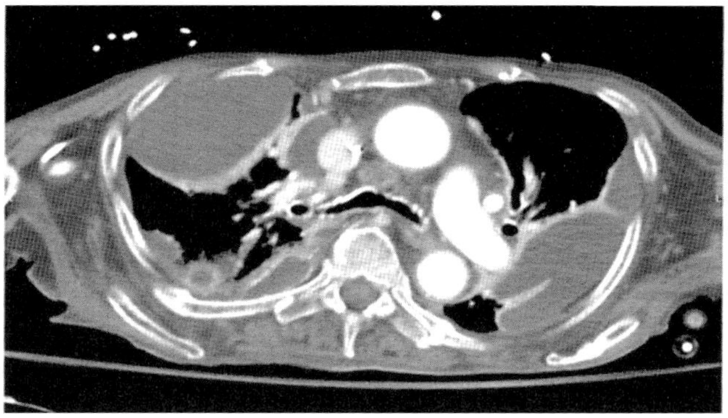

Fig. 19.3 CT scan demonstrating loculated fluid collections suggestive of empyema

Empyema

Empyema refers to the presence of infected fluid within the pleural space. The most common etiology is infection arising in the ipsilateral lung from pneumonia, lung abscess, or bronchiectasis. Other causes include trauma, postsurgical, esophageal perforation, and spread of intra-abdominal infection across the diaphragm. Primary empyema may rarely occur and is most often due to hematogenous spread of bacteria from gingival and upper respiratory tract infections or tuberculosis. Empyema is seen in about 60,000 patients annually and is of particular importance to the geriatric population because it is more common at the extremes of age [11, 14].

Clinical Presentation and Diagnosis

Patients with empyema typically present with pleuritic chest pain, fever, and nonspecific symptoms such as malaise (Fig. 19.2). Chest radiographs are commonly the first-line diagnostic study and can demonstrate pleural effusion and sometimes loculations, but cannot confirm bacterial infection. Similarly, ultrasound can easily demonstrate pleural fluid collections, but does not confirm empyema. Computed tomography is the most useful diagnostic tool. It can demonstrate and quantify pleural fluid collections, loculations, and pleural enhancement or thickening. Though CT findings can be highly suggestive, definitive diagnosis requires aspiration of purulent fluid or gram-stain/culture results [11, 14] (Fig. 19.3).

Management

The treatment of empyema involves drainage of infected fluid with lung re-expansion and antibiotic therapy. The choice of drainage method depends on the phase of the underlying empyema: exudative, fibrinopurulent, or organized. The first two phases can often be managed successfully without surgery [14].

The exudative phase of empyema is characterized by free-flowing fluid with minimal to no loculations. Tube thoracostomy alone is generally sufficient to achieve complete drainage of the empyema. In the fibrinopurulent phase, the fluid is thicker and loculations are common. Sufficient drainage by thoracostomy tube is difficult and may require multiple drains in specific locations. The bedside installation of lytic agents, particularly streptokinase, has been shown to be an effective method to assist the drainage of loculated collections. In many patients, drainage tubes may be required for a prolonged amount of time to prevent reaccumulation. Closed suction drains can be converted to open drains once the lung becomes adherent to the chest wall and gradually backed out over time. If adequate drainage of an early-phase empyema is unsuccessful by percutaneous methods, surgical intervention should be considered [10, 14, 15].

The organized phase of empyema occurs over a period of 4–6 weeks and is characterized by the development of a fibrous "peel" of visceral pleura that prevents lung expansion. Surgical intervention is required to decorticate the lung and remove all infected material. Access to the pleural space can be achieved using VATS or traditional thoracotomy, but minimally invasive approaches are less successful in more advanced cases. Incomplete decortication will not allow full expansion of the lung and obliteration of the infected cavity; thus, reaccumulation will occur. In rare cases in which the pleural cavity cannot be obliterated, an open drainage procedure or muscle rotational flap may be necessary to control the empyema. Patients who cannot tolerate thoracotomy and proper decortication may also be candidates for an open drainage procedure under local anesthetic (assuming the presence of a mature empyema and adherent lung) [10, 11, 14].

Outcome

The mortality rate for empyema depends largely on the underlying etiology and associated comorbidities, but is approximately 15 % overall. Advanced age has not been shown to be an independent risk factor for increased mortality [12, 14].

Spontaneous Pneumothorax

Spontaneous pneumothorax is classified as either primary or secondary, depending upon the presence of underlying lung disease. Primary pneumothorax generally occurs in tall, thin persons between the ages of 10 and 30 years and rarely occurs in individuals over the age of 40. Secondary spontaneous pneumothorax (SSP), however, has a peak incidence between 60 and 65 years of age and is frequently seen among the geriatric population (Fig. 19.4). It is of

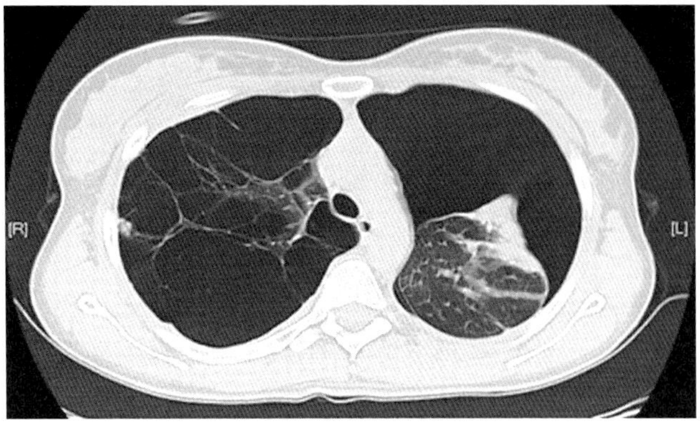

Fig. 19.4 Spontaneous pneumothorax in the presence of significant bleb disease

particular importance because it can frequently be life-threatening, largely due to the underlying lung disease and low cardiopulmonary reserve. The most common cause of SSP among the geriatric population is underlying chronic obstructive pulmonary disease (COPD), representing greater than 70 % of cases. The probability of pneumothorax increases as the severity of COPD worsens. Other etiologies of SSP in the geriatric population include pulmonary fibrosis, autoimmune diseases, and infectious etiologies [16, 17].

Clinical Presentation and Diagnosis

Patients with SSP will present with dyspnea and frequently unilateral chest pain. Severe hypoxemia or hypotension can occur, even with smaller-sized pneumothoraces. Hypercapnia is also extremely common. The diagnosis should always be suspected among patients with known underlying COPD and new onset dyspnea or chest pain. A high index of suspicion is essential, as rapid diagnosis and treatment may be lifesaving [16].

The diagnosis of SSP is usually made with chest x-ray, but can be challenging in patients with large bullous lesions. Radiographically, a pneumothorax should appear as a visceral pleural line that runs parallel to the chest wall. Large bullous lesions that abut the chest wall generally have a concave appearance. If the diagnosis is unclear, computed tomography of the chest can be used for differentiation [16].

Management

Patients with SSP should be treated urgently with chest tube placement with water seal drainage. The chest tube apparatus can be placed to suction for patients with large air leaks or incomplete re-expansion of the lung. A smaller-bore tube (28 french or less) is generally sufficient. Chest tube drainage alone will resolve most SSP, but may require a prolonged time course if there is persistent air leak [16, 18].

Most surgeons would recommend intervention following the first episode of SSP in order to prevent recurrence, as this could be rapidly life-threatening. The least invasive treatment is the installation of sclerosing agents through the chest tube, but this also carries the highest rate of recurrence (up to 25 %). It is even less effective in the presence of an air leak, which is common among SSP. Some patients with SSP may be poor overall surgical candidates, particularly among the geriatric population. In these patients, bedside chemical pleurodesis may be the only viable option to prevent recurrence [16, 18].

Surgical intervention for SSP involves resection of the ruptured bleb and surrounding bullous disease in conjunction with mechanical or chemical pleurodesis. Options for the geriatric patient include standard posterolateral thoracotomy, limited thoracotomy, median sternotomy, and video-assisted thoracoscopic surgery (VATS) approaches. Each approach carries specific advantages and disadvantages, and the decision should be made on an individual basis. Thoracotomy offers the best exposure and has the lowest recurrence rate, but is associated with significant postoperative pain and morbidity. VATS may be less invasive, but has a higher recurrence rate among published series. In addition, VATS generally requires single-lung ventilation of the contralateral lung to allow visualization of the affected lung. Many patients with SSP will not be able to tolerate single-lung ventilation secondary to their underlying pulmonary disease [16–19].

Outcome

The outcome for patients with SSP depends largely on the severity of the underlying lung disease and comorbidities. Overall mortality rates are generally low (<6 %) among geriatric patients with a COPD etiology. Patients with recurrence or who require invasive operative intervention may have prolonged hospital stays and significant morbidity, however.

Aorta

Acute aortic pathology is an important consideration among the elderly, as the major disease processes have an increasing incidence with age. The conditions discussed generally require subspecialized care for definitive management, but initial diagnosis and stabilization may be frequently required of the acute care surgeon.

Acute Aortic Syndrome

Acute aortic syndrome (AAS) is a term used to describe a group of conditions with the common and primary presenting symptom of aortic pain. The conditions that comprise AAS include acute aortic dissection, penetrating aortic ulcer, and intramural hematoma of the aorta. Thoracic aortic aneurysm is a distinct entity, but acute presentations (rupture, expansion, etc.) behave similarly in terms of symptoms and diagnostic workup.

Clinical Presentation and Diagnosis

Patients with AAS typically present with pain that is usually of sudden onset and with maximal initial intensity. It is generally in the substernal area and is classically described as having a "sharp," "tearing," or "ripping" character. The most sensitive description of the pain appears to be the abruptness of onset, as this is present in over 90 % of cases. A careful and thoughtful history is of paramount importance, as up to 30 % of patients ultimately found to have AAS will be initially misdiagnosed [20, 21].

The currently available diagnostic modalities for AAS include computed tomography (CT), transesophageal echocardiography (TEE), magnetic resonance imaging (MRI), and aortic angiography. Contrast-enhanced CT is the most commonly employed as it is readily available and noninvasive. Chest x-ray (CXR) can be suggestive of AAS in up to 85 % of cases, showing a widened mediastinum, pleural effusion, or subtle cardiac contour changes. Electrocardiogram (EKG) tracings in AAS may be abnormal, but are generally nonspecific [20, 21].

AAS is an important consideration among the elderly population because it is predominantly a disease of older people, with at least a third occurring over the age of 70. It is more common among males and is associated with the common comorbidities for atherosclerotic disease such as hypertension and smoking [20, 21].

Acute Aortic Dissection (AAD)

AAD arises from a tear within the intima of the aorta, leading to a flow of blood within the media layer of the aorta. A second or "false" lumen is created as a consequence and can rapidly propagate secondary to the high underlying pressures within the aorta. The diversion of blood flow within the false lumen can lead to ischemia or thrombosis of involved aortic branches. A careful pulse exam is an essential component of the early evaluation, as it may reveal selective deficits that suggest AAD. Dissections of the ascending aorta can have involvement of the coronary ostia and produce cardiac ischemia with associated electrocardiogram changes and enzyme elevations. Consideration of AAD among patients with the appropriate history is important, as confusion with acute coronary syndromes may lead to the premature and potentially disastrous administration of anticoagulation or thrombolytics. Approximately 5 % of AAD is iatrogenic following open cardiac procedures or catheter-based interventions. The iatrogenic AAD population tends to be older and with a higher incidence of underlying vascular disease [20, 22, 23].

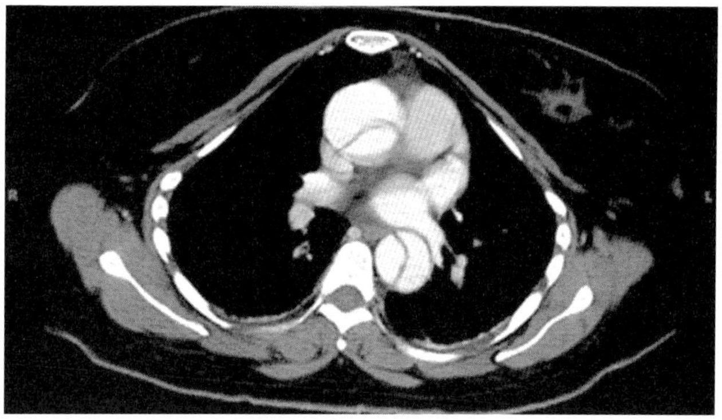

Fig. 19.5 Type A (ascending arch) aortic dissection [23]

Management

The mainstay of medical therapy for AAD is immediate blood pressure control if hypertension is present to try to limit propagation of the dissection. A combination of B-blockers and vasodilators should be employed to reduce the force of ventricular contraction. The goal for systolic blood pressure should be less than 120 mmHg, as long as cerebral and end-organ perfusion is maintained. Surgical interventions vary depending on the type of dissection present. There have been several classification schemes used to describe AAS, but among the most common is the Sanford classification. It describes AAD in terms of its involvement with the ascending aorta (type A) (Fig. 19.5) or the descending aorta (type B) (Fig. 19.6). This division is important, because type A dissections are considered true surgical emergencies. The mortality rate for type A dissections increases significantly with delays to surgical intervention. Factors contributing to mortality include rupture into the pericardium leading to tamponade, coronary vessel involvement and myocardial ischemia, distal organ malperfusion, rupture into the pleural space, or valvular involvement leading to acute cardiac failure [20, 21].

Surgical intervention generally involves resuspension or replacement of the aortic valve with aortic arch replacement and is commonly performed under hypothermic circulatory arrest. Surgery for type A AADs has a mortality rate of 10–35 %, even at the most experienced centers. Most type B dissections can be managed medically with blood pressure control alone. Aortic branch vessel involvement with subsequent end-organ ischemia is the most common reason for surgical intervention among type B dissections. Traditional intervention involves segmental aortic replacement, but endovascular stenting methods have been used successfully [20, 22, 23].

Penetrating Aortic Ulcer (PAU)

PAU is an atherosclerotic plaque that erodes through the intimal layer of the aorta. It may form a pseudoaneurysm, give rise to intramural hematoma, form the initial focus for aortic

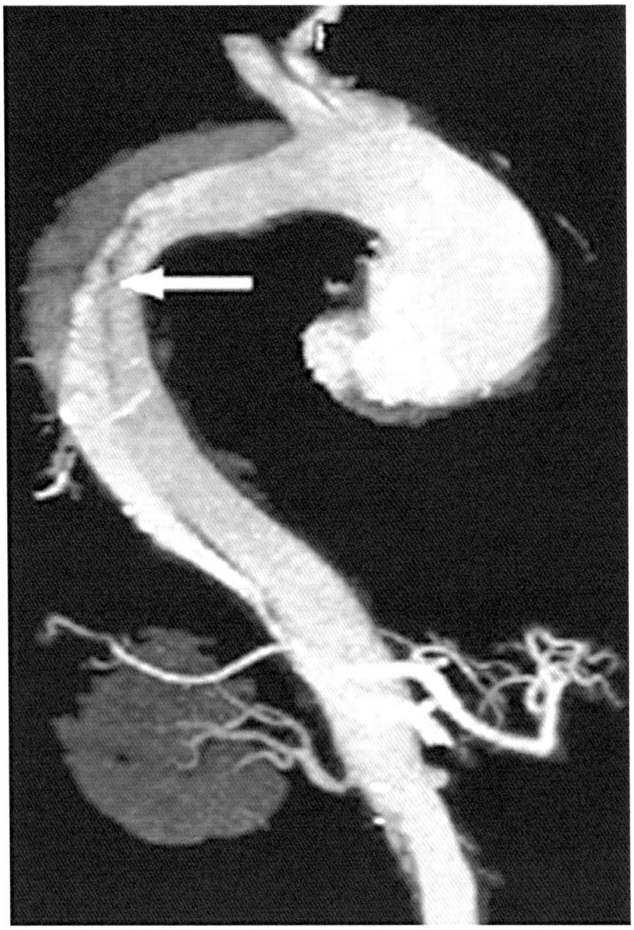

Fig. 19.6 Type B (descending arch) aortic dissection [23]

dissection, erode into adjacent structures, or lead to free rupture. Of the acute aortic syndromes, it has the greatest average age at presentation (>70 years). It is most commonly diagnosed using contrast-enhanced computed tomography (CT) or angiography. It appears as a contrast filled outpouching of the aorta with irregular margins and usually in the background of severe atherosclerotic disease [20, 21].

Management

Definitive management of PAU is surgical and involves either open aortic replacement or endovascular stenting. Patient selection for interventional therapy remains somewhat controversial, particularly since the population of PAU patients tends to be of advanced age and with significant comorbidities. Patients with complications such as erosion or rupture should certainly undergo immediate surgical intervention, but more stable presentations may be managed more conservatively. There are reports of patients undergoing successful medical management of PAU with some even demonstrating radiographic improvement or resolution on follow-up imaging. In general, however, patients presenting with symptomatic PAU should undergo surgical correction if possible. The current preferred approach is via endovascular stent grafting, but specific ulcer location and aortic anatomy may dictate an open approach [20, 21].

Intramural Hematoma (IMH)

IMH is a dissection of blood within the media or subadventitial layers of the aorta. It is distinguished from aortic dissection in that it does not have an associated intimal tear. However, 30–40 % of IMHs convert to classic aortic dissection with highly variable timing ranging from a few hours to several months after the onset of symptoms. The etiology of IMH formation is thought to be hemorrhage from the vasa vasorum or fracture of an atherosclerotic plaque. Its association with underlying atherosclerotic disease may explain the older average age of individuals with IMH as compared to aortic dissection. IMH is best diagnosed using contrast-enhanced computed tomography. Due to the lack of intimal involvement, it may not be appreciated on angiography [20, 21].

Management

The treatment of acute IMH is primarily dictated according to the Sanford classification, with 50–60 % of IMHs occurring in the descending aorta (type B). The current consensus is that uncomplicated type B IMHs may be treated medically with blood pressure control and repeat imaging to ensure stabilization. Spontaneous regression and complete resolution of IMH has been reported with medical therapy alone. The optimal treatment of type A IMH is more controversial, as there are no large reported prospective trials. Type A IMH patients with complications such as pericardial tamponade, cardiac valvular dysfunction, or hemodynamic instability should undergo urgent surgical intervention. Supra-coronary ascending aortic replacement is the most common surgical procedure performed. Stable patients may undergo surgical intervention or medical management with timed surgical intervention based on the development of complications. The overall in-hospital mortality of either approach is less than 20 %. Current work seeks to better characterize those patients at higher risk for progression of stable type A IMH, but progress is hindered by the small overall number of patients with this condition [20, 21].

Thoracic Aortic Aneurysm (TAA)

TAA is a relatively uncommon disease, occurring at a rate of approximately 10.4 per 100,000 person years. However, it is an important diagnostic consideration in the elderly population because the incidence of TAA increases with age. The average age at the time of diagnosis is 69 years. Advancing age is one of the few independent risk factors for TAA rupture. Other risk factors for rupture include aneurysm size (>5 cm), rate of aneurysm expansion, smoking, hypertension, and chronic obstructive pulmonary disease [21, 24].

Management

Patients presenting with symptomatic TAAs should undergo immediate surgical intervention. Traditional open repair involves resection of the aneurysm and replacement with an appropriately sized prosthetic graft. Reimplantation of branch vessels may be necessary depending upon aneurysm location. Involvement of the arch generally requires at least a short period of hypothermic circulatory arrest [21, 25].

Endovascular techniques have been utilized with success in the treatment of TAAs in the elective setting with suggested benefits including decreased early mortality, spinal cord ischemia, and respiratory failure. Specific vascular anatomy, including peripheral access vessels, plays a significant role in defining appropriate candidates for an endovascular approach. Experience in endovascular repair for symptomatic or ruptured TAA is currently limited [21].

Outcome

Most patients with a ruptured TAA do not make it to the hospital alive. The five-year survival rate for patients undergoing emergent surgery is less than 40 %. The prognosis is worse for aneurysms that involve aortic dissections, as this increases the operative complexity [21].

Esophagus/GI Tract

Esophageal Dysmotility/Impaction

Failure of esophageal peristalsis in elderly patients presenting with dysphagia was termed "presbyesophagus" over 40 years ago. It was thought that normal aging leads to changes in esophageal motility in all patients, with some becoming more symptomatic than others. The introduction of modern esophageal manometry techniques has made the concept of presbyesophagus more controversial. The majority of geriatric patients with dysphagia are now diagnosed with one of the established esophageal dysmotility disorders, although some will still be labeled as "nonspecific." Regardless of the etiology, approximately 10 % of people over the age of 50 and 15 % of people over the age of 85 will have dysphagia. This has important implications in terms of acute care surgery because these patients are at risk for esophageal impaction and foreign body aspiration [26].

Esophageal impaction may occur as a result of a variety of ingestions, both accidental and intentional. Impaction of foodstuffs, particularly meat or bones, is the most common etiology among the geriatric population. The presence of a dental appliance is strongly associated with esophageal food impaction in patients over the age of 60. Foreign body impactions of all types may also be seen in the elderly patient, but this phenomenon is more common among children. Among the more common foreign bodies seen in the geriatric population is the accidental ingestion of oral/dental prostheses [27, 28].

Clinical Presentation and Diagnosis

Patients with esophageal impaction will generally present with pain and vomiting with attempted oral intake and a history of recent ingestion. History alone is generally sufficient to suggest the diagnosis. Radiopaque foreign bodies are readily seen on plain x-ray, but food impactions will remain occult. An esophagram may be obtained and will often demonstrate esophageal obstruction, but the diagnosis is usually made via endoscopy. Once an esophageal impaction is diagnosed, it should be cleared as soon as possible. Delay in therapy can lead to inflammatory changes at the point of impaction and increase the risk of perforation.

Management

Esophagoscopy is the usual method of treatment for most esophageal impactions. It can be performed using either a rigid or a flexible scope. Rigid esophagoscopy may be more effective for cervical or very proximal esophageal impactions, but flexible endoscopy is more commonly utilized. Once the impaction is visualized, a variety of techniques may be utilized for clearance. For solitary objects, forceps or graspers may be used to dislodge the object and then remove it. Meat impactions can similarly be removed, but may require a piecemeal approach. The use of an esophageal overtube may facilitate the frequent re-passage of the endoscope in these cases. For food impactions that do not contain bones, the "push" technique may be employed. The endoscope is advanced into the center of the impaction and gently pushed forward until the food bolus is cleared. Regardless of the endoscopic technique used, extreme care must be employed to avoid injury to the esophagus. This is of particular concern for foreign bodies or bone impactions that have sharp edges, as the esophagus may be lacerated during attempted removal. Other techniques to relieve esophageal impaction have been described, but are generally less effective and less commonly utilized than endoscopy [27, 28].

Although rare, surgery may be required to relieve some esophageal impactions. Foreign bodies with significant delays in diagnosis may be difficult or impossible to remove endoscopically in the setting of significant inflammation. Foreign body impactions with sharp edges may be unsuitable for endoscopic removal secondary to a high risk of esophageal laceration. In these cases, surgical exposure of the esophagus with esophagotomy may be necessary for removal of the impaction [27, 28].

Esophageal Perforation

Perforation of the esophagus is an uncommon, but potentially lethal condition. Excluding trauma, the most common causes for esophageal perforation are iatrogenic, spontaneous, and foreign body/ingestion related. The presentation and management for esophageal perforations varies widely depending upon the location and circumstances surrounding the perforation. It is certainly not a disease limited to the geriatric population, but older patients with underlying comorbidities and esophageal disease are at risk. Age in and of itself has not been shown to be an independent risk factor for poor outcome. As such, the evaluation and management of esophageal perforation in the geriatric population does not differ from that of the standard adult population.

Etiologies

Iatrogenic perforation from endoscopy or other instrumentation is the most common overall cause of esophageal perforation, accounting for nearly 60 % of cases. The approximate rate of perforation during routine flexible endoscopy is 0.03 %. Perforations during diagnostic endoscopy most commonly occur at the locations of anatomic narrowing of the esophagus, particularly in the cervical esophagus. The risk of perforation increases when considering therapeutic procedures during endoscopy. Sclerotherapy for varices or bleeding carries a 1–3 % risk of perforation at the site of intervention. Pneumatic dilation for stricture or achalasia carries a risk of perforation of 2–6 %, most commonly in the distal esophagus. Of particular concern for the geriatric population is the risk associated with transesophageal echocardiography, which has an incidence of perforation of 0.18 % [29–31].

Spontaneous esophageal perforation represents approximately 15 % of cases. The purported mechanism for many cases is the Boerhaave's syndrome, in which a rapid increase in intraluminal esophageal pressure through a patent lower esophageal sphincter causes transmural rupture of the esophagus. Described inciting events include forceful vomiting, prolonged coughing or laughing, childbirth, seizures, and weight lifting. Anatomically, this most commonly occurs in the left posterolateral location 2–3 cm proximal to the GE junction. This area is inherently weakened as the longitudinal muscle fibers splay and pass onto the stomach wall. The geriatric population is certainly susceptible to this etiology, with reported cases occurring in individuals over 90 years of age [30, 31].

Foreign body ingestions account for approximately 12 % of cases. Sharp or jagged materials such as fish or chicken bones, partial dentures, and plastic eating utensils are the most common offender among accidentally ingested items. Esophageal perforation usually occurs at points of anatomic narrowing such as the cricopharyngeus muscle, upper esophageal sphincter, aortic arch, left mainstem bronchus, or lower esophageal sphincter. Geriatric patients with underlying esophageal dysmotility such as the previously described presbyesophagus may be at particular risk [30, 31].

The remaining etiologies include eroding carcinoma, reflux ulceration, surrounding infection, and immunodeficiency. Carcinoma of the esophagus is of particular importance in the geriatric population, as greater than 50 % of patients with esophageal cancer are diagnosed after the age of 65 [30–32].

Clinical Presentation

The signs and symptoms of esophageal perforation will vary depending upon the anatomic location, the size of the perforation, degree of contamination, and the time elapsed to presentation. The most common presenting symptoms (in decreasing order) are pain, fever, dyspnea, and crepitus. Perforations in the cervical esophagus commonly present with neck pain and stiffness. Thoracic perforations may progress to rupture of the mediastinal pleura and an associated pleural effusion. Proximal thoracic perforations are more commonly associated with right-sided effusions, while distal esophageal perforations will present with left-sided effusions. With time delay, thoracic perforations may lead to contamination of the mediastinum and subsequent mediastinitis. This may lead to a systemic inflammatory response with associated tachycardia, fluid sequestration, and distributive shock. Perforations near the gastroesophageal (GE) junction may lead to contamination within the abdomen and are associated with epigastric abdominal pain that may progress to diffuse peritonitis [30, 31].

Diagnosis

A variety of studies may aid in the diagnosis of esophageal perforation. Diagnostic algorithms will vary depending on the history and presentation. Iatrogenic perforations commonly present with symptoms shortly following the procedure, and thus the suspicion of esophageal perforation will be high at the outset. Other presentations of esophageal perforation may be more subtle, and patients will undergo a broader workup until suspicion is raised.

Contrast esophagography is the gold standard test for suspected esophageal perforation. The study can be performed with either Gastrografin or barium sulfate. Barium has a higher density and better mucosal adherence, thus allowing it to detect smaller perforations when compared to Gastrografin. However, extravasation of barium may lead to an inflammatory reaction in the mediastinum or peritoneum. As such, it is relatively common to use Gastrografin as the initial contrast agent. This may be followed with barium if a leak is not demonstrated. It should be taken into account that aspiration of Gastrografin is associated with pneumonitis and pulmonary edema. Patients at significant risk for

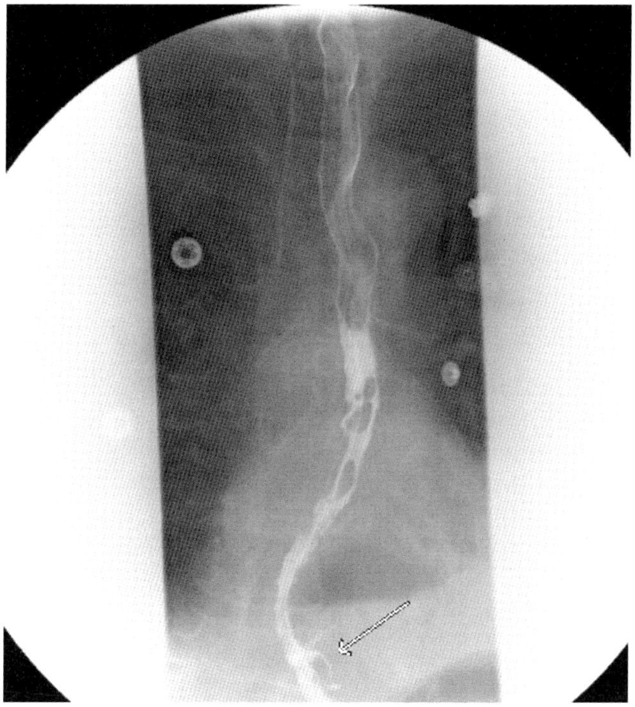

Fig. 19.7 Esophagram showing small area of extravasation in the distal esophagus

aspiration may be best served using barium as the initial contrast agent. Overall, contrast esophagography has a false-negative rate of approximately 10 %. For patients with a high suspicion of esophageal perforation the study may be repeated serially, as initial mucosal inflammation may preclude a positive study [30, 31, 33].

CT scanning has become an important tool in the diagnosis of esophageal perforation. Suggestive findings on CT scan are extraluminal air, esophageal thickening, abscess cavity, or pleural effusions. Small, contained extravasations of contrast not readily visible on esophagography may be seen on CT (Fig. 19.7). Suggestive CT findings, in particular extraluminal air, will be seen in greater than 90 % of cases. For patients with spontaneous perforations, CT findings often raise the initial suspicion for esophageal perforation and lead to esophagography. Conversely, patients undergoing a negative esophagram with continued high suspicion of esophageal perforation (i.e., iatrogenic presentations) may undergo CT scan as an adjunct to identify occult leaks. CT scan is also preferred among patients unable to undergo esophagography [30].

Plain films are less commonly utilized in the workup of esophageal perforation, but may be useful to suggest the diagnosis. Plain films of the lateral neck may show prevertebral air in cervical esophageal perforations. Chest x-ray may demonstrate pneumomediastinum or pleural effusion and suggest thoracic perforation. Abdominal films may show pneumoperitoneum in distal esophageal or GE junction perforation. Importantly, it may take several hours for any associated findings to appear on plain films. Suggestive findings should be confirmed with esophagography or CT scan as appropriate [30].

Flexible endoscopy is generally not recommended in the evaluation of suspected esophageal perforation, but may have a limited role for suspected cases involving foreign bodies, ingestions, or underlying malignancy. The significant drawbacks of endoscopy are that small injuries may be easily missed within the folds of the esophagus and the potential for worsening of the underlying injury through scope trauma or air insufflation [30].

Nonoperative Management

Selected patients may be successfully managed nonoperatively. Proposed criteria include the presence of a contained disruption in the neck or chest, minimal signs of systemic sepsis, early diagnosis, a nonneoplastic etiology, and the lack of underlying obstruction. Nonoperative management includes NPO status, antibiotics covering gastrointestinal flora, and parental nutritional support. The appropriate duration of therapy may vary depending upon specific circumstances of the perforation, but is usually 7–10 days. Importantly, up to 20 % of patients managed nonoperatively will have complications or worsening clinical condition in the first 24 h leading to surgical intervention. Careful and diligent monitoring is essential, as rapid declines in clinical condition are possible. Nonoperative management is most successfully utilized for perforations in the cervical esophagus and in small and early recognized iatrogenic perforations [30, 31, 33].

Surgical Management

The preferred method of surgical treatment is debridement of devitalized tissue, primary closure with or without tissue reinforcement, and wide drainage. Perforations in the neck can be approached via an incision along the anterior border of the sternocleidomastoid muscle (SCM) with lateral retraction of the carotid sheath. High thoracic perforations are approached via a right-sided posterolateral thoracotomy. Low thoracic perforations are approached via a left-sided thoracotomy (Fig. 19.8). Perforations within the abdomen are best approached via a standard laparotomy incision [30].

Once the esophagus is isolated, the full extent of the mucosal defect is generally exposed via a longitudinal esophagomyotomy. The mucosal defect is then closed and the muscular layer re-approximated. When possible, a vascularized pedicle graft is then sutured to buttress the repair. A variety of buttress options have been described depending on the location of the perforation and include muscular flaps (SCM, intercostals, etc.), pleural flaps, pericardial flaps, and diaphragmatic pedicle grafts. Distal esophageal perforations can be buttressed with a gastric fundoplication. The repair

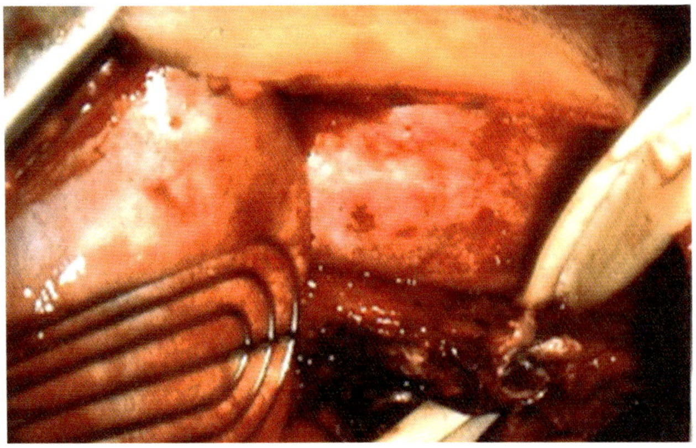

Fig. 19.8 Operative exposure of esophageal perforation via a left thoracotomy (diaphragm left; Penrose around esophagus)

should be widely drained using closed suction drains or chest tubes. Following repair, consideration should be given to the placement of distal enteral feeding access [30, 31, 33].

Patients presenting with esophageal perforation secondary to significant underlying esophageal pathology may not be appropriate candidates for primary surgical repair. The underlying pathology should be addressed or considered at the time of operation. Patients with perforations secondary to malignancy, megaesophagus, caustic ingestions, or chronic stricture should undergo esophagectomy if feasible. Reconstruction can commence immediately or in a delayed fashion, depending upon the clinical condition of the patient [30, 34].

A number of patients will present with significant mediastinal contamination or devitalization of the esophagus associated with hemodynamic instability. In these patients, standard repair techniques may not be feasible, and they may be too unstable for definitive operation. Traditional management of these patients has included cervical esophagostomy, exclusion of the perforated esophageal segment, gastrostomy, jejunostomy, and wide drainage. This approach has significant drawbacks in terms of its morbidity and requirement for extensive reconstruction. A variety of other methods that seek to maintain continuity of the esophagus have been described, including drainage alone or the creation of a controlled fistula through the use of a t-tube. It is important to note that the use of these non-definitive interventions should be based solely on operative findings and overall patient condition and not on time to presentation. Drainage and diversion techniques have previously been emphasized for patients based on significant time delays in diagnosis. However, good results may still be achieved with definitive repair regardless of the amount of delay in diagnosis [30, 35].

Recent series have documented the use of minimally invasive surgery to successfully manage esophageal perforation. Access to the chest is obtained via video-assisted thoracoscopic surgery techniques. Perforations of the distal esophagus within the abdomen may be managed using laparoscopy. The standard principles of debridement, repair, and drainage remain constant when compared to open surgical techniques. These options may be particularly attractive among the elderly patient population, as the significant morbidity of a thoracotomy or laparotomy may be avoided. However, familiarity and technical proficiency with minimally invasive surgery techniques are required [30].

Endoscopic Management

Endoluminal stenting of the esophagus has evolved into a viable treatment option for esophageal perforation, and its use has been documented for a variety of etiologies (Fig. 19.9). Stents utilized for this purpose are generally self-expanding and have a covered central portion that acts to seal the perforation. The stents may then be removed after the perforation has healed. Stenting is an attractive option among patients presenting with terminal disease, such as esophageal cancer. Endoscopic stenting does not allow debridement or drainage and is therefore best suited to those perforations that are diagnosed before there is significant contamination of surrounding tissue [36].

Endoscopic clipping is a technique that has had great success in the control of bleeding, but may also be used to treat small perforations of the esophagus. It was originally described to treat a small injury suffered during pneumatic dilation, but has since been used with success in instrumentation, foreign body, and spontaneous etiologies. Suggested indications include small (<1.5 cm), clean perforations with minimal to no contamination or signs of systemic illness [30].

Endoscopic techniques may be well suited for particularly frail members of the geriatric population, as it potentially avoids the morbidity of major surgery. Advanced age in and of itself is not an indication for endoscopic therapy compared to operative intervention, however. Patients selected for endoscopic management require close observation and diligence, as the possibility of treatment failure and the need for operative intervention always exists.

Outcome

Patients successfully undergoing primary repair have a mortality rate of around 12 %. The mortality rate increases to 17 % for patients requiring esophagectomy and 24 % for the various exclusion and drainage procedures. Patients undergoing drainage alone have an associated mortality of 37 %, though this likely represents a much sicker population of patients. Nonoperative therapy has a published mortality rate of around 18 %, but may be significantly lower with strict adherence to established guidelines [30, 31].

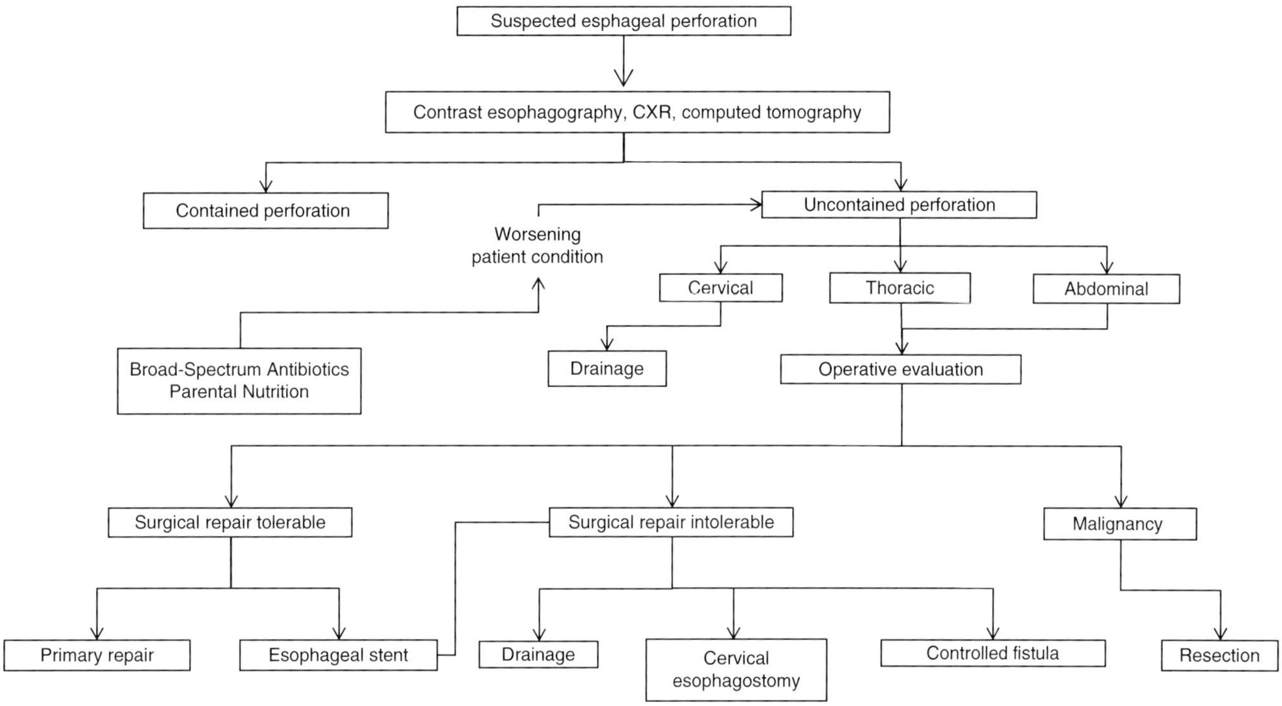

Fig. 19.9 Management of esophageal perforation

Paraesophageal Hernia

Paraesophageal hernia (PEH) is an important consideration in thoracic acute care surgery, particularly in the geriatric population. Long-standing and previously undiagnosed PEH may present acutely with obstruction and often strangulation of herniated abdominal viscera such as stomach, small bowel, or esophagus. Patients with PEH are prone to reflux disease and may therefore also present acutely with complications such as bleeding or perforated ulcerations. Herniated contents may cause direct compression within the thorax leading to acute heart failure or respiratory embarrassment. Tension gastrothorax is a well-described example [37].

Clinical Presentation and Diagnosis

Patients presenting with acute complications of PEH will most often present with upper abdominal or chest pain, often associated with vomiting. Certain complications may additionally present with extreme hemodynamic instability and respiratory compromise. These symptoms may initially be confused for a variety of other more common thoracic pathologies, thus a high index of suspicion must be maintained during the initial workup.

Plain chest or abdominal radiographs can be highly suggestive of the diagnosis of PEH. Intra-abdominal contents can often be readily seen above the diaphragm, particularly in cases of incarceration and obstruction when there may be significant proximal dilatation. CT scan is also extremely useful, with large PEH readily seen, particularly on coronal or sagittal image series. CT may also be highly suggestive of more severe complications such as strangulation or perforation. The presence of pneumatosis intestinalis, extraluminal air, or surrounding fluid may be seen on CT and suggest increased severity. Upper gastrointestinal contrast series is a standard test utilized to diagnose PEH with minimal or no symptoms, but may be difficult or impossible to perform in the setting of an acute complication. In cases involving incarceration of the stomach, flexible endoscopy can be a useful diagnostic aid to assess bowel viability [37].

Management

After addressing potential airway issues, the initial therapeutic intervention in nearly all cases of acute PEH complications is the attempted placement of a nasogastric (NG) tube for decompression. In some cases, decompression may completely resolve the incarceration and lead to a rapid alleviation of symptoms. In cases of tension gastrothorax, decompression is immediately lifesaving. The inability to pass an NG tube generally prompts more urgent surgical intervention to provide decompression.

All patients presenting with a complication of a PEH should undergo consideration for surgical intervention. While there is ongoing debate regarding the optimal treatment and natural history of asymptomatic PEH, patients presenting with acute complications require intervention. Patients with a high suspicion for strangulation and bowel compromise should proceed to the operating room expeditiously. Those that can be initially stabilized with NG decompression may be candidates for delayed intervention in order to undergo a more thorough preoperative evaluation [38, 39].

Repair of the acutely incarcerated PEH has traditionally been accomplished via an abdominal or thoracic approach. Selection depends largely on the comfort level of the operating surgeon. Either approach allows for reduction and assessment of herniated contents, restoration of physiologic esophageal anatomy, and closure of the hiatal defect. Most elective repairs of PEH are currently performed using a laparoscopic abdominal approach with good results. This approach can also be utilized for acute presentations if the operating surgeon is proficient in advanced laparoscopic techniques [37, 39].

Outcome

Early series of patients undergoing emergent surgery for PEH showed a mortality rate of greater than 25 %. This prompted the traditional surgical teaching that all PEH should be fixed following diagnosis to prevent future complications and mortality. More modern series have demonstrated a mortality rate less than 10 %, including a significant number of geriatric patients [38].

Summary

Thoracic surgical emergencies in the elderly represent a complex and diverse group of disease processes. Advanced age in and of itself does not alter the preferred management of these conditions as compared to the general population, but the elderly patient may have significant comorbidities that add to the complexity of treatment. Some etiologies and characteristics also become much more prevalent with or are unique to advancing age. An understanding of these conditions helps clinicians more readily identify them, as confusion and initial misdiagnoses are common. Although definitive management for many of the conditions described requires subspecialist consultation, the acute care general surgeon will commonly be called upon to participate in the care of these patients.

References

1. Dailey RH. Acute upper airway obstruction. Emerg Med Clin North Am. 1983;1(2):261–77.
2. Aboussouan LS, Stoller JK. Diagnosis and management of upper airway obstruction. Clin Chest Med. 1994;15(1):35–53.
3. Lloyd DC, Taylor PM. Calcification of the intrathoracic trachea demonstrated by computed tomography. Br J Radiol. 1990; 63(745):31–2.
4. Jo SH, Choi YJ, Cho GY, Kim HS, Jung KS, Rhim CY. Tracheal calcification. CMAJ. 2008;179(3):291.
5. Swanson KL, Edell ES. Tracheobronchial foreign bodies. Chest Surg Clin N Am. 2001;11(4):861–72.
6. Rafanan AL, Mehta AC. Adult airway foreign body removal. What's new? Clin Chest Med. 2001;22(2):319–30.
7. Jean-Baptiste E. Clinical assessment and management of massive hemoptysis. Crit Care Med. 2000;28(5):1642–7.
8. Karmy-Jones R, Cuschieri J, Vallieres E. Role of bronchoscopy in massive hemoptysis. Chest Surg Clin N Am. 2001;11(4): 873–906.
9. Lenner R, Schilero GJ, Lesser M. Hemoptysis: diagnosis and management. Compr Ther. 2002;28(1):7–14.
10. Schiza S, Siafakas NM. Clinical presentation and management of empyema, lung abscess and pleural effusion. Curr Opin Pulm Med. 2006;12(3):205–11.
11. Wiedemann HP, Rice TW. Lung abscess and empyema. Semin Thorac Cardiovasc Surg. 1995;7(2):119–28.
12. Mwandumba HC, Beeching NJ. Pyogenic lung infections: factors for predicting clinical outcome of lung abscess and thoracic empyema. Curr Opin Pulm Med. 2000;6(3):234–9.
13. Hirshberg B, Sklair-Levi M, Nir-Paz R, Ben-Sira L, Krivoruk V, Kramer MR. Factors predicting mortality of patients with lung abscess. Chest. 1999;115(3):746–50.
14. Christie NA. Management of pleural space: effusions and empyema. Surg Clin North Am. 2010;90(5):919–34.
15. Mansharamani NG, Koziel H. Chronic lung sepsis: lung abscess, bronchiectasis, and empyema. Curr Opin Pulm Med. 2003; 9(3):181–5.
16. Sahn SA, Heffner JE. Spontaneous pneumothorax. N Engl J Med. 2000;342(12):868–74.
17. Nakajima J. Surgery for secondary spontaneous pneumothorax. Curr Opin Pulm Med. 2010;16(4):376–80.
18. Baumann MH, Strange C, Heffner JE, et al. Management of spontaneous pneumothorax: an American College of Chest Physicians Delphi Consensus statement. Chest. 2001;119(2): 590–602.
19. Baumann MH, Strange C. Treatment of spontaneous pneumothorax: a more aggressive approach? Chest. 1997;112(3):789–804.
20. Lansman SL, Saunders PC, Malekan R, Spielvogel D. Acute aortic syndrome. J Thorac Cardiovasc Surg. 2010;140(6 Suppl):S92–7.
21. Ramanath VS, Oh JK, Sundt 3rd TM, Eagle KA. Acute aortic syndromes and thoracic aortic aneurysm. Mayo Clin Proc. 2009; 84(5):465–81.
22. Golledge J, Eagle KA. Acute aortic dissection. Lancet. 2008; 372(9632):55–66.
23. Moon MR. Approach to the treatment of aortic dissection. Surg Clin North Am. 2009;89(4):869–93.
24. Griepp RB, Ergin MA, Galla JD, et al. Natural history of descending thoracic and thoracoabdominal aneurysms. Ann Thorac Surg. 1999;67(6):1927–30.
25. Elefteriades JA. Indications for aortic replacement. J Thorac Cardiovasc Surg. 2010;140(6 Suppl):S5–9.
26. DeVault KR. Presbyesophagus: a reappraisal. Curr Gastroenterol Rep. 2002;4(3):193–9.
27. Brady PG. Esophageal foreign bodies. Gastroenterol Clin North Am. 1991;20(4):691–701.
28. Weissberg D, Refaely Y. Foreign bodies in the esophagus. Ann Thorac Surg. 2007;84(6):1854–7.
29. Kavic SM, Basson MD. Complications of endoscopy. Am J Surg. 2001;181(4):319–32.
30. Wu JT, Mattox KL, Wall Jr MJ. Esophageal perforations: new perspectives and treatment paradigms. J Trauma. 2007;63(5): 1173–84.

31. Brinster CJ, Singhal S, Lee L, Marshall MB, Kaiser LR, Kucharczuk JC. Evolving options in the management of esophageal perforation. Ann Thorac Surg. 2004;77(4):1475–83.
32. Siegel R, Naishadham D, Jemal A. Cancer statistics, 2012. CA Cancer J Clin. 2012;62(1):10–29.
33. Younes Z, Johnson DA. The spectrum of spontaneous and iatrogenic esophageal injury: perforations, Mallory-Weiss tears, and hematomas. J Clin Gastroenterol. 1999;29(4):306–17.
34. Altorjay A, Kiss J, Voros A, Sziranyi E. The role of esophagectomy in the management of esophageal perforations. Ann Thorac Surg. 1998;65(5):1433–6.
35. Richardson JD. Management of esophageal perforations: the value of aggressive surgical treatment. Am J Surg. 2005;190(2):161–5.
36. D'Cunha J. Esophageal stents for leaks and perforations. Semin Thorac Cardiovasc Surg. 2011;23(2):163–7.
37. Landreneau RJ, Del Pino M, Santos R. Management of paraesophageal hernias. Surg Clin North Am. 2005;85(3):411–32.
38. Davis Jr SS. Current controversies in paraesophageal hernia repair. Surg Clin North Am. 2008;88(5):959–78.
39. Stylopoulos N, Rattner DW. Paraesophageal hernia: when to operate? Adv Surg. 2003;37:213–29.

Part III

Traumatic Injury in the Elderly

Epidemiology of Injury in the Elderly

20

Patrick M. Reilly and Nicole J. Krumrei

Introduction

The word epidemiology, derived from Greek, literally meaning "the study of what is upon the people" was coined by Hippocrates, the first person known to have examined the relationships between the occurrence of disease and environmental influences [1]. It is the study of patterns of health and disease occurrence in human population, its effects, and the factors that influence these patterns [2, 3]. The epidemiologic framework typically identifies the factors as relating to the host (intrinsic factors), the agent, and the environment (extrinsic factors). Epidemiology seeks to understand how these multiple factors interact to increase the risk of injury, disease, and poor outcomes.

Although patients are treated as an individual, by studying patterns of occurrence across populations we can learn how to best prevent them, evaluate for them, and treat them when they do occur. The older population (>65 years) is an important growing segment of the US population. In the 2010 census, more people were over the age of 65 than in any previous years, and the rate of increase (15 %) was more than that of the general US population (10 %) [4]. Moreover, the fastest growing segment of the elderly population was those aged 85–94, growing by 29.9 % and increasing to 5.1 million. It is estimated that in the year 2030, one fifth of the US population will be at least 65 years old [5]. It becomes increasingly important to understand this population and its interactions with medicine and traumatic events. This chapter will overview the general epidemiology of injuries in the elderly population and discuss the leading mechanisms of injury.

P.M. Reilly, MD, FACS (✉)
Division of Traumatology, Surgical Critical Care and Emergency Surgery, Department of Surgery, Perelman School of Medicine, University of Pennsylvania, Philadelphia, PA, USA

Department of Surgery, Hospital of the University of Pennsylvania, 3400 Spruce Street, 5 Maloney, Philadelphia, PA 19104, USA
e-mail: reillyp@uphs.upenn.edu

N.J. Krumrei, MD
Division of Traumatology, Surgical Critical Care and Emergency Surgery, Department of Surgery, Perelman School of Medicine, University of Pennsylvania, Philadelphia, PA, USA

Department of Surgery, University of Pennsylvania Medical Center, 3440 Spruce Street, Philadelphia, PA 19104, USA
e-mail: nicole.krumrei@uphs.upenn.edu

Factors that Influence the Pattern of Injury

In the 1960s William Haddon proposed a matrix approach towards delineating the risk factors associated with occurrence and severity of injury [6]. The Haddon Phase-Factor Matrix uses the classic epidemiologic framework of host, agent, and environment in addition to highlighting the dynamic process of injury causation by dividing the timing sequence into pre-event, event, and post-event. Each of the three timing phases interact with the set of host, agent, and environment to determine if an *event* will occur (pre-event), if an *injury* will occur (event), and the *consequences* of the event/injury (post-event). An example is seen in Table 20.1 and illustrates the number of factors that contribute to any injury and can be used to identify strategies for treatment and prevention.

Advanced age is a well-recognized risk factor for morbidity and mortality after trauma [7]. There are many systems-based age-related physiologic changes that have been detailed in the previous chapters that will not be reviewed here, but all play an important role in the decreased physiologic reserve of the elderly trauma patient. They also play a role in increasing the risk of the traumatic event occurring (e.g., deteriorating sight, poor coordination). In general, older adults have more preexisting medical conditions which increase their risk of mortality and are frailer causing more severe injury in response to a given injury [8].

Although the elderly are a special population, the trimodal distribution of traumatic deaths still applies. It states that deaths due to injury occurs in one of three periods [9, 10]. Approximately 50 % of deaths occur within minutes

J.A. Yelon, F.A. Luchette (eds.), *Geriatric Trauma and Critical Care*,
DOI 10.1007/978-1-4614-8501-8_20, © Springer Science+Business Media New York 2014

Table 20.1 Haddon Phase-Factor Matrix: pedestrian hit by a motor vehicle

Phases	Host (individual)	Agent (motor vehicle)	Environment
Pre-event (will event occur)	Age, gender, medications, alcohol use, vision, fatigue, ambulatory aids/ability	Speed, size, ability of driver, brakes	Road design, crosswalk design and timing, weather conditions, visibility, speed restrictions, traffic restrictions
Event (will injury occur)	Age, preexisting conditions (e.g., osteoporosis), medications (e.g., bleeding risk)	Speed, size, brakes	Site of crash, landing zone
Post-event (will consequence occur)	Age, comorbid conditions	Ability to extricate	Availability of EMS, distance from emergency care, quality of trauma system and rehabilitation

Note: Each of the three timing phases interact with the set of host, agent, and environment to determine if an event will occur (pre-event), if an injury will occur (event), and the consequences of the event/injury (post-event). Examples illustrate the number of factors that contribute to any injury and can be used to identify strategies for treatment and prevention

of the injury and are most likely due to severe neurologic (brain, high spinal cord) injury or massive hemorrhage due to rupture of the heart or large blood vessel. These individuals cannot be saved due to the severity of their injuries even in the most mature trauma and EMS systems, and efforts at preventing the occurrence will be effective in reducing this peak of trauma-related deaths. The second peak occurs within minutes to several hours and is usually due to subdural or epidural hematomas or injuries associated with significant blood loss (e.g., splenic or liver laceration, pelvic fractures). These patients require rapid assessment and resuscitation. The third peak occurs several days to weeks, most likely due to sepsis or multisystem organ failure. Efforts at reducing the severity of injury once it has occurred will impact the two later peaks of trauma-related deaths.

Overview of Injury

Unintentional injury is the fifth leading cause of death over all age groups, both sexes, and all races in the United States (which excludes suicides and homicides) [11]. In patients aged 65 or greater, trauma is the seventh leading cause of death. In 2009, over 44,000 people aged 65 or older died from injuries in the United States, which is an average of 120 persons each day or 1 person every 12 min [12]. In those aged 65 years or greater, the leading mechanisms of injury, in rank order, are as follows: falls, motor vehicle crashes, and suicides.

Although the total number of traumatic injuries in the elderly is less than the total number of traumatic injuries in those younger than 45 years of age, the rate (or risk) of injury per age group is just the opposite. The elderly aged 65 and older are at the highest risk of fatal injuries, a risk that increases with each year of age. Using 2010 data, the rate of injury death in 65–74 year olds was 60 per 100,000 population, for persons aged 75–84 it was 124.7 per 100,000 population, and for those 85 and older it was 350 per 100,000 population, which compares to 58 per 100,000 in the general population [13]. The elderly that are older than 65 comprise 13 % of the US population, but account for 33 % of all injury deaths and 32 % of injury-related hospitalizations. The US population continues to age, with those over 65 years of age estimated to be 20 % of the population by 2030 [5]. This has profound implications on health and trauma care with the burden of geriatric injury surely increasing with the aging US population.

Mortality is not the only potential result of a traumatic event. Particularly in the elderly population, the morbidity can be just as serious a complication and have widespread personal, family, and societal repercussions including decreased quality of life and high costs of immediate and long-term medical care. Each year, over 760,000 people older than 65 are hospitalized as the consequence of a traumatic event, while over 2.7 million are treated in the emergency department and released. In this same group, the leading causes of nonfatal injuries are, in rank order, as follows: falls, assault, unintentional overexertion, and motor vehicle crashes. Total lifetime costs associated with *nonfatal* injuries in those aged 65–85 occurring in the year 2005 amount to over $18.5 billion. The costs for nonfatal injuries include direct medical expenditures as well as the value of lost work productivity, but do not include the cost of pain, reduced quality of life, or the reduced quantity of life.

Injury by Mechanism and Intent

Traumatic injuries are classified by their mechanism, their intent, and the place of injury. Mechanism refers to the external agent or activity that caused the injury (e.g., fall, motor vehicle crash, stab wound). Intent is classified as unintentional, intentionally inflicted by someone, or undetermined. The place of injury can be classified as urban, suburban, and rural as well as location in the country.

Falls

Falls are the most common mechanism of fatal injury in the elderly, responsible for 52 % of unintentional injuries in 2009. Falls are also the most common cause of nonfatal injury in the elderly resulting in over 2.2 million emergency department visits and over 580,000 hospitalizations in the year 2009 [13]. In the United States, each year more than 1/3 of individuals over the age of 65 will experience a fall, this increases to 50 % in those who live in an institution [14, 15]. Half of those who do suffer a fall will have at least one more unintentional fall in the next 12 months [16]. Of these, 25 % will be injured and another 25 % will restrict their daily activities for fear of falling [17, 18].

In 2009, 82 % of fall-related deaths were among those aged 65 and older. The rate of falling and becoming injured increases with age. The rate of fall injuries for adults over the age of 85 is four times the rate for adults aged 65–74. Women are 58 % more likely than men to suffer a nonfatal fall injury, with fall-related fractures twice as likely in females than in males. White females are twice as likely as black females to suffer a hip fracture. Up to 30 % of the elderly will suffer a moderate to severe injury such as a laceration, hip fracture, or head injury [17].

Falls are the most common cause of traumatic brain injuries in the geriatric population. In 2000, 46 % of deaths from same height falls in elderly adults were the result of a TBI [19]. Falling from standing is associated with a hip fracture in 5 % of individuals, a risk that increases with age [20]. One half of those who suffer a hip fracture are no longer able to live independently.

Major risk factors for falls among the elderly include those related to the host: advanced age, history of previous falls, hypotension, psychoactive medications, dementia, difficulty with postural stability and gait, visual, cognitive, neurologic, and physical impairments. Environment factors include the following: loose rugs, objects on the floor, ice/slippery surfaces, uneven floors, poor lighting, and stairs without handrails. The risk of falling increases linearly with each additional environmental factor present [20].

Motor Vehicle Crashes

There are 32 million licensed older drivers in the United States [21], 15 % of all drivers. Motor vehicle crashes are the second most common mechanism of fatal injury in persons aged 65 or older, responsible for 34 % of unintentional deaths in 2007 [12] and causing over 170,000 nonfatal injuries (5 % of total nonfatal injuries) in the elderly [13]. These older individuals made up 16 % of all traffic fatalities and 8 % of all people injured in traffic crashes during the year [21].

Although those over the age of 75 have a high risk of dying from their injuries, those in their teens and twenties are actually at the highest risk of fatal and nonfatal injuries due to MVC [22]. However, excluding teens and young adults, drivers older than 85 have a fatality rate that is 7–9 times greater than that of young drivers. In two-vehicle fatal crashes involving an older driver and a younger driver, the vehicle driven by the elder was 1.7 times more likely to be the one that was struck (58 % and 34 %, respectively). In 46 % of these crashes, both vehicles were proceeding straight at the time of the collision. In 24 %, the older driver was turning left—four times more often than the younger driver [21].

In general, older people drive less total miles, less at night, on more familiar roads, and at lower speed limits which results in a majority of elderly traffic fatalities occurring in the daytime (81 %), on weekdays (71 %), and involving other vehicles (69 %) [21].

Injury patterns in the elderly are similar to those that are seen in the general blunt trauma population. Risk factors in the elderly that may contribute to motor vehicle crashes include a larger blind spot (secondary to decreased peripheral vision), limited cervical mobility, slower reaction times, poorer technique for merging into traffic, decreased hearing, and cognitive impairment. Moreover, chronic medical conditions such as dysrhythmias, hypoglycemia (diabetes-related complications), and thromboembolic events such as stroke or myocardial infarction may be the precipitate event resulting in an accident. As with any driver, alcohol and impaired function lead to an increased risk for a crash. Compared to all drivers, older drivers involved in fatal crashes are the least likely to be legally intoxicated defined as a blood alcohol concentration of .08 g/dL or higher (5 % vs. 22 %, respectively) [21].

Major factors contributing to the likelihood of a crash include vehicle speed, vehicle stability, braking deficiencies, inadequate road design, and driver alcohol intoxication. When a collision does occur, important determinants of the likelihood of an injury and its severity include speed at impact, vehicle safety, and the use of restraints. Seventy-nine percent of all older occupants of passenger vehicles involved in fatal crashes were using restraints at the time, compared to 64 % for other adult occupants (18–64 years old) [21].

Pedestrians Hit by Motor Vehicles

In 2009, a total of 4,092 pedestrians were killed, and an estimated 59,000 were injured by vehicles in the United States. In 2009, the fatality rate for older pedestrians (age 65+) was 1.96 per 100,000 population—higher than the rate for all the other ages. On average, a pedestrian was killed every two hours and injured every nine minutes by a motor vehicle.

Pedestrian deaths accounted for 12 % of all traffic fatalities and made up 3 % of all the injuries related to traffic crashes. Older pedestrians (age 65+) accounted for 19 % of all pedestrian fatalities and an estimated 8 % of all pedestrians were injured in 2009 [23]. Moreover, as the pedestrians aged, the risk of mortality increases from a rate of 1.75 per 100,000 population for those aged 65–74 to a rate of 2.29 for those aged 75–84 [12]. Distribution by gender demonstrated that 61 % of elderly pedestrians killed in 2009 were males, with a fatality injury rate of 2.51 per 100,000 compared to 1.33 per 100,000 in females. The male geriatric pedestrian nonfatal rate per 100,000 population was 18 %, twice the rate of 9 % for females.

Seventy-two percent of pedestrian fatalities occurred in an urban setting versus a rural setting. The states with the highest pedestrian fatalities per 100,000 total general population are as follows: District of Columbia (2.33), Florida (2.51), Louisiana (2.38), Mississippi (1.96), and New Mexico (1.94).

For older people, 64 % of pedestrian fatalities in 2009 occurred at non-intersection locations (compared to 78 % for all other pedestrians). Ninety percent of pedestrian fatalities occurred during normal weather conditions, compared to rain, snow, and fog. A majority of the pedestrian fatalities, almost 70 %, occurred at the nighttime. Alcohol involvement—either for the driver or for the pedestrian—was reported in 48 % of the traffic crashes that resulted in pedestrian fatalities. Only 9 % of the elderly pedestrians had a blood alcohol concentration above of 0.08 g/dL which is markedly less than the incidence of 37 % in the general population. The ISS for elderly pedestrians is higher when compared to the younger pedestrians. The geriatric patient is more likely to suffer a severe head injury including subdural hemorrhages, subarachnoid hemorrhages, intraparenchymal contusions, severe thoracic injury with a significant risk for aortic transection, hemothorax, pneumothorax, spinal cord injury, and fractures of the pelvis and tibia [24].

Variables that will impact the injury pattern for a pedestrian struck include the make and model of the vehicle and the environment. Risk factors specific to the elderly pedestrian include comorbid diseases, specifically their cognition, sensory, and ambulatory status. Of interest, 25 % of the elderly were unable to traverse a crosswalk within the posted time limit [25].

Assault and Domestic Abuse

Violence is an increasing cause of injury in the elderly. In 2011, an estimated 25,886 persons over the age of 64 were treated in emergency departments for nonfatal assault-related injuries (rate of 63 per 100,000 population) [12]. The majority of the victims (82 %) were treated in the emergency department and discharged to home, while 16 % required hospitalization. The majority of injuries were contusions or abrasions, lacerations, and fractures [26].

The National Incident-Based Reporting System (NIBRS) is a reporting system used by law enforcement agencies in the United States for collecting and reporting data on crimes. The NIBRS data are not nationally representative, as it is not mandatory in all states. The Bureau of Justice Statistics (BJS) focused on data from Michigan, which was a complete reporting state from 2005 to 2009 to further investigate the epidemiology of violence against older adults [27]. In Michigan, the annual rate of assault incidents for males aged 65 or greater was 247 per 100,000 population which compared to 172 per 100,000 in females in the same age group. Elderly Caucasians and Asians had a similar victimization rate at 145 per 100,000 and 132 per 100,000, respectively, while blacks had the highest rate of at 744 per 100,000. The assailant was more likely to be of the same race than a different race. In Michigan between 2005 and 2009, 85 % of reported violence against the elderly was intra-racial: the majority of victimizations of elderly whites were perpetrated by white offenders (79.6 %), and most attacks of elderly blacks were perpetrated by black offenders (95.8 %). Of note, half (50 %) of elderly victims were assaulted by a family member, such as intimate partners (12.9 %), the victim's own children (22.0 %), grandchildren (8.5 %), or other relatives (6.3 %). The offender was more likely to be a family member in attacks against an elderly female (60.0 %) than an elderly male (38.6 %). Thirty-one percent of incidents involved a nonpersonal weapon (e.g., firearm, knife, or blunt object), while 51 % involved personal weapons (e.g., hands, fists, feet, and teeth), while another 18.1 % involved no weapon or physical force.

According to the National Center on Elder Abuse, elder abuse refers to intentional or negligent acts by a caregiver or "trusted" individual that causes harm to a vulnerable elder. Each state defines elder abuse differently. As noted above, abuse of elderly may take many forms, including physical, sexual, emotional or psychological, financial or material exploitation, neglect, and abandonment. Neglect is the most common type of elder abuse. The National Elder Abuse Incidence Study was the first major investigation into the mistreatment of the elderly in the United States. By soliciting data from the 1996 Adult Protective Service records, they found that 449,924 persons aged 60 or older had been physically abused, neglected, or in some way mistreated [28]. It is believed that the results underestimate the true scope of the problem due to non-reporting and under-identification. An interview survey performed in 2008 found that approximately 11 % of US elders who responded had experienced some type of abuse or potential neglect in the previous year [29].

Abuse should always be considered when evaluating the older trauma patient. Injuries related to falls, or the fall itself, may be the result of abuse or mistreatment. Findings on physical exam that increase the suspicion for elder abuse or neglect include unexplained bruising/trauma/skin tears, injuries not consistent with the mechanism of injury, grooming/hygiene, malnutrition, dehydration, demeanor, pressure ulcers, patient odor, contractures, lice/scabies, fear of examination, and sensory losses. Common risk factors include dementia, social isolation, and poor physical health of the elder as well as a perpetrator with mental health or substance abuse issues [30]. Concerns for elder abuse should prompt further evaluation. Elders who experience abuse, neglect, or self-neglect face considerably higher risk of premature death than elders who have not been mistreated [31, 32].

Penetrating Injuries

In 2010, penetrating injuries (firearms and cut/pierce injuries) were the fourth most common cause of traumatic death in those aged 65 or older, accounting for over 4,900 deaths in the geriatric population (2.7 % overall cause mortality in this age group). Penetrating injuries were the fifth most common cause of traumatic injury with over 140,000 injuries (4 % overall cause of injury). A majority of the deaths from penetrating injuries were related to intentional self-harm or suicide and associated with firearms compared to stab wounds [13].

Firearms were the cause of over 4,700 deaths in 2010 for the geriatric population. Overall, the elderly comprised 14.8 % of all firearm deaths in the United States in 2010. The vast majority (91 %) of the deaths were intentional (suicide), while only 7 % were categorized as homicides. For comparison, when calculated for those aged 20–34, the rate of firearm deaths related to suicide is 40 %. The rate of firearm suicide increased as the population aged with a rate of 13.7 per 100,000 for those aged 65–74 compared to a rate of 17.62 per 100,000 for those aged 85 years or greater. Firearms also accounted for over 1,500 injuries in the elderly population. Of these injuries, 802 were identified as unintentional and 723 were classified as intentional (235 assault vs. 488 self-harm/suicide, respectively).

Although firearms accounted for the majority of penetrating trauma deaths, stab wounds (stabbing, cutting, or piercing) were responsible for the majority of penetrating traumatic injuries in those older than 64. In 2010, 245 deaths were caused by stab wounds (191 intentional, 52 unintentional), and stab wounds resulted in 143,628 injuries (140,823 unintentional, 944 assault, 1,768 self-harm/suicide attempt).

There are relatively few studies of penetrating trauma in the geriatric population. In two studies from large urban level I trauma centers, elderly patients who arrived alive had outcomes equivalent to a younger matched cohort group, but had a significantly longer ICU and hospital length of stay [33, 34]. A more recent study concluded that the mortality rate for penetrating injuries in patients older than 55 years was significantly higher (14.1 % compared to 9.4 % for ages 45–54). When the data was analyzed for patients older than 64 years, the mortality rate of 26.4 % was significantly higher [35]. A study from the National Trauma Database (from 2002 to 2006) demonstrated that within the elderly age group (age 65 and older), all of the following increased with age: ISS, the incidence of self-inflicted injury, and the mortality rate [36]. The most commonly encountered injury was a gunshot wound to the head, which also increased with age. An admission Glasgow Coma Score of less than 9, an Injury Severity Score greater than 15, hypotension on admission, self-inflicted injury, and injury sustained in an assault were factors associated with death in the elderly population.

Summary

As the population ages, the burden of geriatric trauma will markedly increase. While the epidemiology of many traumatic events in this population is similar to that in younger age groups, the elderly present their own unique set of host, agent, and environmental combinations that often put them at excessive risk. Careful understanding of the epidemiology of geriatric trauma can hopefully lead to improved prevention efforts and effective clinical care paradigms to minimize death and disability from injury in this population.

References

1. Merrill RW. Historic developments in epidemiology. In: Introduction to epidemiology. 5th ed. Sudbury: Jones and Bartlett Publishing LLC; 2010. p. 23–46.
2. Lilienfeld AM, Lilienfeld DE. Foundations of epidemiology. New York: Oxford University Press; 1980. p. 3.
3. Porta M. A dictionary of epidemiology. Oxford: Oxford University Press; 2008. p. 10–1.
4. US Bureau of the Census. The 2010 census summary file 1 (SF1). Available at http://www.census.gov/population/www.cen2010/glance/index.html.
5. US Bureau of the Census. US interim projections by age, sex, race, and Hispanic origin. Available at http://www.census.gov/ipc/www/usinterimproj/.
6. Haddon W. The changing approach to epidemiology, prevention, and amelioration of trauma: the transition to approaches etiologically rather than descriptively based. Am J Public Health. 1968;58:1431.
7. Champion HR, Copes WS, Buyer D, et al. Major trauma in geriatric patients. Am J Public Health. 1989;79:1278–82.
8. Milzman DP, Boulanger BR, Rodriquez A, et al. Pre-existing disease in trauma patients: a predictor of fate independent of age and injury severity score. J Trauma. 1992;32(2):236–43.
9. American College of Surgeons Committee on Trauma, editor. Advanced trauma life support student course manual. Chicago: American College of Surgeons; 2008.
10. Demetriades D, Kimbrell B, Salim A, et al. Trauma deaths in a mature urban trauma system: is "trimodal" distribution a valid concept? J Am Coll Surg. 2005;201:343–8.

11. Heron M. Deaths: leading causes for 2009. Nat Vital Stat Rep. 2012;61(7):1–96.
12. Centers for Disease Control and Prevention, National Center for Injury Prevention and Control. WISQARS fatal injuries: mortality reports. Available at: https://webappa.cdc.gov/sasweb/ncipc/mortrate.html.
13. Centers for Disease Control and Prevention, National Center for Injury Prevention and Control. Web-based Injury Statistics Query and Reporting (WISQARS). Available at: http://www.cdc.gov/injury/wisqars/index.html.
14. Hausdorff JM, Rios DA, Edelber HK. Gait variability and fall risk in community-living older adults: a one year prospective study. Arch Phys Med Rehabil. 2001;82:1050.
15. Rubenstein LZ, Josephson KR, Robbins AS. Falls in the nursing home. Ann Intern Med. 1994;121:442.
16. Tinetti ME, Speechley M. Prevention of falls among the elderly. N Engl J Med. 1989;320:1055.
17. Sterling DA, O'Connor JA, Bonadies J. Geriatric falls: injury severity is high and disproportionate to mechanism. J Trauma. 2001; 50:116.
18. Vellas BJ, Wayne SJ, Romero LJ, et al. Fear of falling and restriction of mobility in elderly fallers. Age Aging. 1997;26: 189–93.
19. Stevens JA. Fatalities and injuries from falls among older adults – United States 1993–2003 and 2001–2005. MMWR Morb Mortal Wkly Rep. 2006;55(45):1221–4.
20. Tinetti ME, Speechley M, Ginter SF. Risk factors for falls among elderly persons living in the community. N Engl J Med. 1988; 319:1701.
21. NHTSA Traffic Safety Facts. 2009. Older population. DOT HS 811 391. Available at http://www-nrd.nhtsa.dot.gov/Pubs/811391.pdf.
22. Braver ER, Trempel RE. Are older drivers actually at higher risk of involvement in collisions resulting in deaths or nonfatal injuries among their passengers and other road users? Inj Prev. 2004;10:27.
23. NHTSA Traffic Safety Facts. 2009: pedestrians, DOT HS 811 394. Available at http://www-nrd.nhtsa.dot.gov/Pubs/811394.pdf.
24. Demetriades D, Murray J, Martin M, et al. Pedestrian injured by automobiles: relationship to age to injury type and severity. J Am Coll Surg. 2004;199(3):382–7.
25. Hoxie RE, Rubenstein LA. Are older pedestrians allowed enough time to cross intersections safely? J Am Geriatr Soc. 1994;42:241.
26. Mitchell R, Hasbrouk L, Ingram E, et al. Public health and aging: nonfatal physical assault-related injuries among persons aged >60 years treated in hospital emergency departments – United States, 2001. MMWR Morb Mortal Wkly Rep. 2003;54:812.
27. Smith E. Violent crime against the elderly reported by Law Enforcement in Michigan, 2005–2009 US Department of Justice. 2012. Available at: http://bjs.ojp.usdoj.gov/index.cfm?ty=pbdetail&iid=4352.
28. Tatara T. The national elder abuse incidence study: executive summary. New York: Human Services Press; 1997.
29. Acierno R, et al. Prevalence and Correlates of emotional, physical, sexual, and financial abuse and potential neglect in the United States: the National Elder Mistreatment Study. Am J Public Health. 2010;100:292–7.
30. Harrell R, Toronjo CH, McLaughlin J, et al. How geriatricians identify elder abuse and neglect. Am J Med Sci. 2002;323:34–8.
31. Dong X, et al. Elder self-neglect and abuse and mortality risk in a community-dwelling population. JAMA. 2009;302:517–26.
32. Lachs MS, Williams CS, O'Brien S, et al. The mortality of elder mistreatment. JAMA. 1998;280:428.
33. Nagy KK, Smith RF, Roberts RR, et al. Prognosis of penetrating trauma in elderly patients: a comparison with younger patients. J Trauma. 2000;49:190.
34. Roth BJ, Velmahos GC, Older DB, et al. Penetrating trauma in patients older than 55 years: a case–control study. Injury. 2000;32:551–4.
35. Ottochian M, Salim A, DuBose J, et al. Does age matter? The relationship between age and mortality in penetrating trauma. Injury. 2009;40:254–357.
36. Lustenberger T, Inaba K, Schnuriger B, et al. Gunshot injuries in the elderly: patterns and outcomes. A national trauma databank analysis. World J Surg. 2011;35:528–34.

Geriatric Trauma and Injury Prevention

21

Syed Nabeel Zafar, Edward E. Cornwell III, and Wendy R. Greene

Epidemiology and Background

The elderly population is the fastest growing demographic in industrialized nations. During the past century, the elderly population increased 11-fold as compared a 3-fold increase in the number of people younger than 65 years of age. At the current rate, by the year 2030 one in every five Americans will be aged 65 or older [1].

Trauma is a leading cause of death in the elderly population [2]. Every year approximately 870,000 people aged 65 years and older are involved in some kind of injury and approximately 43,000 die of the injuries. Besides the enormous loss of life, geriatric trauma also poses a huge burden on the economy, accounting for 12 billion dollars per year in medical costs and 25 billion dollars annually in total costs [3]. Elderly trauma patients stay in the hospital twice as long, have three times higher medical expenses, and are twice more likely to die than their younger counterparts.

In a multivariate logistic regression analysis of over 1.6 million patients in the National Trauma Data Bank (NTDB), geriatric trauma patients (394,000; 24 %) in comparison to younger adults were (Zafar et al., Greene et al., 2013, Geriatric trauma, unpublished work):

- Less likely to be a minority race
- Less likely to have alcohol-associated injury
- Less likely to suffer a work-related injury
- More likely to be insured
- More likely to be transported by ambulance
- Have higher injury severity scores
- More likely to be hypotensive at presentation
- More likely to suffer isolated head injuries
- More likely to fall, have a motor vehicular crash, or be a "pedestrian struck by car"
- Less likely to be injured by a firearm or knife

Trauma care for the elderly is improving, and evidence-based management strategies are constantly being developed and revised. However, injury prevention remains the key element in addressing this huge burden.

Implementation of successful injury prevention programs for the elderly is paramount. In this chapter, we discuss injury prevention strategies for three major causes of elderly trauma, i.e., trauma associated with falls, motor vehicle crashes, and elder abuse.

The standard injury control approach devised by William Haddon – which constructs a matrix based on the phase of the trauma (pre-event, injury event, and post-event), as well as the factors such as the host, the vehicle, and the environment – has worthwhile applications in considering prevention of geriatric trauma. The Haddon matrix is described in detail in Chap. 20.

Falls

"I have fallen and I can't get up" is one of the twentieth century's notable quotes, and instantaneously a picture of a frail elderly patient comes to mind. This is unfortunately often the pathway to dependent nursing care and increased healthcare costs. Falls are the leading cause of death in geriatric trauma patients. The injuries resulting from a fall most commonly result in a head injury or hip fractures. Over 25 % of hip fracture patients die within a year after the injury, and recovery in 50 % is limited by a major functional dependence. Studies have evaluated geriatric fall-related injury prevention by studying the effect of bone mineral enhancing agents, use of hip protective devices, exercise programs, physical environment modifications, and screening tool implementation.

S.N. Zafar, MD, MPH • E.E. Cornwell III, MD, FACS, FCCM
W.R. Greene, MD, FACS (✉)
Department of Surgery, Howard University Hospital,
Howard University College of Medicine,
2041 Georgia Avenue NW,
Washington, DC 20060, USA
e-mail: zafar.nabeel@gmail.com; wgreene@howard.edu; ecornwell@howard.edu

J.A. Yelon, F.A. Luchette (eds.), *Geriatric Trauma and Critical Care*,
DOI 10.1007/978-1-4614-8501-8_21,

The recommendation for vitamin D is simple and low cost. It enhances muscle response times, and CNS reaction times and improves balance. Vitamin D facilitates intestinal calcium absorption and mineralization of bone matrix. In the elderly, the decreased levels of vitamin D and calcium lead to increased parathyroid hormone (PTH) secretion at the expense of bone density with an increased risk for fractures. Most studies do not support use of vitamin D and calcium in active, mobile seniors because they do not prevent future fractures [4]. However, vitamin D with calcium is able to reduce the risk of falls and fractures with proper patient selection. Risk reduction for falls is highest in the elderly institutionalized patients [4].

Additional measures to reduce injury during a fall are to use hip protectors. They are only effective in residents of nursing homes. The problem is the reliability of the caretakers to apply the device at all times when the residents are ambulating. One prospective study demonstrated a reduced rate of fracture when a hip protector was used by nursing home residents [5]. However, this was a single-institution study and included only nursing home residents.

Exercise has undeniable benefits for muscles and bones. Balance and strengthening exercises are important to withstanding falls in the elderly [6]. Therefore, strong recommendations are in place for enhancing lower extremity muscle strength, specifically quadriceps strengthening. These exercises improve lower extremity balance, which reduces the rate of falls but not hip fractures if a fall occurs. Dynamic flamingo therapy exercise (which is balancing on one leg for 1 min three times a day) reduces osteoporosis of the femoral neck. Conversely, heavy resistance training in the elderly can lead to more injuries and therefore is not recommended as part of the balance and strengthening regimen to improve balance and reduce the risk of fall.

Environmental modifications have also been shown to be beneficial at reducing falls. The incidence of falls was reduced by 60 % in homes that were renovated by simple measures such as removing clutter and installing grab bars and hand rails [6]. Another study demonstrated installing carpets and adhesives to unsecured rugs could decrease femoral impact forces by up to 50 % without increasing the risk for an unstable gait [7].

For the elderly living at home, outreach activities are associated with decreased falls [8]. The fracture risk index based on bone density can help select patients at risk for low impact fractures and who would benefit from additional prevention tools.

Dementia

While special care is warranted in pursuing trauma prevention for seniors with decreased mental capacity due to dementia, there is legitimate hope that injured demented patients can achieve similar outcomes compared to elderly patients without cognitive impairment.

The largest study to date of trauma outcomes in demented patients demonstrates that dementia is not an independent predictor of in-hospital mortality. Thus, a history of dementia should not be used by clinicians to limit treatment for elderly trauma patients (Greene WR OA, Siram SM, Mellman TA, Cornwell EE, Haider AH, Oyetunji TA, 2013, Brain loss does not equal life loss: acute trauma outcomes in elderly patients is not affected by dementia, unpublished work). This NTDB study of nearly 170,000 seniors with at least moderately severe injury documented a mortality rate of 10 %. Falls were the most common mechanism in 64 % of the elderly patients with a median ISS score of 10 (IQR 9–17). Dementia was diagnosed in 11,823 (4.5 %) patients of whom a significant number (45 % vs. 9 %) with dementia were discharged to nursing homes. In-hospital morbidity and mortality was not associated with the diagnosis of dementia. The authors suggest that evidence-based trauma practice guidelines for the elderly can be applied to the injured geriatric patients diagnosed with dementia.

Motor Vehicle Crash

There are numerous risk factors for traffic collisions in the elderly making it difficult to have a generalized injury prevention strategy. A multipronged approach is often suggested including improvements in human, vehicular, and environmental measures. The approaches are aimed not only at preventing crashes from occurring but also at reducing the energy transferred and thus subsequent injuries that occur once a collision does happen.

A number of differences exist between MVCs involving the elderly when compared to younger drivers. Motor vehicular crashes involving elderly drivers occur at lower speeds, but the elderly passenger is more severely injured than when the passenger is younger. Elderly pedestrians are at increased risk for being struck by a vehicle due to slower mobility and reflexes. Injury prevention strategies are aimed at vehicular factors to make cars safer and human factors to protect drivers and passengers. Additional efforts target identifying behaviors of high-risk drivers. Finally, environmental factors are addressed with highway signage to identify hazardous conditions and engineering design of intersections and crosswalks.

Data from the National Automotive Sampling System – Crashworthiness Data Systems – reveals that elderly front seat-belted occupants are more likely to suffer injuries from low-speed crashes (<25 mph) than their younger counterparts [9]. Most of these injuries involve the chest. Of note, vehicles are not designed for elderly drivers and passenger. Their often shorter stature and frailty make conventional safety measures (air bags and seat belts) inadequate. Also car safety features and crash tests are often designed to prevent injury during a high-speed crash. More emphasis should be placed on low-speed crashes as well. Vehicle modifications such as increased side wall padding, adjusting threshold for airbag deployment, lower steering columns, and special four-point restraint belts designed for elderly passengers in the vehicle are also a consideration to reduce the impact of collisions. However, more research is needed to support these recommendations.

Injuries in elderly pedestrians are a special concern as they are associated with a high mortality and morbidity. In 2008, there were 69,000 pedestrians injured with 4,378 fatalities in the United States. The elderly accounted for 18 % of these deaths and had the highest case fatality rate [10]. The most common setting for the injury is while attempting to cross the road or falling from the curb and being struck by a passing vehicle. Age-related street crossing behavior includes slower decision-making, decreased walking speed, and misjudging oncoming traffic [11]. These problems are heightened on two-way streets and when the approaching vehicle's speed is high.

Interventions addressing these issues include education and training about road crossing and better visualization near the crosswalks. Previous studies demonstrate improved safety when crosswalks used by elderly are marked to notify drivers and improved visibility and orientation near crosswalks for pedestrians. Also speed breakers in the driving surface situated before a marked crosswalk result in higher yield rates to pedestrians [12]. Increasing crossing times for pedestrian is also a viable option for injury prevention. A study of crossing times concluded that 27 % of elderly pedestrians were unable to reach the other side of road before the light changed which put them at an increased risk for being hit by a motor vehicle [13].

A controversial method to reduce elderly crashes deals with screening to identify high-risk elderly drivers. Unfortunately, the published data does not provide enough evidence to support this concept as a method to reduce collision rates for elderly drivers. This is mainly due to the fact that current screening tools used do not effectively determine which elderly drivers are at risk [14]. For example, certain vision tests have been found to be associated with higher rates of crashes; however, optometrists do not routinely perform these tests. Also testing for judgment, insight, rapid decision-making, and reflex times have been controversial. A screening and intervention tool that has shown to be cost-effective is the "speed of processing" intervention [14]. This is a noninvasive moderate-cost intervention that has shown improved driving competence for all seniors including those "at-risk" drivers.

Screening for comorbid conditions has also been a subject of debate. Studies have shown that in general, elderly drivers with chronic medical conditions do have an increased risk for collisions. Elderly drivers with arrhythmias or diabetics are 1.7 and 2.6 times, respectively, more likely to be involved in a crash [15, 16].

Other environmental and behavioral interventions have also been proposed. Some of the low-cost measures include improved signage, adjusted traffic patterns, and use of roundabouts. Studies have also suggested an increased rate of crashes in the early evening. Thus, elderly drivers should avoid driving during this time of day [17]. The general promotion of highway traffic safety measures such as encouragement of seat belt use, speed control, and limiting distractions while driving is also recommended, as these measures are effective in all age groups.

Elder Abuse

An under-recognized and potentially lethal problem is elder abuse. It is estimated that approximately one to two million elderly Americans have been maltreated, injured, or exploited [18]. The CDC recognizes six forms of elder abuse: physical, sexual, emotional, neglect, abandonment, and financial. Elder abuse is often underreported, and some studies estimate that for every reported elder abuse case, there are five that are not [19]. Barriers to addressing elder abuse include lack of complaints by the victims; lack of physician training; reimbursement issues, there are no rewards for identifying or managing abuse; and marginalization of health-care workers actively involved in raising concerns regarding abuse [20].

There is insufficient data supporting routine screening for elder abuse. However, health-care workers should be cognizant of issues pertaining to elder abuse and have a high index of suspicion and refer to the appropriate agency.

The first step in preventing elder abuse is identification. The typical victims of physical abuse and neglect are females over 75 years, primarily Caucasian with a physical or mental impairment. Caregivers, who are found to have perpetrated elder abuse, are more likely to have mental health issues and are dependent on the patient. A careful history and examination often lead to a suspicion of abuse. Certain tools exist to assess the risk for elder abuse, such as the "the Risk of Elder Abuse in the Home" (REAH) tool [21]. The second step is reporting. All abuse cases should be reported even if not mandated by state law. Training of health-care professionals is needed as studies have shown that most physicians are not aware of how to report abuse cases [22]. Preliminary surveys at the state health department have also demonstrated some lack of knowledge and bureaucratic hurdles towards reporting and referral of elder abuse.

Injury prevention practices include social bonding, which allows for less isolation and more resources to keep families connected which empowers the abused and provides them with less perceived isolation. A multidisciplinary approach should be employed with social workers, nurses, physicians, occupational therapists, psychiatrists, and caseworkers.

Some legal interventions can also decrease elder abuse such as guardianship and surveillance.

Future Directions

While injury prevention is the lead consideration of this chapter, the inexact nature of that science has mandated that we expand the discussion to include outcomes of injury. When the latest available analysis of NTDB (2007–2010) is reviewed, the most interesting findings relate to cost and outcome of injuries admitted to centers with variable proportions of geriatric trauma patients. Regression analyses suggest that as the proportion of injured geriatric patients admitted to a trauma center increases, the standardized mortality ratios and cost of care decreases.

Let these data combined with the indisputable evidence of our aging population serve as an early impetus for forward thinking trauma systems to consider the development of geriatric trauma programs.

References

1. Velkoff A. The next four decades, the older population in the United States, 2010 to 2050. Washington, DC: U.S. Census Bureau; 2010.
2. Center for Disease Control. CDC National Center for Health Statistics (NCHS), National Vital Statistics System. http://www.cdc.gov/injury/wisqars/leadingcauses.html. Last accessed Oct. 2013.
3. Center for Disease Control. CDC Data & Statistics (WISQARS™): Cost of Injury Reports Data Source: NCHS Vital Statistics System for numbers of deaths. http://www.cdc.gov/injury/wisqars/index.html. Last accessed Oct. 2013.
4. Law M, Withers H, Morris J, Anderson F. Vitamin D supplementation and the prevention of fractures and falls: results of a randomised trial in elderly people in residential accommodation. Age Ageing. 2006;35(5):482–6.
5. Parkkari J, Heikkila J, Kannus IP. Acceptability and compliance with wearing energy-shunting hip protectors: a 6-month prospective follow-up in a Finnish nursing home. Age Ageing. 1998;27(2): 225–9.
6. Means KM, Rodell DE, O'Sullivan PS. Balance, mobility, and falls among community-dwelling elderly persons: effects of a rehabilitation exercise program. Am J Phys Med Rehabil. 2005;84(4): 238–50.
7. Laing AC, Robinovitch SN. Low stiffness floors can attenuate fall-related femoral impact forces by up to 50% without substantially impairing balance in older women. Accid Anal Prev. 2009;41(3): 642–50.
8. Ziden L, Frandin K, Kreuter M. Home rehabilitation after hip fracture. A randomized controlled study on balance confidence, physical function and everyday activities. Clin Rehabil. 2008;22(12): 1019–33.
9. Augenstein J, Digges K, Bahouth G, Dalmotas D, Perdeck E, Stratton J. Investigation of the performance of safety systems for protection of the elderly. Annu Proc Assoc Adv Automot Med. 2005;49:361–9.
10. NHTSAN. Traffic safety facts 2008: pedestrians. Washington, DC: Department of Transportation (US); 2008.
11. Dommes A, Cavallo V, Vienne F, Aillerie I. Age-related differences in street-crossing safety before and after training of older pedestrians. Accid Anal Prev. 2012;44(1):42–7.
12. Leden L, Garder P, Johansson C. Safe pedestrian crossings for children and elderly. Accid Anal Prev. 2006;38(2):289–94.
13. Hoxie RE, Rubenstein LZ. Are older pedestrians allowed enough time to cross intersections safely? J Am Geriatr Soc. 1994;42(3): 241–4.
14. Viamonte SM, Ball KK, Kilgore M. A cost-benefit analysis of risk-reduction strategies targeted at older drivers. Traffic Inj Prev. 2006;7(4):352–9 [Research Support, N.I.H., Extramural].
15. Gresset J, Meyer F. Risk of automobile accidents among elderly drivers with impairments or chronic diseases. Can J Public Health. 1994;85(4):282–5.
16. Koepsell TD, Wolf ME, McCloskey L, Buchner DM, Louie D, Wagner EH, et al. Medical conditions and motor vehicle collision injuries in older adults. J Am Geriatr Soc. 1994;42(7): 695–700.
17. Renner CH, Heldt KA, Swegle JR. Diurnal variation and injury due to motor vehicle crashes in older trauma patients. Traffic Inj Prev. 2011;12(6):593–8.
18. National Center on Elder Abuse. Elder Abuse Prevalence and Incidence. 2005. http://www.ncea.aoa.gov/Resources/Publication/docs/FinalStatistics050331.pdf. Last accessed Oct. 2013.
19. National Center on Elder Abuse at American Public Human Services Association. National elder abuse incidence study. Washington, DC: Department of Health and Human Services; 1998.
20. Cohen S, De Vos E, Newberger E. Barriers to physician identification and treatment of family violence: lessons from five communities. J Assoc Am Med Coll. 1997;72(1 Suppl):S19–25.
21. Hamilton GP. Prevent elder abuse – using a family systems approach. J Gerontol Nurs. 1989;15(3):21–6.
22. Clark-Daniels CL, Daniels RS, Baumhover LA. Abuse and neglect of the elderly: are emergency department personnel aware of mandatory reporting laws? Ann Emerg Med. 1990;19(9):970–7 [Research Support, Non-U.S. Gov't].

Outcomes for Surgical Care in the Elderly

22

Cathy A. Maxwell, Erin L. Rader, and William F. Fallon Jr.

Introduction

Many older adults in the USA are enjoying the benefits of living longer from excellent health care, with healthier and more active lives. This more active lifestyle can increase risk for injury [1]. Older trauma patients with only minor injury (ISS <9) have a higher mortality rate as compared with younger patients at each level of trauma severity [2]. Although survival is the immediate priority of acute care following trauma, trauma-related injury in older Americans increases disability, and the most significant impact of functional decline is loss of independence.

During the past two decades, *quality* in health care has become increasingly important with a subsequent rise in health services research and a focus on outcomes. Outcomes research examines *results* that can be used to advance evidence-based health care, promote accountability, and guide consumers in making informed decisions [3]. Outcomes research focuses on structures and processes that represent provider- and system-level efforts within a real-world context.

The focus of this chapter is on outcomes following traumatic injury in older adults. Patient characteristics associated with outcomes are addressed first. Next, the importance of functional status as a predictor of outcomes is emphasized through a more in-depth discussion of the definition, risk factors for functional decline, and principles of management. The need for comprehensive geriatric assessment is emphasized, and available instruments for assessment of functional status are presented. Finally, the chapter concludes with a review of treatment characteristics (attributes of the organization and processes of care) within the trauma literature that are associated with outcomes.

Since 1980, over 80 studies have examined outcomes after traumatic injury in older adults. The majority of studies are observational, with a preponderance of retrospective reviews of trauma registry data or other state, regional, or national datasets. Few prospective studies have been conducted, and no randomized controlled trials exist. Inclusion and exclusion criteria for patient samples vary from exclusive (excluded patients based on specific characteristics [e.g., hip fractures, injury severity score <16, admission <48 h]) single-site studies to inclusive (all patients 65 and older admitted with an injury ICD-9 code) multi-institutional studies. The majority of studies examine patient characteristics as predictors of outcomes and few examined structure or process (treatment) variables. In-hospital mortality was the most widely studied outcome. Table 22.1 provides an overview of outcome variables from a sample of published studies in the past 30 years.

Patient Characteristics and Outcomes

Patient characteristics (i.e., clinical characteristics and demographics) represent the patient's baseline status at the outset of treatment or usual status before injury. Patient characteristics are particularly important in older adults in light of increasing age, comorbidities, and declines in physiologic reserve, cognition, and functional ability. Failure to consider all potential risk factors in the data collection process can introduce bias that results in inaccurate conclusions [3]. Table 22.2 summarizes patient characteristic variables examined in a sample of older adult trauma studies.

C.A. Maxwell, RN, PhD
Vanderbilt University School of Nursing, 461 21st Avenue South, Nashville, TN 37240, USA
e-mail: cathy.maxwell@vanderbilt.edu

E.L. Rader, RN, MSN, BSN
Department of Geriatrics, MetroHealth Medical Center, 2500 MetroHealth Drive, Cleveland, OH 44109, USA
e-mail: radere@ccf.org

W.F. Fallon Jr., MD, MBA, FACS (✉)
Department of Surgery, VA New Jersey Healthcare System, East Orange Campus, 385 Tremont Avenue, East Orange, NJ 07018, USA
e-mail: fallonwmd@gmail.com

J.A. Yelon, F.A. Luchette (eds.), *Geriatric Trauma and Critical Care*,
DOI 10.1007/978-1-4614-8501-8_22, © Springer Science+Business Media New York 2014

Table 22.1 Summary of outcome variables in selected older adult trauma studies

Older adult trauma: outcome variables
In-hospital mortality [3–13]
Post-hospitalization mortality [7, 14–17]
Injury severity score (ISS) [8, 18–21]
Length of stay (hospital and ICU) [8, 9, 12, 18, 22–24]
Complications/adverse events [7, 23–26]
Functional status [9, 27–29]
Discharge disposition [8, 26, 30, 31]
Cost/resource utilization [18, 32–34]
Under-triage [35–37]
Likelihood of hospital admission [38]

Table 22.2 Summary of patient characteristic variables in selected older adult trauma studies

Older adult trauma: patient characteristic predictor variables
Age [7, 9, 10, 15, 20, 22, 26–28, 30, 32, 33, 35, 36, 39]
Injury severity [6, 7, 14, 21, 38, 40–47]
Gender [2, 7, 10, 11, 16, 22, 43, 44, 48]
Comorbidities [7, 10, 21, 26, 42, 48–50]
Mechanism of injury [5, 51, 52]
Complications/adverse events [5, 26, 41, 52–54]
Physiologic demise [20–22, 38, 48, 55–59]
Other (addressed in only one or two studies):
Race [10]
Number of injuries [26]
Presence of dementia [17]
Angle of impact [19]
Nonuse of restraints [19]
Injury to other occupants [19]
Post-hospitalization institutionalization [14]
Pre-injury status [14, 60]
Extremity injury [26]

In-Hospital Mortality (IHM)

The association of advancing age and increased IHM is validated in many studies; however, IHM rates within individual studies reflect differing inclusion criteria for study samples. Inclusive, multi-institutional studies report lower IHM than exclusive studies. For example, IHM ranged from 3.2 to 4.3 % in two inclusive multi-institutional studies [7, 10] and 15.8–17 % in exclusive single-center studies [18, 61]. Of note, an increased size and an inclusive scope of patients dilute overall IHM rates.

An increasing injury severity score is consistently associated with higher IHM. In two inclusive multicenter studies, higher injury severity (ISS) resulted in odds ratios for IHM ranging from 1.07 to 2.77 [10, 11]. Other studies [6, 8] compared ISS among different age groups. For example, one study ($N=802{,}211$) included patients with an ISS between 10 and 15 with a mortality rate in young patients (< age 60) of 1.4 % compared with 5.9 % for older patients (≥ age 60) ($p<.001$) [6]. In a second study ($N=7121$), the mortality rate for patients 18–64 years old was 2.6 % compared with 7.4 % for the cohort 65 years and older ($p<.05$) [8].

Several studies demonstrated a relationship between gender and higher IHM rate for males compared with females. For example, in three studies the odds ratios for IHM in males were 1.0 [21], 1.4 [7], and 2.05 [43], as compared with 1.0 [7, 43] and 0.66 [21] for females.

The influence of comorbidities on IHM was examined in several studies with varied results that appear to be dependent on sample inclusion criteria. For example, Pracht et al. [62] found that in patients aged 65–74, the probability of mortality increased as the number of comorbidities increased, while Labib et al. [5] found that in patients 65 years and older with an ISS of greater than 15, preexisting comorbidities were not associated with higher IHM.

Falls are the predominant mechanism of injury (MOI) in older adult trauma but carry a relatively low incidence of IHM. Richmond et al. [26] found that blunt trauma in older adults carried a lower odds ratio of IHM (0.35) compared to penetrating trauma. In other studies, pedestrian injuries and burn injuries were associated with higher mortality rates when compared with other mechanisms of injury [44, 46, 47, 55].

Complications (adverse events) have also been associated with IHM in several studies. Perdue et al. [42] examined infectious complications, Smith et al. [53] examined the number of complications, and Horst et al. [52] examined septic complications. Richmond et al. [26] reported odds ratios of IHM for select complications: cardiovascular complications (2.85), pulmonary complications (2.01), and other complications (2.15). More recently, Labib et al. [5] found that respiratory complications, in contrast to cardiac, renal, and neurologic complications, carried an increased risk for IHM. Adams et al. [25] reported that infectious complications peaked between age 45 and 65 and then declined with increasing age.

Abnormal admission vital signs after traumatic injury including systolic blood pressure, less than 90 mmHg, Glasgow Coma Scale score less than 15, pulse greater than 90, revised trauma score less than 112, and simplified acute physiologic score are associated with higher IHM [20–22, 38, 48, 55–59].

Post-Hospitalization Mortality (PHM)

Post-hospitalization mortality refers to death occurring at any time after discharge from the index hospitalization for injury. Various studies in injured older adults examined PHM at 30, 60, 90, 180, and 365 days post-discharge. The outcome of PMH is particularly important in this population and is perhaps more reflective of the complex interaction between injury and aging. For example, PHM will likely differ in a 79-year-old with significant pre-injury functional limitations and multiple injuries, compared with a highly active 79-year-old with multiple injuries. The effect of injury on the first patient may trigger a rapid decline resulting in death within 2 years, while the second patient may recover to a pre-injury status and survive 10 or more years.

A number of studies have examined the association between increasing age and PHM. Gorra et al. [7] reported IHM ranging from 3.2 to 3.7 % in four geographic regions, while 30-day mortality ranged from 2.8 to 3.5 % in four geographic regions. Clark et al. [16] found a 7.5 % 30-day mortality rate as compared to 3.7 % for IHM. Zarzaur et al. [15] reported a 79.6 % survival rate (20.4 % mortality) at 2 years post-injury in patients 75 and older. Gallagher et al. [63] reported a 2-year mortality rate of 36 % in patients 60 years and older, compared with 7 % in younger patients. More recently, Davidson et al. [14] examined PHM by age and other patient characteristics and found a significant PHM (16 % by 3 years) in injured patients; age was a strong predictor of PHM. These findings indicate that risk of mortality continues beyond hospital discharge. In fact, from a recent study that used Medicare Provider Analysis and Review (MEDPAR) data for the states of Oregon and Washington (2001/2002), Fleischman et al. [64] reported a continued rise in PHM with stabilization occurring at 6 months post-injury and 89 % of change occurring by 60 days. These findings encourage researchers to evaluate both IHM and PHM with caution and call for clinicians to place a greater emphasis on post-discharge care planning [64].

Other Outcomes

Length of stay (hospital and ICU) has been examined in several studies, showing associations among increasing age [8, 18], higher injury severity [31, 59], increased complications [23, 41], and increased length of stay (LOS). Studies have also reported associations between increasing age and *development of complications* [9, 18, 23, 25, 32]. Other studies have reported significant association between higher injury severity and development of complications [7, 26, 41]. Tornetta et al. [41] reported that injury severity predicted the development of acute respiratory distress syndrome, pneumonia, sepsis, and gastrointestinal complications. Bochicchio et al. [23] found that older patients who developed nosocomial infections had higher injury severity scores. Adams et al. [25] reported a significant breakpoint at age 45 for decubitus ulcers and acute renal failure with infectious complications peaking between age 45 and 65 and declining with increasing age. Finally, studies have examined advanced age and *under-triage* [35–37], suggesting that under-triage of injured older adults to non-trauma centers is significantly higher than in younger adults.

Functional Status

Functional status, as an outcome, has been examined in several studies [9, 27–29, 65, 66]. While methods of outcome measurement differed among studies, all studies found significant functional decline after injury in the elderly. Older persons, who are hospitalized for acute illnesses, including surgical interventions, are more prone to develop functional decline and are discharged to institutions for long-term care. While other age groups are recipients of long-term care services, the elderly constitute the largest consumers of long-term care, primarily through nursing home admissions [65]. More than 90 % of geriatric trauma patients required home or institutional nursing care 1 year after injury [47].

While it is important to understand the current and projected growth in numbers of the elderly, it is equally important to note that only a small percentage of this population are actually living in institutionalized care at any given point in time. Even previously independent elders become vulnerable as mobility, cognition, nutrition, and continence can be affected by traumatic injury and operative intervention, resulting in the need for long-term care. As noted previously in this chapter, patients with pre-trauma impairment and cognitive issues are at greatest risk.

Function can best be described as a continuum ranging from complete independence to prediction of death [66]. There is wide variability in the concept of what defines function in an older patient. Functional impairment can simply be defined as a decreased ability to meet one's own needs. Looked at comprehensively, function in older people includes independent performance of basic activities of daily living (ADL), social activities, or instrumental activities of daily living (IADLs), and the assistance needed to accomplish these tasks, as well as sensory ability, cognition, and capacity to ambulate.

Older patients also differ in aging physiology and anatomy compared to the young. Function is different and can be complicated in the older patient. Disease often presents first as functional loss in older persons, and conversely, functional loss can be the result of disease. Epidemiological studies demonstrate that pain, whatever the source, is overlooked as a potential cause of disability. Fall risk is increased with pain [67]. Symptoms from disabling movement disorders such as Parkinson's disease are varied and include tremor, rigidity, bradykinesia, akinesia, postural abnormalities, and dementia. In addition to fractures, osteoporosis can limit mobility by increasing the fear of falling in the elderly, leading to many of the complications associated with immobility [68]. Does identification of morbidity in older people add to understanding of function? Function in the elderly is more than motor ability and the capacity to perform. Do sensory deficits impair communication of needs? Does bladder incontinence contribute to a 70-year-old's social withdrawal?

Cognitive impairment, often underdiagnosed, is a risk factor for medication nonadherence and poor compliance which can lead to further decline in function. The actual reaching distance of an 82-year-old man in a wheelchair with a shoulder injury may be more predictive of function than measuring movement of abduction itself. The combination of arthritis and fractures on movement in navigating a two-story home highlights the need for a holistic understanding of physical function in an older person. Preservation in all spheres of function is critical to restoring independence.

While there are few longitudinal studies evaluating function after injury for older trauma patients, recent research has demonstrated the loss of one ADL in the year following an injury is significant. Limitation in ADL is a stronger predictor of hospital outcomes (functional decline, length of stay, institutionalization, and death) than the admitting diagnosis [69]. Previously injured older persons are at higher risk for recurrent injury when compared to those not previously injured [70].

It is important to recognize all risk factors for functional decline, including injuries, acute illness, medication side effects, pain, depression, malnutrition, decreased mobility, prolonged bed rest (including the use of physical restraints), chronic indwelling Foley catheters, and changes in living environment or routines. Complications that result from functional decline include loss of independence, falls, incontinence, malnutrition, decreased socialization, increased risk for long-term institutionalization, and depression [71]. Even during the recovery phase, common causes of general loss of function such as failure to thrive, weight loss, dehydration, and falls can be difficult to pinpoint. Decline can happen quickly, so prompt identification and treatment of the inciting problem is paramount to a good outcome.

Early identification and management of new or existing medical issues that complicate recovery after injury may improve outcomes for older patients. It is noted in the literature that higher morbidity in the geriatric trauma patient is associated with preexisting medical conditions, a decline in organ function, altered physiologic responses to minor injuries, and atypical symptoms and signs of injury [72]. A useful but *grim triad* offers some measure of predictability. Chronological age plus comorbid disease associated with even moderate injury overwhelms limited physiologic reserve and coping mechanisms for the geriatric trauma patient, which then impairs function [12].

Trauma encompasses the physical, psychological, and spiritual responses that can have an overwhelming impact on the vulnerable or frail older patient. Recent literature concludes that application of aggressive evaluation and resuscitation principles to the geriatric patient improves mortality and morbidity. Although geriatric surgery principles highlight the difference in care between the young and the old in the very early course of recovery, the risks and challenges that older trauma patients present require knowledge and application of principles of geriatric care beyond the acute treatment phase. Consistent utilization of three key principles can move the hospitalized elderly patient towards improved function: (1) treating the individual and not just the injury, (2) the alignment of team resources, and (3) improving function in the context of the care continuum.

Care must be taken to avoid agism. Stereotyping of older patients by health professionals may manifest through discriminatory communication and treatment [73]. Older people are not simply a cross section of a chronically diseased population. Geriatric psychological literature shows that the older a person becomes, the more diverse in personality she/he becomes from peers. To make sense of our world, we categorize; but health-care providers should not assume that older people are all alike. If we see patients as incompetent without assessing them, we will not give them choices or ask the serious questions that need to be answered concerning their care. If patients are seen as feeble and frail, we might assume that their premorbid ADL were minimal. Older patients need respect and a sense that they are viewed as individuals.

A complete history should focus on more than the traumatic event and should include a comprehensive geriatric history and assessment for not only care, but also better outcomes. Diminished pre-injury functional status is a leading predictor of poor outcomes. How well did the older patient function before the injury? How do the patient and family describe the patient's "normal" day-to-day routine? Many older people live with disability, and limited function may be a unique and satisfactory adaptation for them.

The social history is vital information at the time of admission. Documented assessments often contain scant statements such as "lives with spouse" or a social history that is "noncontributory." Knowledge that the elderly patient is a professor of literature at the local college and has been married for 49 years reflects a high functional level of independence. However, an injury which results in multiple rib fractures may significantly affect the patient's ability to return to this pre-injury ADL. After a lifetime of independent decision-making, patients may find themselves completely dependent with uncertain futures. The patient should be approached with respect and dignity as an individual and informed of choices tailored to him.

Assessing fear is critical. Fears, of death, pain, procedures, and the unknown, are more obvious in the hospital setting. Other fears might not be as obvious. If overwhelmed, the patient may become avoidant, resulting in missed therapies and regress back into inactivity. Asking the question: "What is your biggest fear right now?" can be helpful in planning care and in assisting patients who fear falling, nursing home placement, becoming a burden to their loved ones, and the inability to return to a previous level of functioning. Naming the fear out loud lessens its ability to create anxiety and depression that can inhibit healing. Appropriate support can be given to allay these fears and move older patients towards their goals.

Patient motivation as a facilitator of recovery is pivotal. The key to motivation is sharing in one's own goal setting. The older patient should participate in setting obtainable short-term goals and to pursue personal, realistic, and measurable long-term goals, such as attending family celebrations. The trauma team should emphasize function rather than dysfunction and demonstrate hope, optimism, and a sense of humor. The patient and family should be constantly educated regarding the value of independence and the consequences of decline. Recovery is a highly individualized process. By formulating what is desirable and achievable and understanding the older person's unique capacities and limitations, providers can facilitate preservation of as much independence and the sense of dignity as possible.

Continuum of care is a concept describing an integrated system of care that guides and tracks the patient over time through a comprehensive array of health disciplines and services spanning all levels of care. When the older injured patient enters this continuum, the process becomes complex. Although there is great variability in all aspects of presenting needs and care, elderly patients need follow-up through rehabilitation and eventual transition to independent living. The continuum of geriatric care focuses on the individual's functional abilities and resources in the context of the individual's disease or post-trauma state.

Specific changes in the provision of acute hospital care can improve the ability of a heterogeneous group of elderly patients to perform ADLs at the time of discharge from the hospital and can reduce the frequency of discharge to institutions for long-term care [74]. The assessment and treatment plan should be individualized, and it should be assessed and modified frequently throughout hospitalization based on the patient's response to treatment. Assessment tools and geriatric-focused clinical pathways can optimize systematic evaluation.

An argument opposing the use of functional assessment tools is that professionals should have the ability to accurately determine the needs of an older patient based on their years of clinical experience. Members of an interdisciplinary team may not agree on what to treat first and how to maintain the momentum of progress in the face of complications and setbacks that are common in older patients who are susceptible to functional decline.

Assessment Tools

The concept of functional assessment is to "measure change." There are several validated and reliable functional assessment tools used across disciplines for spheres of functionality. Functional assessment should be ongoing throughout hospitalization to make necessary adaptations and to maintain safety and independence.

The Functional Independence Measure (FIM) has been tested for adults of all ages. An analysis of the construct validity and retest reliability of the FIM for persons over age 80 revealed that the motor subscale of the FIM (items A–M) was both valid and stable; the cognitive subscale (items N–R) had construct validity but was less stable; the FIM score could be used to determine a rehabilitation efficiency ratio or the FIM change over the length of stay; and medical comorbidities correlated with lower rehabilitation efficiencies [75].

In the timed "Get up and Go" test, a patient is asked to rise from an armchair, walk 3 m (10 ft), return to the chair, and sit down. The score is the time in seconds it takes to complete this task. This test has significant inter-rater reliability as well as content reliability and predicts whether a patient can walk safely alone outside [76].

The Berg Balance Measure is a 56-point scale that evaluates performance during 14 common activities, including standing, turning, and reaching for an object on the floor. This test has high inter-rater and intra-rater reliability, and while designed to be use as a clinical assessment tool, the Berg Balance test scores were shown to correlate with laboratory test of balance [77].

The Katz Index of Independence in Activities of Daily Living, commonly referred to as the Katz ADL, is the most appropriate instrument to assess functional status as a measurement of the client's ability to perform ADL independently. Clinicians typically use the tool to detect problems in performing ADL and to plan care accordingly. The index ranks adequacy of performance in the six functions of bathing, dressing, toileting, transferring, continence, and feeding. Patients are scored yes/no for independence in each of the six functions. A score of 6 indicates full function, 4 indicates moderate impairment, and 2 or less indicates severe functional impairment [78].

The (Folstein) Mini-Mental State Exam (MMSE) contains questions on orientation, attention, and other cognitive functions. Contrary to popular opinion, it was not created as a diagnostic test for dementia, but is a brief screening tool that allows quantification of cognition over time. It may not detect dementia in people with premorbid high intellectual functioning, and it may inaccurately suggest dementia in cases of the dementia syndrome of depression, previously known as pseudodementia. Screening separately for both dementia and depression is important for determining the patient's ability to return to independent living [79].

The Geriatric Depression Scale – Short Form is a brief (15-item) questionnaire with yes/no answers that the patient can self-administer, and it has been validated in persons over 55 years old [80].

The Confusion Assessment Method (CAM) assesses for delirium and is not specific to the geriatric population. The CAM was designed for use in various clinical settings. It is simple to administer and designed for clinicians who are not psychiatrically trained [81].

There are many assessment tools for other conditions and syndromes in older adults, including falls, pain, and alcohol use. Clinical pathways are intended to address foreseeable aspects of the condition, enhance care, prevent complications, and reduce length of stay and costs. The American College of Emergency Physicians and American College of Surgeons have advocated for the development of evidence-based clinical protocols and pathways for both acute care and ongoing management of geriatric patients to improve functional outcomes [82, 83]. The American Geriatric Society Task Force on the Future of Geriatric Medicine has recommended optimizing the health of older persons by incorporating the principles of geriatric medicine into existing clinical guidelines [84].

Assessing Care Of Vulnerable Elders (ACOVE)

The ACOVE project, developed through expert consensus, assessed the medical conditions prevalent among the elderly that contribute to morbidity, mortality, and functional decline for which effective methods of treatment or prevention exist. For each condition, quality-of-care process indicators were identified to evaluate the care provided to vulnerable elders. ACOVE-3, the third phase of this project, was completed in 2007 and includes 392 quality indicators covering 26 different conditions in four domains of care: screening and prevention, diagnosis, treatment, and follow-up and continuity. Three of these conditions involve the most basic functions of the human body – cognition, ambulation/mobility, and elimination – which are of importance when assessing the decline of a patient's health due to aging. Available training modules focus on educating the providers about geriatric syndromes, including cognitive impairment, falls and mobility disorders, and urinary incontinence [85].

The Vulnerable Elderly Survey-13 (VES-13) is a function-based tool that relies on patient self-reporting living independently in the community to identify older persons at risk for health decline. The VES-13 considers age, self-rated health, limitations in physical function, and functional disabilities. The feasibility of using the VES-13 was tested as part of the ACOVE project, an initiative to develop tools for measuring quality of care for elders at increased risk for a decline in health. The investigators who developed and assessed the ACOVE used the VES-13 to screen 2,200 elders by telephone. The average time to complete the screening was less than 5 min [86]. The VES-13 has been validated on uninjured older populations and has been used to predict risk of death and functional decline in the next 12 months in vulnerable elderly patients [87].

In a recent prospective observational pilot study at a Level I TC, investigators examined whether the VES-13 pre-injury score (the higher the score, the higher the risk) would predict complications or mortality in combination with injury severity. The study controlled for ISS and comorbidity and found that each additional VES-13 point was associated with greater risk of complication or death. The authors suggested that the VES-13 might be a useful tool to predict complications and death in older adults with traumatic injury if utilized early in the hospitalization [88]. The VES-13 may help to identify patients at risk for a decline in health who would benefit from geriatric trauma clinical pathways and a geriatric team approach.

Just as aggressive care and resuscitation after trauma can contribute to better outcomes, optimization of comorbid conditions, prevention of complications, and preservation of function can help towards maintenance of ADL performance. Early recognition of functional, cognitive, and affective impairment through team assessment and utilization of available tools can enable prompt and appropriate management through the use of geriatric principles and care pathways aimed at improving functional outcomes. Utilizing the continuum of care concept, interdisciplinary assessment, and proactive management in providing a framework for delivery of optimal health care to the older patient population may influence a reduction in the incidence and prevalence of functional decline, as well as a decrease in morbidity associated with functional decline.

Treatment Characteristics and Outcomes

Studies that have examined advanced age and *under-triage* [35–37] reveal that under-triage of injured older adults to non-trauma centers is significantly higher than in younger adults. An implication of this finding is that treatment characteristics, including the setting in which care was provided, attributes of the organization itself, and processes of care, are important aspects contributing to outcomes of geriatric trauma [3]. Within the older adult trauma population, treatment characteristics have not been studied as rigorously as in younger patients. Table 22.3 provides a summary of studies that have examined outcomes in geriatric trauma.

Table 22.3 Older adult trauma studies: treatment characteristics and outcome

Study		Outcomes							
Author (year)	Treatment characteristic	In-hospital mortality/ survival	Post-hospitalization Mortality/ Survival	Hospital LOS and (ICU LOS)	DC disposition	Complications	Time to OR	Triage to a trauma center	Reimbursement
Mangram et al. (2012) [24]	Multidisciplinary trauma service model	–	–	X	–	X	X	–	–
Pandya et al. (2011) [4]	Trauma volume – age – ICISS	X	–	–	–	–	–	–	–
Pracht et al. (2011) [62]	Designated trauma centers	X	–	–	–	–	–	–	–
Gorra et al. (2008) [7]	Geographic location	X	X	X	–	–	–	–	–
Clark et al. (2007) [89]	Increased hospital volume	X	–	–	–	–	–	–	–
Fallon et al. (2006) [12]	Geriatric trauma team	X	–	X	X	–	–	–	–
Lane et al. (2003) [37]	Prehospital assessment	–	–	–	–	–	–	X	–
Demetriades et al. (2002) [90]	Trauma team activation policy	X	–	–	–	–	–	–	–
Meldon et al. (2002) [13]	Trauma center care	X	–	–	–	–	–	–	–
Mann et al. (2001) [10]	Presence of trauma system	X	–	–	–	–	–	–	–
Rzepka et al. (2001) [11]	Trauma center care	X	–	–	–	–	–	–	–
Tepas et al. (2000) [91]	Trauma center care	X	–	–	–	–	–	–	–
DeMaria et al. (1988) [32]	DRG payments	–	–	–	–	–	–	–	X

Trauma Centers and Outcomes

From the Major Trauma Outcomes Study (MTOS) [92] data, Meldon et al. [13] examined patients age 80 and older for associations between trauma center (TC) verification and IHM. Comparisons were made between levels I and II trauma centers and non-trauma centers. The mean age of patients was higher in level II centers and non-TCs; ISS was lower in level II centers and non-TCs [13]. The mortality rate was significantly lower in level II TCs (5.2 %) compared with level I TCs (24 %) and non-TCs (9.9 %) [13]. Of note, the MTOS [92] is an exclusive multisite study of all trauma patients from more than 140 hospitals in the USA, Canada, Australia, and the UK. All trauma centers participating in the study submitted data according to one or two sets of inclusion criteria (all hospital admissions related to trauma or all injured patients admitted to intensive care during the hospital stay). The authors acknowledged that conclusions drawn for all injured patients could be inappropriate.

Rzepka et al. [11] examined differences in care at TCs and non-TCs. Level I TCs admitted a greater proportion of younger patients and patients with more severe injuries. Level I TCs were found to have a greater odds ratio for inpatient death (1.49, $p<0.0001$) when compared with levels II and III TCs and non-TCs. Tepas et al. [91] used a computer model to calculate the probability of survival for specific diagnoses using a study population of 698,187 patients. For patients age 55 and older, mortality was 5.5 % in TCs and 3.0 % in non-TCs. The findings were explained by a higher injury severity score for patients admitted to the trauma centers. When probability of survival was included as a variable in the model, the authors concluded that potentially preventable mortality was significantly lower in TCs, but the lower ISS group at the non-trauma centers was not statistically significant.

Pracht et al. [62] analyzed trauma center effectiveness in Florida hospitals. The study indicated that patients admitted to a trauma center with an increased risk for death, i.e., patients aged 65–74 years, had a survival advantage of 7.2 % ($p<.05$) compared to patients taken to a non-trauma center [62]. Differences in mortality rate in patients with lower injury severity were not statistically significant [62].

Trauma Team Activation and Outcomes

Demetriades et al. [90] studied the impact of trauma team activation on outcome for patients older than 70 years. Mortality in patients with an ISS greater than 15 was significantly lower after using age of 70 as an activation criteria (53.8 % vs. 34.2 %, $p=0.003$) [90]. The same benefit in mortality was seen for patients with an ISS greater than 20 (68.4 % vs. 46.9 %, $p=0.01$) [90].

Geographic Location and Outcomes

Gorra et al. [7] studied survival and LOS for injured older adults by the US geographic regions. Females comprised 73 % of the population and 58.7 % were age 80 or older. IHM and 30-day mortality were examined with paradoxical findings. Adjusted odds ratios predicting IHM were West 1.00, Midwest (MW) 1.08, South 1.11, and Northeast (NE) 1.13, while odds ratios for 30-day mortality were West 1.00, MW 1.00, South 0.94, and NE 0.90 ($p<0.05$) [5]. Individual differences in hospital definitions of mortality or early discharge of patients to other facilities prior to death may explain geographic differences [7]. In the same study, hospital LOS was also studied by region. The LOS in days for patients discharged home were West 4.0, Midwest 4.1, South 4.5, and NE 5.2. The hospital LOS for patients discharged to long-term care were West 5.6, Midwest 5.9, South 6.3, and NE 7.1 [7]. For patients who died in the hospital, LOS were West 7.2, Midwest 6.9, South 8.4, and Northeast 9.9 [7]. The authors concluded that the findings were due to differences in access to subacute care facilities and trauma systems in rural versus urban areas [7].

Other Treatment Characteristics and Outcomes

From an analysis of Medicare records, Clark et al. [89] examined survival of older trauma patients with severe injuries to determine whether differences existed by trauma center volume. The study found no difference in 30-day survival between patients taken first to low-volume hospitals compared with patients taken directly to high-volume hospitals. In contrast, Pandya et al. [4] reported a risk-adjusted advantage for geriatric patients injured in a motor vehicle crash (MVC) treated at higher-volume trauma centers in comparison to younger MVC patients and non-trauma geriatric admissions. As noted earlier, differences in inclusion/exclusion criteria of patient samples likely explain these findings.

Mann et al. [10] examined differences in survival between a pre-system phase and an early trauma system implementation phase. No differences in survival within 60 days after injury were found between the two phases. However, for patients with an ISS greater than 15, risk-adjusted survival at 60 days was 5.1 % ($p=0.03$) higher among patients in the trauma system implementation phase [10].

DeMaria et al. [32] studied 82 older injured patients for costs of trauma care and projected DRG reimbursement. Costs dramatically exceeded reimbursement in patients over the age of 80, patients with severe injuries, and patients with complications. The daily costs for patients who died were excessive, reflecting the aggressive care rendered to patients.

Geriatric Consultation and Outcomes

Fallon et al. [12] examined outcomes in older injured adults who received focused attention from a geriatric trauma (consultation) team (GTT) compared with patients who were not seen by the GTT. The study demonstrated marked improvements in management practices for patients seen by a GTT, including advanced care planning, disposition to promote function, medication management, treatment of dementia or delirium, and pain management [12]. Mean age, ISS, and LOS were all higher in patients seen by the GTT. However, the mortality rates were not significantly different for the two groups (4.3 % vs. 18 %). The group without a GTT consultation was younger, predominantly male gender, and had a greater incidence of subdural hematoma [10]. The group who had a GTT had a shorter LOS (7.3 vs. 3.0, $p=0.001$) and were more likely to be discharge home (28 % vs. 40 %, $p=0.001$).

Mangram et al. [24] examined the effectiveness of an inpatient geriatric trauma unit with a multidisciplinary trauma service. Four "time-to-care" goals were established and twice-weekly multidisciplinary rounds were made to address patient care issues. There was a statistically significant reduction in emergency department LOS, time to the operating room, ICU LOS, and hospital LOS as compared to patients cared for prior to establishment of the dedicated geriatric unit [24]. In addition, complications (i.e., urinary tract infections, respiratory failure, and pneumonia) were significantly reduced [24].

The developing body of studies devoted to elder injured *outcomes* validate patient characteristics associated with worse outcomes following hospitalization, including older age, higher ISS, comorbidities, complications, functional impairment, and cognitive impairment. Systematic reviews examining treatment characteristics associated with outcomes among all hospitalized older adults show that interventions addressing geriatric-specific conditions improve outcomes (i.e., functional status, incidence of delirium, and hospital length of stay) [93–97]. Just as aggressive care and resuscitation following trauma can have a dramatic effect in improving outcomes, optimization of care, and comorbid conditions, prevention of complications can all be associated with improvement in ADL performance. Early recognition of functional, cognitive, and affective impairment through team assessment and tools can enable prompt and appropriate management utilizing geriatric principles and care pathways to improve functional outcomes. Utilizing the continuum of care concept in providing a framework for delivery of optimal health care to the geriatric population along with evidence of continued interdisciplinary assessments, proactive management, and evaluation of care related to function may influence a reduction in incidence and prevalence of function decline and a decrease in morbidity associated with functional decline.

References

1. Callaway D, Wolfe R. Geriatric trauma. Emerg Med. 2007;25(3):837–60.
2. Clark D, Chu M. Increasing importance of the elderly in a trauma system. Am J Emerg Med. 2002;20(2):108–11.
3. Kane R. Understanding health care outcomes research. 2nd ed. Boston: Jones & Bartlett Publishers; 2006.
4. Pandya SR, Yelon JA, Sullivan TS, Risucci DA. Geriatric motor vehicle collision survival: the role of institutional trauma volume. J Trauma. 2011;70(6):1326–30.
5. Labib N, Nouh T, Winocour S, Deckelbaum D, Banici L, Fata P, et al. Severely injured geriatric population: morbidity, mortality, and risk factors. J Trauma. 2011;71(6):1908–14.
6. Schifflette V, Lorenzo M, Mangram A, Truitt M, Amon J, Dunn E. Should age be a factor to change from a level II to a level I trauma activation? J Trauma. 2010;69(1):88–92.
7. Gorra A, Clark D, Mullins R, DeLorenzo M. Regional variation in hospital mortality and 30-day mortality for injured Medicare patients. World J Surg. 2008;32(6):954–9.
8. Sharma O, Oswanski M, Sharma V, Stringfellow K, Raj S. An appraisal of trauma in the elderly. Am Surg. 2007;73(4):354–8.
9. Grossman M, Scaff D, Miller D, Reed J, Hoey B, Anderson H. Functional outcomes in octogenarian trauma. J Trauma. 2003;55(1):26–32.
10. Mann C, Calm R, Mullins R, Brand D, Jurkovich G. Survival among injured geriatric patients during construction of a statewide trauma system. J Trauma. 2001;50(6):1111–6.
11. Rzepka SG, Malangoni MA, Rimm AA. Geriatric trauma hospitalization in the United States: a population-based study. J Clin Epidemiol. 2001;54(6):627–33.
12. Fallon W, Rader E, Zyzanski S, Mancuso C, Martin B, Breedlove L, et al. Geriatric outcomes are improved by a geriatric trauma consultation service. J Trauma. 2006;61(5):1040–6.
13. Meldon S, Reilly M, Drew B, Mancuso C, Fallon W. Trauma in the very elderly: a community-based study of outcomes at trauma and non-trauma centers. J Trauma. 2002;52(1):79–84.
14. Davidson GH, Hamlat CA, Rivara FP, Koepsell TD, Jurlovich GJ, Arbabi S. Long-term survival of adult trauma patients. JAMA. 2011;305(10):1001–7.
15. Zarzaur B, Magnotti L, Croce M, Haider A, Fabian T. Long-term survival and return on investment after nonneurologic injury: implications for the elderly trauma patient. J Trauma. 2010;69(1):93–8.
16. Clark D, DeLorenzo M, Lucan F, Weinberg D. Epidemiology and short-term outcomes of injured Medicare patients. J Am Geriatr Soc. 2004;52(12):2023–30.
17. Battistella F, Din A, Perez L. Trauma patients 75 years and older: long-term follow-up results justify aggressive management. J Trauma. 1998;44(4):618–24.8.
18. Newell M, Rotondo M, Toschlog E, Waibel B, Savraves S, Schenarts P, et al. The elderly trauma patient: an investment for the future? J Trauma. 2009;67(2):337–40.
19. Scheetz L. Using crash scene variables to predict the need for trauma center care in older persons. Res Nurs Health. 2007;30(4):399–412.
20. Hannan E, Waller C, Farrell L, Rosati C. Elderly trauma inpatients in New York State: 1994–1998. J Trauma. 2004;56(6):1297–304.
21. Grossman M, Miller D, Scaff D, Arcona S. When is an elder old? Effect of preexisting conditions on mortality in geriatric trauma. J Trauma. 2002;52(2):242–6.
22. Taylor M, Tracy K, Meyer W, Pasquale M, Napolitano L. Trauma in the elderly: intensive care unit resource use and outcome. J Trauma. 2002;53(3):407–14.
23. Bochicchio G, Hoshi M, Knorr K, Scalea T. Impact of nosocomial infections in trauma: does age make a difference? J Trauma. 2001;50(4):612–9.
24. Mangram AJ, Mitchell CD, Shifflette VK, Lorenzo M, Truitt MS, Goel A, et al. Geriatric trauma service: a one-year experience. J Trauma. 2012;72(1):119–22.
25. Adams SD, Cotton BA, McGuire MF, Dipasupil E, Podbielski JM, Zaharia A, et al. Unique pattern of complications in elderly trauma patients at a level I trauma center. J Trauma. 2012;72(1):112–8.
26. Richmond T, Kauder D, Strumpf N, Meredith T. Characteristics and outcomes of serious traumatic injury in older adults. J Am Geriatr Soc. 2002;50(2):215–22.
27. Richmond T, Thompson H, Kauder D, Robinson K, Strumpf N. A feasibility study of methodological issues and short-term outcomes in seriously injured older adults. Am J Crit Care. 2006;15(2):158–65.
28. McGwin G, Melton S, May A, Rue L. Long-term survival in the elderly after trauma. J Trauma. 2000;49(3):470–6.
29. DeMaria E, Kenney P, Merriam M, Casanova L, Gann D. Aggressive trauma care benefits the elderly. J Trauma. 1987;27(11):1200–6.
30. Bennett K, Scarborough J, Vaslef S. Outcomes and health care resource utilization in super-elderly trauma patients. J Surg Res. 2010;163(1):127–31.
31. Nagy K, Smith R, Roberts R, Joseph K, Bokhari R, Barrett J. Prognosis of penetrating trauma in elderly patients: a comparison with younger patients. J Trauma. 2000;49(2):190–4.
32. DeMaria E, Merriam M, Casanova L, Gann D, Kenney P. DRG payments adequately reimburse the costs of trauma care in geriatric patients? J Trauma. 1988;28(8):1244–9.
33. Osler T, Hales K, Back B, Bear K, Hsi K, Pathak D, et al. Trauma in the elderly. Am J Surg. 1988;156(6):537–43.
34. Weingarten M. Trauma and aging effects on hospital costs and length of stay. Ann Emerg Med. 1988;17(1):34–7.
35. Hsia RY, Wang E, Saynina O, Wise P, Perez-Stable EJ, Auerbach A. Factors associated with trauma center use for elderly patients with trauma. Arch Surg. 2011;146(5):585–92.
36. Chang D, Bass R, Cornwell E, MacKenzie E. Undertriage of elderly trauma patients to state-designated trauma centers. Arch Surg. 2008;143(8):776–81.
37. Lane P, Sorondo B, Kelly J. Geriatric trauma patients – are they receiving trauma center care? Acad Emerg Med. 2003;10(3):244–50.
38. Peschman J, Neideen T, Brasel K. The impact of discharging minimally injured trauma patient: does age play a role in trauma admission? J Trauma. 2011;70(6):1331–6.
39. Demetriades D, Sava J, Alo K, Newton E, Velhamos G, Murray J, et al. Old age as a criterion for trauma team activation. J Trauma. 2001;51(4):754–7.
40. Ferrera P, Bartfield J, D'Andrea C. Outcomes of admitted geriatric trauma victims. Am J Emerg Med. 2000;18(5):575–80.

41. Tornetta P, Mostafavi J, Riina J, Turen C, Reimer B, Levine R, et al. Morbidity and mortality in elderly trauma patients. J Trauma. 1999;46(4):702–6.
42. Perdue P, Watts D, Kaufmann C, Trask A. Differences in mortality between elderly and younger adult trauma patients: geriatric status increases risk of delayed death. J Trauma. 1998;45(4):805–10.
43. Gubler K, Davis R, Koepsell T, Soderberg R, Maier R, Rivara F. Long-term survival of elderly trauma patients. Arch Surg. 1997; 132(9):1010–4.
44. Knudson M, Lieberman J, Morris J, Cushing B, Stubbs H. Mortality factors in geriatric blunt trauma patients. Arch Surg. 1994;129(4): 448–53.
45. Van Aalst J, Morris J, Yates K, Miller R, Bass S. Severely injured geriatric patients return to independent living: a study of factors influencing function and independence. J Trauma. 1991;31(8):1096–102.
46. Sklar D, DeMarest G, McFeeley P. Increased pedestrian mortality among the elderly. Am J Emerg Med. 1989;7(4):387–90.
47. Oreskovich M, Howard J, Copass M, Carrico J. Geriatric trauma: injury patterns and outcome. J Trauma. 1984;24(7):565–72.
48. Nirula R, Gentilello L. Futility of resuscitation criteria for the "young' old and the "old" old trauma patient: a national trauma data bank analysis. J Trauma. 2004;63(5):965–71.
49. Milzman D, Boulanger B, Rodriguez A, Soderstrom C, Mitchell K, Magnant C. Pre-existing disease in trauma patients: a predictor of fate independent of age and injury severity score. J Trauma. 1992;32(2):236–44.
50. Morris J, MacKenzie E, Edelstein S. The effect of pre-existing conditions on mortality in trauma patients. JAMA. 1990;263(14): 1942–6.
51. Zautcke J, Coker S, Morris R, Stein-Spencer L. Geriatric trauma in the state of Illinois: substance use and injury patterns. Am J Emerg Med. 2002;20(1):14–7.
52. Horst H, Obeid F, Sorensen V, Bivins B. Factors influencing survival of elderly trauma patients. Crit Care Med. 1986;14(8): 681–4.
53. Smith D, Enderson B, Maull K. Trauma in the elderly: determinants of outcome. South Med J. 1990;83(2):171–7.
54. DeMaria E, Kenney P, Merriam M, Casanova L, Gann D. Survival after trauma in geriatric patients. Ann Surg. 1987;206(6):738–43.
55. Hui T, Avital I, Soukiasian H, Margulies D, Shabot M. Intensive care unit outcome of vehicle-related injury in elderly trauma patients. Am Surg. 2002;68(12):1111–4.
56. Davis J, Kaups K. Base deficit in the elderly: a marker of severe injury and death. J Trauma. 1998;45(5):873–7.
57. Shabot M, Johnson C. Outcome from critical care in the "oldest old" trauma patients. J Trauma. 1995;39(2):254–60.
58. Johnson C, Margulies D, Kearney T, Hiatt J, Shabot M. Trauma in the elderly: an analysis of outcomes based on age. Am Surg. 1994;60(11):899–902.
59. Pellicane J, Byrne K, DeMaria E. Preventable complications and death from multiple organ failure among geriatric trauma victims. J Trauma. 1992;33(3):440–4.
60. McGwin G, May A, Melton S, Reiff D, Rue L. Recurrent trauma in elderly patients. Arch Surg. 2001;136(2):197–203.
61. Young J, Cephas G, Blow O. Outcome and cost of trauma among the elderly: a real life model of a single-payer reimbursement system. J Trauma. 1998;45(4):800–4.
62. Pracht EE, Langland-Orban B, Flint L. Survival advantage for elderly trauma patients treated in a designated trauma center. J Trauma. 2011;71(1):69–77.
63. Gallagher S, Williams B, Gomez C, DesJardins C, Swan S, Durham M, et al. The role of cardiac morbidity in short- and long-term mortality in injured older patients who survive initial resuscitation. Am J Surg. 2003;185(2):131–4.
64. Fleischman RJ, Adams AL, Hedges JR, Ma OJ, Mullins RJ, Newgard CD. The optimum follow-up period for assessing mortality outcomes in injured older adults. J Am Geriatr Soc. 2010; 58(10):1843–9.
65. Institute of Medicine. Improving the quality of care in nursing homes. Washington, DC: National Academy Press; 2000. www.ncbi.nlm.nih.gov/books.
66. Pearson V. Assessment of function. In: Kane RL, Kane RA, editors. Assessing older persons: measures, meaning, and practical applications. New York: Oxford University Press; 2000. p. 17–48.
67. American Geriatrics Society, British Geriatrics Society, & American Academy of Orthopaedic Surgeons on Falls Prevention. Guidelines for the prevention of falls in older persons. J Am Geriatr Soc. 2001;49:664–72.
68. Lim P, Brander V, Kaelin D, et al. Rehabilitation of orthopedic and rheumatologic disorders. Arch Phys Med Rehabil. 2000;8 Suppl 1: 55–9.
69. Kelly-Quon L, et al. Functional status after injury: a longitudinal study of geriatric trauma. Am Surg. 2010;76(10):1055–8.
70. Rue L, Reiff D, Melton S, et al. Recurrent trauma in elderly patients. Arch Surg. 2001;136(2):197–203.
71. Kresevic D, et al. A patient-centered model of acute care for elder. Nurs Clin North Am. 1998;3:515–27.
72. Campbell J, DeGolia P, Fallon W, Rader E. In harm's way: moving the older trauma patient toward a better outcome. Geriatrics. 2009;64(1):8–13, 28.
73. Zebrowitz L, Montepare J. Too young, too old: stigmatizing adolescents and elders. In: Heatherton T, Kelck R, Hebl M, Hull J, editors. The social psychology of stigma. New York: Guilford Press; 2000. p. 334–73.
74. Williams S, Jones P, Pofahl W. Preoperative management of the older patient-a surgeon's perspective: part II. Clin Geriatr. 2006; 14(7):24–8.
75. Pollak N, et al. Reliability and validity of the FIM for persons aged 80 years and above from a multilevel continuing care retirement community. Arch Phys Med Rehabil. 1996;77(10):1056–61.
76. Podsiadlo D, Richardson S. The timed "Up & Go": a test of basic functional mobility for frail elderly persons. J Am Geriatr Soc. 1991;39(2):142–8.
77. Berg K, Maki B, Williams J, et al. Clinical and laboratory measures of postural balance in an elderly population. Arch Phys Med Rehabil. 1992;73(11):1073–80.
78. Katz S. Assessing self-maintenance: activities of daily living, mobility and instrumental activities of daily living. J Am Geriatr Soc. 1983;31(12):721–6.
79. Tombaugh T, McIntyre N. The mini-mental state examination: a comprehensive review. J Am Geriatr Soc. 1992;40(9):922–35.
80. Yesavage J, Brink T, Rose T, et al. Development and validation of a geriatric depression screening scale: a preliminary report. J Psychiatr Res. 1982–1983;17(1):37–49.
81. Inouye S, VanDyck C, Alessi C, et al. Clarifying confusion: the confusion assessment method. A new method for detection of delirium. Ann Intern Med. 1990;113(12):941–8.
82. American College of Emergency Physicians. Report on the future of geriatric care in our nation's emergency departments: impact and implications. Irving: American College of Surgeons; 2008. apps.acep.org.
83. American College of Surgeons, Committee on Trauma. Resources for optimal care of the injured patient. Chicago: American College of Surgeons; 2006. www.facs.org/trauma.
84. American Geriatrics Society. Comprehensive geriatric assessment position statement. Ann Long Term Care. 2006;14(3):34–6.
85. Wenger N, Roth C, Shekelle P. Introduction to the assessing care of vulnerable elders-3 quality indicator measurement set. J Am Geriatr Soc. 2007;55(S2):247–52.
86. Saliba S, Elliott M, Rubenstein L, et al. The vulnerable elders survey (VES-13): a tool for identifying vulnerable elders in the community. J Am Geriatr Soc. 2001;49:1691–9.

87. Min L, Elliot M, Wenger N, et al. Higher vulnerable elders survey scores predict death and functional decline in vulnerable older people. J Am Geriatr Soc. 2006;54(3):507–11.
88. Min L, Ubhayakar N, Saliba D, et al. The vulnerable elders survey-13 predicts hospital complications and mortality in older adults with traumatic injury: a pilot study. J Am Geriatr Soc. 2011;59(8):1471–6.
89. Clark D, DeLorenzo M, Lucas F, Cushing B. Initial presentation of older injured patients to high-volume hospitals is not associated with lower 30-day mortality in Medicare data. Crit Care Med. 2007;35(8):1829–36.
90. Demetriades D, Karaiskakis M, Velmahos G, Alo K, Newton E, Murray J, et al. Effect on outcome of early intensive management of geriatric trauma patients. Br J Surg. 2002;89(10):1319–22.
91. Tepas J, Veldenz H, Lottenberg L, Romig L, Pearman A, Hamilton B, et al. Elderly injury: a profile of trauma experience in the sunshine (retirement) state. J Trauma. 2000;48(4):581–6.
92. Champion H, Copes W, Sacco W, Lawnick M, Keast S, Bain L, et al. The major trauma outcome study: establishing national norms for trauma care. J Trauma. 1990;30(11):1356–65.
93. Campbell S, Seymour G, Primrose W. A systematic literature review of factors affecting outcome in older medical patients admitted to hospital. Age Ageing. 2004;33(2):110–5.
94. McCusker J, Kakuma R, Abrahamowicz M. Predictors of functional decline in hospitalized elderly patients: a systematic review. J Gerontol A Biol Sci Med Sci. 2002;57(9):M569–77.
95. Hoogerduijn J, Schurmans M, Duijnstee M, Rooij S, Grypdonck M. A systematic review of predictors and screening instruments to identify older hospitalized patients at risk for functional decline. J Clin Nurs. 2006;16(1):46–57.
96. Hickman L, Newton P, Halcomb E, Chang E, Davidson P. Best practice interventions to improve the management of older people in acute care settings: a literature review. J Adv Nurs. 2007;60(2):113–26.
97. Bachmann S, Finger C, Huss A, Egger M, Stuck A, Clough-Gorr K. In-patient rehabilitation specifically designed for geriatric patients: systematic review and meta-analysis of randomized controlled trials. BMJ. 2010;340:c1718. doi:10.1136/bmj.cl1718.

Geriatric Neurotrauma

23

Jack Wilberger and Diana J. Jho

Introduction

> The ageing process is, of course, a biological reality which has its own dynamic, largely beyond human control. However, it is also subject to the constructions by which each society makes sense of old age. In the developed world, chronological time plays a paramount role. The age of 60 or 65 years, roughly equivalent to retirement ages in most developed countries, is said to be the beginning of old age. In many parts of the developing world, chronological time has little or no importance in the meaning of old age. Other socially constructed meanings of age are more significant, such as the roles assigned to older people; in some cases it is the loss of roles accompanying physical decline which are significant in defining old age. Thus, in contrast to the chronological milestones which mark life stages in the developed world, old age in many developing countries is seen to begin at the point when active contribution is no longer possible. [1]

Geriatric trauma patients represent a unique subset of the trauma population and require special considerations in evaluation and treatment. As the years in age increases, so does the number of comorbidities. The elderly also have less physiologic reserve than their younger counterparts. As the body matures, physiologic changes occur that make it more likely to sustain injuries such as decreased visual acuity, diminished hearing, loss of proprioception, slower reflexes, and atrophy of muscles. Atrophy of the brain, adherence of the dura to the skull, arthritic changes of the spine are some of the physiologic changes that occur to make the elderly more susceptible to greater injuries with minor forces. The mechanism of injury differs in the elderly with falls and motor vehicle accidents accounting for the majority of head injuries [2–5].

Traumatic brain injury (TBI) has been extensively studied in order to better understand its pathophysiology and prolonged neurological and behavioral effects. It has been defined by various groups as recently as 2010 as "an alteration in brain function or other evidence of brain pathology caused by an external force" [6]. Overwhelming evidence suggest that those at highest risk for associated TBI morbidity and mortality are the geriatric population, especially those patients 65 years and older [7–16]. This increased mortality is not necessarily dependent on the injury or its severity, but rather elderly patients with mild injuries do not recover as well as a younger counterpart with more severe trauma [7, 10, 11, 13, 17–19].

Normal physiologic changes with aging may contribute to the worse outcomes in this patient population following trauma. As a result, it is necessary to evaluate, treat, and manage these patients as a unique patient group in an attempt to optimize outcomes in emergency, inpatient, and rehabilitation settings. Indeed, however, there is very little literature on age-appropriate care, and optimal care may be difficult to achieve. For example, TBI may not be suspected in an elderly patient who presents with symptoms of delirium, dementia, or psychosis, yet head injuries may cause similar cognitive and behavioral signs [20]. Care may be further compromised in the elderly due to medical comorbidities, especially those associated with anticoagulation therapy.

This chapter will review the unique injuries that the geriatric population may sustain, the physiologic changes that occur that make the elderly population more susceptible to certain injury patterns, and the special considerations necessary to effectively treat the geriatric TBI patient.

Epidemiology

In general, the geriatric population is considered to be those aged 65 and over, although there is no uniform consensus. In Britain, the Friendly Societies Act enacted the definition of old age as "any age after 50," but pension plans mostly used ages 60 or 65 years for eligibility [21]. In specific areas of Africa, the World Health Organization (WHO) has proposed ages greater than 50 to be considered the elderly population.

J. Wilberger, MD, FAANS, FACS (✉)
Department of Neurosurgery, Allegheny General Hospital,
420 East North Avenue, Suite 302, Pittsburgh, PA 15212, USA
e-mail: jwilberg@wpahs.org

D.J. Jho
Department of Neurosurgery, Allegheny General Hospital,
320 East North Street, Suite 302, Pittsburgh, PA 15212, USA
e-mail: djho@wpahs.org

J.A. Yelon, F.A. Luchette (eds.), *Geriatric Trauma and Critical Care*,
DOI 10.1007/978-1-4614-8501-8_23, © Springer Science+Business Media New York 2014

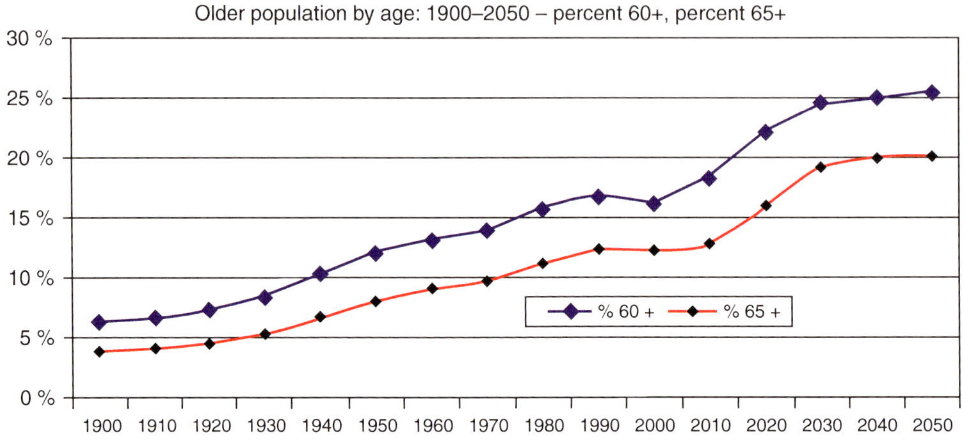

Fig. 23.1 Data and projections for the US population from the US Census Bureau [24]

Within the United States, the geriatric population is increasing in number as the "baby-boomer" generation ages. The 2010 US census predicts that the older population in the USA will double from the current 35 million to 70 million by 2030 and 86 million in 2050 [22]. This increase in the geriatric population has been observed worldwide. For example, the elderly constitutes about 15 % of the population in the United Kingdom [23]. In 2010, the United States census estimated that 13 % of the population were 65 years and older. By 2050, the census predicts that over 20 % of the US population will fall in that age group [24]. Costs to the healthcare system are high with estimates exceeding 2.2 billion total in 2003 [12] and $70,000, per person per year in 2005 [25].

The Centers for Disease Control (CDC) regards traumatic brain injury as a public health problem (Fig. 23.1). The CDC reports 1.7 million people of all ages sustain traumatic brain injury (TBI) every year [26]. In the geriatric population, emergency room visits, hospitalization rates, and deaths significantly increased between 2002 and 2006 [26]. TBI is responsible for more than 80,000 emergency department visits each year in people aged 65 and older, approximately three-quarters of which result in hospitalization [12]. In the elderly, falls are the leading cause of TBI for older adults (51 %), and motor vehicle traffic crashes are second (9 %). Assaults account for 1 % of TBIs in older adults, and all other known causes account for 17 %, although more than 21 % of TBIs in older adults are from unknown causes [12, 26, 27].

In Pennsylvania, the incidence of moderate-to-severe TBI in those aged 65–90 increased by 87 % between 1992 and 2009 [28]. On a global scale, it has been posited that TBI will be the third leading cause of death and disability by 2020 [29, 30]. Given the increasing trend of TBI in the growing geriatric population, adequate knowledge of the mechanism of injury and associated outcomes becomes increasingly important for physicians.

Although the hospital course varies with severity of injury and associated comorbidities, the in-hospital mortality rate or discharge to a residential home correlates positively with age [4]. Indeed the literature almost universally shows an increasing likelihood of poor outcome with increasing age. Jennett showed that less than 5 % of patients greater than 65 years of age who remain in coma for greater than 6 h had a good outcome or recovered to moderate disability [31].

Some studies have found a higher incidence of TBI in older females which opposes the trend seen in younger populations in which males more frequently present with TBI [9, 32]. Mechanism of injury is an additional difference found in older patient populations; falls are the most common reason for TBI in geriatric patients [4, 8–10, 28, 33, 34]. After falling, the most common brain injury is intracranial hemorrhage, especially chronic subdural hematoma (CSDH). Alcohol abuse is increasingly seen in this population and obviously predisposes to falls [35]. Other disorders predisposing to falls include increased frailty in bone and musculature [36–40] and comorbid conditions such as diabetes [41].

Pathophysiology of the Aging Brain

Following a traumatic brain injury, damage occurs in two phases, primary and secondary. Primary injury refers to the initial insult to the brain resulting in immediate cellular perturbation or death. This results in neurological deficits dependent upon the type of injury and specific location within the brain as well as vascular damage which results in immediate hemorrhage. Secondary injury is a consequence of primary injury and includes changes in the microenvironment, altered cellular metabolism, diminished vascular response, hypoxia, edema, and inflammation. In the context of a geriatric patient, these mechanisms may be enhanced due to the normal physiologic changes that occur with increased age [42].

Primary Injury

Neuronal change and glial cell loss are expected occurrences in the aging brain. Beginning in the fifth decade of life, normal brains begin to undergo some degree of degeneration [43, 44]. Nerve cells mainly experience death secondary to Wallerian degeneration, apoptosis, or decreased efficiency due to diminished synaptic potential [45]. Consequently, aging reduces plasticity and repair mechanisms [9, 43, 46, 47]. Although the natural reduction in cell number and plasticity has been studied in the context of diminished memory [48, 49], plasticity plays an important role following traumatic brain injury. For instance, Yager et al. showed decreased plasticity measured by functional outcome following a cerebrovascular accident in immature versus mature mice [47].

Evidence from animal studies suggests marked differences in the morphology, number, and/or organization in the supportive cells of the central nervous system. Astrocytes appear to undergo hypertrophy with advanced age without increasing in number [50–56]. Studies indicating increased staining with glial fibrillary acidic protein (GFAP) support this hypothesis [57, 58]. Additionally, the gap junctions by which astrocytes communicate and maintain the blood–brain barrier appear to undergo reorganization. The changes in microglial cells during the normal aging process are not fully understood. Some studies report an increased phagocytic activity of these protective cells. There is conflicting evidence as to whether these cells proliferate, particularly in female versus male. Further studies suggest that microglia undergo "dystrophy," in which morphological changes occur due to the increased age of the cells. The third type of neuroglial cell, oligodendrocytes appear to undergo both proliferation and reorganization of cellular alignment [53, 59–61]. Evidence of remyelination of nerve fibers in the CNS supports the need for increased numbers of oligodendrocytes with increasing age [62]. Although little is known about the fourth type of neuroglial cell, which stains to NG2 antibodies, these cells have been suggested to be precursors to oligodendrocytes and their proliferation during the aging process [63, 64]. Demyelination in the aging brain is thought to occur due to the degenerative processes that have been studied in animals and a consequential nerve fiber loss quantified in humans. Studies have shown that changes in myelin include dense cytoplasmic accumulations, areas of myelin ballooning, and changes in the lipid composition [65–69]. As a result of myelin degeneration, studies have shown that white matter loss also occurs during aging. Additional imaging studies support the loss of white matter in the normal aging brain [45].

Traumatic brain injury in the elderly contributes to the cellular loss of the natural aging process and may further enhance any pathological diseases in these patients. Immediate cell death in the brain following traumatic brain injury is dependent upon the type of injury. For example, a penetrating injury or localized impact initially causes focal damage, whereas a rotational head injury or greater impact may cause diffuse brain injury. When mechanical damage occurs, it has been shown that axonal damage can be primary from direct injury or secondary from death following initial swelling [70]. In either case, axonal injury leads to cell death and eventually to coma and increased mortality [71].

Another main mechanism of primary injury in TBI results from direct damage to blood vessels in the context of naturally changing and weaker vasculature. Geriatric patients are more susceptible to immediate vascular damage. Due to the decreased brain volume associated with age and decreased neuronal density, the brains of elderly patients allow for more space in which the subdural veins are located [34, 72, 73]. As such, they are less protected and more prone to rupture causing a subdural hematoma. Additionally, the inherent strength of the cellular composition of blood vessels with age is diminished increasing the incidence of leakage and rupture following less intense mechanical disruptions that might cause hemorrhage in younger patients [73].

Another important aspect of vascular changes with increased age is a natural decrease in cerebral blood flow (CBF) and altered vascular reactivity [74–77]. Studies suggest that decreased intracranial blood flow with age is associated with arteriolar rarefaction with conflicting evidence regarding capillary density [76, 78]. A combination of factors is most likely responsible from hormonal to structural changes of the vessels; in addition, changes in blood flow decrease metabolism and affect signaling, neuronal plasticity, and neurogenesis [77].

Decreased CBF with age and following injury leads to hypoxia and further damage. A study in rats following fluid percussion injury showed decreased heart rate in aged subjects while increased heart rate in younger rats. The aged rats showed significantly increased damage using histopathology and mortality endpoint [79]. Czosnyka et al. studied whether a failure of cerebral autoregulation might contribute to poor outcomes in the elderly [80]. Measures of autoregulation and pressure reactivity worsened with age. Older patients were found to have worse outcomes after brain trauma than younger patients despite having higher initial GCS scores. Interestingly, the intracranial pressure was lower and the cerebral perfusion pressure higher in the elderly patients, which typically are associated with improved outcomes [80, 81].

Secondary Injury

Mechanical perturbation from direct injury results in the release of ions, toxins, and neurotransmitters. Damaged cells experience metabolic changes, which contribute to the toxic metabolites in the microenvironment of the injured brain tissue. Both mechanisms further contribute to secondary cellular loss and subsequent injury mechanisms such as edema and inflammation in the aging brain.

One of the first ions to be released following increased membrane permeability or cell death is intracellular calcium [82]. The significant calcium release sets in motion a prolonged apoptotic and immediate necrotic pathways via caspase and calpain proteases, respectively [83–85]. In aged animals, there is significantly altered calcium regulation resulting in prolonged after hyperpolarization of cells, both of which may exacerbate the apoptotic process.

Glutamate is the main excitatory neurotransmitter in the central nervous system as well as the main neurotransmitter responsible for increasing damage following TBI in geriatric patients [83, 86, 87]. Hamm et al. suggests this effect is particularly harmful in an aged brain due to the increased density of receptors with age due to a natural loss of neurons [79]. Lactate is also released into the microenvironment and increasingly taken up by the brain following traumatic injury [88–100]. The increased concentrations of lactate can lead to edema via breakdown of the blood–brain barrier or ischemia [88, 101–104]. As previously noted, the blood–brain barrier is naturally compromised in the elderly brain, further exacerbating this issue.

Numerous studies have concluded that the formation of free radicals contributes to secondary cell damage and death following TBI [83, 105, 106]. The pertinent free radicals in this context include superoxide anion (O2), nitric oxide (NO), and peroxynitrite (ONOO). These substances are formed immediately following the rise of extracellular calcium ions [106] as well as in response to altered neuronal metabolism, vascular changes, and the other mechanisms of secondary injury following TBI [105, 107]. Free radicals increase the damage following TBI by interfering with vasodilatation [108], subcellular components, and particularly mitochondria [109, 110] in addition to creating oxidative stress [111].

Another mechanism of secondary injury following TBI are the resulting inflammation and edema of brain tissue [112]. In addition to hemorrhage, inflammation and edema contribute to increased intracranial pressure (ICP). The decreased ability of the aged brain to compensate for the changes in volume may be another reason for the increased mortality and morbidity in this patient population. Evidence suggests inflammation results in release of pro-inflammatory cytokines and mediators [113, 114]. Onyszchuk et al. reported the edema that develops in the aged rats requires a longer time to subside and affects a larger area of the brain [115].

Lastly, studies have reported the formation of thrombin and plasmin following TBI [116, 117]. These coagulation mediators become particularly important in a patient population that is frequently prescribed anticoagulation therapy for atrial fibrillation, ischemic heart disease, and peripheral vascular disease. One study showed the injection of the thrombin into the caudate of mice correlated with increased infiltration of inflammatory cells, angiogenesis, and reactive gliosis [118].

Medical Management of Geriatric TBI

While the medical management/neurocritical care of TBI has been codified through the Guidelines for the Management of Severe TBI for greater than 10 years, their application to geriatric patients remains unclear.

After several iterations, there remain only four class I evidence-based recommendations [119]:

1. Avoidance of hyperventilation
2. Utilization of anticonvulsants in the first week after injury
3. Avoidance/correction of hypoxia and hypotension
4. Avoidance of the use of steroids for treatment of the TBI

While the general principles put forth in the guidelines would seem to hold true for any adult patient of any age, there are some areas which might require special consideration given the unique pathophysiology of the aging brain.

As previously described, there is evidence that autoregulation worsens with age. The impact of hyperventilation in the elderly might be attenuated with respect to decreasing cerebral blood flow [81]. However, there is also evidence that CBF naturally decreases with age [74, 75, 77, 84]. Thus, avoidance of hypoperfusion from hyperventilation and maintenance of adequate fluid resuscitation would appear to be an extremely important component of geriatric neurocritical care of TBI.

While not specifically studied in elderly patients, the avoidance/minimization of hypoxia or hypotension is particularly important. The blood pressure issue requires consideration of the fact that many geriatric patients have longstanding hypertension. Thus, they may require a higher blood pressure to maintain adequate cerebral blood flow and oxygenation as a result of vascular noncompliance. It thus may be reasonable to allow blood pressure to remain higher than normal or if known the same as that of the pre-injury status in elderly patients.

In general, ICP issues are not of paramount importance in elderly patients unless there is an associated significant intracranial hemorrhage, which may or may not be treated surgically. Given the overall reduced brain volume and the high incidence of low velocity injuries from falls, the likelihood of diffuse axonal injury is quite low; the occurrence of significant brain swelling is minimal, and thus the need for aggressive and escalating ICP control is rare.

While mannitol for the control of ICP has the highest level of evidence in the guidelines, there may be an advantage for hypertonic saline in elderly patients. As previously described, there is a reorganization of the astrocytic gap junctions with a resultant "opening" of the blood–brain barrier with normal aging [57, 58, 120–124]. This lack of normal "tightness" in the BBB in elderly patients may allow for greater egress of mannitol into the extracellular space potentially exacerbating cerebral edema and ICP.

While there are no randomized controlled clinical trials regarding the use of hypertonic saline in this setting, it has become a generally accepted treatment principle across all age groups. In addition, hypertonic saline may assist in overall fluid management, as fluid overload in the elderly patient is a frequent and significant issue. In this population, it is recommended that heart ejection fraction be established to guide fluid management. In general, 3 cc/kg of hypertonic saline provides the same level of volume expansion as 10 cc/kg of other resuscitative fluids.

As elderly patients for the most part have been excluded from the phase III neuroprotective clinical trials that took place in the 1990s and are now reemerging, it is unknown whether any of the previous or current agents might be more beneficial in geriatric patients than they were in the younger patients.

Recent information, however, has become available that statins may improve outcomes in geriatric TBI [125–129]. Statins are common medications used to treat hyperlipidemia in elderly patients with or without comorbid cardiovascular disease. Statin use in patients without concomitant cardiovascular disease showed a decreased risk in incidence of in-hospital mortality as well as improved 12-month functional outcome in geriatric patients with TBI [125]. It is important to note that these patients were already being treated with statins, and there is no indication that post TBI use of statins might have a similar effect [130].

Surgical Management of Geriatric TBI

While guidelines have been developed for the surgical management of traumatic brain injury, there is no class I evidence and all "guidelines" are put forward as "recommendations" [119]. The recommendations for surgical management of acute subdural hematoma are as follows: "In acute SDH with a thickness greater than 10 mm and/or midline shift greater than 5 mm on computed tomographic (CT) scan should be surgically evacuated regardless of the patient's Glasgow coma score (GCS)" [119].

One would expect that such a recommendation needs to be tempered in elderly patients. The surgical literature is quite contradictory in this regard. Lau et al. recently posed the following question on craniotomy for hematoma in elderly patients: "do elder patients continue to suffer higher morbidity and mortality than younger patients." One-hundred and three patients (27 older than 80; 76 younger than 80) were studied. Age was not associated with any significant difference in return to baseline, 30-day mortality or postoperative ICU length of stay. However, there was no stratification of age versus GCS score which was 13–15 in almost 50 % of patients [131]. In stark contradistinction, Cagetti et al. in a retrospective study of 28 patients aged 80–100 demonstrated an 88 % mortality rate. All 19 patients with a GCS less than 9 died [132]. It must be acknowledged that the Cagetti paper is 20 years old and since that time neurocritical care has significantly improved. Nonetheless, the majority of the literature on this subject points to an unfortunately dismal prognosis in the setting of severe TBI associated with intracranial hemorrhage in patients older than 65 years.

However, the majority of posttraumatic intracranial hematomas in the elderly are chronic subdural hematomas (CSDH). The incidence of CSDH increases from 1.72 per 100,000 per year in those less than 70 years old to 7.35 per 100,000 per year in those greater than 70 [133]. These patients may present solely with headache and subtle mental status changes. Less than 10 % present with significant neurological symptoms.

CSDH has generally been felt to be a benign lesion. While there are a variety of treatment methodologies, the literature has uniformly shown good outcomes from both medical and surgical treatment. The overall in-hospital mortality ranges from less than 5 % to approximately 16 % [130].

Recent literature, however, indicates that CSDH is not necessarily a "benign" disease/injury. Miranda et al. recently studied the 6-month and 1-year outcomes of 209 patients treated surgically for CSDH in patients 65–96 years of age [134]. Mortality rates were 26.3 % at 6 months and 32 % at 12 months. The follow-up period extended for up to 8.3 years (median 1.45 years). Comparison of survival with anticipated actuarial survival demonstrated a twofold increase in mortality in those patients who had suffered a CSDH. Similar outcomes have been found in long-term follow-up after hip fracture [135–137]. Miranda postulates that CSDH "unmasks" underlying medical conditions and exacerbates them [134].

Obviously, the decision/recommendation to operate or not operate cannot be based on guidelines or prior nonclass I evidence. Increasingly, patients are providing more and more specific living will and potential end-of-life instructions which must be respected. Nevertheless, families will look to the neurosurgeon to guide final decisions. (See section "Palliative Care".)

Outcomes

Although overwhelming evidence suggests poor outcome with increased age following TBI, there is discord about whether this trend is stepwise with an age threshold beyond which outcome is significantly worse versus continuously increasing poor outcomes with increasing age. A number of reports provide evidence showing increased mortality as well as a 4–6 fold higher probability for unfavorable outcome [8, 9, 80, 81, 132, 138, 139]. Thomas et al. retrospectively showed hospital and death rates after nonfatal TBI to increase with the near-geriatric age group in both men and women [140]. Diminished functioning in all areas – cognitive, motor, and memory – has also been reported [9, 141].

Many studies have been conducted to investigate risk factors for worse outcomes following TBI specific to the geriatric population. It has been shown that gender plays a role; females typically have better outcomes [142–145] although this has been contended [146]. This suggests a possible role of estrogen or progesterone in the reparation process following a TBI. The ProTECT trial found that the patients that received progesterone had a lower 30-day mortality rate that those that received placebo [147]. Moderate traumatic brain injury survivors who received progesterone were more likely to have a moderate-to-good outcome than those randomized to placebo. The specific type of injury has been shown to be another factor. Improved outcomes with progesterone have been shown in other randomized controlled trials [148, 149].

The mainstay of understanding the pathophysiology and risk factors for worse outcomes in the geriatric population rests in potential optimization of treatment and prevention of TBI. Researchers have identified varied reasons for the worse outcomes in these patients. For instance, older patients do not receive the same intensity of care as younger patients [150]. There is a delay in getting geriatric patients to neurosurgical intervention when compared to younger patients with TBI [14, 150]. This suggests that improvements in timing and logistical care within hospitals may be the first step toward improving outcomes.

Prevention targets the patient before they arrive at the hospital. Given that the most common reason for TBI in these patients is falls, it is imperative to work toward the prevention of falls. One way in which this might be possible is to monitor medications that may contribute to falls [151]. Another way is to emphasize bone health and exercise. If patients have appropriate bone density, fracture might be prevented thus preventing falls. Additionally, if a patient does fall, an improved muscular response may prevent head impact or injury.

Special Considerations

Unfortunately, the care in this patient population is unique given their medications and comorbidities at the time of brain injury. This complicated medical picture requires more research to improve knowledge regarding how common medications and pathological processes in elderly patients may affect the treatment needed following TBI.

A particular challenge in management is anticoagulation. A significant number of patients greater than 65 years of age are on some sort of anticoagulation or antiplatelet medication given the well-known vascular processes that predispose older patients to cardiovascular disease. However, the data on the effect of this therapy in TBI is very conflicting. Some studies have shown that anticoagulation therapy has a significant effect on outcome. One study showed increased mortality in those on warfarin (trade name Coumadin) who fall from standing [152]. In a retrospective study of 384 patients 55 years or older, warfarin use before a closed head injury was associated with more serious injuries and increased mortality [153]. Yet, other studies have not been able to show a significant effect of anticoagulation therapy on outcome. Fortuna et al. found no significant effect of clopidogrel, aspirin, or warfarin on outcome in those with blunt head trauma [154]. Another study analyzed 3 age groups within the geriatric population without taking into account mechanism of head injury with nonsignificant CT findings between pre-injury warfarin use and worsened outcome [155].

Pieracci et al. further evaluated this question by retrospectively grouping the geriatric patients with TBI based on warfarin use with INR greater or less than 2 and those who did not take warfarin [156]. The group with an INR greater than 2 showed significant likelihood for GCS below 13 and increased mortality. In those with an INR less than 2 and those who were on no pre-injury anticoagulation, the difference in mortality rates was not significant [156]. This study suggests that TBI might be affected not merely by anticoagulation therapy but more so by the degree of anticoagulation at the time of injury.

Additional studies used this data to evaluate the effect of anticoagulation on current therapy in elderly patients.

Some have suggested repeating normal CT scans in patients with GCS of 14 or 15 and supratherapeutic INRs within 6 h after presentation whereas others suggest emergency CT is not necessary in those with GCS of 15 irrespective of coagulation status [157, 158].

Recently, direct thrombin inhibitors have been introduced in the United States. These anticoagulants exert their effect at the end of the coagulation cascade. Thus, there is currently no method of reversal. Serum half-life of these drugs is 12–17 h. Their level can be monitored by checking a thrombin time.

The Re-Ly trial showed that low doses of the direct thrombin inhibitor dabigatran (trade name Pradaxa) were associated with less risk of ICH when compared with warfarin while high doses had a similar risk [159]. However, this was not a head injury study.

A recent case report demonstrated fatal progressive bilateral ICH over the course of 6 h in an 83-year-old after a ground level fall and a GCS of 15 on admission [160]. These authors suggested that hemodialysis be used to clear the drug as factor VIIa and fresh frozen plasma are ineffective in reversing the effects of the dabigatran; however, only approximately 35–60 % of the drug can be removed within 23 h.

Since there is little purpose served by supratherapeutic anticoagulation, there is little argument that patients who present with TBI even with good GCS and normal CT scans should have their warfarin "reversed" to levels of normal anticoagulation for their medical condition.

When it is otherwise felt best to reverse the patient's anticoagulation with warfarin, the first step is the use of intravenous or intramuscular vitamin K. However, this is rarely sufficient to accomplish a normalization of INR, and fresh frozen plasma has been the mainstay of therapeutic reversal. While fresh frozen plasma is quite effective in this regard, in the elderly population, one has to be particularly vigilant for volume overload. The issue of volume overload may be addressed by the use of Prothrombin Complex Concentrates (PCC). While there is no literature to support its use, in desperate situations, recombinant factor VIIa may be brought into play.

The primary reversal agent for the platelet inhibitors is the administration of platelets. However, because of the half-life of these drugs, it is frequently necessary to administer platelets over a prolonged period of time. DDAVP has shown some promise in effecting more rapid normalization of platelet function.

As noted previously, at this time, there is no means or mechanism of reversing the effects of the direct thrombin inhibitors (Table 23.1).

Aside from anticoagulation, the most common comorbid conditions include diabetes, hypertension, cardiac arrhythmias, chronic pulmonary disease, congestive heart failure, and electrolyte disorders.

Palliative Care

The issue of palliative care in the neurotrauma patient is of increasing importance – especially with the ever-increasing geriatric population.

Obviously, the neurosurgeon's first priority is to "do no harm." However, this has been liberally interpreted as not needlessly prolonging suffering – even in a comatose patient – when moral responsibility dictates otherwise.

Thus, it is incumbent upon the neurosurgeon and trauma surgeon to keep abreast of the ever-increasing literature on geriatric neurotrauma to be in the optimal position to answer the very frequent question of "what would you do if this were your family member."

While neurosurgical technical advances in neurocritical care have in many cases been lifesaving, at the same time it has brought forth conundrums in initiating and withholding care. Heifitz focuses on the concept of beneficence and justice – "the equal treatment of all and privacy or the freedom to make a choice of what is not wanted."

Decisions are typically made on ranking values and principles. A physician must guide patients and families through these difficult decisions while at the same time taking care not to make decisions for the patient or family based on the physician's moral and ethical beliefs.

Decisions on not initiating or withholding care should be considered in the context of prognosis, poor quality of life before the TBI or poor quality of life anticipated after TBI.

As previously noted, today about 15 % of the population are over 65, while by 2030 this would double. Unfortunately many live with a limited quality. Two million are in nursing homes. While at some point in their lives over 65 years, seven million will spend some time in a nursing home with 80 % having mental impairment.

These societal issues cannot be overlooked in end-of-life TBI decisions.

Table 23.1 Commonly used anticoagulants, their brand names, mechanism of action, and reversal agents

	Brand name	Mechanism of action	Reversal agents
Warfarin	Coumadin	Vitamin K antagonist (inhibits factors II, VII, IX, and X)	Fresh frozen plasma (FFP), vitamin K, prothrombin complex concentrate (PCC)
Aspirin		Antiplatelet: thromboxane inhibitor	DDAVP, platelets may give temporary reversal
Clopidogrel	Plavix	Antiplatelet: ADP receptor/P2Y12 inhibitors	
Prasugrel	Effient		
Ticlopidine	Ticlid		
Abciximab	ReoPro	Antiplatelet: glycoprotein IIb/IIIa inhibitors	
Eptifibatide	Integrilin		
Tirofiban	Aggrastat		
Fondaparinux	Arixtra	Heparin group/glycosaminoglycans/(binds antithrombin)	Protamine sulfate (not as effective as with heparin)
Enoxaparin	Lovenox		
Dabigatran	Pradaxa	Direct thrombin (II) inhibitor	None known

References

1. Gorman M. Development and the rights of older people. In: Randel J et al., editors. The ageing and development report: poverty, independence and the world's older people. London: Earthscan Publications, Ltd; 1999. p. 3–21.
2. Guerrero JL, Thurman DJ, Sniezek JE. Emergency department visits associated with traumatic brain injury: United States, 1995–1996. Brain Inj. 2000;14(2):181–6.
3. Jager TE, Weiss HB, Coben JH, Pepe PE. Traumatic brain injuries evaluated in U.S. emergency departments, 1992–1994. Acad Emerg Med. 2000;7(2):134–40.
4. Coronado VG, Thomas KE, Sattin RW, Johnson RL. The CDC traumatic brain injury surveillance system: characteristics of persons aged 65 years and older hospitalized with a TBI. J Head Trauma Rehabil. 2005;20(3):215–28.
5. Fletcher AE, Khlaed S, Mallonee S. The epidemiology of severe traumatic brain injury among persons 65 years of age and older in Oklahoma, 1992–2003. Brain Inj. 2007;21(7):691–9.
6. Menon DK, Schwab K, Wright DW, Maas AI, Demographics and Clinical Assessment Working Group of the International and Interagency Initiative toward Common Data Elements for Research on Traumatic Brain Injury and Psychological Health. Position statement: definition of traumatic brain injury. Arch Phys Med Rehabil. 2010;91(11):1637–40.
7. Susman M, DiRusso SM, Sullivan T, Risucci D, Nealon P, Cuff S, Haider A, Benzil D. Traumatic brain injury in the elderly: increased mortality and worse functional outcome at discharge despite lower injury severity. J Trauma. 2002;53(2):219–23; discussion 223–4.
8. Tokutomi T, Miyagi T, Ogawa T, Ono J, Kawamata T, Sakamoto T, Shigemori M, Nakamura N. Age-associated increases in poor outcomes after traumatic brain injury: a report from the Japan Neurotrauma Data Bank. J Neurotrauma. 2008;25(12):1407–14.
9. Stocchetti N, Paternò R, Citerio G, Beretta L, Colombo A. Traumatic brain injury in an aging population. J Neurotrauma. 2012;29(6):1119–25.
10. Hukkelhoven CW, Steyerberg EW, Rampen AJ, Farace E, Habbema JD, Marshall LF, Murray GD, Maas AI. Patient age and outcome following severe traumatic brain injury: an analysis of 5,600 patients. J Neurosurg. 2003;99(4):666–73.
11. Mushkudiani NA, Engel DC, Steyerberg EW, Butcher I, Lu J, Marmarou A, Slieker F, McHugh GS, Murray GD, Maas AI. Prognostic value of demographic characteristics in traumatic brain injury: results from the IMPACT study. J Neurotrauma. 2007;24(2):259–69.
12. Thompson HJ, McCormick WC, Kagan SH. Traumatic brain injury in older adults: epidemiology, outcomes, and future implications. J Am Geriatr Soc. 2006;54(10):1590–5.
13. Mosenthal AC, Lavery RF, Addis M, Kaul S, Ross S, Marburger R, Deitch EA, Livingston DH. Isolated traumatic brain injury: age is an independent predictor of mortality and early outcome. J Trauma. 2002;52(5):907–11.
14. Munro PT, Smith RD, Parke TR. Effect of patients' age on management of acute intracranial haematoma: prospective national study. BMJ. 2002;325(7371):1001.
15. Mohindra S, Mukherjee KK, Gupta R, Chhabra R. Continuation of poor surgical outcome after elderly brain injury. Surg Neurol. 2008;69(5):474–7.
16. Bruns Jr J, Hauser WA. The epidemiology of traumatic brain injury: a review. Epilepsia. 2003;44 Suppl 10:2–10.
17. Rothweiler B, Temkin NR, Dikmen SS. Aging effect on psychosocial outcome in traumatic brain injury. Arch Phys Med Rehabil. 1998;79(8):881–7.
18. Richardson 3rd NS, Paysinger BD. Outcome of acute subdural and epidural hematomas in a level I trauma center in South Carolina. J S C Med Assoc. 1990;86(11):573–6.
19. Pennings JL, Bachulis BL, Simons CT, Slazinski T. Survival after severe brain injury in the aged. Arch Surg. 1993;128(7):787–93.
20. Flanagan SR, Hibbard MR, Riordan B, Gordon WA. Traumatic brain injury in the elderly: diagnostic and treatment challenges. Clin Geriatr Med. 2006;22(2):449–68; x.
21. Roebuck J. When does old age begin? The evolution of the English definition. J Soc Hist. 1979;12(3):416–28.
22. Vincent GK, Velkoff VA. The next four decades, the older population in the United States: 2010 to 2050. Current population reports. Washington, DC: U.S. Census Bureau, Editor; 2010.
23. Le Roux AA, Nadvi SS. Acute extradural haematoma in the elderly. Br J Neurosurg. 2007;21:16–20.
24. US Bureau of the Census, US Administration of Aging. Older population by age, 1900–2050. 11 Aug 2005. Available from online: http://www.aoa.gov/AoARoot/Aging_Statistics/future_growth/future_growth.aspx#age.
25. Thompson HJ, Weir S, Rivara FP, Wang J, Sullivan SD, Salkever D, Mackenzie EJ. Utilization and costs of health care after geriatric traumatic brain injury. J Neurotrauma. 2012;29(10):1864–71.
26. Faul M, Xu L, Wald MM, Coronado VG. Traumatic brain injury in the United States: emergency department visits, hospitalizations, and deaths, 2002–2006. Atlanta: US Department of Health and Human Services, Centers for Disease Control and Prevention, National Center for Injury Prevention and Control; 2010.
27. Langlois JA, Rutland-Brown W, Thomas KE. Traumatic brain injury in the United States: emergency department visits, hospitalizations, and deaths. Atlanta: US Department of Health and Human Services, Centers for Disease Control and Prevention, National Center for Injury Prevention and Control; 2004.
28. Ramanathan DM, McWilliams N, Schatz P, Hillary FG. Epidemiological shifts in elderly traumatic brain injury: 18-year trends in Pennsylvania. J Neurotrauma. 2012;29(7):1371–8.
29. Povlishock JT, Katz DI. Update of neuropathology and neurological recovery after traumatic brain injury. J Head Trauma Rehabil. 2005;20(1):76–94.
30. Murray CJ, Lopez AD. Alternative projections of mortality and disability by cause 1990–2020: Global Burden of Disease Study. Lancet. 1997;349(9064):1498–504.
31. Jennett B. Head injuries in elderly. In: Caird FL, editor. Neurological disorders of the elderly. Bristol: Wright and Sons; 1982. p. 779–83.
32. Adekoya N, Thurman DJ, White DD, Webb KW. Surveillance for traumatic brain injury deaths – United States, 1989–1998. MMWR Surveill Summ. 2002;51(10):1–14.
33. Langlois JA, Kegler SR, Butler JA, Gotsch KE, Johnson RL, Reichard AA, Webb KW, Coronado VG, Selassie AW, Thurman DJ. Traumatic brain injury-related hospital discharges. Results from a 14-state surveillance system, 1997. MMWR Surveill Summ. 2003;52(4):1–20.
34. Schönberger M, Ponsford J, Reutens D, Beare R, O'Sullivan R. The Relationship between age, injury severity, and MRI findings after traumatic brain injury. J Neurotrauma. 2009;26(12):2157–67.
35. Sinha VD, Gupta V, Singh DK, Chopra S, Gupta P, Bagaria H. Geriatric head injuries – experience and expectations. Indian J of Neurotrauma. 2008;5(2):69–73.
36. Frankel JE, Marwitz JH, Cifu DX, Kreutzer JS, Englander J, Rosenthal M. A follow-up study of older adults with traumatic brain injury: taking into account decreasing length of stay. Arch Phys Med Rehabil. 2006;87(1):57–62.
37. McLean RR, Jacques PF, Selhub J, Tucker KL, Samelson EJ, Broe KE, Hannan MT, Cupples LA, Kiel DP. Homocysteine as a predictive factor for hip fracture in older persons. N Engl J Med. 2004;350(20):2042–9.
38. Dhonukshe-Rutten RA, Pluijm SM, de Groot LC, Lips P, Smit JH, van Staveren WA. Homocysteine and vitamin B12 status relate to

bone turnover markers, broadband ultrasound attenuation, and fractures in healthy elderly people. J Bone Miner Res. 2005;20(6): 921–9.
39. van Meurs JB, Dhonukshe-Rutten RA, Pluijm SM, van der Klift M, de Jonge R, Lindemans J, de Groot LC, Hofman A, Witteman JC, van Leeuwen JP, Breteler MM, Lips P, Pols HA, Uitterlinden AG. Homocysteine levels and the risk of osteoporotic fracture. N Engl J Med. 2004;350(20):2033–41.
40. Dhonukshe-Rutten RA, Lips M, de Jong N, Chin A, Paw MJ, Hiddink GJ, van Dusseldorp M, De Groot LC, van Staveren WA. Vitamin B-12 status is associated with bone mineral content and bone mineral density in frail elderly women but not in men. J Nutr. 2003;133(3):801–7.
41. Kennedy RL, Henry J, Chapman AJ, Nayar R, Grant P, Morris AD. Accidents in patients with insulin-treated diabetes: increased risk of low-impact falls but not motor vehicle crashes – a prospective register-based study. J Trauma. 2002;52(4):660–6.
42. Powers R. Neurobiology of aging. In: Cummings J, Coffey CE, editors. Textbook of geriatric neuropsychiatry. Washington, DC: American Psychiatric Press; 2000. p. 33–79.
43. Peters A. The effects of normal aging on nerve fibers and neuroglia in the central nervous system. In: Riddle DR, editor. Brain aging: models, methods, and mechanisms. Boca Raton: CRC Press; 2007. Chapter 5.
44. Povlishock JT, Erb DE, Astruc J. Axonal response to traumatic brain injury: reactive axonal change, deafferentation, and neuroplasticity. J Neurotrauma. 1992;9 Suppl 1:S189–200.
45. Kumar A, Foster TC. Neurophysiology of old neurons and synapses. In: Riddle DR, editor. Brain aging: models, methods, and mechanisms. Boca Raton: CRC Press; 2007. Chapter 10.
46. Kovacs EJ. Aging, traumatic injury, and estrogen treatment. Exp Gerontol. 2005;40(7):549–55.
47. Yager JY, Wright S, Armstrong EA, Jahraus CM, Saucier DM. The influence of aging on recovery following ischemic brain damage. Behav Brain Res. 2006;173(2):171–80.
48. Smith DE, Rapp PR, McKay HM, Roberts JA, Tuszynski MH. Memory impairment in aged primates is associated with focal death of cortical neurons and atrophy of subcortical neurons. J Neurosci. 2004;24(18):4374–81.
49. Morrison JH, Hof PR. Life and death of neurons in the aging brain. Science. 1997;278(5337):412–9.
50. Vaughn JE, Peters A. Electron microscopy of the early postnatal development of fibrous astrocytes. Am J Anat. 1967;121(1):131–52.
51. Diamond MC, Johnson RE, Gold MW. Changes in neuron number and size and glia number in the young, adult, and aging rat medial occipital cortex. Behav Biol. 1977;20(4):409–18.
52. Pakkenberg B, Pelvig D, Marner L, Bundgaard MJ, Gundersen HJ, Nyengaard JR, Regeur L. Aging and the human neocortex. Exp Gerontol. 2003;38(1–2):95–9.
53. Sandell JH, Peters A. Effects of age on the glial cells in the rhesus monkey optic nerve. J Comp Neurol. 2002;445(1):13–28.
54. Berciano MT, Andres MA, Calle E, Lafarga M. Age-induced hypertrophy of astrocytes in rat supraoptic nucleus: a cytological, morphometric, and immunocytochemical study. Anat Rec. 1995;243(1):129–44.
55. Long JM, Kalehua AN, Muth NJ, Calhoun ME, Jucker M, Hengemihle JM, Ingram DK, Mouton PR. Stereological analysis of astrocyte and microglia in aging mouse hippocampus. Neurobiol Aging. 1998;19(5):497–503.
56. Hansen LA, Armstrong DM, Terry RD. An immunohistochemical quantification of fibrous astrocytes in the aging human cerebral cortex. Neurobiol Aging. 1987;8(1):1–6.
57. Colombo JA. Interlaminar astroglial processes in the cerebral cortex of adult monkeys but not of adult rats. Acta Anat (Basel). 1996;155(1):57–62.
58. Nichols NR, Day JR, Laping NJ, Johnson SA, Finch CE. GFAP mRNA increases with age in rat and human brain. Neurobiol Aging. 1993;14(5):421–9.
59. Peters A. Age-related changes in oligodendrocytes in monkey cerebral cortex. J Comp Neurol. 1996;371(1):153–63.
60. Peters A, Sethares C. Oligodendrocytes, their progenitors and other neuroglial cells in the aging primate cerebral cortex. Cereb Cortex. 2004;14(9):995–1007.
61. Peters A, Josephson K, Vincent SL. Effects of aging on the neuroglial cells and pericytes within area 17 of the rhesus monkey cerebral cortex. Anat Rec. 1991;229(3):384–98.
62. Peters A, Sethares C. Is there remyelination during aging of the primate central nervous system? J Comp Neurol. 2003;460(2): 238–54.
63. Levison SW, Young GM, Goldman JE. Cycling cells in the adult rat neocortex preferentially generate oligodendroglia. J Neurosci Res. 1999;57(4):435–46.
64. Levine JM, Reynolds R, Fawcett JW. The oligodendrocyte precursor cell in health and disease. Trends Neurosci. 2001;24(1):39–47.
65. Feldman ML, Peters A. Ballooning of myelin sheaths in normally aged macaques. J Neurocytol. 1998;27(8):605–14.
66. Peters A, Moss MB, Sethares C. Effects of aging on myelinated nerve fibers in monkey primary visual cortex. J Comp Neurol. 2000;419(3):364–76.
67. Peters A, Sethares C. Aging and the myelinated fibers in prefrontal cortex and corpus callosum of the monkey. J Comp Neurol. 2002;442(3):277–91.
68. Malone MJ, Szoke MC. Neurochemical studies in aging brain. I Structural changes in myelin lipids J Gerontol. 1982;37(3): 262–7.
69. Sloane JA, Hinman JD, Lubonia M, Hollander W, Abraham CR. Age-dependent myelin degeneration and proteolysis of oligodendrocyte proteins is associated with the activation of calpain-1 in the rhesus monkey. J Neurochem. 2003;84(1):157–68.
70. Cervós-Navarro J, Lafuente JV. Traumatic brain injuries: structural changes. J Neurol Sci. 1991;103(Suppl):S3–14.
71. Johnson VE, Stewart W, Smith DH. Axonal pathology in traumatic brain injury. Exp Neurol. 2013;246:35–43.
72. Kim E. Elderly. In: Silver JM, McAllister TW, Yudofsky SC, editors. Textbook of traumatic brain injury. Arlington: American Psychiatric Association; 2011. p. 451–9.
73. Cummings JL, Bensen DF. Dementia: a clinical approach. 2nd ed. Boston: Buttersworth; 1992.
74. Martin AJ, Friston KJ, Colebatch JG, Frackowiak RS. Decreases in regional cerebral blood flow with normal aging. J Cereb Blood Flow Metab. 1991;11(4):684–9.
75. Moeller JR, Ishikawa T, Dhawan V, Spetsieris P, Mandel F, Alexander GE, Grady C, Pietrini P, Eidelberg D. The metabolic topography of normal aging. J Cereb Blood Flow Metab. 1996;16(3):385–98.
76. Farkas E, Luiten PG. Cerebral microvascular pathology in aging and Alzheimer's disease. Prog Neurobiol. 2001;64(6):575–611.
77. Sonntag WE, Eckman DM, Ingraham J, Riddle DR. Regulation of cerebrovascular aging. In: Riddle DR, editor. Brain aging: models, methods, and mechanisms. Boca Raton: CRC Press; 2007. p. 279–304.
78. Kalaria RN. Cerebral vessels in ageing and Alzheimer's disease. Pharmacol Ther. 1996;72(3):193–214.
79. Hamm RJ, Jenkins LW, Lyeth BG, White-Gbadebo DM, Hayes RL. The effect of age on outcome following traumatic brain injury in rats. J Neurosurg. 1991;75(6):916–21.
80. Czosnyka M, Balestreri M, Steiner L, Smielewski P, Hutchinson PJ, Matta B, Pickard JD. Age, intracranial pressure, autoregulation, and outcome after brain trauma. J Neurosurg. 2005;102(3): 450–4.

81. Yam AT, Lang EW, Lagopoulos J, Yip K, Griffith J, Mudaliar Y, Dorsch NW. Cerebral autoregulation and ageing. J Clin Neurosci. 2005;12(6):643–6.
82. Fineman I, Hovda DA, Smith M, Yoshino A, Becker DP. Concussive brain injury is associated with a prolonged accumulation of calcium: a 45Ca autoradiographic study. Brain Res. 1993;624(1–2):94–102.
83. McAllister TW. Neurobiological consequences of traumatic brain injury. Dialogues Clin Neurosci. 2011;13(3):287–300.
84. Farkas O, Povlishock JT. Cellular and subcellular change evoked by diffuse traumatic brain injury: a complex web of change extending far beyond focal damage. Prog Brain Res. 2007;161:43–59.
85. Raghupathi R. Cell death mechanisms following traumatic brain injury. Brain Pathol. 2004;14(2):215–22.
86. Katayama Y, Becker DP, Tamura T, Hovda DA. Massive increases in extracellular potassium and the indiscriminate release of glutamate following concussive brain injury. J Neurosurg. 1990;73(6):889–900.
87. Bullock R, Zauner A, Woodward JJ, Myseros J, Choi SC, Ward JD, Marmarou A, Young HF. Factors affecting excitatory amino acid release following severe human head injury. J Neurosurg. 1998;89(4):507–18.
88. Madikiansn A, Giza CC. A clinicain's guide to the pathophysiology of traumatic brain injury. Indian J Neurotrauma. 2006;3(1):9–17.
89. Biros MH, Dimlich RV. Brain lactate during partial global ischemia and reperfusion: effect of pretreatment with dichloroacetate in a rat model. Am J Emerg Med. 1987;5(4):271–7.
90. Kawamata T, Katayama Y, Hovda DA, Yoshino A, Becker DP. Lactate accumulation following concussive brain injury: the role of ionic fluxes induced by excitatory amino acids. Brain Res. 1995;674(2):196–204.
91. Richards TL, Keniry MA, Weinstein PR, Pereira BM, Andrews BT, Murphy EJ, James TL. Measurement of lactate accumulation by in vivo proton NMR spectroscopy during global cerebral ischemia in rats. Magn Reson Med. 1987;5(4):353–7.
92. Nilsson B, Pontén U, Voigt G. Experimental head injury in the rat. Part 1: mechanics, pathophysiology, and morphology in an impact acceleration trauma model. J Neurosurg. 1977;47(2):241–51.
93. Yang MS, DeWitt DS, Becker DP, Hayes RL. Regional brain metabolite levels following mild experimental head injury in the cat. J Neurosurg. 1985;63(4):617–21.
94. Meyer JS, Kondo A, Nomura F, Sakamoto K, Teraura T. Cerebral hemodynamics and metabolism following experimental head injury. J Neurosurg. 1970;32(3):304–19.
95. Corbett RJ, Laptook AR, Nunnally RL, Hassan A, Jackson J. Intracellular pH, lactate, and energy metabolism in neonatal brain during partial ischemia measured in vivo by 31P and 1H nuclear magnetic resonance spectroscopy. J Neurochem. 1988;51(5):1501–9.
96. Magistretti PJ, Sorg O, Yu N, Martin JL, Pellerin L. Neurotransmitters regulate energy metabolism in astrocytes: implications for the metabolic trafficking between neural cells. Dev Neurosci. 1993;15(3–5):306–12.
97. Pellerin L, Magistretti PJ. Glutamate uptake into astrocytes stimulates aerobic glycolysis: a mechanism coupling neuronal activity to glucose utilization. Proc Natl Acad Sci U S A. 1994;91(22):10625–9.
98. Pellerin L, Magistretti PJ. Neuroenergetics: calling upon astrocytes to satisfy hungry neurons. Neuroscientist. 2004;10(1):53–62.
99. Prins ML, Lee SM, Fujima LS, Hovda DA. Increased cerebral uptake and oxidation of exogenous betaHB improves ATP following traumatic brain injury in adult rats. J Neurochem. 2004;90(3):666–72.
100. Glenn TC, Kelly DF, Boscardin WJ, McArthur DL, Vespa P, Oertel M, Hovda DA, Bergsneider M, Hillered L, Martin NA. Energy dysfunction as a predictor of outcome after moderate or severe head injury: indices of oxygen, glucose, and lactate metabolism. J Cereb Blood Flow Metab. 2003;23(10):1239–50.
101. Gardiner M, Smith ML, Kågström E, Shohami E, Siesjö BK. Influence of blood glucose concentration on brain lactate accumulation during severe hypoxia and subsequent recovery of brain energy metabolism. J Cereb Blood Flow Metab. 1982;2(4):429–38.
102. Kalimo H, Rehncrona S, Söderfeldt B, Olsson Y, Siesjö BK. Brain lactic acidosis and ischemic cell damage: 2. Histopathology J Cereb Blood Flow Metab. 1981;1(3):313–27.
103. Myers RE. A unitary theory of causation of anoxic and hypoxic brain pathology. Adv Neurol. 1979;26:195–213.
104. Siemkowicz E, Hansen AJ. Clinical restitution following cerebral ischemia in hypo-, normo- and hyperglycemic rats. Acta Neurol Scand. 1978;58(1):1–8.
105. O'Connell KM. The role of free radicals in traumatic brain injury. Biol Res Nurs. 2013;15(3):253–63.
106. Bains M, Hall ED. Antioxidant therapies in traumatic brain and spinal cord injury. Biochim Biophys Acta. 2012;1822(5):675–84.
107. Park E, Bell JD, Baker AJ. Traumatic brain injury: can the consequences be stopped? CMAJ. 2008;178(9):1163–70.
108. Faraci FM. Reactive oxygen species: influence on cerebral vascular tone. J Appl Physiol. 2006;100(2):739–43.
109. Besson VC, Margaill I, Plotkine M, Marchand-Verrecchia C. Deleterious activation of poly(ADP-ribose)polymerase-1 in brain after in vivo oxidative stress. Free Radic Res. 2003;37(11):1201–8.
110. Rohn TT, Hinds TR, Vincenzi FF. Ion transport ATPases as targets for free radical damage. Protection by an aminosteroid of the Ca2+ pump ATPase and Na+/K+ pump ATPase of human red blood cell membranes. Biochem Pharmacol. 1993;46(3):525–34.
111. Ansari MA, Roberts KN, Scheff SW. Oxidative stress and modification of synaptic proteins in hippocampus after traumatic brain injury. Free Radic Biol Med. 2008;45(4):443–52.
112. Yang GY, Betz AL, Chenevert TL, Brunberg JA, Hoff JT. Experimental intracerebral hemorrhage: relationship between brain edema, blood flow, and blood–brain barrier permeability in rats. J Neurosurg. 1994;81(1):93–102.
113. Shohami E, Novikov M, Bass R, Yamin A, Gallily R. Closed head injury triggers early production of TNF alpha and IL-6 by brain tissue. J Cereb Blood Flow Metab. 1994;14(4):615–9.
114. Sandhir R, Puri V, Klein RM, Berman NE. Differential expression of cytokines and chemokines during secondary neuron death following brain injury in old and young mice. Neurosci Lett. 2004;369(1):28–32.
115. Onyszchuk G, He YY, Berman NE, Brooks WM. Detrimental effects of aging on outcome from traumatic brain injury: a behavioral, magnetic resonance imaging, and histological study in mice. J Neurotrauma. 2008;25(2):153–71.
116. Xue M, Del Bigio MR. Acute tissue damage after injections of thrombin and plasmin into rat striatum. Stroke. 2001;32(9):2164–9.
117. Stein SC, Chen XH, Sinson GP, Smith DH. Intravascular coagulation: a major secondary insult in nonfatal traumatic brain injury. J Neurosurg. 2002;97(6):1373–7.
118. Nishino A, Suzuki M, Ohtani H, Motohashi O, Umezawa K, Nagura H, Yoshimoto T. Thrombin may contribute to the pathophysiology of central nervous system injury. J Neurotrauma. 1993;10(2):167–79.
119. Brain Trauma Foundation; American Association of Neurological Surgeons; Congress of Neurological Surgeons; Joint Section on Neurotrauma and Critical Care, AANS/CNS, Bratton SL, Chestnut RM, Ghajar J, McConnell Hammond FF, Harris OA, Hartl R, Manley GT, Nemecek A, Newell DW, Rosenthal G, Schouten J, Shutter L, Timmons SD, Ullman JS, Videtta W, Wilberger JE, Wright DW. Guidelines for the management of severe traumatic brain injury. J Neurotrauma. 2007;24 Suppl 1:S7–95.
120. O'Callaghan JP, Miller DB. The concentration of glial fibrillary acidic protein increases with age in the mouse and rat brain. Neurobiol Aging. 1991;12(2):171–4.

121. Kohama SG, Goss JR, Finch CE, McNeill TH. Increases of glial fibrillary acidic protein in the aging female mouse brain. Neurobiol Aging. 1995;16(1):59–67.
122. Amenta F, Bronzaetti E, Sabbatini M, Vega JA. Astrocyte changes in aging cerebral cortex and hippocampus: a quantitative immunohistochemical study. Microsc Res Tech. 1998;43(1):29–33.
123. Colombo JA, Yáñez A, Puissant V, Lipina S. Long, interlaminar astroglial cell processes in the cortex of adult monkeys. J Neurosci Res. 1995;40(4):551–6.
124. Sloane JA, Hollander W, Rosene DL, Moss MB, Kemper T, Abraham CR. Astrocytic hypertrophy and altered GFAP degradation with age in subcortical white matter of the rhesus monkey. Brain Res. 2000;862(1–2):1–10.
125. Schneider EB, Efron DT, MacKenzie EJ, Rivara FP, Nathens AB, Jurkovich GJ. Premorbid statin use is associated with improved survival and functional outcomes in older head-injured individuals. J Trauma. 2011;71(4):815–9.
126. Efron DT, Sorock G, Haut ER, Chang D, Schneider E, Mackenzie E, Cornwell 3rd EE, Jurkovich GJ. Preinjury statin use is associated with improved in-hospital survival in elderly trauma patients. J Trauma. 2008;64(1):66–73; discussion 73–4.
127. Indraswari F, Wang H, Lei B, James ML, Kernagis D, Warner DS, Dawson HN, Laskowitz DT. Statins improve outcome in murine models of intracranial hemorrhage and traumatic brain injury: a translational approach. J Neurotrauma. 2012;29(7):1388–400.
128. Wible EF, Laskowitz DT. Statins in traumatic brain injury. Neurotherapeutics. 2010;7(1):62–73.
129. Tapia-Pérez JH, Sanchez-Aguilar M, Schneider T. The role of statins in neurosurgery. Neurosurg Rev. 2010;33(3):259–70.
130. Lee S, Jadhav V, Lekic T, Hyong A, Allard M, Stier G, Martin R, Zhang J. Simvastatin treatment in surgically induced brain injury in rats. Acta Neurochir Suppl. 2008;102:401–4.
131. Lau D, El-Sayed AM, Ziewacz JE, Jayachandran P, Huq FS, Zamora-Berridi GJ, Davis MC, Sullivan SE. Postoperative outcomes following closed head injury and craniotomy for evacuation of hematoma in patients older than 80 years. J Neurosurg. 2012;116(1):234–45.
132. Cagetti B, Cossu M, Pau A, Rivano C, Viale G. The outcome from acute subdural and epidural intracranial haematomas in very elderly patients. Br J Neurosurg. 1992;6(3):227–31.
133. Fogelholm R, Heiskanen O, Waltimo O. Chronic subdural hematoma in adults. Influence of patient's age on symptoms, signs, and thickness of hematoma. J Neurosurg. 1975;42(1):43–6.
134. Miranda LB, Braxton E, Hobbs J, Quigley MR. Chronic subdural hematoma in the elderly: not a benign disease. J Neurosurg. 2011;114(1):72–6.
135. Tarazona-Santabalbina FJ, Belenguer-Varea A, Rovira-Daudi E, Salcedo-Mahiques E, Cuesta-Peredó D, Doménech-Pascual JR, Salvador-Pérez MI, Avellana-Zaragoza JA. Early interdisciplinary hospital intervention for elderly patients with hip fractures: functional outcome and mortality. Clinics (Sao Paulo). 2012;67(6):547–56.
136. Leslie WD, Lix LM, Wu X, On behalf of the Manitoba Bone Density Program. Competing mortality and fracture risk assessment. Osteoporos Int. 2013;24(2):681–8.
137. Shoda N, Yasunaga H, Horiguchi H, Matsuda S, Ohe K, Kadono Y, Tanaka S. Risk factors affecting inhospital mortality after hip fracture: retrospective analysis using the Japanese Diagnosis Procedure Combination Database. BMJ Open. 2012;2(3):1–7.
138. Howard 3rd MA, Gross AS, Dacey Jr RG, Winn HR. Acute subdural hematomas: an age-dependent clinical entity. J Neurosurg. 1989;71(6):858–63.
139. Livingston DH, Lavery RF, Mosenthal AC, Knudson MM, Lee S, Morabito D, Manley GT, Nathens A, Jurkovich G, Hoyt DB, Coimbra R. Recovery at one year following isolated traumatic brain injury: a Western Trauma Association prospective multicenter trial. J Trauma. 2005;59(6):1298–304.
140. Thomas KE, Stevens JA, Sarmiento K, Wald MM. Fall-related traumatic brain injury deaths and hospitalizations among older adults–United States, 2005. J Safety Res. 2008;39(3):269–72.
141. Teasdale G, Jennett B. Assessment and prognosis of coma after head injury. Acta Neurochir (Wien). 1976;34(1–4):45–55.
142. Bayir H, Marion DW, Puccio AM, Wisniewski SR, Janesko KL, Clark RS, Kochanek PM. Marked gender effect on lipid peroxidation after severe traumatic brain injury in adult patients. J Neurotrauma. 2004;21(1):1–8.
143. Wagner AK, Fabio A, Puccio AM, Hirschberg R, Li W, Zafonte RD, Marion DW. Gender associations with cerebrospinal fluid glutamate and lactate/pyruvate levels after severe traumatic brain injury. Crit Care Med. 2005;33(2):407–13.
144. Roof RL, Duvdevani R, Stein DG. Gender influences outcome of brain injury: progesterone plays a protective role. Brain Res. 1993;607(1–2):333–6.
145. Slewa-Younan S, Baguley IJ, Heriseanu R, Cameron ID, Pitsiavas V, Mudaliar Y, Nayyar V. Do men and women differ in their course following traumatic brain injury? A preliminary prospective investigation of early outcome. Brain Inj. 2008;22(2):183–91.
146. Farace E, Alves WM. Do women fare worse? A metaanalysis of gender differences in outcome after traumatic brain injury. Neurosurg Focus. 2000;8(1):e6.
147. Wright DW, Kellermann AL, Hertzberg VS, Clark PL, Frankel M, Goldstein FC, Salomone JP, Dent LL, Harris OA, Ander DS, Lowery DW, Patel MM, Denson DD, Gordon AB, Wald MM, Gupta S, Hoffman SW, Stein DG. ProTECT: a randomized clinical trial of progesterone for acute traumatic brain injury. Ann Emerg Med. 2007;49(4):391–402.
148. Xiao G, Wei J, Yan W, Wang W, Lu Z. Improved outcomes from the administration of progesterone for patients with acute severe traumatic brain injury: a randomized controlled trial. Crit Care. 2008;12(2):R61.
149. Junpeng M, Huang S, Qin S. Progesterone for acute traumatic brain injury. Cochrane Database Syst Rev. 2011;19(1):CD008409.
150. Thompson HJ, Rivara FP, Jurkovich GJ, Wang J, Nathens AB, MacKenzie EJ. Evaluation of the effect of intensity of care on mortality after traumatic brain injury. Crit Care Med. 2008;36(1):282–90.
151. Woolcott JC, Richardson KJ, Wiens MO, Patel B, Marin J, Khan KM, Marra CA. Meta-analysis of the impact of 9 medication classes on falls in elderly persons. Arch Intern Med. 2009;169(21):1952–60.
152. Howard 2nd JL, Cipolle MD, Horvat SA, Sabella VM, Reed 3rd JF, Fulda G, Tinkoff G, Pasquale MD. Preinjury warfarin worsens outcome in elderly patients who fall from standing. J Trauma. 2009;66(6):1518–22; discussion 1523–4.
153. Lavoie A, Ratte S, Clas D, Demers J, Moore L, Martin M, Bergeron E. Preinjury warfarin use among elderly patients with closed head injuries in a trauma center. J Trauma. 2004;56(4):802–7.
154. Fortuna GR, Mueller EW, James LE, Shutter LA, Butler KL. The impact of preinjury antiplatelet and anticoagulant pharmacotherapy on outcomes in elderly patients with hemorrhagic brain injury. Surgery. 2008;144(4):598–603; discussion 603–5.
155. Kennedy DM, Cipolle MD, Pasquale MD, Wasser T. Impact of preinjury warfarin use in elderly trauma patients. J Trauma. 2000;48(3):451–3.
156. Pieracci FM, Eachempati SR, Shou J, Hydo LJ, Barie PS. Degree of anticoagulation, but not warfarin use itself, predicts adverse outcomes after traumatic brain injury in elderly trauma patients. J Trauma. 2007;63(3):525–30.
157. Reynolds FD, Dietz PA, Higgins D, Whitaker TS. Time to deterioration of the elderly, anticoagulated, minor head injury patient who presents without evidence of neurologic abnormality. J Trauma. 2003;54(3):492–6.

158. Gittleman AM, Ortiz AO, Keating DP, Katz DS. Indications for CT in patients receiving anticoagulation after head trauma. AJNR Am J Neuroradiol. 2005;26(3):603–6.
159. Eikelboom JW, Wallentin L, Connolly SJ, Ezekowitz M, Healey JS, Oldgren J, Yang S, Alings M, Kaatz S, Hohnloser SH, Diener HC, Franzosi MG, Huber K, Reilly P, Varrone J, Yusuf S. Risk of bleeding with 2 doses of dabigatran compared with warfarin in older and younger patients with atrial fibrillation: an analysis of the randomized evaluation of long-term anticoagulant therapy (RE-LY) trial. Circulation. 2011;123(21):2363–72.
160. Garber ST, Sivakumar W, Schmidt RH. Neurosurgical complications of direct thrombin inhibitors–catastrophic hemorrhage after mild traumatic brain injury in a patient receiving dabigatran. J Neurosurg. 2012;116(5):1093–6.

Chest Wall Injury

24

Eileen M. Bulger

Introduction

Thoracic injury accounts for up to 25 % of fatalities among injured patients. Chest wall injuries are common with rib fractures identified in approximately 10–26 % of patients presenting to a trauma center and sternal fractures in <1 % [1–3]. Elderly patients are at increased risk for both rib and sternal fractures when compared to younger patients [4, 5]. Several studies have reported that these injuries are associated with increased morbidity and mortality in this patient cohort [4, 6–10]. The purpose of this chapter is to review the current literature regarding the patterns of chest wall injury in the geriatric population, evaluate the factors contributing to worse outcome, and discuss injury prevention and management strategies for patients with these injuries.

Epidemiology

A recent report from the National Trauma Data Bank noted that 9 % of patients in this database carried a diagnosis of one or more rib fractures with an overall mortality rate of 10 % [1]. The incidence of rib fractures in the elderly has been reported at 60 per 100,000 persons per year [11]. Elderly patients are thought to be at greater risk for rib fractures due to loss of cortical bone mass, which allows the bones to fracture with less kinetic energy than is required in younger patients. In the study by Bergeron et al., more than 50 % of elderly patients presenting with rib fractures had suffered a fall from standing [6]. The second most common etiology is motor vehicle crashes (MVC). A recent report from the Crash Injury Research and Engineering Network (CIREN) database noted that the majority of rib and sternal fractures occurring in elderly patients following MVCs result from compression of the thorax by the seat belt system [5]. They suggest that with the increasing number of elderly drivers, attention should be paid to the design of these safety systems relative to the increased fragility of older patients.

Several studies report increased morbidity and mortality among older patients subjected to chest wall injury compared to a younger cohort. Most studies evaluating disparity in outcome between younger and older patients focus on the population >65 years of age; however, some studies have noted impaired outcome beginning at age 45 [8]. Mortality reports range from 2 to 22 % and are likely heavily influenced by inclusion of patients with multisystem injury. Bulger et al. reported that mortality for elderly patients (>65 years) was more than twofold higher than the younger cohort (22 % vs. 10 %) [7]. The risk of mortality increased 19 % and the risk of pneumonia by 27 % for each additional rib fracture. Several others have noted increased morbidity with increasing number of ribs fractures. A recent meta-analysis, which evaluated the risk factors associated with poor outcome, reported a combined odds ratio for mortality of 1.98 (95 % CI: 1.86–2.11) for age >65 years and 2.02 (95% CI: 1.89–2.15) for three or more rib fractures [12]. Another report noted a significant increase in mortality for 6 or more fractured ribs [1].

Another contributing factor to impaired outcome in the elderly is likely the increased rate of associated medical comorbidities. Bergeron et al. reported a nearly threefold increased risk of mortality for patients with a preexisting medical condition (OR 2.98, 95 % CI 1.1–8.3) [6]. In a recent multicenter study, focusing on elderly patients with isolated blunt chest injury, 19.9 % of patients had coexisting coronary artery disease, 13.5 % lung disease, and 7.1 % congestive heart failure [13]. Preexisting congestive heart failure was one of the strongest predictors of mortality in this series. Similarly, Brasel et al. reported an adjusted odds ratio of 2.62 (95 % CI:1.93–3.55) for mortality following blunt chest trauma in patients with congestive heart failure [14].

E.M. Bulger, MD
Department of Surgery, Harborview Medical Center, University of Washington, 325 Ninth Avenue, 359796, Seattle, WA 98104-2499, USA
e-mail: ebulger@u.washington.edu

J.A. Yelon, F.A. Luchette (eds.), *Geriatric Trauma and Critical Care*,
DOI 10.1007/978-1-4614-8501-8_24, © Springer Science+Business Media New York 2014

The primary complication which develops in these patients after hospitalization is pneumonia. Pneumonia rates vary depending on the population studied. For the entire population hospitalized with one or more rib fractures, the rate of pneumonia is reported to be 6 % [14]. However, when one reviews patients admitted to a trauma center, reports range from 11 to 17 % for patients younger than 65 years to 31–34 % for patients older than 65 years [6, 7]. Bulger et al. reported that elderly patients had a risk of pneumonia exceeding 30 % [7]. The impact of pneumonia on mortality is debated. Bergeron noted a nearly fourfold increase in mortality risk for patients who developed a pneumonia (OR 3.8 (95 % CI: 1.5–9.7) [6]. However, Brasel et al. reported that pneumonia was associated with increased mortality among those with no associated injuries but was not a major factor for those with multisystem injury [14]. Regardless, the development of pneumonia has been associated with increased duration of mechanical ventilation and prolonged ICU stay, thus significantly impacting the resources required to care for these patients.

Injury Prevention

The leading causes of chest wall injury in the elderly are falls and motor vehicle crashes. There are several programs which have been proposed for elderly fall prevention which are beyond the scope of this review. However, recent data also supports consideration for specific injury prevention strategies associated with chest wall fractures resulting from motor vehicle collisions. Bansal et al. reported an analysis of 287 elderly patients with rib and sternal fractures after MVCs and noted that the primary source of these injuries in frontal impacts was compression from the seat belts or contact with the rim of the steering wheel [5]. For side impact crashes, contact with the side interior (door panel) was the primary etiology. For seat belt-related injuries, they suggest that a four-point safety belt system or wider shoulder straps may allow more even distribution of the force to the chest and thus have the potential to reduce these injuries. For side impact crashes, advances in side airbags/torso bags should be investigated. The use of "elderly," more fragile, crash test dummies might be needed to test these innovations.

Treatment

Hospital Admission

The first question to address in the management of elderly patients with rib fracture is which patients will benefit from hospital admission. This is an issue for the elderly patient with isolated chest wall injury, which can occur after even a minor fall from standing. Several authors have advocated that based on the increased risk of poor outcome in this patient cohort, patients over age 65 with >3 rib fractures should be admitted to the hospital and those with >6 rib fractures should be admitted to an intensive care unit for monitoring even without evident respiratory compromise on admission [10].

Pain Management

The cornerstone of management for multiple rib fractures is attention to pain control. Patients with inadequate pain control will minimize their chest wall motion by reducing their tidal volume and coughing and as a result are at significant risk of developing nosocomial pneumonia. The options for initial inpatient pain control include intravenous narcotics and regional anesthetics. These may be supplemented with injectable or oral NSAIDS as indicated, with eventual transition to oral narcotics prior to discharge. There have been a number of studies, which have investigated pain control strategies for these patients. These are discussed for each option below. Regardless of the approach selected, involving a dedicated pain relief service to monitor the effectiveness of the strategy chosen is critical. Development of a multidisciplinary pathway for management of these patients has been associated with improved outcome [15–17]. Todd et al. recently reported on a pathway for patient with four or more rib fractures over the age of 45 years [15]. In this study pathway patients were monitored closely for pain and cough scores and incentive spirometry volume. Based on this assessment a pain service was consulted to optimize pain control, respiratory therapy was consulted for a volume expansion protocol, physical therapy was consulted to increase patient mobility, and attention was paid to nutritional support and medical comorbidities. Patients managed with this clinical pathway were found to have a shorter ICU and hospital stay and lower mortality.

Oral Pain Medications

Oral narcotics are generally reserved for patients with minimal rib fractures who may be managed as outpatients. Patients on intravenous or regional medications may be transitioned to oral agents several days after injury in anticipation of discharge. Nonsteroidal anti-inflammatory drugs may be given in concert with narcotics to reduce the opioid need, although there are no studies specific to rib fracture pain management. NSAID use is limited by bleeding concerns and potential renal toxicity, so should be avoided in trauma patients with significant early bleeding risk, such as ongoing hemothorax or solid organ injury, and in those with renal insufficiency.

Intravenous Narcotics

Intravenous narcotics are usually the first method of pain control employed for patients with multiple rib fractures. This route of administration is preferred over subcutaneous or intramuscular injection, as the onset of action is more rapid and more predictable. Patients must be closely monitored for excessive sedation or depression of respiratory drive, especially among the elderly. Patient-controlled analgesia is a good option for patients who are alert as they can control the delivery of the medication, which may provide a more timely response and diminish excessive sedation. Excessive sedation of elderly patients is associated with a significant increased risk of aspiration, which can further compromise pulmonary function. Thus, for patients who are particularly sensitive to narcotics, regional analgesia regimen should be considered.

Regional Anesthetics

There are several approaches to the administration of regional anesthetics/narcotics. These include continuous epidural infusion of local anesthetics and/or narcotics, paravertebral or intrapleural infusion of local anesthetic, intermittent intercostal nerve blocks, and continuous local anesthetic infusion in the subcutaneous space following thoracotomy.

The most widely studied approach is the use of epidural catheters for infusion of local anesthetics, with or without narcotics. Previous studies have shown that the use of epidural catheters results in improved pulmonary function tests and better pain scores when compared to intravenous narcotics [18–22]. These studies have generally included all adults and have not focused specifically on the elderly population. In the trial by Bulger et al., patients were randomized to receive intravenous narcotics vs. epidural catheter. There was a significant reduction in the risk of pneumonia and a 2-day reduction in the average duration of mechanical ventilation for the epidural group [23]. A recent systematic review of the literature failed to identify a clear impact of epidural analgesia on mortality or ICU length of stay, but did suggest a benefit on the duration of mechanical ventilation [24]. Use of epidural catheters for pain control after severe blunt chest wall injury is a Level 1 recommendation in the 2004 EAST guidelines [25].

Epidural catheter use is limited in some cases due to the many contraindications to catheter placement in patients with multisystem injury. The most common contraindications are associated spine fractures and coagulopathy. In a recent survey of pain service directors at major trauma centers in the USA, it was evident that there remains considerable controversy in this area and better definition of the absolute and relative contraindications is needed to weigh against the potential benefit of this approach [26]. A common side effect of epidural infusion is systemic hypotension, which thus mandates close monitoring especially in the elderly patient population. One retrospective series noted a higher rate of complications among elderly patients receiving epidural analgesia; however, this analysis was limited due to significant differences in the baseline characteristics between the treatment groups [27].

Three recent studies have evaluated the use of paravertebral infusion of local anesthetics and found this approach to be as effective as epidural infusion (need ref). This approach is effective only in patients with unilateral rib fractures and was associated with a lower rate of systemic hypotension. The authors also note that placement of these catheters is technically easier than epidural catheters. The sample size for these studies was small so more work needs to be done in this area [28–30].

Another option is the placement of intrapleural catheters for infusion of local anesthetics directly into the pleural space. In some cases these are placed adjacent to a thoracostomy tube. One study, which was placebo controlled, failed to find clear benefit with this approach [31]. Another study which compared intrapleural to epidural analgesia found the epidural approach associated with better pain relief [32].

Intermittent injection of local anesthetics to block the intercostal nerves has been reported as one approach to pain management for these patients. This approach is limited by the duration of the block and thus requires repeated injections to achieve continuous relief. This is very labor intensive, and as a result, this approach has largely been replaced by the continuous infusion strategies noted above. There is also a device available that can be placed in the subcutaneous tissue after thoracotomy for continuous infusion of local anesthetic, but it has not been evaluated in patients who do not require thoracotomy [33].

Respiratory Therapy

The second cornerstone of management of patients with multiple rib fractures is to provide close attention to respiratory function and encourage deep breathing through incentive spirometry and coughing to clear secretions. Use of chest physiotherapy may be limited by chest wall pain. The indications for mechanical ventilation are based on the underlying pulmonary physiology and traditional signs of respiratory failure including increased work of breathing, hypercapnia, and hypoxia [34]. In general, adequate attention to pain control is key to reducing pulmonary collapse and thus avoiding intubation. For intubated patients, there was one study that suggested that intermittent recruitment maneuvers may improve oxygenation, but it is not clear if this will affect outcome [35].

Operative Stabilization of Rib Fractures

The operative stabilization of rib fractures has been controversial, and the procedure has evolved as better technology has become available to stabilize the ribs with a minimally invasive approach. A recent survey of trauma and thoracic surgeons in the USA suggested that the majority felt that rib fracture fixation was appropriate for selected patients, yet only 26 % of these surgeons had performed this procedure [36]. One generally accepted indication is the stabilization of significantly displaced ribs identified at the time of a thoracotomy for other reasons, known as "on the way out fixation." Other potential indications for primary rib fixation include as follows: flail segment with failure to wean from mechanical ventilation, unstable ribs refractory to conventional pain management, chest wall deformity/defect, and rib fracture nonunion [37].

Several single-center studies have suggested that rib fracture stabilization may facilitate ventilator weaning and thus shorten the duration of mechanical ventilation. There have been two small, randomized trials. Tanaka et al. randomized 37 patients with flail chest, requiring mechanical ventilation to surgical stabilization vs. nonoperative management [38]. Patients in the surgical group spent fewer days on the ventilator, had a lower incidence of pneumonia, and had better pulmonary function at 1 month. Granetzny et al. randomized 40 patients with flail chest to operative stabilization vs. external splinting with adhesive plaster [39]. The operative group had a shorted duration of mechanical ventilation and a lower rate of pneumonia. A case-controlled study by Nirula et al. was consistent with these results [40]. Patients with significant pulmonary contusions are less likely to benefit [41]. The guideline from the Eastern Association for the Surgery of Trauma recognizes surgical fixation as a Level III recommendation for management of flail chest given the small numbers of patients randomized and the lack of comparison with more recent care pathways for these patients including the use of epidural analgesia [42]. Another area of ongoing investigation involves the potential impact of operative fixation on long-term morbidity for this patient population [43]. There are no studies which focus specifically on the risks and benefits of rib fracture fixation in the elderly population. These patients may face greater surgical risks due to medical comorbidities, and the poor bone quality may also limit the success of fixation. Further studies are needed to determine the optimal use of this approach in the elderly population.

Summary

In summary, elderly patients not only are at greater risk to have chest wall fractures even with minor mechanisms of injury but also suffer from significantly increased risks of morbidity and mortality. As a result, care protocols should focus on a low threshold for hospital and ICU admission and close attention to pain management and respiratory therapy. The role of operative fixation in this population requires further study.

References

1. Flagel BT, Luchette FA, Reed RL, et al. Half-a-dozen ribs: the breakpoint for mortality. Surgery. 2005;138(4):717–23; discussion 723–15.
2. Recinos G, Inaba K, Dubose J, et al. Epidemiology of sternal fractures. Am Surg. 2009;75(5):401–4.
3. Ziegler DW, Agarwal NN. The morbidity and mortality of rib fractures [see comments]. J Trauma. 1994;37(6):975–9.
4. Stitzel JD, Kilgo PD, Weaver AA, Martin RS, Loftis KL, Meredith JW. Age thresholds for increased mortality of predominant crash induced thoracic injuries. Ann Adv Automot Med. 2010;54:41–50.
5. Bansal V, Conroy C, Chang D, Tominaga GT, Coimbra R. Rib and sternum fractures in the elderly and extreme elderly following motor vehicle crashes. Accid Anal Prev. 2011;43(3):661–5.
6. Bergeron E, Lavoie A, Clas D, et al. Elderly trauma patients with rib fractures are at greater risk of death and pneumonia. J Trauma. 2003;54(3):478–85.
7. Bulger EM, Arneson MA, Mock CN, Jurkovich GJ. Rib fractures in the elderly. J Trauma. 2000;48(6):1040–6; discussion 1046–7.
8. Holcomb JB, McMullin NR, Kozar RA, Lygas MH, Moore FA. Morbidity from rib fractures increases after age 45. J Am Coll Surg. 2003;196(4):549–55.
9. Elmistekawy EM, Hammad AA. Isolated rib fractures in geriatric patients. Ann Thorac Med. 2007;2(4):166–8.
10. Sharma OP, Oswanski MF, Jolly S, Lauer SK, Dressel R, Stombaugh HA. Perils of rib fractures. Am Surg. 2008;74(4):310–4.
11. Palvanen M, Kannus P, Niemi S, Parkkari J, Vuori I. Epidemiology of minimal trauma rib fractures in the elderly. Calcif Tissue Int. 1998;62(3):274–7.
12. Battle CE, Hutchings H, Evans PA. Risk factors that predict mortality in patients with blunt chest wall trauma: a systematic review and meta-analysis. Injury. 2012;43(1):8–17.
13. Harrington DT, Phillips B, Machan J, et al. Factors associated with survival following blunt chest trauma in older patients: results from a large regional trauma cooperative. Arch Surg. 2010;145(5):432–7.
14. Brasel KJ, Guse CE, Layde P, Weigelt JA. Rib fractures: relationship with pneumonia and mortality. Crit Care Med. 2006;34(6): 1642–6.
15. Todd SR, McNally MM, Holcomb JB, et al. A multidisciplinary clinical pathway decreases rib fracture-associated infectious morbidity and mortality in high-risk trauma patients. Am J Surg. 2006;192(6):806–11.
16. Wilson S, Bin J, Sesperez J, Seger M, Sugrue M. Clinical pathways – can they be used in trauma care. An analysis of their ability to fit the patient. Injury. 2001;32(7):525–32.
17. Winters BA. Older adults with traumatic rib fractures: an evidence-based approach to their care. J Trauma Nurs. 2009;16(2):93–7.
18. Mackersie RC, Karagianes TG, Hoyt DB, Davis JW. Prospective evaluation of epidural and intravenous administration of fentanyl for pain control and restoration of ventilatory function following multiple rib fractures. J Trauma. 1991;31(4):443–9; discussion 449–51.
19. Mackersie RC, Shackford SR, Hoyt DB, Karagianes TG. Continuous epidural fentanyl analgesia: ventilatory function improvement with routine use in treatment of blunt chest injury. J Trauma. 1987;27(11):1207–12.

20. Moon MR, Luchette FA, Gibson SW, et al. Prospective, randomized comparison of epidural versus parenteral opioid analgesia in thoracic trauma. Ann Surg. 1999;229(5):684–92.
21. Govindarajan R, Bakalova T, Michael R, Abadir AR. Epidural buprenorphine in management of pain in multiple rib fractures. Acta Anaesthesiol Scand. 2002;46(6):660–5.
22. Wisner DH. A stepwise logistic regression analysis of factors affecting morbidity and mortality after thoracic trauma: effect of epidural analgesia. J Trauma. 1990;30(7):799–804; discussion 804–5.
23. Bulger EM, Edwards T, Klotz P, Jurkovich GJ. Epidural analgesia improves outcome after multiple rib fractures. Surgery. 2004;136(2):426–30.
24. Carrier FM, Turgeon AF, Nicole PC, et al. Effect of epidural analgesia in patients with traumatic rib fractures: a systematic review and meta-analysis of randomized controlled trials. Can J Anaesth. 2009;56(3):230–42.
25. Simon BJ, Cushman J, Barraco R, et al. Pain management guidelines for blunt thoracic trauma. J Trauma. 2005;59(5):1256–67.
26. Bulger EM, Edwards WT, de Pinto M, Klotz P, Jurkovich GJ. Indications and contraindications for thoracic epidural analgesia in multiply injured patients. Acute Pain. 2008;10(1):15–22.
27. Kieninger AN, Bair HA, Bendick PJ, Howells GA. Epidural versus intravenous pain control in elderly patients with rib fractures. Am J Surg. 2005;189(3):327–30.
28. Karmakar MK, Critchley LA, Ho AM, Gin T, Lee TW, Yim AP. Continuous thoracic paravertebral infusion of bupivacaine for pain management in patients with multiple fractured ribs. Chest. 2003;123(2):424–31.
29. Mohta M, Verma P, Saxena AK, Sethi AK, Tyagi A, Girotra G. Prospective, randomized comparison of continuous thoracic epidural and thoracic paravertebral infusion in patients with unilateral multiple fractured ribs–a pilot study. J Trauma. 2009;66(4): 1096–101.
30. Truitt MS, Murry J, Amos J, et al. Continuous intercostal nerve blockade for rib fractures: ready for primetime? J Trauma. 2011;71(6):1548–52; discussion 1552.
31. Short K, Scheeres D, Mlakar J, Dean R. Evaluation of intrapleural analgesia in the management of blunt traumatic chest wall pain: a clinical trial. Am Surg. 1996;62(6):488–93.
32. Luchette FA, Radafshar SM, Kaiser R, Flynn W, Hassett JM. Prospective evaluation of epidural versus intrapleural catheters for analgesia in chest wall trauma. J Trauma. 1994;36(6):865–9; discussion 869–70.
33. Wheatley 3rd GH, Rosenbaum DH, Paul MC, et al. Improved pain management outcomes with continuous infusion of a local anesthetic after thoracotomy. J Thorac Cardiovasc Surg. 2005;130(2):464–8.
34. Barone JE, Pizzi WF, Nealon Jr TF, Richman H. Indications for intubation in blunt chest trauma. J Trauma. 1986;26(4):334–8.
35. Schreiter D, Reske A, Stichert B, et al. Alveolar recruitment in combination with sufficient positive end-expiratory pressure increases oxygenation and lung aeration in patients with severe chest trauma. Crit Care Med. 2004;32(4):968–75.
36. Mayberry JC, Ham LB, Schipper PH, Ellis TJ, Mullins RJ. Surveyed opinion of American trauma, orthopedic, and thoracic surgeons on rib and sternal fracture repair. J Trauma. 2009;66(3): 875–9.
37. Nirula R, Diaz Jr JJ, Trunkey DD, Mayberry JC. Rib fracture repair: indications, technical issues, and future directions. World J Surg. 2009;33(1):14–22.
38. Tanaka H, Yukioka T, Yamaguti Y, et al. Surgical stabilization or internal pneumatic stabilization? A prospective randomized study of management of severe flail chest patients. J Trauma. 2002;52(4): 727–32; discussion 732.
39. Granetzny A, Abd El-Aal M, Emam E, Shalaby A, Boseila A. Surgical versus conservative treatment of flail chest. Evaluation of the pulmonary status. Interact Cardiovasc Thorac Surg. 2005; 4(6):583–7.
40. Nirula R, Allen B, Layman R, Falimirski ME, Somberg LB. Rib fracture stabilization in patients sustaining blunt chest injury. Am Surg. 2006;72(4):307–9.
41. Voggenreiter G, Neudeck F, Aufmkolk M, Obertacke U, Schmit-Neuerburg KP. Operative chest wall stabilization in flail chest–outcomes of patients with or without pulmonary contusion. J Am Coll Surg. 1998;187(2):130–8.
42. Management of pulmonary contusion and flail chest. 2006; http://www.east.org/tpg.asp. Accessed 22 Jun 2012.
43. Mayberry JC, Kroeker AD, Ham LB, Mullins RJ, Trunkey DD. Long-term morbidity, pain, and disability after repair of severe chest wall injuries. Am Surg. 2009;75(5):389–94.

Thoracic

25

Robert K. Parker and David T. Harrington

General Considerations

Thoracic trauma is a significant contributor to the morbidity and mortality in trauma patients regardless of age. Though protected by the bony skeleton, once this rigid protective envelope is breached, the vital contents of the thorax, the heart and lungs, can manifest significant physiologic derangements. Many chest injuries may be managed effectively and definitively by simple bedside procedures that most physicians involved in trauma care should be able to perform, whereas other chest injuries require urgent, major operative repair. Rib fractures, flail chest, sternal fracture, blunt cardiac injury, and blunt aortic injury may require attention in specialized centers. Some straightforward injuries, such as pneumothorax and hemothorax, do not require different management based on age; however because of increased underlying comorbidities and decreased physiologic reserve in the geriatric population, the severely injured elderly patient requires intensive monitoring, aggressive cardiopulmonary management, and comprehensive care [1–3].

Blunt chest trauma is caused by various mechanisms, but motor vehicle collision is the most common [4]. In MVCs, multiple rib fractures, higher injury severity score, and increased age are associated with increased morbidity and mortality. Other risk factors associated with significant injury include high-speed collision, lack of seat belt use, front seat occupancy, and steering wheel deformity. Falls are also significant sources of trauma in the elderly. Even a fall from standing can cause serious injury in the elderly population. Penetrating injury from stab wounds or gunshot wounds is very uncommon in the over 65-year-old trauma patient.

Increased age is associated with a decrease in organ function. Respiratory function declines with aging. As chest wall compliance decreases secondary to structural changes, such as vertebral collapse and kyphosis, inspiratory capacity decreases. Progressive decline in muscle strength results in loss of up to 50 % in inspiratory and expiratory force. Decreased lung elasticity and increased alveolar collapse result in air trapping and ventilation-perfusion mismatching. This leads to a decline of 0.3–0.4 mmHg annually in arterial oxygen tension. The cardiovascular system has a limited response to metabolic demand due to a lower maximum heart rate, insufficient cardiac output, and increased peripheral vascular resistance. Physiologic deterioration places the elderly trauma patient at increased risk for complications and death following blunt thoracic trauma.

Though there is a steady decline in physiologic reserve of all organ systems with aging, the major driver of poor outcomes in the elderly are the chronic health conditions that may also develop in some patients with age. A long list of home medications have been shown to correlate with both increased risk of injury and worse outcomes once injured [5, 6]. Practitioners should evaluate not chronologic age, but physiologic age when assessing risk for a poor outcome from trauma. Decreased physiologic reserve can be assessed not only by a patient's response to the initial injury but also by the patient's ability to weather the complications that develop following the initial trauma or surgical procedure. An elderly patient with comorbidities may tolerate an operation, but if a complication occurs, then that patient's outcome suffers significantly. The mortality rate in patients at Veteran Affairs Hospitals undergoing noncardiac surgery rose from 4 to 26 % in patients who developed any complication. In this population, the American Society of Anesthesiologist (ASA) class, poor baseline function and emergency surgery were the strongest predictors of mortality, but age alone increased risk of mortality by 5 % for every additional year after age 80 [7].

Declining organ function with aging has a negative effect on patient outcomes. Isolated chest trauma in the elderly can result in significant morbidity with reported adverse outcomes ranging from 16 to 33 % [8, 9]. Patient variables that

R.K. Parker, MD • D.T. Harrington, MD, FACS (✉)
Department of Surgery, Rhode Island Hospital,
Providence, RI 02903, USA
e-mail: robert.k.parker@gmail.com; dharrington@usasurg.org,
dharrington@lifespn.org

J.A. Yelon, F.A. Luchette (eds.), *Geriatric Trauma and Critical Care*,
DOI 10.1007/978-1-4614-8501-8_25, © Springer Science+Business Media New York 2014

predict a worse prognosis include increased age (>85 years), decreased initial systolic blood pressure (<90 mmHg), three or more unilateral rib fractures, or the presence of hemothorax, pneumothorax, or pulmonary contusion [8]. In the geriatric population, underlying comorbidities, such as congestive heart failure, may significantly compromise recovery [10]. Thoracic trauma directly accounts for one fourth of all injury-related deaths and is a contributing factor in the demise of one half of all trauma death. After sustaining blunt chest trauma, elderly patients have a higher mortality and morbidity than younger patients with similar injuries [11, 12]. At our institution thoracic trauma and its pulmonary sequelae are the second most common cause of mortality, following head injury, and represents 30 % of deaths in the geriatric (>65 years) population [13].

Primary Survey: Initial Evaluation and Management

Blunt chest trauma can result in the injury of multiple, significant structures. As described in Advanced Trauma Life Support, life-threatening conditions must be addressed first: airway, breathing, circulation, disability, and exposure. Establishing a secure airway is the first priority. Special attention must be given to the cervical spine due to high incidence of preexisting abnormalities and high rates of vertebral injury in the elderly [14]. Second, ventilation must be ensured. Physical exam of the chest should focus on the presence of breath sounds (often difficult to distinguish in a loud trauma bay), tracheal deviation, chest wall movement, and presence of crepitus. If a pneumothorax is present, this injury should be addressed by needle decompression or chest tube placement. Circulation can then be assessed clinically by assessment of mental status, skin perfusion, strength of peripheral pulses, and blood pressure. Circulatory deficits need to be addressed and the source of blood loss identified and stopped. Cardiac and pulmonary contusions should not delay definitive treatment for other injuries. The primary survey should be continued to assess disability, with an awareness of the baseline neurological status of the elderly, and ensuring full exposure of the whole patient to avoid missed injuries while promoting normothermia.

The initial assessment of an elderly trauma patient should be approached very carefully, for standard triage criteria may not properly identify the gravity of their condition [15]. For example, standard physiologic triage variables, such as heart rate and systolic blood pressure, may be misleading in identifying severe injury in geriatric patients. For heart rate, an increase in mortality is seen in elderly patients once presenting heart rate is greater than 90. This same mortality effect is not seen in the 17–35-year-old trauma population until heart rates exceed 130. For systolic blood pressure, the inflection point for mortality appears to be 110 in the elderly, but 95 in the younger population [13]. While a heart rate of 92 and a systolic blood pressure of 105 usually indicates smooth sailing in the young trauma patient, it may indicate shock in the elderly trauma patient.

In blunt chest trauma, emergent ED thoracotomy is rarely successful. Reported rates of neurologically intact survival for all patients are less than 5 % if the patient is in shock and less than 1 % in those with no measureable blood pressure. Most series report no survivors in patient greater than 65 years of age [16]. At our institution, emergent ED thoracotomy for blunt trauma is not performed in the elderly due to the lack of meaningful survival and the risks to all involved.

Diagnostic Imaging

CxR

The chest radiograph (CxR) may be the single most essential test for the blunt trauma victim, and its usage is recommended for all trauma patients. CxR is not invasive, low cost, easily obtainable, and can reveal a great deal of information. The CxR should be interpreted immediately and certainly prior to transfer from the trauma bay with attention to life-threatening injuries to the airway, evidence of pneumothorax, hemothorax, or blunt aortic injury.

Ultrasound

Bedside ultrasound is increasingly used in the evaluation of blunt trauma patients. The focused assessment with sonography for trauma (FAST) exam, which examines the hepatorenal and splenorenal spaces and the pelvis, may be performed while other resuscitative interventions occur in a hypotensive patient. A FAST exam's true utility is the assessment for intra-abdominal fluid in the hypotensive patient, where it can reliably detect 100–150 cc of fluid [17]. FAST has less utility in the normotensive patient and cannot be reliably used to detect solid or hollow viscus injuries. At most centers an evaluation for pericardial effusion is included in the FAST exam. Collapse of the right atrium by a pericardial effusion is a sensitive indicator for cardiac tamponade. Some authors have advocated an extended FAST exam as the primary diagnostic modality for hemothorax and pneumothorax [18, 19].

Chest CT

Computed tomography (CT) scans are often utilized in the evaluation of blunt trauma and have had increased usage over the last two decades. Driving this increased utilization is the desire to reduce missed traumatic injury thereby reducing complications from delayed diagnosis [20]. Increased utilization is seen not just during initial workup but also throughout the hospital course. This trend of high utilization of CT scanning is most pronounced in the elderly patient [21]. Plurad et al. question the clinical utility of the increased utilization of this expensive test. The majority of chest CT scans in their study were performed after an initial normal CxR, and although a number of occult pneumothoraces and hemothoraces were identified, few patients were identified who had significant injury requiring treatment [22]. Significant traumatic mechanism, abnormal CxR, or patterns of associated injuries should prompt a chest CT scan in order to diagnose injuries such as blunt aortic injury or diaphragmatic hernia.

Tube Thoracostomy

Tube thoracostomy has been in the medical armamentarium since it was first described by Hippocrates. Initially a metal tube used in the treatment of empyema, it has evolved into its modern form and been used for many different medical conditions. Tube thoracostomy is often used as initial and definitive management (75–80 %) of blunt chest trauma. Pneumothorax and hemothorax are the most common indications. To place a chest tube, the chest should be prepped and draped with sterile technique and full barrier precautions: caps, gown, mask, glove, and full barrier sheet. A local anesthetic, such as lidocaine, should be infiltrated in the subcutaneous tissues and around the perineural tissue and pleura. An incision, in the fourth or fifth intercostal space in the anterior axillary line, should be carried down through skin and subcutaneous tissue down to muscle. A blunt clamp should be inserted over the top of the rib into the pleural cavity and entry confirmed with insertion of a finger. A large-bore chest tube (>28 French) should be placed and directed posterior and toward the apex [23]. The tube should be connected initially to a 20-cm wall suction with a water seal and collection system. Despite the simplicity of the procedure, it is not without complications. These complications can be classified as insertional (bleeding, parenchymal lung injury), positional (retained fluid or blood), and infective (empyema) with rates as high as 30 % in trauma victims. Routine antibiotic prophylaxis is not recommended for tube thoracostomy, particularly given the morbidity of antibiotic-associated Clostridium difficile colitis in elderly patients [24, 25].

Specific Injuries

Pulmonary Contusion

Pulmonary contusion is the most common of the potentially lethal chest injuries and is often associated with other traumatic injuries. It is caused by trauma to the lung parenchyma typically adjacent to the site of impact; however, it may also occur in a countercoup fashion. The initial diagnosis is usually made on chest radiograph or computed tomography, but these evaluations often miss the true severity, for contusions often blossom over the first 24–36 h after injury. Although contusion occurs in 75 % of all patients with significant chest trauma, the incidence may be less in the elderly patient population with a less compliant thorax. The less compliant thorax dissipates the force of the trauma within the elderly skeleton through fractures instead of transmitting the energy to the lung parenchyma. Parenchymal injury causes ventilation-perfusion inequalities with right-to-left shunt and hypoxia, which is often exacerbated by hypoventilation secondary to splinting. If pulmonary contusion is not complicated by infection, large resuscitation, or volutrauma from mechanical ventilation, contusion resolves in 3–5 days. Pulmonary contusion is a risk factor for development of ARDS and has a significant impact on mortality across all age ranges [26–28]. Treatment of pulmonary contusion includes supportive therapy and aggressive pulmonary hygiene. There is no role for prophylactic antibiotics, steroids, or diuretics in this injury.

Pneumothorax

Pneumothorax is one of the most common sequelae of blunt chest trauma. Pneumothorax is caused by trauma disrupting the lung parenchyma or tracheobronchial structures resulting in air escaping into the thoracic space. The leak of air into the thoracic cavity results in partial or complete lung parenchymal collapse. In healthy people with intact pulmonary reserve, a partial collapse may be asymptomatic. In the elderly, who often have compromised baseline pulmonary function, tachypnea and declining systemic oxygenation can occur. Continued leak of air into the chest cavity can result in increased intrathoracic pressure that decreases cardiac venous return and causes hypotension and shock. Although classic signs of tension pneumothorax, tracheal deviation, unilateral decreased breath sounds, and jugular venous distention may not be appreciable in the trauma bay, suspicion should be high and needle decompression or tube thoracostomy should be utilized liberally in hemodynamically compromised patients.

Reliance on CT scanning during the diagnostic workup of trauma has revealed a significant rate of occult pneumothoraces. These small pneumothoraces, not visible on plain film, may be observed clinically. Positive pressure ventilation is not a contraindication for observation of an occult pneumothorax, though it is critical that the diagnosis of occult pneumothorax is passed between care teams during sign-outs and hand-offs. Progression of these pneumothoraces and the need for chest tube placement is required in less than 10 % of patients. In hospitalized patients daily chest radiographs should be utilized to follow progression. Visible pneumothorax on CxR, which is a sign of continued air leak, should prompt the placement of a chest tube [29, 30].

Hemothorax

All hemothoraces visible on plain chest radiograph should be drained by tube thoracostomy. In elderly patients with a history of trauma, the practice of ascribing a pleural fluid collection to their underlying cardiac or pulmonary condition and not placing a chest tube should be discouraged. The majority of hemothoraces following blunt trauma are easily treated by drainage and re-expansion of the lung. If bleeding continues, underlying factors such as coagulopathy, acidosis, and hypothermia should all be sought and addressed. Particular attention should be paid to the elderly on various forms of anticoagulation. Initial chest tube output of >1,500 mL and ongoing bleeding (>200 mL × 4 h) indicate injury to structures such as diaphragm, intercostal artery, or cardiac injury and requires thoracotomy. Retained hemothorax, occurring in roughly 10 % of hemothoraces, is a complication of misplaced or inadequate chest tube drainage. The blood of retained hemothorax may provide a nidus for infection that results in empyema and should be evacuated completely either by further tube thoracostomies or operative intervention – video-assisted thoracoscopy (VATS) or open thoracotomy. A retained hemothorax significantly increases the risk of formation of an empyema [31]. VATS is not contraindicated even in the very elderly (although one-lung ventilation is required) and should be utilized for posttraumatic hemothorax [32]. Open thoracotomy is indicated in ongoing bleeding, persistent large-clotted hemothorax refractory to tube thoracostomy and VATS, empyema, or need for definitive repair of injury.

Empyema

Empyema is a significant complication following chest trauma, occurring in 4–5 % patients who have a traumatic hemothorax. Empyemas can be caused by multiple sources: bronchopleural fistula, parapneumonic effusion, pulmonary abscess, retained hemothorax, esophageal injury, or diaphragmatic hernia with contamination from abdominal contents. CxR is generally not useful in diagnosing an empyema because it cannot differentiate between fluid, contusion, or atelectasis. A chest CT with IV contrast is a valuable diagnostic test since it may identify a rim-enhancing lesion or visualize a loculated collection. Antibiotic therapy is an important component of treatment, but source control through drainage and/or decortication is most important.

Tracheal/Bronchial Injury

Blunt tracheobronchial injury occurs in less than 1 % of trauma patients presenting to trauma centers, though it is a common cause of prehospital mortality with these patients dying of asphyxia. While significant disruption of the tracheal/bronchial tree can present in a dramatic manner with massive subcutaneous air and continuous air leaks from chest tubes, minor injuries are often missed initially and present late with a median time to diagnosis of 6 months [33, 34]. Shear force to the intrathoracic trachea occurs at the fixed points of the carina and cricoid and most tracheobronchial injuries occur within 2.5 cm of the carina. Injury confined to the mediastinal space presents as pneumomediastinum. Injuries into the pleural space present as a pneumothorax, which may cause a persistent large air leak after tube thoracostomy. Pneumomediastinum, persistent subcutaneous emphysema without other etiology, or persistent large air leak should prompt a rigid or flexible bronchoscopy looking for a tracheobronchial injury. Minor injuries, such as mucosa injuries only and injuries in the membranous portion of the airway, can often be managed nonoperatively [35]. Even if these injuries require delayed operative intervention, good outcome can be obtained [34]. Increased age is associated with increased mortality for tracheobronchial injuries [35]. Massive, continuous air leaks or massive subcutaneous emphysema poses a significant treatment challenge. Careful fiber-optic-assisted intubation below the level of the injury can stabilize patients with injuries near the cricoid. Patients with lower injuries can be very difficult to ventilate, oxygenate, or to keep their lung expanded. In this situation, the chest tube should be removed from suction to water seal in order to decrease air leak, potentially increase tidal volumes, and provide a window to stabilize the patient prior to operative repair. Upper airway injuries can be approached surgically through a collar incision, and injuries to the carina and main stem bronchi are best approached through a right thoracotomy incision. For injuries to the left main stem bronchus greater than 1 cm away from the carina, a left thoracotomy incision may be the best approach.

Blunt Cardiac Injury

Blunt cardiac injury (BCI) ranges from cardiac contusion to cardiac disruption. Often resulting from direct force to the chest from MVC or fall, BCI is often associated with a fractured sternum or ribs. The right ventricle, the most anterior portion of the heart, is the most common location of injury. Myocardial damage from contusion may result in arrhythmias or mechanical dysfunction [36]. Identifying 100 % of blunt cardiac injuries with an exhaustive diagnostic workup is unnecessary. An appropriate diagnostic strategy is to identify patients who are at risk for cardiac complications requiring treatment: dysrhythmia, cardiogenic shock, or structural injury. Workup should include a 12-lead electrocardiogram. Cardiac enzyme panels are unnecessary. If the ECG is normal, no further diagnostic tests or monitoring is necessary. If the ECG shows nonspecific abnormalities, the patient may be observed in a cardiac-monitored bed for 12–24 h and discharged once the ECG returns to normal and if asymptomatic. ECG findings such as dysrhythmia, heart block, or ST elevation warrant a 24–48-h admission with further workup dependent upon the clinical course of the patient. Cardiac injury generally manifests within the first 24 h of admission and further monitoring beyond that period is generally not warranted [37]. Dysrhythmias should be managed with rate control and correction of electrolytes. Contusions are not a vascular-based disease and therefore are not managed like myocardial infarction (aspirin and rate control with beta-blockade). Treatment of cardiac contusion consists of observation of the hemodynamically normal patient and inotropic support and decreasing right ventricular afterload in patients with hemodynamic perturbations. Pericardial tamponade can be diagnosed on ultrasound and prompt surgical drainage of the pericardial sac will provide profound hemodynamic improvement. However, pericardial tamponade in blunt injury often arises from a significant underlying cardiac injury, which can be difficult to repair. Tears at the level of the IVC and right atrium junction are difficult to isolate, will probably require cardiopulmonary bypass (CPB) to repair, but often are non-survivable. Burst injuries of the atrial appendages are fairly straightforward and can be repaired directly. Ventricular disruption is associated with a significant surrounding zone of injury, most often require CPB for attempted repair, but often are non-survivable.

Blunt Aortic Injury

Blunt aortic injury (BAI) is the second most common cause of death due to blunt trauma. The incidence of aortic injury in blunt chest trauma is between 1 and 2 %, but less than 20 % of these patients survive to be treated in hospitals [38] Sudden deceleration, most often due to motor vehicle collision, results in injury to the aorta at areas of fixation to the bony skeleton – aortic root, ligamentum arteriosum, or aortic hiatus. The force of injury creates a tear through the intimal and medial layers leaving just the adventitia of the aortic wall containing the systolic pressures in the intravascular space. This unstable condition may last anywhere from seconds to years. The rupture of the adventitia results in exsanguination and death. Though three potential areas of injury exist, the injury most commonly seen in patients who survive to hospital evaluation is the injury at the ligamentum arteriosum. Survival to the hospital does not ensure survival, for some patients die soon after arrival or are unable to have definitive management of aortic repair due to concomitant intra- and or extrathoracic injuries [39].

Diagnostic testing for BAI is based on mechanism of injury and initial CxR. An upright CxR is a reasonable screening test for BAI and may reveal widened mediastinum (supine CxR >8 cm, upright CxR >6 cm), right tracheal deviation and/or left main stem depression, left hemothorax, left apical capping, an obscured aortic knob, and rightward deviation of a nasogastric tube. With a low-velocity mechanism and non-deceleration injury, a normal CxR reliably excludes BAI; however a normal CxR in patients with these high-risk mechanisms is not adequate. Helical CT scan is the diagnostic test of choice in these patients because of its high sensitivity and specificity. Aortography and MRI are less commonly used diagnostic modalities for this injury.

Once BAI is diagnosed, antihypertensive therapy with beta-blockade for SBP of 110–120 should be instituted as plans for operative repair are made. In patients who have minimal associated injuries, operative repair should be done early within the first or second hospital day, though longer observation periods with appropriate blood pressure control have been shown to be well tolerated [40]. Operative management has traditionally involved left posterolateral thoracotomy with clamp and sew repair. This approach is associated with significant rates of morbidity, paraplegia (19 %), and mortality (16 %). Improvements in bypass techniques have demonstrated some progress with paraplegia rates of approximately 5 %, but require systemic heparinization [41]. Reports of mortality rates up to 80 % in the elderly patient following operative repair led some to advocate nonsurgical management of elderly patients [42]. Given the high rates of morbidity and mortality following open repair, the use of endovascular techniques is being utilized more frequently. Garcia-Toca et al. reported the successful use of thoracic endovascular aortic repair (TEVAR) for blunt thoracic aortic injury without the need for systemic anticoagulation [43] Endovascular repair appears to have lower rates of cardiac and pulmonary complications, paraplegia, and a lower mortality rate [44]. It remains unclear if TEVAR will be a safe long-term approach in the young trauma patient with BAI and a long life expectancy, but for the elderly patient with blunt aortic injury, it has great promise [45]. There are patients with severe pulmonary contusions and complex head injuries who are not candidates for open or endovascular repair. Several series have shown that these patients can be managed with rigorous blood pressure control for prolonged periods [38, 46, 47].

The use of high resolution CT scans for diagnosing BAI has led to the diagnosis of a new injury termed "minimal aortic injury" [48]. The management of these injuries is evolving, but there is a growing body of experience that patients with small intimal flaps and minimal aortic wall hematoma can be managed with blood pressure control and observation. Most of these injuries resolve on their own and only a small percentage of patients eventually require an operative intervention.

Diaphragm Injury

Injury to the diaphragm has been reported in approximately 1 % of patients hospitalized for blunt trauma and up to 8 % of trauma surgical explorations. Diaphragmatic hernias are more common in the elderly population and they have higher associated mortality than younger age groups [49, 50]. Diagnosing a diaphragmatic rupture after trauma is a challenge to the clinician [50]. The initial CxR can be diagnostic; however in one series of elderly patients with traumatic hernias, 50 % of initial CxR were normal. A normal admission CxR can result in delays in diagnosis and delay to operative repair which increases rates of surgical complications such as time of ventilatory support and death [51]. Even CT scanning can be nondiagnostic. Atelectasis, pulmonary contusions, hemothorax, and intra-abdominal pathology can mask diaphragmatic injury. Operative approach to these injuries depends on the timing of presentation. Acute hernias are best approached through the abdomen so any associated intra-abdominal injuries can be addressed. Primary repair of these hernias is often possible. With large rents where primary repair is not possible, the diaphragm must sometimes be detached from the rib cage and replanted onto a higher rib. Delayed presentations of diaphragmatic injuries are easily approached through the chest, which affords excellent exposure. These repairs most often need a synthetic implant for repair. Despite its association with significant morbidity and mortality, diaphragmatic injury is rarely the sole injury, and mortality is often related to the associated injuries.

Thoracic Duct Injury

Injury to the thoracic duct is rare after blunt chest trauma [52]. When present, patients typically have other chest or skeletal injuries. Diagnosis is confirmed after drainage of pleural effusion reveals chyle with analysis showing high numbers of chylomicrons and triglycerides. Often with high output (approximately 1 L daily), the patient suffers from nutritional and immunologic deficiencies, which leads to an associated high mortality. Nonoperative therapy either consisting of medium-chain fatty acid oral diet or NPO with TPN can be considered. Both have been shown to be efficacious. Octreotide may be used to decrease chylous output. If nonoperative management fails, the thoracic duct should be ligated above and below the injury.

Esophageal Injury

Traumatic esophageal injury is rare, and the majority of cases are caused by penetrating trauma. The left side of the gastroesophageal junction is the most common site of blunt esophageal rupture – similar to the pathology of Boerhaave syndrome. Delay in diagnosis and injury to adjacent structures are associated with increased morbidity and mortality. Most patients are without symptoms at presentation and a high degree of suspicion must be present to promptly diagnose and treat this condition. Although pneumomediastinum may be present in esophageal injury, other more common injuries, such as bronchial injury, usually get worked up first. Pleural effusion, mediastinitis, or intraperitoneal air demand a thorough evaluation of the esophagus by esophagoscopy and contrast esophagography. Operative repair requires debridement, primary mucosal repair, buttress of the repair with pleural or intercostal muscle flap, and drainage.

Conclusion

Thoracic trauma is a significant contributor to the morbidity and mortality in trauma patients regardless of age. Blunt chest trauma is caused by various mechanisms, but motor vehicle collisions and falls are the most common. Compromised baseline organ function often seen in the elderly can make management of traumatic injury challenging. Even fall from standing can be a fatal event in a frail elderly patient. Management of thoracic trauma in the injured elderly patient has not changed much over the last 30 years, but technology is driving changes from discovering new conditions such as minimal aortic injury to endovascular repair of blunt aortic injury.

References

1. Victorino GP, Chong TJ, Pal JD. Trauma in the elderly patient. Arch Surg. 2003;138:1093–8.
2. Demetriades D, Karaiskakis M, Velmahos G, et al. Effect on outcome of early intensive management of geriatric trauma patients. Br J Surg. 2002;89:1319–22.
3. Gregg SC, Heffernan DS, Legere JT, et al. The multiply injured trauma patient: resuscitation, rehabilitation, recovery. Med Health R I. 2010;93(4):112, 115–6.
4. McGwin Jr G, Reiff DA, Moran SG, Rue 3rd LW. Incidence and characteristics of motor vehicle collision-related blunt thoracic aortic injury according to age. J Trauma. 2002;52:859.
5. Bauer TK, Lindenbaum K, Sroka MA, Engel S, Linder R, Verheyen F. Fall risk increasing drugs and injuries of the frail elderly – evidence from administrative data. Pharmacoepidemiol Drug Saf. 2012;21(12):1321–7. doi:10.1002/pds.3357.
6. Ferraris VA, Bernard AC, Hyde B. The impact of antiplatelet drugs on trauma outcomes. J Trauma Acute Care Surg. 2012;73(2):492–7.
7. Hamel MB, Henderson WG, Khuri SF, Daley J. Surgical outcomes for patients aged 80 and older: morbidity and mortality from major noncardiac surgery. J Am Geriatr Soc. 2005;53:424–9.
8. Lotfipour S, Kaku SK, Vaca FE, et al. Factors associated with complications in older adults with isolated blunt chest trauma. West J Emerg Med. 2009;10(2):79–84.

9. Bulger EM, Arneson MA, Mock CN, Jurkovich GJ. Rib fractures in the elderly. J Trauma. 2000;48:1040–7.
10. Harrington DT, Phillips B, Machan J, et al. Factors associated with survival following blunt chest trauma in older patients: results from a large regional trauma cooperative. Arch Surg. 2010;145(5):432–7.
11. Shorr RM, Rodriguez A, Indeck MC, Crittenden MD, Hartunian S, Cowley RA. Blunt chest trauma in the elderly. J Trauma. 1989; 29(2):234–7.
12. Perdue PW, Watts DD, Kaufmann CR, Trask AL. Differences in mortality between elderly and younger adult trauma patients: geriatric status increases risk of delayed death. J Trauma. 1998;45(4):805–10.
13. Heffernan DS, Thakkar RK, Monaghan SF, et al. Normal presenting vital signs are unreliable in geriatric blunt trauma victims. J Trauma. 2010;69(4):813–20.
14. Hasler RM, Exadaktylos AK, Bouamra O, Benneker LM, Clancy M, Sieber R, Zimmermann H, Lecky F. Epidemiology and predictors of cervical spine injury in adult major trauma patients: a multicenter cohort study. J Trauma Acute Care Surg. 2012;72(4):975–81.
15. Lehmann R, Beekley A, Casey L, et al. The impact of advanced age on trauma triage decisions and outcomes: a statewide analysis. Am J Surg. 2009;197(5):571–5.
16. Moore EE, Knudson MM, Burlew CC, Inaba K, Dicker R, Biffle WL, Malhotra AK, et al. Defining the limits of resuscitative emergency department thoracotomy: a contemporary western trauma association perspective. J Trauma. 2011;70(2):334–9.
17. Von Kuenssberg Jehle D, Stiller G, Wagner D. Sensitivity in detecting free intraperitoneal fluid with the pelvic views of the FAST exam. Am J Emerg Med. 2003;21(6):476–8.
18. Kirkpatrick AW, Sirois M, Laupland KB, et al. Hand-held thoracic sonography for detecting post-traumatic pneumothoraces: the Extended Focused Assessment with Sonography for Trauma (EFAST). J Trauma. 2004;57:288–95.
19. Alrajhi K, Woo MY, Vaillancourt C. Test characteristics of ultrasonography for the detection of pneumothorax: a systematic review and meta-analysis. Chest. 2012;141(3):703–8.
20. Trupka A, Waydhas C, Hallfeldt KK, et al. Value of thoracic computed tomography in the first assessment of severely injured patients with blunt chest trauma: results of a prospective study. J Trauma. 1997;43(3):405–11.
21. Roudsari B, Psoter KJ, Fine GC, Jarvik JG. Falls, older adults, and the trend in utilization of CT in a level I trauma center. AJR Am J Roentgenol. 2012;198(5):985–91.
22. Plurad D, Green D, Demetriades D, Rhee P. The increasing use of chest computed tomography for trauma: is it being overutilized? J Trauma. 2007;62(3):631–5.
23. Inaba K, Lustenberger T, Recinos G, et al. Does size matter? A prospective analysis of 28–32 versus 36–40 French chest tube size in trauma. J Trauma Acute Care Surg. 2012;72(2):422–7.
24. Maxwell RA, Campbell DJ, Fabian TC, et al. Use of presumptive antibiotics following tube thoracostomy for traumatic hemopneumothorax in the prevention of empyema and pneumonia–a multicenter trial. J Trauma. 2004;57(4):742–8.
25. Bosman A, de Jong MB, Debeij J, et al. Systematic review and meta-analysis of antibiotic prophylaxis to prevent infections from chest drains in blunt and penetrating thoracic injuries. Br J Surg. 2012;99(4):506–13.
26. Watkins TR, Nathens AB, Cooke CR, et al. Acute respiratory distress syndrome after trauma: development and validation of a predictive model. Crit Care Med. 2012;40(8):2295–303.
27. Miller PR, Croce MA, Kilgo PD, et al. Acute respiratory distress syndrome in blunt trauma: identification of independent risk factors. Am Surg. 2002;68(10):845–50.
28. Stitzel JD, Kilgo PD, Weaver AA, et al. Age thresholds for increased mortality of predominant crash induced thoracic injuries. Ann Adv Automot Med. 2010;54:41–50.
29. Wolfman NT, Myers WS, Glauser SJ, Meredith JW, Chen MY. Validity of CT classification on management of occult pneumothorax: a prospective study. AJR Am J Roentgenol. 1998;171:1317–20.
30. Collins JC, Levine G, Waxman K. Occult traumatic pneumothorax: immediate tube thoracostomy versus expectant management. Am Surg. 1992;58:743–6.
31. DuBose J, Inaba K, Demetriades D, Scalae TM, O'Connor J, Menaker J, Morales C, et al. Management of post-traumatic retained hemothorax: a prospective, observational, multicenter AAST study. J Trauma Acute Care Surg. 2012;72(1):11–22; discussion 22–4; quiz 316.
32. Schweigert M, Beron M, Dubecz A, et al. Video-assisted thoracoscopic surgery for posttraumatic hemothorax in the very elderly. Thorac Cardiovasc Surg. 2012;60(7):474–9.
33. Kiser AC, Obrien SM, Detterbeck FC. Blunt tracheobronchial injuries: treatment and outcomes. Ann Thorac Surg. 2001;71(6):2059–65.
34. Glazer ES, Meyerson SL. Delayed presentation and treatment of tracheobronchial injuries due to blunt trauma. J Surg Educ. 2008;65(4):302–8.
35. Gomez-Caro A, Ausin P, Moradiellos FJ, et al. Role of conservative medical management of tracheobronchial injuries. J Trauma. 2006; 61(6):1426–34.
36. Ismailov RM, Ness RB, Redmond CK, et al. Trauma associated with cardiac dysrhythmias: results from a large matched case–control study. J Trauma. 2007;62(5):1186–91.
37. Keough V, Letizia M. Blunt cardiac injury in the elderly trauma patient. Int J Trauma Nurs. 1998;4:38–43.
38. Neschis DG, Scalea TM, Flinn WR, Griffith BP. Blunt aortic injury. N Engl J Med. 2008;359(16):1708–16.
39. Arthurs ZM, Starnes BW, Sohn VY, et al. Functional and survival outcomes in traumatic blunt thoracic aortic injuries: an analysis of the National Trauma Databank. J Vasc Surg. 2009;49:988.
40. Fabian TC, Davis KA, Gavant ML, et al. Prospective study of blunt aortic injury: helical CT is diagnostic and antihypertensive therapy reduces rupture. Ann Surg. 1998;227(5):666–76.
41. Fabian TC, Richardson JD, Croce MA, et al. Prospective study of blunt aortic injury: multicenter trial of the American Association for the Surgery of Trauma. J Trauma. 1997;42(3):374–80.
42. Camp Jr PC, Rogers FB, Shackford SR, et al. Blunt traumatic thoracic aortic laceration in the elderly: an analysis of outcome. J Trauma. 1994;37:418–23.
43. Garcia-Toca M, Naughton PA, Matsumura JS, et al. Endovascular repair of blunt traumatic thoracic aortic injuries seven-year single-center experience. Arch Surg. 2010;145(7):679–83.
44. Riesenman PJ, Brooks JD, Farber MA. Acute blunt traumatic injury to the descending thoracic aorta. J Vasc Surg. 2012;56(5):1274–80. doi:10.1016/j.jvs.2012.04.035. Epub 2012 Jun 23.
45. Demetriades D, Velmahos GC, Scalea TM, Jurkovich GJ, Karmy-Jones R, Teixeira PG, Hemmila MR, et al. Diagnosis and treatment of blunt thoracic aortic injuries: changing perspectives. J Trauma. 2008;64(6):1415–8; discussion 1418–9.
46. Hirose H, Gill IS, Malangoni MA. Nonoperative management of traumatic aortic injury. J Trauma Acute Care Surg. 2006;60(3):597–601.
47. Caffarelli AD, et al. Early outcomes of deliberate nonoperative management for blunt thoracic aortic injury in trauma. J Thorac Cardiovasc Surg. 2010;140(3):598–605.
48. Kidane B, et al. Natural history of minimal aortic injury following blunt thoracic aortic trauma. Can J Surg. 2012;55(6):377–81.
49. Lewis JD, Starnes SL, Pandalai PK, et al. Traumatic diaphragmatic injury: experience from a level I trauma center. Surgery. 2009;146(4):578–83; discussion 583–4.
50. Hanna WC, Ferri LE, Fata P, Razek T, Mulder DS. The current status of traumatic diaphragmatic injury: lessons learned from 105 patients over 13 years. Ann Thorac Surg. 2008;85(3):1044–8.
51. Hsu YP, Chen RJ, Fang JF, Lin BC. Blunt diaphragmatic rupture in elderly patients. Hepatogastroenterology. 2005;52(66):1752–8.
52. Apostolakis E, Akinosoglou K, Koletsis E, Dougenis D. Traumatic chylothorax following blunt thoracic trauma: two conservatively treated cases. J Card Surg. 2009;24(2):220–2.

Pelvic Fracture

26

Sharon M. Henry

Introduction

The presence of a pelvic fracture has special significance to trauma surgeons. Pelvic bones are considered the strongest in the body. Therefore, significant kinetic energy is required to fracture them. Such forceful trauma frequently is associated with injury to other organ systems and the extremities. The injury itself can also result in significant mortality related to hemorrhage and morbidity resulting from imperfect healing and/or nerve injury. There are differences in the mechanism of injury and associated injuries expected between younger and older patients with pelvic fractures. Younger patients typically sustain injury through high-energy mechanisms (motor vehicle collision), while older patients' injuries occur in the context of osteoporosis and from low-energy mechanisms (fall from standing).

Trauma is the fifth leading cause of death in patients over the age of 65 years. They account for 28 % of deaths due to trauma, though only representing 12 % of the population [1]. For each year increase in age over 65, the risk of dying following trauma increases by 6 % [2]. The US population over the age 50 years is predicted to increase by 60 % between 2000 and 2025 [3]. As of 2010 there were 40.3 million persons aged 65 or older, representing 13.0 % of the US population [4]. By the year 2030 it is estimated that those aged 65 and older will represent 19 % of the population. The average life expectancy of those reaching the age of 65 years is an additional 18.8 years [5]. Over a third (37 %) of elder Americans report some type of disability, ranging from major to minor. A study of Medicare beneficiaries over the age of 65 found 27 % reported difficulties with activities of daily living (ADL) [6]. Despite this, the vast majority of older Americans are living independently. The percentage of older adults (age 65 and older) living in nursing homes declined from 4.2 % in 1985 to 3.6 % in 2004 according to the National Nursing Home Survey (NNHS) [7]. Clearly injury that occurs with pelvic fracture has the potential to worsen the disability that many older adults are successfully coping with. There is substantial likelihood that such an injury could lead to increasing dependency and result in the need for institutionalized care.

Epidemiology

The incidence of pelvic fracture is 9.3 % among patients who have suffered major blunt trauma. A high-energy mechanism is associated with 13–18 % of all pelvic fractures. Fractures involving the pelvis account for 3–8 % of all skeletal injuries [8]. Pelvic fractures display a bimodal age and gender distribution. Young males are overly represented in the early peak and elderly females in the later peak. Pelvic fractures vary significantly in initial presentation. Two subgroups can be recognized. There are mechanically stable minimally displaced fractures that occur after simple falls, or high kinetic energy-associated injuries that occur in patients with multiple injuries with potential for hemorrhage from pelvic ring disruptions. A population-based study from England found the incidences of both high-energy and low-energy pelvic fractures to be 10 cases per 100,000 persons per year. The incidence of pelvic fracture with prehospital death occurred in 3 persons per 100,000 person years [9]. Among older patients, the incidence and rates of pelvic fracture increase after the age of 55 years in females and 65 years in males. By age 85 years 2 % of white females will have suffered a pelvic fracture (Fig. 26.1) [10]. A Finnish study documented a 23 % per year increase in the age-adjusted incidence of pelvic fracture from 1970 to 1997 [11].

A 2009 retrospective review found the mechanism of injury associated with pelvic fracture in patients younger than 65 years was motor vehicle collision (MVC) in 86.7 % and fall in 13.3 %; however, in those over the age of 65

S.M. Henry, MD
Department of Surgery, Program in Trauma, R. Adams Cowley Shock Trauma Center,
University of Maryland School of Medicine,
22 South Greene Street, Baltimore, MD 21201, USA
e-mail: shenry@umm.edu

J.A. Yelon, F.A. Luchette (eds.), *Geriatric Trauma and Critical Care*,
DOI 10.1007/978-1-4614-8501-8_26, © Springer Science+Business Media New York 2014

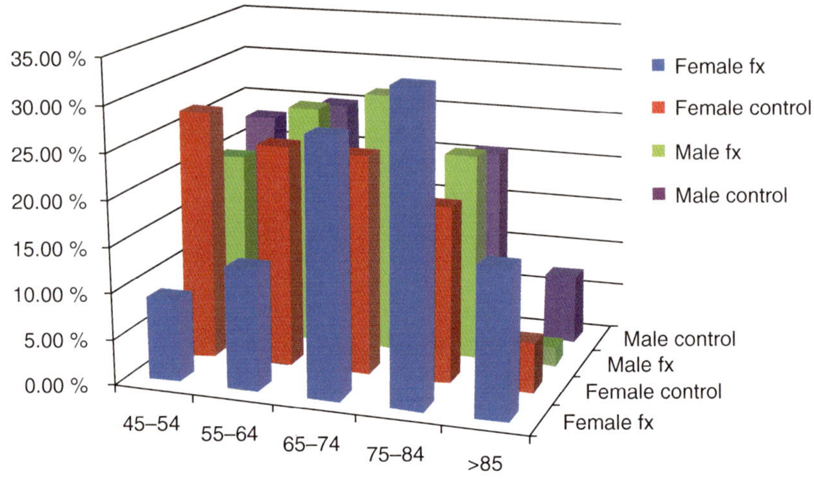

Fig. 26.1 Distribution of pelvic fracture cases and controls by age and gender [10] (Reprinted, with permission, from Oxford University Press)

years, nearly 30 % had a fall as the mechanism of injury [12]. Another study of pelvic fractures in patients over the age of 65 years found 83 % suffered injury from low-energy trauma as a result of fall from standing or transferring [13]. These fractures continue to present treatment dilemmas and can be a major source of morbidity and mortality.

Risk Factors

The older population is disproportionally impacted by falls. Patients older than 65 years represent 43 % of those injured by falls. Ground-level falls are traditionally thought to be a low-impact mechanism associated with inconsequential injuries. However, age greater than 55 years is independently predictive of significant injury in patients with low-energy mechanisms of injury [14]. Ground-level falls are the immediate cause of injury in nearly 80 % of elder patients with a pelvic fracture. Since falls are a significant mechanism for the disruption of the pelvic ring, it stands to reason that the risk factors for falls (Table 26.1) would be similar for pelvic fracture. Osteoporosis is an important comorbidity affecting elderly patients. It is estimated that 64 % of fractured pelvis are osteoporotic and in patients over the age of 60 years, the incidence increases to 94 % [15]. Seely et al. in a prospective cohort study demonstrated that pelvic fractures among others were related to reduced bone mass [16]. Fractures of the pelvic bones represent 7 % of all osteoporosis-related fractures in people 50 years or older in the United States. Several other associations have been suggested (Table 26.2) [10].

Table 26.1 Contributing factors to injuries in elderly patients

Chronic medical condition	Environmental factors	Acute medical conditions	Other
Osteoarthritis	Rugs	Syncope	Older age
Osteoporosis	Lighting	Dysrhythmias	Female gender
CVA	Stairs	CVA, TIA	Alcohol and drug use
Ischemic heart disease	Bathtubs/ showers	Acute MI	Elder abuse
Anemia	Footwear	Seizure	
DM	Uneven ground	Acute renal failure	
HTN	Weather	Infection	
Gait and balance disturbances	Walking aids	Hypoglycemia	
Visual impairment	Acute fractures	AAA	
Depression	Self-inflicted injury	New medications	
Polypharmacy		Dehydration	
Parkinson's disease			
Dementia			

From Aschkenasy and Rothenhaus [2]

Anatomy

The pelvis is composed of five bones, the ilium, the ischium, the pubis, the sacrum, and coccyx. The bones are connected to each other by several strong ligaments that resist transverse and longitudinal rotational forces to maintain pelvic stability. In general high energy is required to disrupt these strong bones and ligaments. However, in the elderly complex fracture can occur through low-energy impacts due to the presence of osteoporosis. The lumbosacral and coccygeal nerve plexuses are anterior to the sacrum and coccyx. These nerves arise from the T12 to S4 spinal nerves. Somatic and autonomic nerve injury is a real threat with injury to the pelvis. A thin-walled venous plexus is intimately attached to the sacrum and pubic bones. A rich blood supply arising from the iliac arteries supplies the soft tissues of the pelvis. These structures are all at risk for injury when the bones and ligaments in the region are injured. When the skin and superficial fascia are degloved as result with a closed shearing injury between the skin and superficial fascia, a Morel-Lavallee injury is produced [17]. In the elderly patient these injuries can result in enormous blood loss compared to a younger patient where the bleeding is self limiting. With the loss of tissue elasticity and the loss of blood vessel compliance, this kind of injury can result in ongoing hemorrhage leading to hemodynamic instability. The pelvis contains the lower genitourinary viscera and injury to the pelvis may also result in injury to these organs by proximity.

Table 26.2 Associations with pelvic fracture in the elderly

Potential risk factors for pelvic fracture
History of previous fracture after age of 45 years[a]
Maternal history of hip fracture[a]
Cigarette smoking[a]
History of hysterectomy[a]
History of seizure[a]
History of Parkinson's disease
Caucasian female[a]
Use of assistive devices
Low body weight[a]
Need for assistance with ADL[a]
History of stroke
Wearing corrective lenses
Frequent use of hearing aid
Increased height
Left handedness
Use of walking aids

[a]Statistically significant in multivariant analysis

Classification

Several classification systems to describe pelvic fractures exist. Initially fractures are assessed for stability. Stable fractures are characterized by single fractures of the pelvic ring, pure acetabular factures, straddle fractures of the pubic rami, and chip fractures or avulsion factures. Unstable fractures, on the other hand involve disruption of the pelvic rim in more than one place, such as the posterior pelvis, sacrum and sacroiliac complex. This includes the so-called Malgaigne (fractures of both rami and a posterior fracture of the sacroiliac complex) and open-book fractures (diastasis of the symphysis pubis and external rotation of one or both iliac bones). Arguably the most widely used classification system is the Young and Burgess system (see Table 26.3) [18]. Such classifications guide surgical intervention for fixation of these fractures. They are dependent on knowledge of direction of injury force in addition to the anatomic site of injury. Many investigators have tried to correlate injury classification with likelihood of associated injury and transfusion needs with variable results. Many

Table 26.3 Young and Burgess pelvic fracture classification

Fracture type	Common characteristic	Differentiating characteristic	Avg EBL 24 h
Lateral compression (LC)	Anterior transverse fracture of the pubic rami		2.4
Type I	Anterior transverse fracture of the pubic rami	Sacral compression on side of impact	2.8
Type II	Anterior transverse fracture of the pubic rami	Crescent (iliac wing) fx	
Type III	Anterior transverse fracture of the pubic rami	Contralateral open-book (anterior posterior compression) APC injury	5.7
Anterior posterior compression (APC)	Symphyseal diastasis		
Type I	Symphyseal diastasis	Slight widening of pubic symphysis and/or sacroiliac (SI) joint; stretched but intact anterior and posterior ligaments	
Type II	Symphyseal diastasis or anterior vertical fx	Widened (SI) joint; disrupted anterior ligaments; intact posterior ligaments	6.4
Type III	Symphyseal diastasis	Complete hemipelvis separation, but no vertical displacement; complete SI joint disruption; complete anterior and posterior ligament disruption	20.5
VS	Symphyseal diastasis or anterior vertical fx	Vertical displacement anteriorly and posteriorly, usually through SI joint, occasionally through iliac wing and/or sacrum	7.8
Combined mechanism	Anterior and/or posterior, vertical and/or transverse components	Combination of other injury patters LC/VS or LC/APC	7.1

From Burgess et al. [19]

Table 26.4 Physical findings seen in severe pelvic injury

Acronym	Finding	Significance
Destot's sign	Superficial hematoma above the inguinal ligament or in the scrotum or thigh	
	Leg length discrepancy with leg fracture	
Earle's sign	Bony prominence or large hematoma and tenderness on digital rectal examination	Pelvic hematoma
Grey-Turner's sign	Bruising on the flank	Retroperitoneal hematoma
Morel-Lavallee lesion	Closed internal degloving injury over the greater trochanter	High-energy injury
	Subcutaneous tissue avulsed from underlying fascia creating a cavity and hematoma	Acetabular fracture
	May be delayed in appearance	
Roux's sign	Decreased distance form greater trochanter to the pubic spine	Lateral compression pelvic fracture

studies of patients with pelvic fracture conclude that patients with disrupted ligaments and high-grade fracture patterns are at highest risk of arterial bleeding. The patterns identified include APC II, APC III, LC III, and vertical shear (VS). Angiographic embolization has been noted to be required more frequently in patients with APC, VS, or combined fracture patterns. It was required in 20 % of the former, while necessary in only 2 % of patients with lateral compression injuries (Table 26.3) [19]. A 2002 study of 234 patients with pelvic fracture found that lateral compression mechanisms were most common in patients over the age of 55 years, with 80 % classified as LC1. Despite this, patients with lateral compression fractures that were over the age of 55 were 3.9 times as likely to require blood transfusion as those younger than 55 [20]. Metz et al. found older patients with stable fracture patterns demonstrated more vascular injury than would be predicted. The average age of patients in the older group was 67 years. They postulated that these patients had decreased vascular compliance making them more vulnerable to shearing injury to blood vessels [21].

Diagnostics

Patients are initially assessed clinically. The hallmark of injury is pain. A non-tender pelvis in a neurologically normal patient is unlikely to be fractured. Palpation should include the symphysis pubis, the iliac crest, and sacroiliac region. Patients with severe fractures may have other findings on physical examination such as hematoma, abrasions, and lacerations (see Table 26.4). Leg length discrepancy may be seen and rotational or vertical instability may be elicited on physical examination. Bimanual compression and distraction of the iliac wings can discern vertical or rotational instability but can also recreate bleeding from a stabilized hematoma so should be performed with care and only once when an abnormality is elicited.

In patients with suspected osteoporotic fractures, levels of thyroid-stimulating hormone (TSH), parathyroid hormone (PTH), calcium, phosphorous, albumin, 25-hydroxyvitamin D, creatinine, full blood count, liver function tests, C-reactive protein (CRP), and erythrocyte sedimentation rate (ESR) may be useful in addition to routine trauma laboratory studies.

Radiographic evaluation begins with an anterior posterior pelvic x-ray. These may be supplemented with inlet, outlet, and Judet views. There are those who would argue that pelvic x-rays are sufficiently insensitive to render them unnecessary in patients who are going to undergo computed tomography [22]. Pelvic films are most useful in the evaluation of the hemodynamically abnormal patient who has suffered high-energy blunt trauma. Diagnosing pelvic fracture based on x-ray may be challenging in the osteopenic patient especially when compounded by overlying bowel gas. This is a common finding in the elderly patient population. Bowel contrast may also limit the ability to interpret pelvic x-rays as well as computed tomography. When computed tomography is equivocal, magnetic resonance imaging may aid the diagnosis. This may be particularly helpful in patients with stable fractures and low-impact mechanisms associated with osteoporosis. Advanced radiography may also be necessary in patients who are unable to provide history because of cognitive limitations. Elderly patients with their low-energy mechanism frequently present with hemodynamic normalcy but remain at risk for decompensation and subsequent death. It is important to maintain vigilance in their reassessment.

Treatment

The management of the geriatric patient with pelvic fracture injury depends on the patient's clinical presentation. In patients presenting with hemodynamic instability following moderate- and high-energy mechanisms, the priority is to identify and control the site of hemorrhage. The danger with

Table 26.5 Complications following pelvic fractures

Time scale	Life threatening	Increased morbidity disability or deformity
Acute (hours)	Hemorrhage, hypotension, tissue hypoxia	Neurological: lumbar and sacral root avulsion, autonomic nerve disruption (bladder sphincter control, erectile dysfunction, and incontinence), sciatic, obturator or superior gluteal nerve injury, pain Open injury: degloving skin injury, perineal, urinary vaginal, or rectal injury
Subacute (days, weeks)	Pelvic hematoma, open injury, sepsis, multiorgan dysfunction syndrome (MODS), systemic inflammatory response syndrome (SIRS), pulmonary embolism (PE)	Secondary wound drainage or debridement, deep venous thrombosis, postphlebitic syndrome Urinary or fecal diversion
Late (months, years)		Bony malunion or nonunion: leg length discrepancy, sitting disturbance, gait disturbance (foot drop), muscle weakness, disuse osteoporosis, chronic pain Genitourinary: incontinence, impotence, dyspareunia, rectovaginal, or rectovesical fistula

Modified from Gillespie P. [28]

these patients is the risk of bleeding that comes from multiple sites. External blood loss and internal bleeding in the thorax, abdomen or retroperitoneal space, and multiple long-bone fractures may be present. In severe pelvic injury there is a high incidence of combined intra-abdominal trauma, which will influence the therapeutic interventions. As often as 1/3 of the time, bleeding will be identified from a non-pelvic source [23]. Rapid identification of intra-abdominal source begins with the use of focused abdominal sonography for trauma (FAST). Thoracic, head, and long-bone and vertebral fracture or injuries should also be considered and identified and treated or stabilized. When the pelvis is the source of hemorrhage, the site of bleeding needs to be determined. Bleeding from the fracture site or from torn veins or soft tissue is controlled by stabilizing and immobilizing the fracture site or performing pelvic packing. When an AP compression pelvic fracture is identified, the placement of a pelvic wrap or binder can be life saving. More permanent stabilization with external or internal fixation may be necessary. Loose, inelastic skin combined with antiplatelet and anticoagulant use can produce major blood loss from lower-grade injury. Arterial injury is more uncommon and less likely to be controlled with immobilization, angioembolization or surgical control may be necessary. Noncompressible blood vessels may require angioembolization or even operative ligation or repair. Concomitant injuries must be identified and treated. Early correction of coagulopathy is imperative. Correction with fresh frozen plasma can be time-consuming and result in high infusion volume to produce the desired international normalized ratio (INR). Use of clotting factor complexes or factor VIIa may result in more rapid correction, lower infused volume without substantively increasing the cost of therapy [24]. When patients are taking antiplatelet therapy, correction can only be accomplished through replacement with functioning platelets despite a normal platelet count. Patients with chronic kidney disease who are uremic may benefit from the administration of 1-deamino-8-D-arginine vasopressin (ddAVP) [25].

The nonurgent management of pelvic fracture in the elderly patients requires thoughtful assessment of their physiologic reserve and healing capacity. Compromise of these factors, which occur commonly in the elderly, results in less favorable outcome. Osteoporosis is prevalent in this population and may limit the treatment options available. The clinical presentations of the fracture in the elderly range from high energy to low energy and insufficiency fractures resulting from extreme frailty. Treatment includes conservative measures such as bed rest, percutaneous or minimally invasive procedures, open reduction and fixation, and total hip arthroplasty. When determining the management of high-energy pelvic fracture in the elderly patient, the patient's comorbidities must be weighed against the benefits of improved reduction, more rapid mobilization, easier nursing care, decreased pain, decreased blood loss, decreased pneumonia, decreased decubitus ulcer formation, and decreased deep venous thrombosis.

Low-energy injuries in the elderly are typically stable fractures. These injuries are most often treated with bed rest until the patient is able to tolerate increased mobility. Pain medication is often necessary. Medication interactions must be prevented and dosage decreased to avoid lethargy and confusion. Complications related to immobility and to the provision of pain medication may be seen (Table 26.5). LC 1 and AP 1 injuries can be managed with pain medication and bed rest with weight bearing and ambulation progressing as tolerated. Early rehabilitation and moderate weight bearing may increase bone formation. Prolonged immobilization can result in bone reabsorption, not to mention the increased risk of deep venous thrombosis, pulmonary embolus, increased pulmonary complications, increased gastrointestinal complications, and decreased muscle strength. Unstable fractures require operative intervention. Insufficiency fractures are frequently of the sacrum and occur predominately in elderly women. Risk factors include osteoporosis, corticosteroid use, a history of radiotherapy to the area, rheumatoid arthritis, and fluoride treatment (see Table 26.6). Trauma is causative in only 30 % of these types of fractures. Incapacitating pain and neurologic symptoms are the presenting complaints [26]. These injuries are most frequently treated with bed rest, though percutaneous fixation may also be utilized. The osteoporosis seen in the majority of these elderly patients should also be addressed. Table 26.7 lists the possible treatments. These injuries can be challenging for a variety of reasons. Osteoporosis can make the operative intervention challenging and increase the likelihood of nonunion. Older patients are more likely to have comorbidities that lessen their ability to tolerate general anesthesia and operative intervention.

Outcome

Pelvic fractures are associated with significant morbidity in older patients. Deaths can be related to hemorrhage from the associated soft tissue injury to complications related to the fracture, from other injuries suffered as a result of the trauma, or from underlying comorbidities. The mortality is four times higher than in younger patients. A retrospective review of patients hospitalized for pelvic fracture that were over the age of 65 years found the mortality to be 7.6 %. Those patients were found to have a 1-year mortality of 27 % and all-cause mortality at 3 years of 50 %. The length of hospital stay for these patients was 21.4 days [13].These patients seldom return to their preoperative mobility status. Following discharge most required walking assistance with at least a cane and more than half required the assistance of another person. One third of patients required institutional care. Furthermore, a retrospective review of German nursing home patients demonstrated an increased risk of death in the first 2 months following pelvic fracture in women and up to a year following pelvic fracture in men [27].

Table 26.6 Risk factors for osteoporosis

Hyperparathyroidism
Osteomalacia
Renal osteodystrophy
Lumbosacral fusion
Paget's disease
Reconstructive surgery of the lower limb
Transplantation of the lung, heart-lung, kidney, and liver
Rheumatoid arthritis
Radiation therapy
Vitamin D deficiency
Pregnancy and lactation

Summary

The population is aging and many are maintaining active life styles that place them at risk for a traumatic injury. Pelvic fractures are sustained by the elderly through two predominate mechanisms. High-energy mechanisms common in the younger patient, such as motor vehicle crashes, or low-energy mechanisms seen strictly in the elderly ground-level falls. Declining physiology, medical comorbidities, and medications affect the response to injury in high- and low-energy mechanisms. The expected mortality in the elderly is higher for a given injury severity than in the younger patient. Low-energy mechanisms commonly result in mechanically stable fracture patterns. Nonetheless these injuries can have significant impact on the older patient's ability to live independently or ambulate unassisted. Though representing only 12 % of the injured population, the elderly account for 28 %

Table 26.7 Possible treatments for osteoporosis

Agent			Action	Cautions
Vitamin D			Increase vitamin D to improve calcium absorption	
Bisphosphonates	Alendronate	Fosamax	Inhibit bone reabsorption	Oversuppression of bone turnover
	Ibandronate	Boniva	Can reduce incidence of new fractures in patients with osteoporosis	Paradoxical inhibition of bone formation reduced osteoblastic activity
	Risedronate	Actonel, Atelvia	Increase bone mineral density (BMD)	Gastrointestinal discomfort, acute influenza-like illness, renal insufficiency, osteonecrosis of the jaw, and atypical stress fractures
	Zoledronic acid	Reclast	Most beneficial during first 5 years of therapy	
Calcitonin	Fortical, Miacalcin		Increases bone mass by reducing turnover	Use in postmenopausal osteoporosis
			Analgesic for bone pain	
Anabolic agents	Teriparatide (Forteo) (recombinant human PTH) and selective estrogen receptor modulators (SERMS)		Increases BMD	Increased risk of osteosarcoma

of the deaths [2]. Vigilance and anticipating decompensation are important in assuring optimal outcome when treating this population.

References

1. Kochanek K, Xu J, Murphy S, Minino A, Kung H. Deaths: preliminary data for 2009. Natl Vital Stat Rep. 2011;59:1–51.
2. Aschkenasy MT, Rothenhaus TC. Trauma and falls in the elderly. Emerg Med Clin North Am. 2006;24:413–32.
3. Burge R, Dawson-Hughes B, Solomon D, Wong J, King A, Tosteson A. Incidence and economic burden of osteoporosis-related fractures in the United States, 2005–2025. J Bone Miner Res. 2007; 22:465–75.
4. Werner C. The Older Population: 2010 in the 2010 Census Briefs. http://www.census.gov/prod/cen2010/briefs/c2010br-09.pdf. Accessed 19 July 2012.
5. A Profile of Older Americans: 2011. Department of Health and Human Services Administration on Aging. http://www.aoa.gov/aoaroot/aging_statistics/profile/index.aspz. Accessed 18 July 2012.
6. Manton KG, Gu X, Lamb VL. Change in chronic disability from 1982 to 2004/2005 as measured by long-term changes in function and health in the U.S. elderly population. Proc Natl Acad Sci U S A. 2006;103(48):18374–9.
7. Nursing Home use by "Oldest Old" Sharply Declines. http://www.globalaging.org/elderrights/us/2006/oldestold.pdf. Accessed 18 July 2012.
8. Lorich D, Gardener M, Helfet D. Trauma to the pelvis and extremities. In: Norton J, Barie P, Bollinger R, Chang A, Lowry S, Mulvihill S, et al., editors. Surgery basic science and clinical evidence. New York: Springer Science and Business Media, LLC; 2008. p. 505–20.
9. Balogh Z, King KL, Mackay P, McDougall D, Mackenzie S, Evans JA, Lyons T, Deane SA. The epidemiology of pelvic ring fractures: a population-based study. J Trauma. 2007;63:1066–107.
10. Kelsey J, Prill M, Keegan T, Quesenberry C, Sideney S. Risk factors for pelvis fracture in older persons. Am J Epidemiol. 2005; 162:879–86.
11. Kannus P, Palvanen M, Niemi S, Parkkari J, Järvinen M. Epidemiology of osteoporotic pelvic fractures in elderly people in Finland: sharp increase in 1070–1997 and alarming projections for the new millennium. Osteoporos Int. 2000;11:443–8.
12. Dechert T, Duane T, Frykberg B, Aboutanos M, Malhotra AJ, Ivatury R. Elderly patients with pelvic fracture: interventions and outcomes. Am Surg. 2009;75:291–5.
13. Morris RO, Sonibare A, Green DJ, Masud T. Closed pelvic fractures: characteristics and outcomes in older patients admitted to medical and geriatric wards. Postgrad Med J. 2000;76:646–50.
14. Velmahos GC, Jindal A, Chan LS, et al. "Insignificant" mechanism of injury: not to be taken lightly. J Am Coll Surg. 2001;192:147–52.
15. Krappinger D, Kammerlander C, Hak D, Blauth M. Low energy osteoporotic pelvic fractures. Arch Orthop Trauma Surg. 2010; 130:1167–75.
16. Seeley D, Browner W, Nevitt M, Genant H, Scott J, Cummings S. Which fractures are associated with low appendicular bone mass in elderly women? Ann Intern Med. 1991;1125:837–42.
17. Trikha V, Gupta H. Current management of pelvic fractures. J Clin Orthop Trauma. 2011;2:12–8.
18. McCormack R, Strauss E, Alwattar B, Tejwani N. Diagnosis and management of pelvic fractures. Bull NYU Hosp Jt Dis. 2010;68(4):281–91.
19. Burgess A, Eastridge B, Young J, Ellison S, Ellison S, Poka A, Bathon H, Burmback R. Pelvic disruptions: effective classification system and treatment protocols. J Trauma. 1990;30:848–56.
20. Henry S, Pollak A, Jones A, Boswell S, Scalea T. Pelvic fracture in geriatric patients: a distinct clinical entity. J Trauma. 2002;53:15–20.
21. Metz C, Hak D, Goulet J, Williams D. Pelvic fracture patterns and their corresponding angiographic sources of hemorrhage. Orthop Clin North Am. 2004;35:431–7.
22. Duane T, Tan B, Golay D, Cole F, Weireter L, Britt LD. Blunt trauma and the role of routine pelvic radiographs: a prospective analysis. J Trauma. 2002;53:463–8.
23. White C, Hsu J, Holcomb J. Hemodynamically unstable pelvic fractures. Injury. 2009;40:1023–30.
24. Armand R, Hess J. Treating coagulopathy in trauma patients. Transfus Med Rev. 2003;17:223–31.
25. Mannucci P. Decompression in the treatment of bleeding disorders: the first 20 years. Blood. 1997;90:2515–21.
26. Tsiridis E, Upadhyay P, Giannoudis V. Sacral insufficiency fractures: current concepts of management. Osteoporos Int. 2006;17:1716–25.
27. Rapp K, Cameron ID, Kurrle S, Klenk J, Kleiner A, Heinrich S, König HH, Becker C. Excess mortality after pelvic fractures in institutionalized older people. Osteoporos Int. 2010;21:1835–9.
28. Gillespie P. Pelvic Fracture. Surgery. 2009;27:292–296.

27 Extremity Injury

Scott P. Ryan, Olivia Kates, and Charles Cassidy

Prevention of Osteoporotic Fractures

Osteoporosis is a condition of fragile bone defined by a bone density, as measured by dual-energy X-ray absorptiometry (DXA), of more than 2.5 standard deviations below the average for healthy adults. Regardless of the absolute DXA score, geriatric patients with a fragility fracture (a fracture during normal activities, particularly a fall from standing height or less) can be considered to have fragile, osteoporotic bone [1]. The incidence of fragility fracture has risen exponentially in the last century, leading to considerable cost, morbidity, and mortality [2–4]. Prevention of osteoporotic fractures must address risk factors in two major categories – those associated with trauma or falls and those associated with bone strength [5–7].

Non-pharmacologic Interventions

Fall is one of the most common risk factors associated with fragility fracture, with 33 % of elderly in the community and up to 60 % of institutionalized patients falling each year [7–10]. Fractures occur in 3–12 % of falls, with hip fracture occurring in less than 1 % [6]. However, for patients who fall frequently, the annual prevalence of hip fracture is 14 % [11]. Fall prevention is a primary target of non-pharmacologic interventions for the prevention of osteoporotic fractures.

Fall prevention can be achieved through improvements in strength and balance, through assistive devices, or through environment modification. Strength training and weight-bearing exercise improve muscle tone, balance, and agility as well as bone density [12]. Some patients may require orthotics, a cane, or a walker in order to ambulate safely. Patients at risk for falls should avoid uneven ground or strenuous activities that increase their risk [13].

To improve skeletal health, nutritional counseling can address dietary calcium and vitamin D needs as well as general dietary needs for peak health and performance. However, many North-American patients will require supplementation to achieve desired serum levels [14–17].

Perhaps the most crucial first-line intervention for patients at risk for fragility fracture is effective management of comorbid conditions. A wide range of neurological, cardiac, gastrointestinal, metabolic, and other conditions can be counterproductive for both fall prevention and skeletal health maintenance. Furthermore, significant comorbidities affecting gait, cognition, and nutrition are common among the elderly. The risk of polypharmacy is an additional consideration for these patients and must be addressed [18, 19].

Pharmacological Interventions

The American College of Physicians strongly recommends that physicians offer pharmacologic treatment to patients with osteoporosis [20]. Drugs with good or fair evidence for preventing hip fractures are alendronate, risedronate, estrogen, and zoledronic acid. Drugs with good or fair evidence for preventing vertebral fractures are alendronate, etidronate, ibandronate, risedronate, zoledronic acid, estrogen, teriparatide, raloxifene, and calcitonin [21]. Physicians should assess risks and benefits on an individual basis to determine a pharmacological program for each patient [20].

Calcium and Vitamin D

Calcium and Vitamin D supplementation are at the forefront of pharmacological interventions for the prevention of osteoporotic fractures. Calcium supplementation is generally prescribed in 500–1,200 mg/day doses to slow the rate of bone loss in the elderly. Although conflicting evidence exists about its effects in fracture prevention, vitamin D levels remain an important target for many physicians treating

S.P. Ryan, MD • O. Kates, MD • C. Cassidy, MD (✉)
Department of Orthopaedic Surgery, Tufts Medical Center, 800 Washington Street, #306, Boston, MA 02111, USA
e-mail: ccassidy@tuftsmedicalcenter.org; syran3@tuftsmedicalcenter.org

J.A. Yelon, F.A. Luchette (eds.), *Geriatric Trauma and Critical Care*,
DOI 10.1007/978-1-4614-8501-8_27,

patients at risk for osteoporotic fractures [22]. Doses of 700–1,000 IU daily are known to be safe and do not require monitoring [23].

Estrogen and Estrogen-Related Compounds

Estrogen reduces bone loss in postmenopausal women, particularly in combination with adequate calcium supplementation. Estrogen reduces the risk of hip and vertebral fractures and is effective at maintaining bone mineral density for as long as the drug is taken. When estrogen is stopped, bone loss proceeds at the high rates characteristic of menopause [24–26]. Hormone replacement is a broadly acting therapy with long-term risks such as stroke, MI, breast cancer, and venous thromboembolism [27].

Raloxifene (Vista) is a selective estrogen receptor modulator with antagonistic effects in the breast and endometrium but agonistic effects in the bone. Raloxifene has been shown to decrease risk of vertebral fractures and of breast cancer, but is associated with a risk of venous thrombosis and pulmonary embolism at a similar rate to estrogen hormone replacement therapy [28–30].

The synthetic steroid Tibolone acts on estrogen, progesterone, and androgen receptors and has been shown to prevent bone loss in postmenopausal women. A 2008 study showed reduction in vertebral fracture and breast cancer with an increased risk of stroke in Tibolone vs. placebo. Tibolone is not FDA approved for the treatment of osteoporosis and is not available in the USA [27].

Bisphosphonates

The bisphosphonates are a diverse class of compounds that bind strongly to hydroxyapatite crystals in bone with a half-life of several years. Bisphosphonates reduce the recruitment of osteoclasts and induce their apoptosis, limiting bone resorption and decreasing turnover. As a class of drugs, bisphosphonates are supported by the greatest body of evidence indicating reduced fracture rates among osteoporotic patients. They are available in oral and intravenous administrations given daily, weekly, monthly, biannually, or annually [31–35].

Side effects of oral bisphosphonates include esophagitis, dyspepsia, diarrhea, and abdominal pain, which are sometimes severe. Oral bisphosphonates should be taken fasting with a full glass of water, with instructions to remain upright for 30–60 min. Intravenous bisphosphonates may cause a brief period of flu-like symptoms, particularly following the first dose [32, 33]. Rare but serious possible complications of bisphosphonates exist, including aseptic osteonecrosis of the jaw and atypical subtrochanteric fractures of the femur. The long-term effects of bisphosphonate use are not yet studied, despite half lives of many years in bone. Patients with an extensive history of bisphosphonate use or a history of fracture despite bisphosphonates should be considered for other therapies [31].

Bisphosphonates approved for the treatment of osteoporosis include alendronate (Fosamax, generic), ibandronate (Boniva, generic), risedronate (Actonel, Atelvia), and zoledronic acid (Zometa, Reclast, Aclasta) [31].

Calcitonin

Calcitonin is an osteoclast-inhibiting hormone produced by the C cells of the thyroid. FDA-approved formulations of salmon calcitonin (Miacalcin, Fortical) for the treatment of osteoporosis in postmenopausal women are administered by nasal puff and have shown fair effectiveness in reduction of vertebral fractures. Nasally administered calcitonin is not associated with any serious side effects but may cause irritation of the nasal mucous membranes [35, 36].

Parathyroid Hormone

Long-term exposure to parathyroid hormone (PTH) ultimately leads to increased bone turnover and decreased bone mineral density. However, in the short term, PTH can be used to stimulate new bone formation and prevent resorption [37, 38]. Teriparatide (Forte) is a biosynthetic PTH fragment administered daily by subcutaneous injection into the thigh or abdominal wall for up to 2 years. Teriparatide has been shown to be effective in reducing vertebral and nonvertebral fractures in postmenopausal women with a history of fracture and may be more effective than alendronate for this purpose. The safety of teriparatide beyond 2 years has not been established. The drug carries a black box warning because of possible increased risk of osteosarcoma as demonstrated in rats. Teriparatide is contraindicated in patients with any elevated risk of osteosarcoma, Paget's disease of bone, open epiphyses, cancer of the bone, metastases of other cancers to the bone, or prior radiation therapy affecting the skeleton. Common side effects of teriparatide include hypercalcemia, transient orthostatic hypotension, pain, gastrointestinal symptoms, and flu-like symptoms [37, 39].

Teriparatide can be administered in combination with bisphosphonates for a greater potential increase in bone mineral density. Trials considering combination therapy with a single zoledronic acid infusion and with daily alendronate both showed increased bone mineral density of the lumbar spine relative to either therapy alone [40, 41].

Denosumab

Denosumab (Prolia) is a human monoclonal antibody which binds receptor activator of nuclear factor kappa-B ligand (RANKL), a key part of the osteoclast activation cascade. Denosumab was approved by the FDA in 2010 for use in women with osteoporosis and at high risk for fracture [42]. Based on a randomized controlled trial of 7,868 osteoporotic women, denosumab showed decreased risk of vertebral fractures and nonvertebral fractures including hip fractures specifically. Denosumab was associated with increased risk of flatulence, eczema, and severe adverse events of cellulitis and may be contraindicated in patients with a history of severe rash or cellulitis [43]. A later systematic review of additional Denosumab trials confirmed these findings, including the risk of serious adverse events of cellulitis [44].

Strontium

Strontium ranelate (Protelos, Protos) takes advantage of the chemical similarity between calcium and strontium to achieve good uptake into bone, where it decreases resorption and may increase formation. Strontium ranelate is not FDA approved and not available in the USA, but a review of four controlled trials has demonstrated a decrease in vertebral fractures relative to placebo. Adverse effects were rare but included diarrhea, venous thromboembolism, pulmonary embolism, headache, seizure, memory loss, and altered consciousness [45]. Strontium therapy has also raised concerns about cost-effectiveness and is not believed to have any advantage over bisphosphonates in this category [46].

Fluoride

Fluoride therapy is controversial and is not approved by the FDA for the treatment of osteoporosis. Although fluoride incorporated into bone and may stimulate osteoblast activity to increase bone mineral density in the spine, systematic reviews have shown no fracture protection. Furthermore, fluoride may be associated with an increased risk of nonvertebral fractures at higher doses [47–49].

Summary and Conclusions

Management of elderly patients at risk for fragility fracture must address the two major risk categories of fall risk and skeletal health. A crucial first step is careful review of comorbid conditions and medications to minimize counterproductive effects on function and nutrition. Weight-bearing exercise has favorable effects on both fall risk and skeletal health. Many elderly patients, particularly in institutional settings, are candidates for supplementation with calcium and vitamin D. Patients at an increased risk should consider FDA-approved drugs with demonstrated effectiveness at reducing vertebral and nonvertebral fractures. Among these, bisphosphonates are the most common and the most affordable. However, their long-term use has not been adequately studied and serious adverse events have been reported. Alternatives include Raloxifene, Calcitonin, PTH, and Denosumab, each with a different profile of costs, risks, and benefits. Ultimately, each patient should receive a personalized multifaceted therapy combining pharmacologic and non-pharmacologic approaches as needed.

While prevention is not often the province of a trauma surgeon, in the emergency room setting, it is the responsibility of the trauma surgeon and acute care surgeon to identify possible osteoporotic fractures and ensure appropriate referral for long-term management.

Consideration in Treatment of Osteoporotic Bone

The goals of treating elderly patients with lower extremity fractures are to control pain and to assist with early mobilization and weight bearing. This is done by providing stable fracture fixation. Achieving such stability can be difficult in the elderly due to poor bone quality and more comminuted and complex fracture patterns. Osteoporosis is a contributing factor in 75 % of fractures caused by low-energy falls [50]. In addition, fractures around implants such as total hip or knee replacements can turn a simple fracture into a much more complicated operation if it affects the stability of the prosthesis. Nonoperative care can result in complications from being immobile, such as pressure sores, respiratory problems, deconditioning, and a diminished likelihood of full recovery [51]. Other objectives in treating elderly patients with fractures include minimizing surgical morbidity by performing the safest operation and decreasing the chance of reoperation from a failed initial surgery. Ultimately, the surgeon's goal is to return the patient to pre-injury functional activity.

Advances in implants (i.e., locking screws and plates) and augments such as polymethylmethacrylate have aided in the ability to provide stable fixation in poor-quality bone [52, 53]. This is paramount, as the ability to heal fractures correlates negatively with age [54]. It is important to preserve the biology of the fracture to aid in healing. Some newer implants are designed to be inserted percutaneously, thereby minimizing additional soft tissue disruption. With the improvement in implants, failure of operative fixation is typically through cutout of the implant construct due to poor-quality bone, rather than by implant breakage [51].

Intramedullary nail fixation of long bone fractures is preferred to plate and screw fixation as it is biomechanically superior and can permit immediate weight bearing. These prostheses are load-sharing devices and allow the surrounding bone to experience some stress, which encourages bone healing [23]. Plate and screw constructs are considered to be load-bearing devices, since the weight is transferred from the bone to the plate, bypassing the fracture site. With either type of fixation, full weight bearing should be allowed within several weeks of fixation if not appropriate immediately [55]. Elderly patients have difficulty regulating weight-bearing status after lower extremity operations. Physical therapy should assess the patient's ability to ambulate with weight bearing as tolerated or for non-weight bearing with a mobility aid.

Treatment of most geriatric fractures in the lower extremity is similar to younger patients. This section will focus on the perioperative management of the most common types of fractures (i.e., hip fractures), controversial fractures (i.e., acetabular fractures), and care of fractures specific to this population (i.e., periprosthetic fractures).

Preoperative Evaluation and Considerations

Caring for elderly patients with fractures requires a multidisciplinary approach. This involves constant communication with orthopedics; the acute care surgery service, medical service, or geriatric service; and anesthesiology since these patients typically have multiple medical comorbidities. Medical problems, which may have been stable prior to the injury, may resurface as a result of the physiologic stress from a fractured long bone. When a long bone fractures, it not only results in blood loss into the extremity that can effect the cardiac status but also causes the release of inflammatory cells that can cause a stress response affecting other organ systems [56]. During the initial history and physical, it is important to ask about the pre-ambulatory status and living situation of the patient. This is predictive of how likely the patient is to return to their baseline function and living arrangements [57].

Most of the studies on preoperative evaluation of elderly patients with lower extremity fractures come from the hip fracture literature. The role of the acute care surgery service or geriatric service is to assess the risk stratification of the patient and medically optimize the patient's cardiovascular function prior to surgery. Risk stratification is important to know in order to have an informed discussion with the patient and their family regarding nonoperative versus operative fracture care. Advanced age is not an independent risk factor for complications after surgery, but medical comorbidities are. Patients with an ASA of III or IV have nine times higher mortality than patients with an ASA of I or II [58]. The American College of Cardiology and the American Heart Association have recommended a preoperative echocardiogram for patients with a history of angina or decreased left ventricular dysfunction. This information can be useful for perioperative fluid management and risk stratification. In addition, they recommend a preoperative cardiac stress test for patients with new-onset angina or a change in the pattern of angina.

The appropriate admitting service for a geriatric patient with a lower extremity fracture is often an issue of debate. Vidin et al. [59] performed a randomized controlled trial of over 300 patients who were admitted with a hip fracture. One group was admitted to an orthopedic surgery service with a medical consultation as needed, and the other group was admitted to a geriatric service with the orthopedic service as a consultant. The primary outcomes were medical complications, mortality, and functional status. There was a significant decrease in mortality, medical complications, and improved functional status at 3 months when hip fracture patients were admitted to a geriatric service. The authors concluded that early geriatric intervention during the acute phase of hip fracture in the elderly reduces the in-hospital mortality and medical complications.

We recommend a protocol for preoperative evaluation of these patients in the emergency room. Whichever service is primarily taking care of these patients, they require medical management or consultation throughout the perioperative period.

Timing of Surgery

The timing of surgery has also been extensively studied in the hip fracture population. It is commonly extrapolated to other long bone fractures in the lower extremity in this population because the complications from delay are from being bedbound and in pain. The decision of when to take an elderly patient to the operating room is a balance between medical stabilization and mobilization. Kenzora et al. [60] studied over 400 patients with hip fractures and found that patients operated on less than 24 h after admission had a 34 % 1-year mortality rate. Those patients operated on hospital day 2–5 had a 6 % 1-year mortality rate, and those operated on after 5 days had a 35 % 1-year mortality. They rationalized this by stating that the patients who underwent surgery early may not have been medically optimized. Sexson et al. [61] found that those patients with less than 2 medical comorbidities had a higher survival if they were operated on less than 24 h following admission, and those that had more than 3 comorbidities had a higher mortality if operated on early. They recommended taking healthier patients to the operating room as soon as possible and waiting for medical optimization on sicker patients. Moran et al. [62], in a prospective study of over 2,600 patients, found that a surgical delay of greater than 4 days increased mortality in hip fracture patients. Egol and Strauss [63], in a review of the literature on hip fractures, recommended operative fixation of hip fractures within 48 h in the majority of patients and medical optimization and delay no longer than 4 days in patients with more than 3 medical comorbidities.

Type of Anesthesia

Best evidence is lacking in determining whether regional (spinal) or general anesthesia is safer for these patients. There are risks and benefits to both and the anesthetic plan should be discussed with all services involved with care, as well as the patient. In a meta-analysis of 15 randomized controlled trials of regional versus general anesthesia in hip fracture patients [64], regional anesthesia had the benefits of a decreased 30-day mortality rate and a lower DVT rate. The long-term mortality rate was, however, the same. Regional anesthesia should be considered in patients with severe pulmonary disease. The risk of regional anesthesia is hypotension, which increases the risk of stroke. The patients in the general anesthesia group had a trend for a lower incidence of stroke and fewer episodes of intra operative hypotension. Parker et al. had similar results in a *Cochrane Database Systematic Review* [65].

Treatment of Specific Fracture Types

The goals of treatment of lower extremity fractures in the elderly patient population are to provide pain control and early mobility and return the patient as close as possible to their baseline function and living situation. This section will review the treatment options for fractures specific to the elderly patient population.

Hip Fractures

The general term of hip fractures describes three different types of fractures that require a variety of treatment options: femoral neck, intertrochanteric, and subtrochanteric. These fractures are typically sustained in low-energy falls. All elderly patients with hip fractures should undergo a preoperative evaluation as described previously.

Epidemiology

Fractures of the hip are common, with lifetime incidence of hip fracture ranging from 40 to 50 % in women and 13 to 22 % in men [66]. Multiple factors contribute to the epidemiologic trends in hip fractures. While increased life expectancies and demographic shift raise valid concerns about a growing population at risk, medical management of risk factors, specifically osteoporosis, is improving [67]. Thus, the age-adjusted incidence of hip fracture fell between 1995 and 2005, while the total number of hip fractures remains high. The patients at highest risk are elderly, as incidence increases exponentially with age. Females are at greater risk than males, due to increased risk factors such as osteoporosis and different anatomy of the hip joint [68]. There is some racial variation in incidence, with increased incidence in Caucasians relative to African-Americans [69]. The vast majority of cases are treated surgically, comprising 20 % of the operative workload of an orthopedic trauma unit [70].

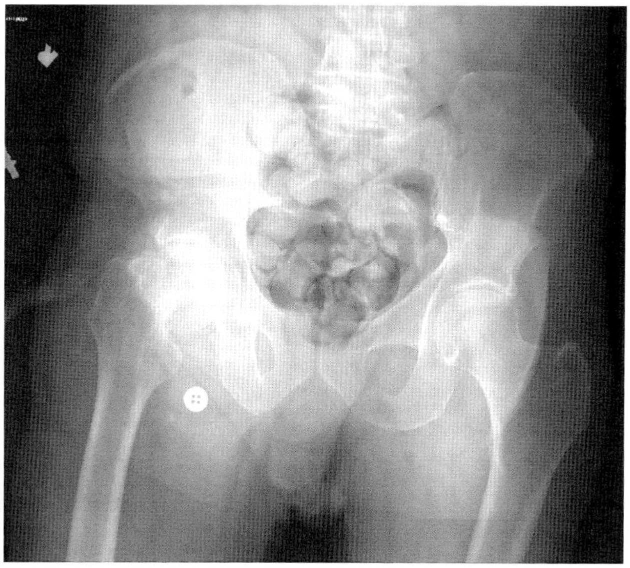

Fig. 27.1 AP pelvis X-ray of a right displaced femoral neck fracture

Femoral Neck Fractures

Fractures of the femoral neck are typically sustained during a simple fall on the trochanteric region (Fig. 27.1). The greater trochanter transmits the force of the fall along the femoral neck, which fractures [71]. Other mechanisms of injury include high-trauma events, stress fracture, and pathologic fracture, which together account for less than 10 % of these fractures among geriatric patients [72, 73].

Plain radiographs with anteroposterior and lateral are sufficient to diagnose fracture in 98 % of cases. MRI is a low-radiation, high-sensitivity and high-specificity alternative when there is a high suspicion of fracture without conclusive findings on X-ray [74]. Treatment plan and outcome measures are correlated with displaced vs non-displaced fracture features [75]. Eighty-five percent of femoral neck fractures are displaced at the time of diagnosis [23].

Non-displaced [76] or valgus-impacted femoral neck fractures are generally treated with percutaneous pinning using a cannulated screw system (Fig. 27.2) [77]. Patients can bear weight as tolerated after surgery and should be followed with serial radiographs to evaluate union [78, 79].

There is a high risk of complications treating non-displaced fractures nonoperatively. Rates of subsequent displacement range from 19 to 46 % [80–82]. Ultimately, these complications lead to worse outcomes overall than operative treatment. Thus, nonoperative treatment should be reserved for those patients whose comorbidities make them very poor candidates for surgery or nonambulatory patients in a palliative care setting. Additionally, patients may elect to try non-operative treatment, but should be made aware of the alternatives [83].

Displaced femoral neck fractures are typically treated with hemiarthroplasty or total hip arthroplasty (Fig. 27.3).

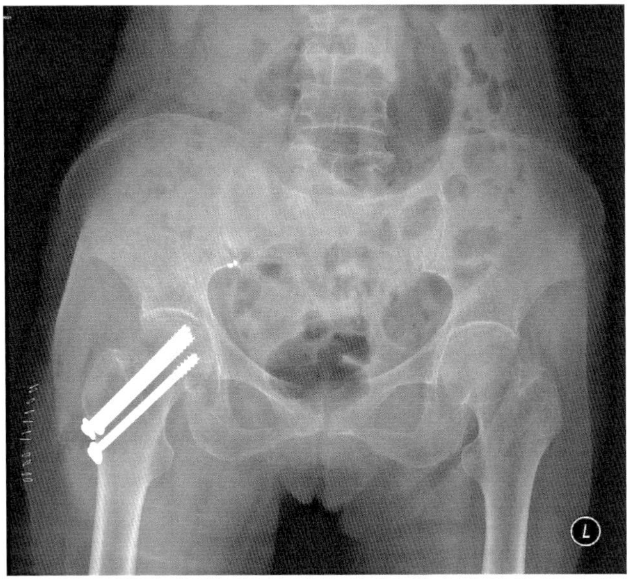

Fig. 27.2 AP pelvis X-ray of percutaneous screws for fixation of a valgus-impacted femoral neck fracture

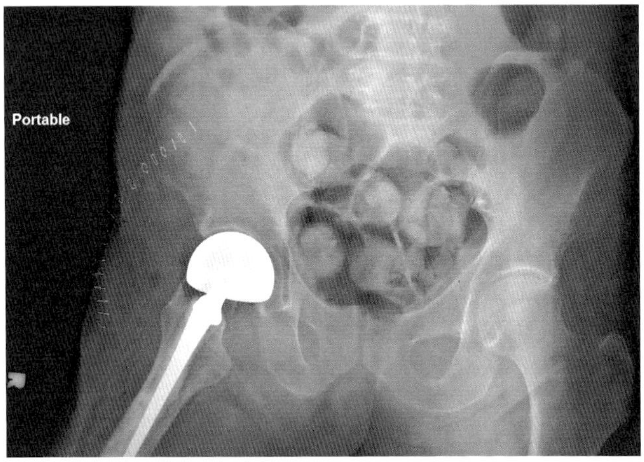

Fig. 27.3 AP pelvis X-ray of a bipolar hemiarthroplasty for treatment of a displaced femoral neck fracture

These procedures eliminate the risk of nonunion and fixation failure by using a prosthesis to bridge the joint space. Prostheses may be cemented or uncemented. Cemented femoral components may offer a decreased risk of intraoperative fracture and improved postoperative function over many uncemented components; however, comparative studies are not available for current generation uncemented systems [84–87]. These procedures are performed with the patient in a lateral position through either the lateral or posterior approach to the hip. The posterior approach preserves abductor strength better, but the lateral approach gives a lower risk of postoperative dislocation. The selection of procedure and implant type depends on patient demographics, baseline function, and functional goals.

In unipolar hemiarthroplasty, the femoral neck and head are replaced by a non-modular implant. The modularity of bipolar hemiarthroplasty is thought to provide an advantage over the unipolar design. In bipolar hemiarthroplasty, an inner head articulates with a shell that in turn articulates with the acetabulum. In theory, this reduces wear and acetabular protrusion (femoral head migration into the pelvis) [88–91]. The modularity of a bipolar system allows the surgeon to test a variety of head/neck options in order to optimize stability. Despite these theoretical advantages, results are comparable with unipolar hemiarthroplasty [92, 93].

Total hip arthroplasty has been shown to have better outcomes for treatment of displaced femoral neck fractures in cognitively intact patients [94]. This comes at a risk of a higher dislocation rate [95]. Total hip arthroplasty is a longer and more complex procedure, and may have higher cost [96]. Although the procedure is more complex than hemiarthroplasty or percutaneous screws, 30-day mortality is low at 2.4 % [97]. Long-term mortality and reoperation are low at 12 and 5 %, respectively. All of these data compare favorable to other methods of treatment. Rates of complication are understandably higher for secondary total hip arthroplasty to revise failed internal fixation [86, 98–100].

In conclusion, non-displaced femoral neck fractures should be treated with percutaneous screw fixation. Displaced femoral neck fractures in the elderly should be treated with replacement, either hemi- or total hip arthroplasty. This decision is based on age, activity level, and cognitive status of the patient [101–105]. Patients with preexisting hip arthritis may also benefit from total hip arthroplasty [106, 107].

Intertrochanteric Fractures

Intertrochanteric fractures are extracapsular, proximal metaphyseal fractures between the greater and lesser trochanter. In older patients, these injuries are predominantly due to low-energy trauma such as falls from standing height [108, 109]. The greater and lesser trochanters and the intertrochanteric region are sites of extensive muscle attachment, and fractures in this region are subject to considerable stress. Stable anatomic reduction and fixation are the paramount challenges of treating fractures in this functionally essential region [110, 111].

Nonoperative treatment is reserved for patients with very low baseline function or very short life expectancies where medical palliation is adequate to control pain. Patients should be quickly mobilized to an upright position to minimize the risks of prolonged bedrest [112].

Operative fixation of intertrochanteric hip fractures is the standard of care. For stable fractures, which are either nondisplaced or displaced but a stable fracture pattern, a sliding hip screw is often preferred (Fig. 27.4a, b) [113, 114]. Sliding hip screws are designed to provide dynamic compression across the fracture to enhance stability and healing. If addi-

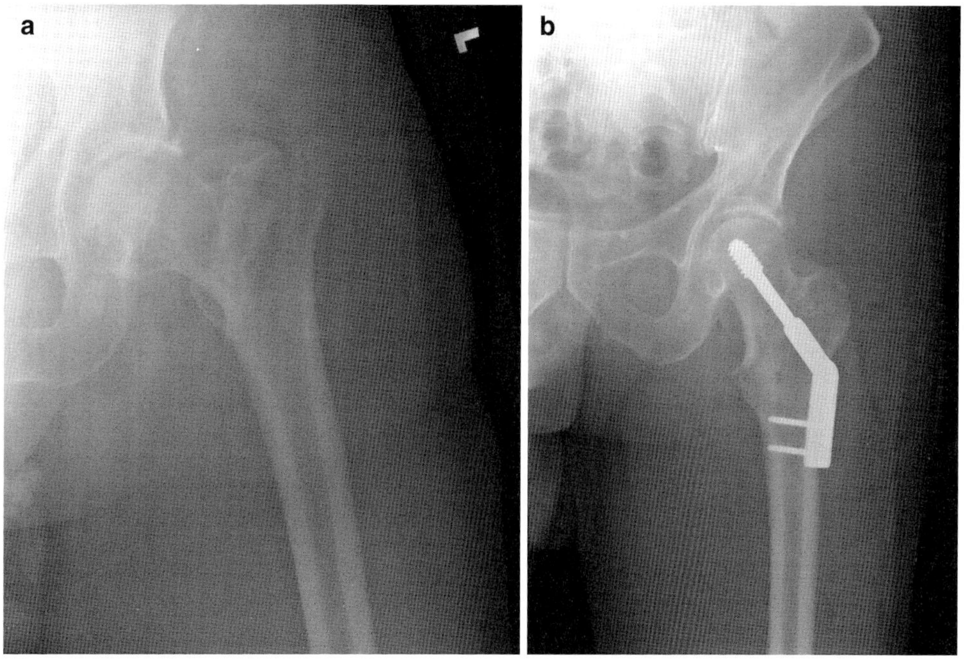

Fig. 27.4 Pre- (**a**) and post- (**b**) operative radiograph of a stable intertrochanteric hip fracture fixed with a sliding hip screw

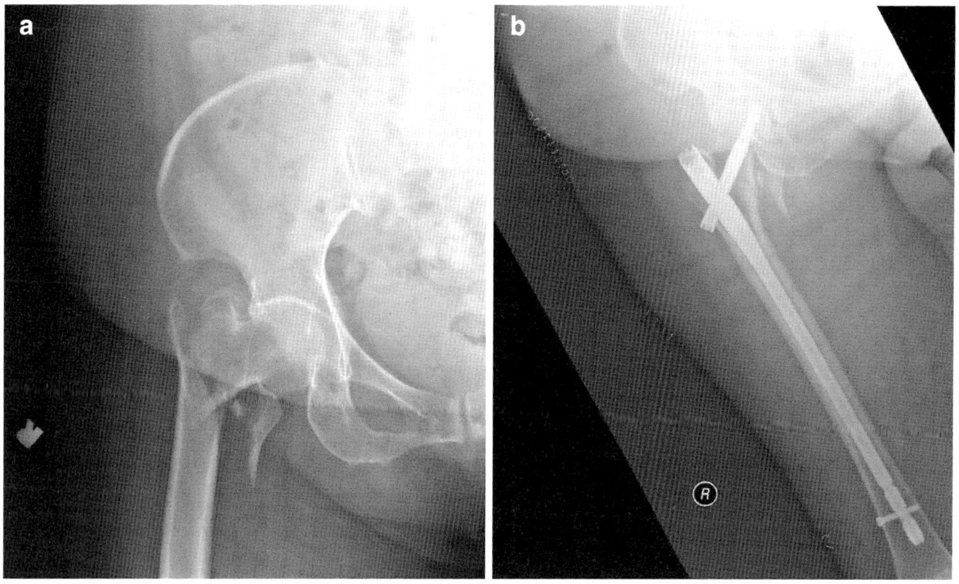

Fig. 27.5 Pre- (**a**) and post- (**b**) operative radiograph of a stable intertrochanteric hip fracture fixed with a sliding hip screw

tional rotational stability is required, an additional screw can be placed in the femoral neck, parallel to the sliding screw system [115]. If possible, a closed reduction to anatomic position is achieved under fluoroscopy. Otherwise, open reduction is performed. The sliding screw system is placed using a lateral approach to the proximal femur. Guide wires placed under fluoroscopy are used to direct the screw in the correct position, and a plate is placed over the screw and secured to the femur [23, 116]. The typical mode of failure is cutout, which occurs in 4–7 % of patients. Reoperation is required in around 4 % of patients [23].

For unstable fractures, an intramedullary device should be chosen to avoid excessive settling of the fracture (Fig. 27.5a, b) [117, 118]. The intramedullary approach requires a small incision over the proximal femur, marked with a guide wire under fluoroscopy. The nail is stabilized by an interlocking screw or blade extending into the femoral neck and head [119, 120]. This design provides linear compression across the fracture, and the nail itself provides a buttress for the fracture to settle against. Nails vary in length, curvature, and diameter. Care must be taken to select the implant that will optimally reduce and stabilize the patient's fracture [23].

After fixation of both stable and unstable intertrochanteric fractures, patients can begin weight bearing as tolerated with a walker or crutches [121].

Subtrochanteric Fractures

Subtrochanteric fractures are less common than femoral neck and intertrochanteric fractures, but are a significant surgical challenge. These fractures occur in the proximal femur, distal to the lesser trochanter by up to 5 cm (Fig. 27.6). In elderly patients, the majority of subtrochanteric fractures are due to a simple fall [122, 123]. Due to enormous compressive, tensile, and torsional stresses in the region, deformation of the fracture segments is common. Often the proximal segment is deformed by the action of the hip flexors and abductors. The distal segment is subject to the action of adductors and knee extensors. Furthermore, the region is poorly vascularized, posing another obstacle to successful union [23].

A unique pattern of subtrochanteric fractures associated with bisphosphonate therapy has emerged in recent years. These are short, oblique fractures of the metaphyseal junction showing lateral cortical thickening and a medial cortical spike (Fig. 27.6). Patients can report prodromal symptoms prior to the fracture event. The proposed mechanism behind this is impaired healing of a stress reaction in the subtrochanteric region due to the bisphosphonate-induced inhibition of osteoclasts, which are normally required for fracture remodeling [124].

All subtrochanteric fractures are treated operatively unless a severe comorbidity precludes this. Operative treatment is typically with intramedullary nail (Fig. 27.7) [122, 125]. The same percutaneous approach for intramedullary nailing is used as was described for intertrochanteric fractures. Reduction is achieved under fluoroscopy and the nail inserted in the prepared canal. Most nailing systems will offer a choice of locking mechanisms, with a cephalomedullary locking device preferred in an unstable, osteoporotic fracture or any fracture without an intact lesser trochanter. A single large lag screw or 2 smaller screws directed into the femoral head may offer added protection of the femoral neck in osteoporotic patients [126]. Otherwise, a standard greater to lesser oblique trochanteric-locking screw can be placed through the nail [127].

Patients are made weight bearing as tolerated after fixation with an intramedullary nail. Subtrochanteric hip fractures, as with other fractures around the hip joint, are associated with significant morbidity and mortality. Although they make up a small minority of proximal femoral fractures in the orthopedic trauma unit, these fractures are typically complex to treat and may be associated with an underlying pathologic cause.

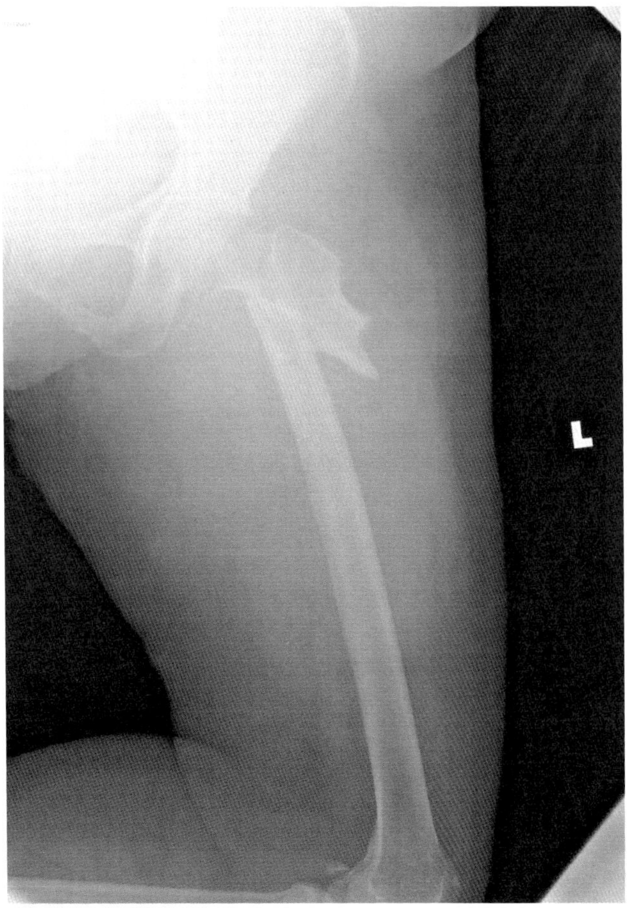

Fig. 27.6 AP femur X-ray of a left subtrochanteric hip fracture

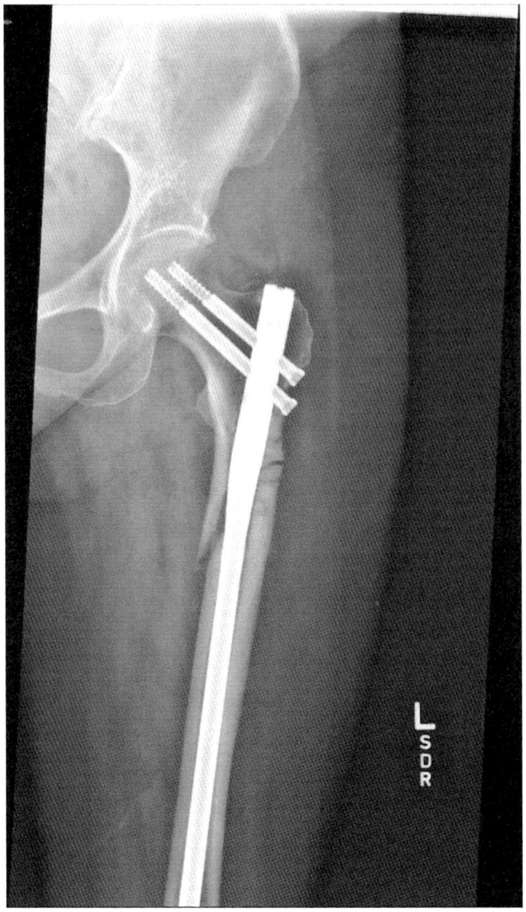

Fig. 27.7 AP femur X-ray of an intramedullary nail for treatment of a left subtrochanteric hip fracture

Mortality After Hip Fractures

Unfortunately, mortality after hip fracture is surprisingly high. It is clear that hip fractures are truly a surgical problem as the early mortality is almost double compared to nonoperative treatment of hip fractures [128]. Richmond et al. [129] reviewed 830 patients with hip fractures and found the highest mortality was within the first 3 months. Younger patients (age <85) also had a higher mortality, as were patients with a higher ASA classification. The in-hospital mortality was 3 %. The one year mortality rates in multiple studies are varied, but estimate a 30 % 1-year mortality. This is higher for cognitively impaired patients (50 %) and lower for cognitively intact patients (12 %) [23].

More than the fracture itself, the broken hip is a marker for declining functional and physiologic status. This is evident because the most common causes of death after hip fracture is not a complication from the broken bone, but circulatory disease, followed by complications of dementia. The risk of mortality in hip fracture patients is 3 times higher than in the general population [130].

Return to Functional Status

Return to baseline ambulatory status and living situation is dismal after hip fracture. Sixty percent of patients lose a level of ambulatory mobility at 1 year, i.e., community ambulators return as household ambulators after hip fracture surgery. Patients who are younger than 85 years, have lower ASA, or have a lower preoperative ambulatory status (low demand) are more likely to return to their baseline function [131]. Seventy-five percent of independent community ambulators are able to return to their pre-injury living status [57].

Acetabular Fractures

The dogma states that nonoperative management of displaced acetabular fractures in the elderly gives poor results. This is true for the younger population, but it is not necessarily true for the older population, that has less functional demands. Operative treatment of acetabular fractures in the elderly generally gives good results, but it is unclear whether there is an improvement over conservative management. There are currently no published data on operative versus nonoperative treatment of acetabular fractures in the elderly.

The fracture patterns in the elderly are different and often more complicated than in the younger population (Fig. 27.8). This is because of poor bone quality, which leads to more comminution and femoral head impaction, both of which can impact the ability to accurately repair these fractures [132]. In certain instances, fracture characteristics are predictive of early failure, such as impaction of the superior acetabular dome [133].

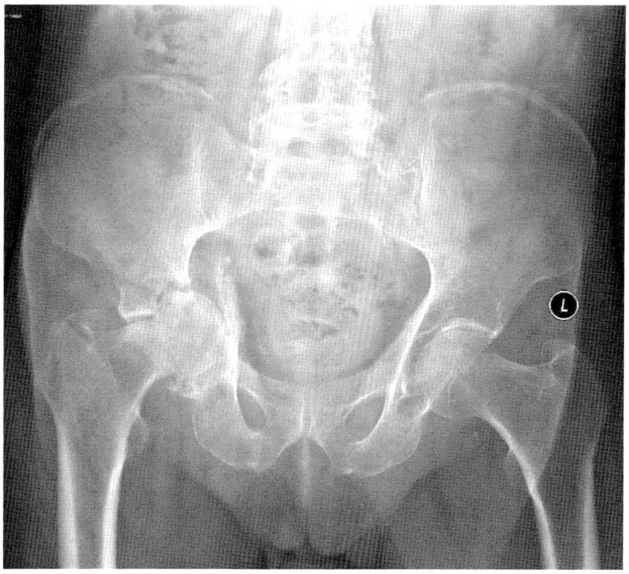

Fig. 27.8 AP pelvis X-ray of a displaced right acetabular fracture

Evaluation of these patients in the emergency department should parallel the evaluation of the hip fracture patient. Radiographic studies should include an AP pelvis and Judet (obturator and iliac oblique) radiographs, as well as a CT scan with coronal and sagittal reconstructions. The technology of 3-dimensional imaging has improved our understanding of these fractures and can be a useful teaching tool.

The decision whether to operate should be based on patient physiologic age, activity level, medical comorbidities, preexisting arthritis, and whether the operation can be preformed safely. Conservative management for most acetabular fractures in the elderly can be considered, with the exception of fracture patterns with posterior instability. Despite having relatively poor results with operative management, posteriorly dislocated or subluxated hips should be surgically stabilized [134]. Other fracture patterns, including those with medial wall protrusion into the pelvis, can be managed nonoperatively. Operations for acetabular fractures are significantly more complex than surgery for hip fractures.

Nonoperative Management

Spencer et al. [135] retrospectively evaluated 23 patients treated nonoperatively with radiographic and functional outcomes. This study is often quoted as having "poor results," but the authors' outcomes are not validated and the measures do not stand up to today's standards. Letournel and Judet, the pioneers of acetabular surgery, reported on their results with operative fixation of acetabular fractures [136]. Although they did use validated functional outcomes, they only reported on 10 patients over the age of 70 years and could not make any conclusions about patients in this age group (fractures of the acetabulum).

Operative Management

Several authors have reported good results with operative management of these fractures. Carroll et al. [132] suggested an algorithm for treatment of this patient population. They recommended all patients with displaced fractures that would require less 3–4 h of operative time should be fixed with primary open reduction internal fixation. If the surgery was expected to take longer than 4 h, they recommended acute total hip arthroplasty. They reported good functional results with primary fixation of the fracture, but 30 % went onto total hip arthroplasty at 2.5 years. They did not report on a nonoperative cohort. Obviously, there is much variability in how much a given surgeon can accomplish within a 4-h window.

Leflamme et al. [137] recently reported their cohort of 21 patients stabilized using a slightly different approach, but nonetheless primary fixation of the fracture. They also reported good functional results comparable to previous studies, but reported anatomic reduction in only half of their patients, which has been correlated to functional results.

Traditional approaches and fixation methods can result in significant blood loss and potentially increased morbidity. Gary et al. [138] have reported on percutaneous fixation of these fractures. Since anatomic reduction is only possible in approximately half of the patients, this group advocates getting general alignment of the columns of the acetabulum and fixation with percutaneous screws (Fig. 27.9). In a retrospective review of 43 patients, they reported similar functional results and conversion rates to total hip arthroplasty as standard open reduction internal fixation, with fewer medical complications.

There are no studies comparing standard open reduction internal fixation to closed or limited reduction and fixation.

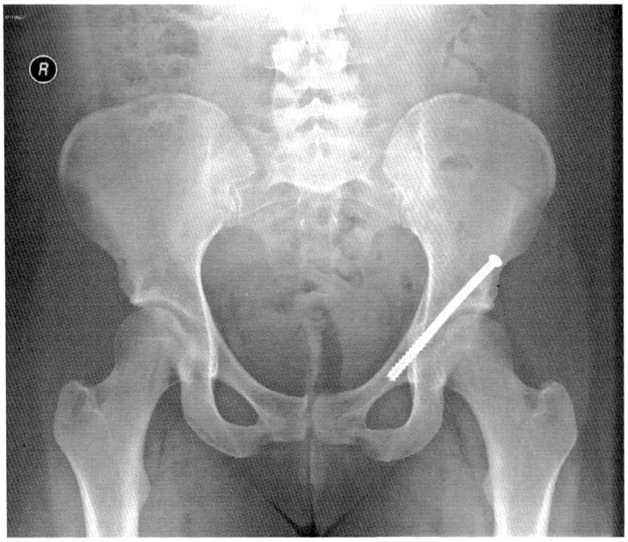

Fig. 27.9 AP pelvis X-ray of a percutaneously treated acetabular fracture

The option of percutaneous fixation of acetabular fractures in the elderly may also provide pain relief and improved mobilization, which is critical in this population. However, objective data is lacking.

Comparison of Operative Versus Nonoperative Care

Several studies have been presented (but not published) on operative versus nonoperative care for these patients. Lucas et al. [139], in a retrospective study, reported that the 1-year mortality was less for the nonoperative group (15 % vs. 35 %) and the return to baseline living arrangements better in the nonoperative group. There was no difference in the ability of either group to return to baseline ambulation. Only 40 % of patients in either group were able to return to their baseline ambulatory status.

Ryan et al. presented data suggesting that hip function scores and general health scores are equivalent when comparing operative versus nonoperative treatment. The results continued to be not statistically significant when controlling for fracture pattern. A flaw of this study was that the conservatively treated patients were significantly older and had more medical comorbidities, which may mean they were lower demand [140].

Total Hip Arthroplasty

There are certain fracture patterns in the patient population, which are prone to failure, as defined by the need for conversion to total hip arthroplasty [133]. Some surgeons question whether the best operation for these patients should be immediate total hip arthroplasty to avoid a second surgery.

Mears and Velyvis [141] reported on 57 patients who underwent acute hip replacement, and 80 % had good-to-excellent outcomes at 8 years of follow-up. Herscovici et al. [142] reported complication rates, surgical times, blood loss, and length of stay were similar to primary fixation.

There are no reports directly comparing the spectrum of options including standard surgical treatment, percutaneous fixation, acute total hip arthroplasty, and nonoperative management.

Periprosthetic Fractures

With the increasing number of total hip and total knee replacements being performed, the incidence of periprosthetic fractures is increasing [143]. These fractures are difficult to manage secondary to poor bone quality and the presence of a prosthesis already in the bone, which may or may not be well fixed.

Preoperative workup should mirror that done for a hip fracture patient previously described. It is important to obtain operative notes from the replacement surgery in order to plan for any revision of the components if necessary.

Imaging should include radiographs of the entire extremity, being sure to include the prosthesis. If possible, it is important to compare previous radiographs of the extremity before injury to see if there are any subtle changes in the prosthesis, which would indicate loosening of the implant.

The principles of management are based on whether the prosthesis is stable or loose. Sometimes it is not possible to know whether a prosthesis is loose until testing it in the operating room, so one should be prepared to both fix the fracture and revise the prosthesis if necessary.

Fractures Around a Total Hip Replacement

The most useful classification is the Vancouver classification, which is both reliable and valid [144]. Fractures around the greater or lesser trochanters (Vancouver A) are typically minimally or non-displaced and can be managed nonoperatively [23]. If the fracture affects the stability of the prosthesis, fixation of the fracture or revision of the prosthesis is required.

Fracture at or around the shaft of the prosthesis is classified as a Vancouver Type B. Fractures can either involve a stable prosthesis (Fig. 27.10) or an unstable prosthesis. Fractures with well-fixed prostheses can undergo primary bone fixation with retention of the prosthesis (Fig. 27.11), while those that have loose prosthesis require revision.

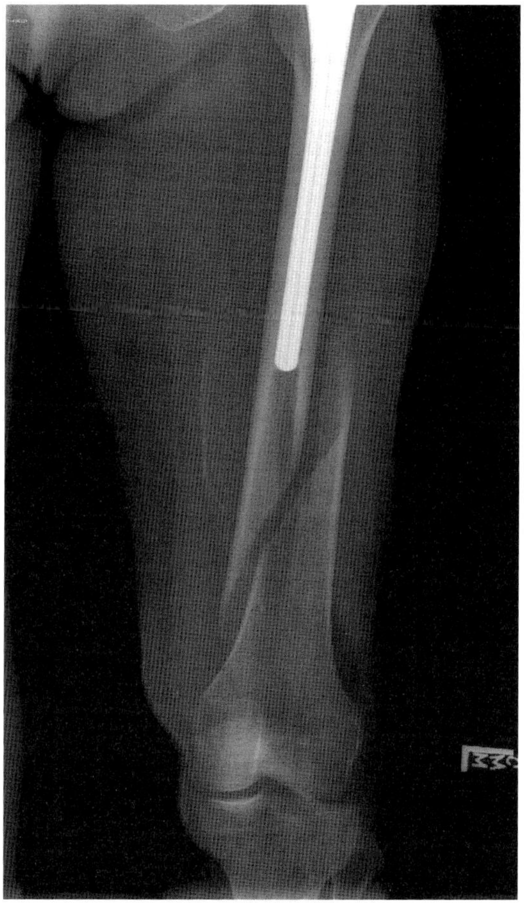

Fig. 27.10 AP femur X-ray of a fracture around a hip prosthesis with a stable implant

There is limited data on comparisons of techniques, but general principles include using implants with sufficient length and stability and preserving the biology of the fracture if possible [143]. There are multiple options for fixation of these types of fractures, which include plate and screw fixation [145], cable plates [146], and with or without allograft struts for support [147].

Postoperative care should involve immediate mobilization. Unfortunately, restricted weight bearing is usually necessary given the poor bone quality and limited fixation around a prosthesis.

Union rates have been reported as high as 85–100 % [148, 149]. Ricci reported 75 % of patients returned to baseline functional status [147]. Mortality after periprosthetic fracture has not been extensively studied as in the hip fracture population, but the 1-year mortality has been reported at 11 % [150].

Fractures that are distal to the prosthesis are classified as a Vancouver Type C . Without the hip prosthesis, these fractures are typically treated with an intramedullary nail. With the prosthesis in place, this is not an ideal construct as it leaves a stress riser between the nail and the prosthesis. Thus,

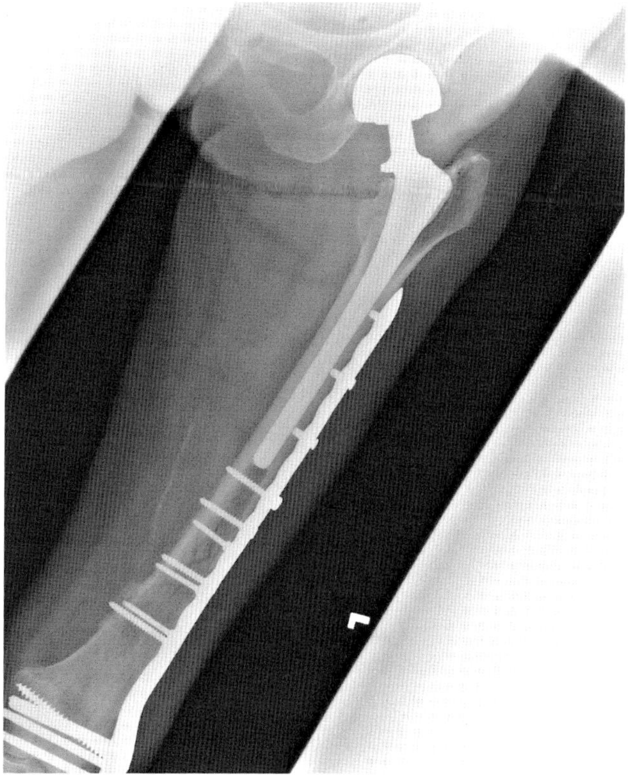

Fig. 27.11 AP femur X-ray of fixation of a periprosthetic fracture

the treatment should be with a laterally based plate that spans the hip prosthesis proximally (Fig. 27.11).

Fractures Around a Total Knee Replacement

Fractures around a total knee replacement happen twice as frequently around the femoral prosthesis than the tibial or patellar (Fig. 27.12). Risk factors for fracture include osteopenia, osteolysis (wear of the prosthesis), and technical errors such as notching of the anterior femur [23]. Treatment of supracondylar femur fractures around a total knee prosthesis is also based on whether the component is stable or unstable.

The goals of treatment include restoration of alignment and early return to function Non-displaced, stable supracondylar femur fractures can be managed nonoperatively in low-demand patients [151]. Operative fixation gives the advantages of immediate range of motion, earlier weight bearing, and less risk of late displacement. All displaced distal femur fractures are indicated for surgical stabilization.

Displaced fractures can be treated with either lateral locked plating (Fig. 27.13) or intramedullary nailing. Results were similar in a comparison of a small group of patients [152].

Intramedullary nailing of these fractures is challenging. Meticulous preoperative planning is necessary, as the surgeon must be familiar with the type and dimensions of the implant to ensure that the nail will pass [153]. There must also be enough bone stock in the distal segment in order to support the interlocking screws. In addition, placement of additional fixation (i.e., blocking screws) may be necessary in order to achieve and maintain alignment [23].

Lateral locked plating has also been reported to successfully treat these fractures [154]. Because of osteoporotic bone, supplemental fixation may be necessary to help avoid varus collapse (Fig. 27.13).

If the implant is loose, revision total knee surgery is required. This surgery is technically challenging and is often best accomplished by an experienced arthroplasty surgeon. Revision involves not only fixing the fracture but also ensuring stability and alignment to the knee [151].

Upper Extremity Fractures

Although upper extremity fractures in the elderly are not typically life-threatening, the resultant impairment may be

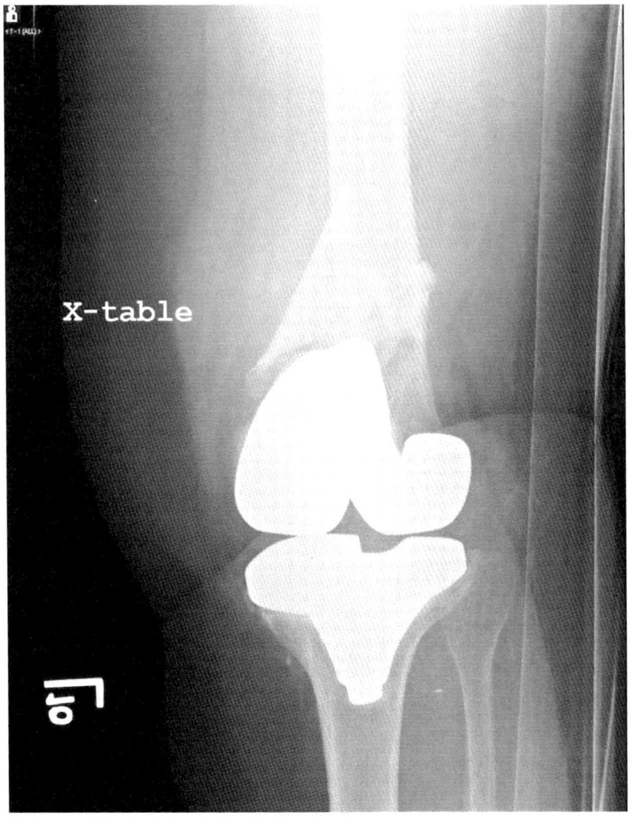

Fig. 27.12 AP knee X-ray of a periprosthetic femur fracture above a knee replacement

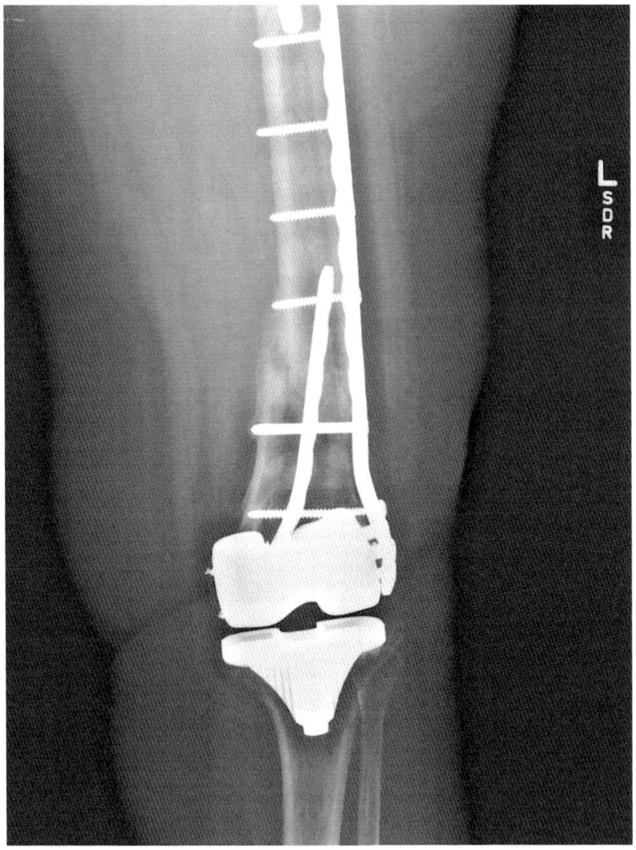

Fig. 27.13 AP knee X-ray of fixation with lateral plating of a periprosthetic femur fracture. In this instance, a second (intramedullary) plate was used for added stability

so functionally debilitating that the injured patient can no longer manage independently. The majority of such upper extremity fractures may be treated nonoperatively. However, the physician must be aware of the potential consequences of prolonged immobilization on the entire limb. Locking plate technology is particularly suitable for providing stable fixation in poor bone, permitting early mobilization, and functional recovery.

Distal Radius Fractures

Distal radius fractures in the elderly are quite common. The incidence rate increases with age and is highest in patients 80 years and older. These typically occur as isolated, low-energy injuries resulting from a fall onto the outstretched hand. However, a neurovascular examination is essential, focusing on the median nerve. Preexisting carpal tunnel syndrome may be exacerbated by the energy of injury and/or the displacement of the distal radius. Concomitant progressive or severe median nerve dysfunction is an indication for urgent carpal tunnel release; in such instances, the fracture is usually stabilized with plate fixation.

The method of treatment of displaced distal radius fractures in the elderly population remains controversial. While restoration of anatomy is a goal of treatment in the younger patient, the relevance of such an approach in the elderly is unclear. A prospective, randomized study [155] comparing closed reduction and cast treatment with open reduction and internal fixation using a volar locking plate demonstrated better grip strength in the operatively treated group; however, there was no difference in wrist motion, pain, or function at 1 year between the two groups. Although 78 % of nonoperatively treated patients had a visible deformity (prominent ulnar head), none of them was dissatisfied with the clinical appearance or the result. The complication rate in the surgical group was 36 %, including tendon ruptures. Similar results have been reported retrospectively in an analogous patient population [156].

Interestingly, the patients treated surgically reported better function during the first 3 months following injury. This is not surprising, since nonoperatively treated distal radius fractures are casted for approximately 6 weeks, whereas patients may be placed into a removable splint soon after plate fixation. This highlights the importance of patient factors in the decision-making process. Older patients who are living alone may be able to retain their independence if treated surgically.

When the decision is made to operate, a number of options are available for fixation. As a rule, percutaneous pin fixation is unreliable when the bone quality is poor. Volar locking plates, in which the screws thread into the plate itself, are ideal for managing osteoporotic fractures [157]. Equivalent results may be obtained with external fixation. Surgeon experience is a principal determinant in the type of implant selected.

Distal Humeral Fractures

One of the most challenging fractures to treat are articular fractures of the distal humerus, particularly in the setting of osteoporosis. With rare exception, these fractures require surgery. A 1984 study demonstrated good-to-excellent results in 76 % of operatively treated fractures compared with 9 % for those treated nonoperatively [158]. These injuries require anatomic reduction and stable fixation in order to allow for early motion, as prolonged casting (>14 days) results in permanent stiffness. The advent of locked, pre-contoured plates has simplified the surgery to some extent. For the elderly, low-demand patient, primary total elbow arthroplasty may be a better alternative.

The initial evaluation should include an assessment of associated soft tissue injuries, such as an open fracture, and neurovascular status, with particular attention to the ulnar nerve which rests in close proximity to the elbow joint. Ipsilateral orthopedic injuries, such as fractures of the distal radius, are not uncommon; the entire limb should be examined and radiographed if necessary. History should include specific inquiry as to the pre-injury status of the elbow, since preexisting arthritis may influence the decision-making process. Radiographic evaluation must include AP, lateral, and oblique views of the elbow; these may be difficult to interpret because of fracture displacement and patient positioning. On occasion, traction views performed in the emergency department may provide additional detail regarding the complexity of the fracture. Virtually all patients with distal humeral fractures will require a non-contrast CT scan of the affected elbow as an element of preoperative planning. In the absence of an open fracture, these injuries are managed semi-electively in order to ensure that appropriate equipment is available.

Surgical repair of distal humeral fractures involves multiple steps; on many occasions, exposure includes ulnar nerve transposition and olecranon osteotomy for exposure. Surgery is performed under tourniquet control to limit blood loss and enhance visualization. Typical fixation includes a minimum of two plates in order to maximize stability and permit early motion. Locking plates have decreased the likelihood of failure of fixation. Nevertheless, complications are not uncommon and include ulnar nerve injury, stiffness, heterotopic ossification, and infection. Pain relief is fairly predictable, with one study reporting 83 % of patients having no or mild pain [159].

In the 1990s, dissatisfaction with the results of surgical repair of distal humeral fractures in the elderly using nonlocking plates led Morrey to manage some of these injuries in a way analogous to femoral neck fractures – total elbow arthroplasty [160]. A more recent review of these patients at the Mayo Clinic showed an average range of motion of 24–132° and a high degree of patient satisfaction. The reoperation rate was 12 % [161]. Two distal humeral fracture studies comparing repair and total elbow arthroplasty in patients older than 65 years of age have come to similar conclusions [162, 163]. Elbow arthroplasty was associated with shorter surgical times, better elbow scores, less disability (as measured by DASH scores) than open reduction internal fixation. Range of motion was at least equivalent. However, given concerns about wear, the typical postoperative restrictions include lifting no more than 10 lb as a single lift or 2 lb repetitively with the affected arm. Consequently, total elbow arthroplasty is reserved for low-demand, elderly patients with preexisting arthritis or with comminuted low articular fractures with limited bone for fixation.

Proximal Humerus Fractures

In the elderly population, fractures of the proximal humerus typically are the result of a fall from standing height. These fractures are about half as common as hip fractures in this population, accounting for 10 % of fractures in people >65 years of age. Associated injuries, such as head trauma and rib fractures, should be excluded. Displaced proximal humerus fractures may be associated with neurovascular injury, including subclavian artery and brachial plexus injuries. If pulses are diminished, Doppler studies should be performed, and the blood pressure recording should be compared with the other arm. If the pulses remain altered following gentle realignment of the limb, an urgent vascular consult must be obtained. The neurologic status of the extremity may be difficult to assess due to pain; the examiner should check for altered sensation in the deltoid area to assess for axillary nerve dysfunction. Other relatively painless maneuvers include assessment of sensation in the median (index finger), radial (first web space), and ulnar (little finger) distributions and motor function, including elbow flexion (musculocutaneous), wrist and digital extension (radial), thumb flexion (anterior interosseous branch of median nerve), and ability to cross fingers (ulnar).

Radiographs must include a shoulder trauma series, which consists of an AP of the shoulder, a lateral "Y" view, and a supine axillary view. The latter view may be difficult to obtain because of patient discomfort, but orthogonal views are necessary to exclude a dislocation. An alternative view, termed a Velpeau lateral, may be obtained with the patient sitting comfortably in a sling.

The Neer classification [155] is commonly used as a guide for treatment. The proximal humerus is considered as four components: the head, the greater tuberosity, the lesser tuberosity, and the shaft. To be considered a part, the component must be displaced more than 1 cm or rotated more than 45° [164]. Between 45 and 80 % of proximal humerus, fractures are non-displaced and may be managed in a simple sling. For non-displaced two-part distal humerus fractures, early mobilization appears to result in less pain and faster and potentially better recovery than 3 weeks of immobilization [165]. Nevertheless, at least 40 % of these elderly patients will require pain control and basic care [166].

For displaced fractures, fracture factors and patient factors are critically important in deciding whether to operate. A prospective study [167] of internal fixation versus nonoperative treatment for 3-part proximal humerus fractures in the elderly demonstrated slightly improved motion and function (although most parameters did not reach statistical significance). However, 30 % of the surgically treated patients required additional surgery. Fracture comminution and poor bone quality make fixation somewhat tenuous in spite of locking plate technology. Disruption of the blood supply to the humeral head is common with four-part fractures; this poses a relative indication for primary hemiarthroplasty in the elderly patient. However, the data is not compelling enough to convincingly argue for surgery in patients with significant medical comorbidities. In fact, a recent prospective, randomized study showed no demonstrable benefit of hemiarthroplasty over nonoperative treatment in patients older than 65 years of age [168].

Conclusion

Caring for elderly patients with osteoporotic fractures is challenging and requires a multidisciplinary approach. Treatment of hip fractures is typically a surgical problem, while the optimal treatment of displaced acetabular fractures is still unknown. Periprosthetic fractures around hip or knee replacements often require unconventional surgical techniques. Surgical management of these fractures often decreases morbidity and mortality compared to nonoperative management, even faced with multiple medical comorbidities. Upper extremity fractures can often be treated without surgery. However, seemingly minor fractures may seriously affect the functional status of the elderly patient. Although not always possible, the goal is to return the patient to their baseline functional status, living situation, and decrease pain.

References

1. WHO. Assessment of fracture risk and its application to screening for postmenopausal osteoporosis. Report of a WHO Study Group. World Health Organ Tech Rep Ser. 1994;843:1–129.
2. Benger U. Epidemiological changes over 30 years in an urban population. Thesis, Lund University, Lund, 1987.
3. Kannus P, Niemi S, Parkkari J, et al. Hip fractures in Finland between 1970 and 1997 and predictions for the future. Lancet. 1999;353:802–5.
4. Obrant KJ, Bengner U, Johnell O, et al. Increasing age-adjusted risk of fragility fractures: a sign of increasing osteoporosis in successive generations? Calcif Tissue Int. 1989;44:157–67.

5. Greenspan SL, Myers ER, Maitland LA, et al. Fall severity and bone mineral density as risk factors for hip fracture in ambulatory elderly. JAMA. 1994;271:128–33.
6. Tinetti ME, Doucette J, Claus E, et al. Risk factors for serious injury during falls by older persons in the community. J Am Geriatr Soc. 1995;43:1214–21.
7. Tinetti ME, Speechley M, Ginter SF. Risk factors for falls among elderly persons living in the community. N Engl J Med. 1988;319:1701–7.
8. Luukinen H, Koski K, Honkanen R, et al. Incidence of injury-causing falls among older adults by place of residence: a population-based study. J Am Geriatr Soc. 1995;43:871–6.
9. Ryynanen OP, Kivela SL, Honkanen R, et al. Incidence of falling injuries leading to medical treatment in the elderly. Public Health. 1991;105:373–86.
10. Tinetti ME. Factors associated with serious injury during falls by ambulatory nursing home residents. J Am Geriatr Soc. 1987;35:644–8.
11. Rice D, MacKenzie E, Associates. Cost of injury in the United States: a report to congress. San Francisco: University of California; 1989.
12. Howe TE, Shea B, Dawson LJ, Downey F, Murray A, Ross C, et al. Exercise for preventing and treating osteoporosis in postmenopausal women. Cochrane Database Syst Rev. 2011;7, CD21735380.
13. Feldstein AC, Vollmer WM, Smith DH, Petrik A, Schneider J, Glauber H, et al. An outreach program improved osteoporosis management after a fractures. J Am Geriatr Soc. 2007;55:1464–9.
14. Shea B, Wells G, Cranney A, et al. Meta-analyses of therapies for postmenopausal osteoporosis. VII. Meta-analysis of calcium supplementation for the prevention of postmenopausal osteoporosis. Endocr Rev. 2002;23:552–9.
15. Shea B, Wells G, Cranney A, et al. Calcium supplementation on bone loss in postmenopausal women. Cochrane Database Syst Rev. 2004;1:CD004526. Review. Update in: Cochrane Database Syst Rev. 2006;1:CD004526.
16. Chapuy MC, Arlot ME, Delmas PD, et al. Effect of calcium and cholecalciferol treatment for three years on hip fractures in elderly women. BMJ. 1994;308:1081–2.
17. Chapuy MC, Arlot ME, Duboeuf F, et al. Vitamin D3 and calcium to prevent hip fractures in elderly women. N Engl J Med. 1992;327:1637–42.
18. Province MA, Hadley EC, Hornbrook MC, et al. The effects of exercise on falls in elderly patients. A preplanned meta-analysis of the FICSIT trials. Fragility and injuries: cooperative studies of intervention techniques. JAMA. 1995;273:1341–7.
19. Tinetti ME, McAvay G, Claus E. Does multiple risk factor reduction explain the reduction in fall rate in the Yale FICSIT trial? Frailty and injuries cooperative studies of intervention techniques. Am J Epidemiol. 1996;144:389–99.
20. Qaseem A, Snow V, Shekelle P, Hopkins Jr R, Forciea MA, Owens DK, et al. Pharmacologic treatment of low bone density or osteoporosis to prevent fractures: a clinical practice guideline from the American College of Physicians. Ann Intern Med. 2008;149:404–15.
21. MacLean C, Newberry S, Maglione M, McMahon M, Ranganath V, Suttorp M, et al. Systematic review: comparative effectiveness of treatments to prevent fractures in men and women with low bone density or osteoporosis. Ann Intern Med. 2001;148:197–213.
22. Avenell A, Gillespie WJ, Gillespie LD, O'Connell D. Vitamin D and vitamin D analogues for preventing fractures associated with involutional and postmenopausal osteoporosis. Cochrane Database Syst Rev. 2009;2, CD19370554.
23. Rockwood CA, McQueen MM, et al. Rockwood and Green's fractures in adults. Karlsson KM, Josefsson OJ, editors. 7th ed. Philadelphia: Lippincott Williams and Wilkins; 2010, pp. 492–517.
24. Christiansen C, Christensen MS, Transbol I. Bone mass in postmenopausal women after withdrawal of oestrogen/gestagen replacement therapy. Lancet. 1981;1:459–61.
25. Felson DT, Zhang Y, Hannan MT, et al. The effect of postmenopausal estrogen therapy on bone density in elderly women. N Engl J Med. 1993;329:1141–6.
26. Lindsay R, Hart DM, Fogelman I. Bone mass after withdrawal of oestrogen replacement. Lancet. 1981;1:729.
27. Cummings SR, Ettinger B, Delmas PD, Kenemans P, Stathopoulos V, Verweij P, et al. The effects of tibolone in older postmenopausal women. N Engl J Med. 2008;359:697–708.
28. Ettinger B, Black DM, Mitlak BH, et al. Reduction of vertebral fracture risk in postmenopausal women with osteoporosis treated with raloxifene: results from a 3-year randomized clinical trial. Multiple Outcomes of Raloxifene (MORE) Investigators. JAMA. 1999;282:637–45.
29. Cauley JA, Norton L, Lippman ME, et al. Continued breast cancer risk reduction in postmenopausal women treated with raloxifene: 4-year results from the MORE trial. Multiple outcomes of raloxifene evaluation. Breast Cancer Res Treat. 2001;65:123–34.
30. Cummings SR, Black DM, Thompson DE, et al. Effect of alendronate on risk of fracture in women with low bone density but without vertebral fractures: results from the fracture intervention trial. JAMA. 1998;280:2077–82.
31. Fleisch H. Bisphosphonates in bone disease: from the laboratory to the patient. 4th ed. San Diego: Academic; 2000.
32. De Groen PC, Lubbe DF, Hirsch LJ, et al. Esophagitis associated with the use of alendronate. N Engl J Med. 1996;335:1016–21.
33. Black DM, Delmas PD, Eastell R, et al. Once-yearly zoledronic acid for treatment of postmenopausal osteoporosis. N Engl J Med. 2007;356:1809–22.
34. Schnitzer T, Bone HG, Crepaldi G, et al. Therapeutic equivalence of alendronate 70 mg once-weekly and alendronate 10 mg daily in the treatment of osteoporosis. Alendronate Once-Weekly Study Group. Aging (Milano). 2000;12:1–12.
35. Chesnut 3rd CH, Silverman S, Andriano K, et al. A randomized trial of nasal spray salmon calcitonin in postmenopausal women with established osteoporosis: the prevent recurrence of osteoporotic fractures study. PROOF Study Group. Am J Med. 2000;109:267–76.
36. Cranny A, Tugwell P, Zytaruk N, et al. Meta-analyses of therapies for postmenopausal osteoporosis. VI. Meta-analysis of calcitonin for the treatment of postmenopausal osteoporosis. Endocr Rev. 2002;23:540–51.
37. Neer RM, Arnaud CD, Zanchetta JR, et al. Effect of parathyroid hormone (1–34) on fractures and bone mineral density in postmenopausal women with osteoporosis. N Engl J Med. 2001;344:1434–41.
38. Seeman E, Delmas PD. Reconstructing the skeleton with intermittent parathyroid hormone. Trends Endocrinol Metab. 2001;12:281–3.
39. Greenspan SL, Bone HG, Ettinger MP, et al. Effect of recombinant human parathyroid hormone (1–84) on vertebral fracture and bone mineral density in postmenopausal women with osteoporosis: a randomized trial. Ann Intern Med. 2007;146:326–39.
40. Cosman F, Eriksen EF, Recknor C, Miller PD, Guañabens N, Kasperk C, et al. Effects of intravenous zoledronic acid plus subcutaneous teriparatide [rhPTH(1–34)] in postmenopausal osteoporosis. J Bone Miner Res. 2011;26:503–11.
41. Cosman F, Nieves J, Zion M, Woelfert L, Luckey M, Lindsay R. Daily and cyclic parathyroid hormone in women receiving alendronate. N Engl J Med. 2005;353:566–75.
42. FDA approves new injectable osteoporosis treatment for postmenopausal women. http://www.fda.gov.ezproxy.library.tufts.edu/NewsEvents/Newsroom/PressAnnouncements/ucm214150.htm. Accessed 20 June 2012.
43. Cummings SR, San Martin J, McClung MR, Siris ES, Eastell R, Reid IR, et al. Denosumab for prevention of fractures in postmeno-

pausal women with osteoporosis. N Engl J Med. 2009;361: 756–65.
44. Anastasilakis AD, Toulis KA, Goulis DG, Polyzos SA, Delaroudis S, Giomisi A, et al. Efficacy and safety of denosumab in postmenopausal women with osteopenia or osteoporosis: a systematic review and a meta-analysis. Horm Metab Res. 2009;41:721–9.
45. Meunier PJ, Roux C, Seeman E, Ortolani S, Badurski JE, Spector TD, et al. The effects of strontium ranelate on the risk of vertebral fracture in women with postmenopausal osteoporosis. N Engl J Med. 2004;350:459–68.
46. O'Donnell S, Cranney A, Wells GA, Adachi J, Reginster JY. Strontium ranelate for preventing and treating postmenopausal osteoporosis. Cochrane Database Syst Rev. 2008;4, CD16856092.
47. Meunier PH, Sebert JL, Reginster JY, et al. Fluoride salts are no better at preventing new vertebral fractures than calcium-vitamin D in postmenopausal osteoporosis: the FAVO Study. Osteoporos Int. 1998;8:4–12.
48. Riggs BL, Hodgson SF, O'Fallon WM, et al. Effect of fluoride treatment on the fracture rate in postmenopausal women with osteoporosis. N Engl J Med. 1990;322:802–9.
49. Haguenauer D, Welch V, Shea B, et al. Fluoride for treating postmenopausal osteoporosis. Cochrane Database Syst Rev. 2000;4:CD002825. Review.
50. Lucas TS, Einhorn TA. Osteoporosis: the role of the orthopaedist. J Am Acad Orthop Surg. 1993;1:48–56.
51. Cornell CN. Internal fixation in patients with osteoporosis. J Am Acad Orthop Surg. 2003;11(2):109–18.
52. Koval KJ, Hoehl JJ, Kummer FJ, Simon JA. Distal femoral fixation: a biomechanical comparison of the standard condylar buttress plate, a locked buttress plate and the 95-degree blade plate. J Orthop Trauma. 1997;11:521–4.
53. Welch RD, Zhang H, Bronson DG. Experimental tibial plateau fractures augmented with calcium phosphate cement or autologous bone graft. J Bone Joint Surg Am. 2003;85A:222–3.
54. Silver JJ, Einhorn TA. Osteoporosis and aging: current update. Clin Orthop. 1995;316:10–20.
55. Dorotka R, Schoechtner H, Buchinger W. The influence of immediate surgical treatment of proximal femoral fractures on mortality and quality of life. Operation within 6 hours of the fracture versus later than 6 hours. J Bone Joint Surg Br. 2003;85:1107–13.
56. Pape HC, Grimme K, van Griensven M, et al. Impact of intramedullary instrumentation versus damage control for femoral fractures on immunoinflammatory parameters: prospective randomized analysis by the EPOFF Study Group. J Trauma. 2003;55:7–13.
57. Koval KJ, et al. Dependency after hip fracture in geriatric patients: a study of predictive factors. J Orthop Trauma. 1996;10(8):531–5.
58. Michel JP, Klopfenstein C, Hoffmeyer P, Stern R, Grab B. Hip fracture surgery: is the pre operative American Society of Anesthesiologists (ASA) score a predictor of functional outcome? Aging Clin Exp Res. 2002;14(5):389–94.
59. Vidan M, Serra JM, Moreno C, Riquelme G, Ortiz J. Efficacy of a comprehensive geriatric intervention in older patients hospitalized for hip fracture: a randomized controlled trial. J Am Geriatr Soc. 2005;53:1476–82.
60. Kenzora JE, McCarthy RE, Lowell JD, Siedge CB. Hip fracture mortality. Relation to age, treatment, preoperative illness, time of surgery and complications. Clin Orthop Relat Res. 1984;186:15–25.
61. Sexson SB, Lehner JT. Factors affecting hip fracture mortality. J Orthop Trauma. 1987;1:298–305.
62. Moran CG, Wenn RT, Sikand M, Taylor AM. Early mortality after hip fracture: is delay before surgery important? J Bone Joint Surg Am. 2005;87:483–9.
63. Egol KA, Strauss EJ. Perioperative considerations in geriatric patients with hip fracture: what is the evidence? J Orthop Trauma. 2009;23:386–94.
64. Urwin SC, Fox GS. Anaesthesia for hip fracture surgery in the elderly. Can J Anaesth. 1989;36(3 Pt 1):311–9.
65. Parker MJ, Handoll HH, Griffiths R. Anaesthesia for hip fracture surgery in adults. Cochrane Database Syst Rev. 2004;4, CD000521.
66. Brauer CA, Coca-Perraillon M, Cutler DM, Rosen AB. Incidence and mortality of hip fractures in the United States. JAMA. 2009;302:1573–9.
67. Dennison E, Mohamed MA, Cooper C. Epidemiology of osteoporosis. Rheum Dis Clin North Am. 2006;32(4):617–29.
68. Piirtola M, Vahlberg T, Isoaho R, et al. Incidence of fractures and changes over time among the aged in a Finnish municipality: a population-based 12-year follow-up. Aging Clin Exp Res. 2007;19(4):269–76.
69. Solomon L. Osteoporosis and fracture of the femoral neck in the South African Bantu. J Bone Joint Surg. 1968;50B:2–13.
70. Singer BR, McLauchlan GJ, Robinson CM, et al. Epidemiology of fractures in 15,000 adults: the influence of age and gender. J Bone Joint Surg Br. 1998;80(2):243–8.
71. Linten P. Type of displacement in fractures of the femoral neck and observations on impaction of fractures. J Bone Joint Surg. 1949;34B:184–9.
72. Farooq MA, Orkazai SH, Okusanya O, Devitt AT. Intracapsular fractures of the femoral neck in younger patients. Ir J Med Sci. 2005;174(4):42–5.
73. Freeman MAR, Todd RC, Pirie CJ. The role of fatigue in the pathogenesis of senile femoral neck fractures. J Bone Joint Surg. 1974;56B:698–702.
74. Fairclough J, Colhoun E, Johnston D, et al. Bone scanning for suspected hip fractures. A prospective study in elderly patients. J Bone Joint Surg. 1987;69B:251–3.
75. Rajan DT, Parker MJ. Does the level of an intracapsular femoral fracture influence fracture healing after internal fixation? A study of 411 patients. Injury. 2001;32(1):53–6.
76. Raaymakers EL, Marti RK. Non-operative treatment of impacted femoral neck fractures. A prospective study of 170 cases. J Bone Joint Surg Br. 1991;73(6):950–4.
77. Krastman P, van den Bent RP, Krijnen P, et al. Two cannulated hip screws for femoral neck fractures: treatment of choice or asking for trouble? Arch Orthop Trauma Surg. 2006;126(5): 297–303.
78. Clark DI, Crofts CE, Saleh M. Femoral neck fracture fixation. Comparison of a sliding screw with lag screws. J Bone Joint Surg. 1990;72B:797–800.
79. Lee YS, Chen SH, Tsuang YH, et al. Internal fixation of undisplaced femoral neck fractures in the elderly: a retrospective comparison of fixation methods. J Trauma. 2008;64(1): 155–62.
80. Chua D, Jaglal SB, Schatzker J. Predictors of early failure of fixation in the treatment of displaced subcapital hip fractures. J Orthop Trauma. 1998;12:230–4.
81. Shuqiang M, Kunzheng W, Zhichao T, et al. Outcome of non-operative management in Garden I femoral neck fractures. Injury. 2006;37(10):974–8.
82. Verheyen CC, Smulders TC, van Walsum AD. High secondary displacement rate in the conservative treatment of impacted femoral neck fractures in 105 patients. Arch Orthop Trauma Surg. 2005;125(3):166–8.
83. Heim M, Adunski A, Chechick A. Nonoperative treatment of intracapsular fractures of the proximal femur. Clin Orthop Relat Res. 2002;399:35–41.
84. Weinrauch PC, Moore WR, Shooter DR, et al. Early prosthetic complications after unipolar hemiarthroplasty. ANZ J Surg. 2006;76(6):432–5.
85. Faraj AA, Branfoot T. Cemented versus uncemented Thompson's prostheses: a functional outcome study. Injury. 1999;30(10): 671–5.
86. Parker MJ, Gurusamy K. Arthroplasties (with and without bone cement) for proximal femoral fractures in adults. Cochrane Database Syst Rev. 2006;3, CD001706.

87. Singh GK, Deshmukh RG. Uncemented Austin-Moore and cemented Thompson unipolar hemiarthroplasty for displaced fracture neck of femur – comparison of complications and patient satisfaction. Injury. 2006;37(2):169–74.
88. Bochner RM, Pellicci PM, Lyden JP. Bipolar hemiarthroplasty for fracture of the femoral neck. Clinical review with special emphasis on prosthetic motion. J Bone Joint Surg Am. 1988;70: 1001–10.
89. Eiskjaer S, Boll K, Gelineck J. Component motion in bipolar cemented hemi-arthroplasty. J Orthop Trauma. 1989;3(4):313–6.
90. Hodgkinson JP, Meadows TH, Davies DR, et al. A radiological assessment of interprosthetic movement in the Charnley-Hastings hemiarthroplasty. Injury. 1988;19(1):18–20.
91. Phillips TW. The Bateman bipolar femoral head replacement. J Bone Joint Surg. 1987;69B:761–4.
92. Brueton RN, Craig JS, Hinves BL, et al. Effect of femoral component head size on movement of the two-component hemi-arthroplasty. Injury. 1993;24(4):231–5.
93. Parker MJ, Gurusamy K. Arthroplasties (with and without bone cement) for proximal femoral fractures in adults. Cochrane Database Syst Rev. 2004;2, CD001706.
94. Hedbeck CJ, Enocson A, Lapidus G, Blomfeldt R, Törnkvist H, et al. Comparison of bipolar hemiarthroplasty for displaced femoral neck fractures: a concise four-year follow-up of a randomized controlled trial. J Bone Joint Surg Am. 2011;93(5):445–50.
95. Burgers PT, Van Geene AR, Van den Bekerom MP, Van Lieshout EM, Blom B, et al. Total hip arthroplasty versus hemiarthroplasty for displaced femoral neck fractures in the healthy elderly: a meta-analysis and systematic review of randomized trials. Int Orthop. 2012;36(8):1549–60.
96. Bilgen O, Karaeminogullari O, Kulecioglu A. Results of conversion total hip prosthesis performed following painful hemiarthroplasty. J Int Med Res. 2000;28:307–12.
97. Parvizi J, Ereth MH, Lewallen DG. Thirty-day mortality following hip arthroplasty for acute fracture. J Bone Joint Surg Am. 2004;86-A(9):1983–8.
98. Bhandari M, Devereaux PJ, Swiontkowski MF, et al. Internal fixation compared with arthroplasty for displaced fractures of the femoral neck: a meta-analysis. J Bone Joint Surg Am. 2005;87(9):2122–30.
99. Lu Yao GL, Keller RB, Littenberg B, et al. Outcomes after displaced fractures of the femoral neck. A meta-analysis of one hundred and six published reports. J Bone Joint Surg. 1994;76A:15–25.
100. Rogmark C, Johnell O. Orthopaedic treatment of displaced femoral neck fractures in elderly patients. Disabil Rehabil. 2005; 27:1143–9.
101. Blomfeldt R, Törnkvist H, Eriksson K, et al. A randomised controlled trial comparing bipolar hemiarthroplasty with total hip replacement for displaced intracapsular fractures of the femoral neck in elderly patients. J Bone Joint Surg Br. 2007;89(2):160–5.
102. Keating JF, Grant A, Masson M, et al. Displaced intracapsular hip fractures in fit older people: a randomised comparison of reduction and fixation, bipolar hemiarthroplasty and total hip arthroplasty. Health Technol Assess. 2005;9(41):iii–iV, ix–x, 1–65.
103. Patel KK, Ashford RU, Frasquet-Garcia A, et al. Müller straight stem total hip arthroplasty for fractured neck of femur. Injury. 2006;37(8):727–33.
104. Rogmark C, Carlsson A, Johnell O, Sembo I. A prospective randomised trial of internal fixation versus arthroplasty for displaced fractures of the neck of the femur. Functional outcome for 450 patients at 2 years. J Bone Joint Surg Br. 2002;84(2): 183–8.
105. Tidermark J, Zethraeus N, Svensson O, et al. Quality of life related to fracture displacement among elderly patients with femoral neck fractures treated with internal fixation. J Orthop Trauma. 2002;16(1):34–8.
106. Stephen IBM. Subcapital fractures of the femur in rheumatoid arthritis. Injury. 1979;11:233–41.
107. Strömqvist B, Brismar J, Hansson LI, et al. Technetium 99 m-methylenediphosphonate scientimetry after femoral neck fracture. A 3 year follow-up study. Clin Orthop Relat Res. 1984;182:177–89.
108. Hwang LC, Lo WH, Chen WM, et al. Intertrochanteric fractures in adults younger than 40 years of age. Arch Orthop Trauma Surg. 2001;121(3):123–6.
109. Hopkinson-Woolley JA, Parker MJ. Fractures of the hip: does the type of fall really affect the site of fracture? Injury. 1998;29(8):585–7.
110. Lambotte A. L'intervention opératoire dans les fractues recenes et anciennes envisagéc particulierement au point de vue de l'osteosynthese avec la description des plusiers techniques nouvelles. Paris; 1907.
111. Lambotte A. Chiugie opératoire des fractures. Paris: Mason et Cie; 1913.
112. Bick E. Source book of orthopaedics. New York: Hafner; 1968.
113. Parker MJ, Handoll HH. Gamma and other cephalocondylic intramedullary nailes versus extramedullary implants for extracapsular hip fractures in adults. Cochrane Database Syst Rev. 2008;3, CD000093.
114. Parker MJ, Handoll HH. Intramedullary nails for extracapsular hip fractures in adults. Cochrane Database Syst Rev. 2006;3, CD000093.
115. Gotfried Y, Cohen B, Rotem A. Biomechanical evaluation of the percutaneous compression plating system for hip fractures. J Orthop Trauma. 2002;16(9):644–50.
116. Tronzo RG. Use of an extramedullary guide pin for fractures of the upper end of the femur. Orthop Clin North Am. 1974;5(3): 525–7.
117. De Grave PW, Tampere T, Byn P, Van Overschelde J, Pattyn C, Verdonk R. Intramedullary fixation of intertrochanteric hip fractures: a comparison of two implant designs. A prospective randomised clinical trial. Acta Orthop Belg. 2012; 78(2):192–8.
118. Butler M, Forte M, Joglekar S, Swiontkowski MF, Kane RL. Evidence summary: a systematic review of surgical treatments for geriatric hip fractures. J Bone Joint Surg Am. 2011;93(12): 1104–15.
119. Russell TA, Mir HR, Stoneback J, et al. Avoidance of malreduction of proximal shaft fractures with the use of a minimally invasive nail insertion technique (MINIT). J Orthop Trauma. 2008;22(6):391–8.
120. Robinson CM, Houshian S, Khan L. Trochanteric-entry long cephalomedullary nailing of subtrochanteric fractures caused by low energy trauma. J Bone Joint Surg Am. 2005;87-A: 2217–26.
121. Kamel H, Iqbal M, Mogallapu R, et al. Time to ambulation after hip fracture surgery: relation to hospitalization outcomes. J Gerontol A Biol Sci Med Sci. 2003;58:1042–5.
122. Bedi A, Toanle T. Subtrochanteric femur fractures. Orthop Clin North Am. 2004;35(4):473–83, review.
123. Fielding JW, Magliato HJ. Subtrochanteric fractures. Surg Gynecol Obstet. 1966;122:555–69.
124. Goh SK, Yang KY, Koh JS, et al. Subtrochanteric insufficiency fractures in patients on alendronate therapy: a caution. J Bone Joint Surg. 2007;89B(3):349–53.
125. Sims SH. Subtrochanteric femur fractures. Orthop Clin North Am. 2002;33(1):113–26, review.
126. Kitajima I, Tachibana S, Mikama Y, et al. Insufficiency fracture of femoral neck after intramedullary nailing. J Orthop Sci. 1999;4: 304–6.
127. Dora C, Leunig M, Beck M, et al. Entry point soft tissue damage in antegrade femoral nailing: a cadaver study. J Orthop Trauma. 2001;15(7):488–93.
128. Sherk HH, Snape WJ, Loprete FL. Internal fixation versus nontreatment of hip fractures in senile patients. Clin Orthop Relat Res. 1979;141:196–8.

129. Richmond J, Aharonoff GB, Zuckerman JD, Koval KJ. Mortality risk after hip fracture. J Orthop Trauma. 2003;17(1):53–6.
130. Panula J, Pihlamjamak H, Mattila VM, Jaatinen P, Vahlberg T, Aarnio P, et al. Mortality and cause of death in hip fracture patients aged 65 or older: a population based study. BMC Musculoskeletal Disord. 2011;12:105.
131. Koval KJ, Skovron ML, Aharonoff GB, Meadows SE, Zukerman JD. Ambulatory ability after hip fracture. A prospective study in geriatric patients. Clin Orthop Relat Res. 1995; 310:150–9.
132. Carroll EA, Huber FG, Goldman AT, Virkus WW, Pagenkopf E, Lorich DG. Treatment of acetabular fractures in an older population. J Orthop Trauma. 2010;24(10):637–44.
133. Anglen JO, Burd TA, Hendricks KJ, Harrison P. The "Gull Sign": a harbinger of failure for internal fixation of geriatric acetabular fractures. J Orthop Trauma. 2003;17(9):625–34.
134. Tile M. Fractures of the pelvis and acetabulum. Baltimore: Williams and Wilkins; 1984.
135. Spencer RF. Acetabular fractures in older patients. J Bone Joint Surg Br. 1989;710-B:774–6.
136. Letournel E, Judet R, editors. Fractures of the acetabulum (trans: Elson RA). 2nd ed. Berlin: Springer; 1993.
137. Leflamme GY, Herbert-Davies J, Rouleau D, Benoit B, Leduc S. Internal fixation of osteoporotic acetabular fractures involving the quadrilateral plate. Injury. 2011;42:1130–4.
138. Gary JL, VanHal M, Gibbons SD, Reinert CM, Starr AJ. Functional outcomes in elderly patients with acetabular fractures treated with minimally invasive reduction and percutaneous fixation. J Orthop Trauma. 2012;26(5):278–83.
139. Lucas J, Chacko AT, Rodriguez EK, Appleton P. Comparison of outcomes of operative versus non operative treatment of acetabular fractures in the elderly and severely comorbid patients. In: Presented Orthopaedic Trauma Association, Denver, 2008.
140. Ryan SP, Manson TT, Lebrun CT, Nascone JW, Sciadini MF, Castillo RC. Functional outcomes of non operative treatment of geriatric acetabular fractures meeting operative criteria. In: Presented Orthopaedic Trauma Association, San Antonio, 2011.
141. Mears DC, Velyvis JH. Acute total hip arthroplasty for selected displaced acetabular fractures: two to twelve-year results. J Bone Joint Surg Am. 2002;84A:1–9.
142. Herscovici D, Lindvall E, Bolhofner B, Scaduto JM. The combined hip procedure: open reduction internal fixation combined with total hip arthroplasty for the management of acetabular fractures in the elderly. J Orthop Trauma. 2010;24(5):291–6.
143. Pike J, Davidson D, Garbuz D, Duncan CP, O'Brien PJ, Bassam MA. Principles of treatment for periprosthetic femoral shaft fractures around well fixed total hip arthroplasty. J Am Acad Orthop Surg. 2009;17(11):677–88.
144. Duncan CP, Masri BA. Fractures of the femur after hip replacement. Instr Course Lect. 1995;44:293–304.
145. Buttaro MA, Farfalli G, Paredes NM, Comba F, Piccaluga F. Locking compression plate fixation of Vancouver type B-1 periprosthetic femoral fractures. J Bone Joint Surg Am. 2007;89(9):1964–9.
146. Haddad FS, Marston RA, Muirhead-Allwood SK. The Dall-Miles cable and plate system for periprosthetic femoral fractures. Injury. 1997;28:445–7.
147. Ricci WM, Bolhofner BR, Lofts T, Cox C, Mitchell S, Borrelli J. Indirect reduction and plate fixation, without grafting, for periprosthetic femoral shaft fractures about a stable intramedullary implant: surgical technique. J Bone Joint Surg Am. 2006;88(Suppl 1 pt 2):275–82.
148. Sen R, Prasad P, Kumar S, Nagi O. Periprosthetic femoral fractures around well fixed implants: a simple method of fixation using LC-DCP with trochanteric purchase. Acta Orthop Belg. 2007;73:200–6.
149. Abhaykumar S, Elliott DS. Percutaneous plate fixation for periprosthetic femoral fractures: a preliminary report. Injury. 2000;31: 627–30.
150. Bhattacharyya T, Chang D, Meigs JB, Estok II DM, Malchau H. Mortality after periprosthetic fracture of the femur. J Bone Joint Surg Am. 2007;89:2658–62.
151. Dennis DA. Periprosthetic fractures following total knee arthroplasty. J Bone Joint Surg. 2001;83A(1):120–30.
152. Wick M, Muller EJ, Kurscha-Lissberg F, et al. Periprosthetic supracondylar femoral fractures: LISS or retrograde intramedullary nailing? Problems with the use of minimally invasive technique. Unfallchirurgie. 2001;107:181–8.
153. Su ET, DeWal H, Di Cesare PE. Periprosthetic femoral fractures above total knee replacements. J Am Acad Orthop Surg. 2004;12:12–20.
154. Ricci WM, Borrelli Jr J. Operative management of periprosthetic femur fractures in the elderly using biological fracture reduction and fixation techniques. Injury. 2007;38 suppl 3:553–8.
155. Arora R, Lutz M, Deml C, Krappinger D, et al. A prospective randomized trial comparing nonoperative treatment with volar locking plate fixation for displaced unstable distal radial fractures in patients sixty-five years of age and older. J Bone Joint Surg Am. 2011;93:2146–53.
156. Egol KA, Walks M, Romo-Cardoso S, Dorsky S, Paksima N. Distal radial fractures in the elderly: operative compared with nonoperative treatment. J Bone Joint Surg Am. 2010;92:1851–7.
157. Jupiter JB, Ring D, Weitzel PP. Surgical treatment of redisplaced fractures of the distal radius in patients older than 60 years. J Hand Surg Am. 2002;27:714–23.
158. Zagorski JB, Jennings JJ, Burkhalter WE, et al. Comminuted intraarticular fractures of the distal humeral condyles: surgical vs. nonsurgical treatment. Clin Orthop Relat Res. 1986;202:197–204.
159. Sanchez-Sotelo J, Torchia ME, O'Driscoll SW. Complex distal humeral fractures: internal fixation with a principle-based parallel-plate technique. J Bone Joint Surg Am. 2007;89:961–9.
160. Cobb TK, Morrey BF. Total elbow arthroplasty as primary treatment for distal humeral fractures in elderly patients. J Bone Joint Surg Am. 1997;79(6):826–32.
161. Kamineni S, Morrey BF. Distal humeral fractures treated with noncustom total elbow replacement. J Bone Joint Surg Am. 2004;86:940–7.
162. Frankle MA, Herscovici Jr D, DiPasquale TG, Vasey MB, Sanders RW. A comparison of open reduction and internal fixation and primary total elbow arthroplasty in the treatment of intraarticular distal humerus fractures in women older than age 65. J Orthop Trauma. 2003;17:473–80.
163. McKee MD, Veillette CJ, Hall JA, Schemitsch EH, Wild LM, McCormack R, et al. A multicenter, prospective, randomized, controlled trial of open reduction–internal fixation versus total elbow arthroplasty for displaced intra-articular distal humeral fractures in elderly patients. J Shoulder Elbow Surg. 2009;18:3–12.
164. Neer II CS. Displaced proximal humerus fractures, I: classification and evaluation. J Bone Joint Surg Am. 1970;52(6): 1077–89.
165. Handoll HHG, Madhok R. Interventions for treating proximal humeral fractures in adults (review). The Cochrane Collaboration. Hoboken: Wiley; 2008.
166. Roux A, Decroocq L, El Batti S, Bonnevialle N, Moineau G, Trojani C, et al. Epidemiology of proximal humerus fractures managed in a trauma center. Orthop Traumatol Surg Res. 2012;98(6):715–9. pii:S1877-0568(12)00157-0.
167. Olerud P, Ahrengart L, Ponzer S, Saving J, Tidermark J. Internal fixation versus nonoperative treatment of displaced 3-part proximal humeral fractures in elderly patients: a randomized controlled trial. J Shoulder Elbow Surg. 2011;20(5):747–55.
168. Boons HW, Goosen JH, van Grinsven S, van Susante JL, van Loon CJ. Hemiarthroplasty for humeral four-part fractures for patients 65 years and older: a randomized controlled Trial. Clin Orthop Relat Res. 2012;470(12):3483–91.

Penetrating Injury in the Elderly

28

Nicholas Melo, Kenji Inaba, and Demetrios Demetriades

Although penetrating trauma in the elderly is fairly rare, it accounts for a significant number of deaths in this age group. Due to reduced physiological reserves and the presence of comorbid conditions, the prognosis is much worse when compared with younger age groups. For these reasons, it is important that elderly patients with penetrating trauma are evaluated, monitored, and treated much more aggressively than younger victims.

Epidemiology

The leading causes of death in the population over the age of 65 in the United States are heart disease, cancer, and strokes. Trauma is the fifth leading cause and is mainly blunt, due to falls, motor vehicle injuries, and auto-versus-pedestrian injuries, in this order. In an analysis of 2,016 trauma deaths due to penetrating trauma in the county of Los Angeles, 137 (6.8 %) involved victims over 60 years old. However, review of the 699 trauma deaths from all causes in this age group showed that a penetrating mechanism was responsible for 137 (19.6 %) deaths [1].

In a National Trauma Data Bank (NTDB) study of 98,242 hospital admissions with gunshot wounds, only 1,514 (1.5 %) were ≥65 years old, but the overall mortality in this age group was 39.9 % (604 deaths) (Fig. 28.1) [2]. These figures underestimate the magnitude of the problem because fatalities at the scene or admissions at non-trauma hospitals are not captured by the NTDB.

Suicides play a major role in penetrating trauma in the elderly, and the incidence increases with age. Self-inflicted gunshot wounds are responsible for 29.2 % of firearm injuries in the age group 55–64 years, 46.2 % in the group of 65–74 years, and 51.5 % in the group ≥75 years old [2] (Table 28.1). Attempted suicide in the elderly is a well-known public health problem in western societies. Reasons include chronic illness and depression. The Center of Disease Control and Prevention reports an overall incidence of suicides of 11/100,000 in the general population and 14/100,000 in the age group ≥65 years [3]. In urban settings the suicide rate is even higher. Demetriades et al. [4] in an analysis of trauma deaths in the county of Los Angeles reported that in Caucasian males ≥65 years of age, the suicide rate by penetrating trauma was 29.5/100,000. The suicide rate by a penetrating mechanism was 9.5/100,000 in the age group >60 years, as compared to 5.0/100,000 in the age group 15–34 years. Firearms were used in more than 80 % of suicides [4]. The body area injured in penetrating trauma in elderly patients is determined to a significant extent by the intent of the injury. In self-inflicted gunshot wounds in the age group ≥65 years, the head is the most commonly injured anatomical area (54.2 %), followed by the chest (13.5 %) and the abdomen (8.2 %). In patients with assault-related injuries, the abdomen and chest are the most commonly injured anatomical areas (21.6 and 21.4 %, respectively), followed by the extremities (16.9 %) and head (15.9 %) [2].

Physiological Changes of Aging

Significant physiological changes which occur with aging may affect the clinical presentation of the elderly patient with penetrating trauma. The cardiovascular system becomes

N. Melo, MD, MS
Department of Surgery, Cedars-Sinai Hospital,
8700 Beverly Blvd., Saperstein Tower, 5837,
Los Angeles, CA 90068, USA
e-mail: nicolas.melo@cshs.org, melon@usc.edu

K. Inaba, MD, FACS, FRCSC
Division of Trauma and Critical Care, University of Southern California Medical Center, 2051 Marengo Street,
Los Angeles, CA 90033, USA
e-mail: kenji.Inaba@med.usc.edu

D. Demetriades, MD, PhD (✉)
Department of Surgery, Los Angeles County & University of Southern California Medical Center, 1200 North State Street,
Los Angeles, CA 90033, USA
e-mail: demetri@usc.edu

J.A. Yelon, F.A. Luchette (eds.), *Geriatric Trauma and Critical Care*,
DOI 10.1007/978-1-4614-8501-8_28,

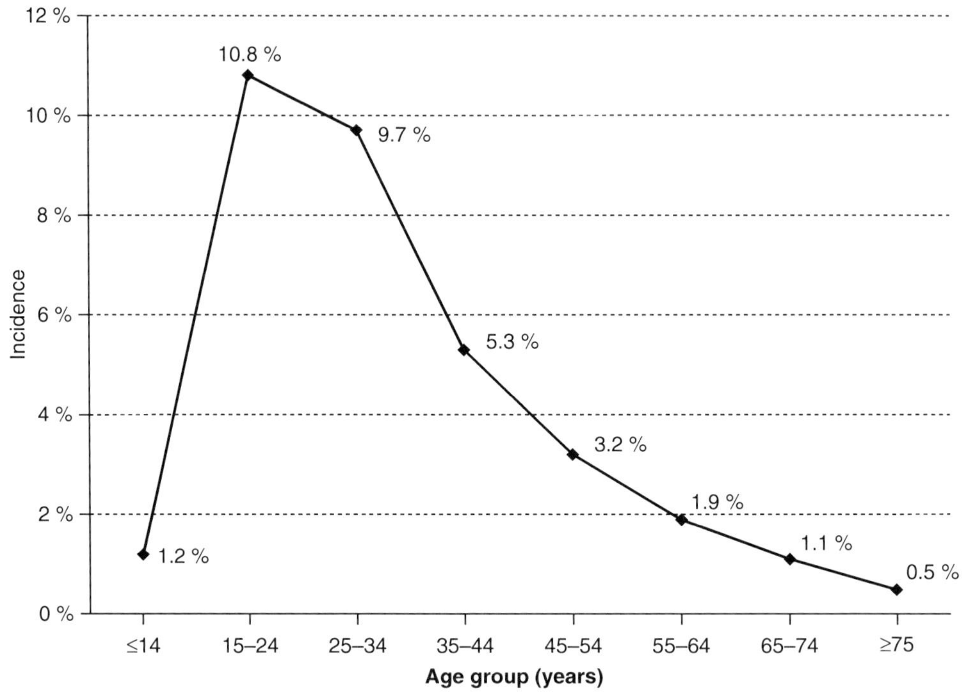

Fig. 28.1 Incidence of gunshot wounds stratified by age groups in 98,242 hospital admissions with gunshot injuries (Reproduced, with permission, from the author)

Table 28.1 Intent of injury in gunshot wounds stratified by age

	66–64 years	65–74 years	≥75 years	
Intent of injury	*N*=1,676	*N*=727	*N*=787	*p*-value
Assault	804 (48.0 %)	336 (46.2 %)	444 (56.4 %)	<0.001
Self-inflicted	489 (29.7 %)	232 (31.9 %)	225 (28.6 %)	<0.001
Unintentional	268 (16.0 %)	117 (16.1 %)	77 (9.8 %)	<0.001

Lustenberger et al. [2]

less responsive to endogenous catecholamines, which normally increase in response to traumatic stress. In addition, many elderly patients are on beta blockers or cardiac medications, which blunt the tachycardic response following blood loss and may result in hypotension and tissue hypoperfusion much earlier than in younger patients. The commonly used definition of hypotension as a systolic blood pressure <90 mmHg is highly inaccurate in the elderly, who are often normally hypertensive. A "low normal" blood pressure in these patients may be a hypoperfusion condition and may give a false sense of security to the inexperienced physician.

Heffernan et al. [7] demonstrated increased mortality in elderly trauma patients (≥65 years) when the systolic blood pressure was less than 110 mmHg, while in young patients, the increased mortality was observed only when the systolic blood pressure was <95 mmHg.

Many elderly patients are on diuretic medications, and many patients have a contracted intravascular volume. Modest blood loss in these patients may cause severe hypotension. Finally, due to the limited cardiac reserve and atherosclerotic disease, the safety margin between hypovolemia and fluid overload with cardiac failure is narrow. Early, advanced cardiac monitoring is essential in order to avoid this problem. Injured atherosclerotic vessels cannot constrict effectively, and bleeding may be more severe and last longer compared to younger injured patients.

The respiratory physiological reserve also deteriorates with aging, and these changes include increased dead space and decreased compliance and PaO_2. Elderly trauma patients with even modest chest trauma may decompensate rapidly and unexpectedly, often during CT scan evaluation or while being transported. Therefore, early intubation is advisable in patients with borderline respiratory function or hemodynamic instability.

Aging also results in a reduction of the kidney mass, as well as the efficiency of the glomerulus and ability to concentrate urine. Elderly patients are at increased risk of acute kidney injury from hypotension, intravenous radiological contrast, and nephrotoxic drugs.

Finally, loss of effective thermoregulation is another significant physiological change which occurs with aging.

Elderly trauma patients become hypothermic even after modest trauma, especially with head injury or blood loss. Hypothermia aggravates bleeding due to coagulopathy which then increases mortality.

Initial Evaluation and Management

Due to the major physiological changes observed with aging, often impacted by cardiac medications, elderly patients need to be monitored closely and carefully resuscitated. The usual hemodynamic criteria used for trauma team activation (systolic BP <90 mmHg or heart rate >120/min) are unreliable in the elderly. Patients who meet the criteria for trauma team activation receive the highest level expert consultation early with continuous monitoring and should have priority for radiological investigations, admission to the ICU, and operative interventions. Thus, misleading admission vital signs in the elderly may delay the activation of the trauma team with negative consequences on outcome.

The poor sensitivity of the initial vital signs as a criterion for activating the highest level of trauma response was demonstrated in a large study from Los Angeles [5]. In a study of 883 trauma patients ≥70 years old, 63 % of victims with severe trauma (ISS >15) and 25 % of victims with critical injuries (ISS >30) did not meet the usual blood pressure and heart rate criteria for the highest level of trauma team activation. The mortality rate in the 660 patients who did not meet the activation criteria was 16 %. The study concluded that (a) elderly trauma patients have a high mortality, even with minor and moderate injuries; (b) a significant number of elderly patients with severe trauma do not meet the standard criteria for trauma team activation; and (c) age ≥70 years alone should be a criterion for trauma team activation, irrespective of vital signs [5]. These findings resulted in a change of the trauma team activation protocol at the LAC + USC Trauma Center, to include age ≥70 years. In addition, the new protocol required early, advanced cardiac monitoring, early endotracheal intubation in the emergency department, and ICU admission after even minor injury in all patients older than 70 years. A follow-up study showed that the new protocol improved survival and functional outcomes. The mortality in patients with ISS >15 was reduced from 54 to 34 % ($p=0.003$), and there was a trend toward lower permanent disability (17 % vs. 12 %, NS) [6].

In a recent study from Rhode Island Hospital, the authors concluded that "normal presenting vital signs are unreliable in geriatric blunt trauma victims." The study reported that mortality increased considerably with systolic blood pressure <110 mmHg in the geriatric patients but not until a systolic blood pressure of <95 mmHg in the young patients. Similarly the mortality increased for heart rate >90 beats per minute in the elderly but not until a heart rate >130 in young patients [7].

A recent study from the state of Florida showed that elderly trauma patients transported to a trauma center had significantly higher survival than patients transported to non-trauma centers [8].

In the emergency department a detailed history should be obtained, if necessary by calling a close family member or their nursing facility. Many medications, often taken by the elderly, such as beta blockers, cardiac medications, diuretics, anticoagulants, and antiplatelet agents, can affect the clinical presentation, the degree of bleeding, and ultimately the outcome. Reversal of anticoagulation or antiplatelet therapy may be needed even before any laboratory results become available.

The primary survey described in the ATLS manual should be followed, but more aggressively than in younger patients. The airway should be protected early, even after moderately injury with normal vital signs and SaO_2, because of the frequent unexpected respiratory deterioration in many of these patients. Dentures should be removed. Airway establishment in the elderly may be technically more challenging than in young patients, because of degenerative changes in the cervical spine.

The cardiovascular evaluation should always include an EKG to assess for any underlying cardiac problems. Modern methods of noninvasive cardiac monitoring are now available and can be used in the emergency department to monitor the cardiac output and tissue perfusion. Bioimpedance technology has been shown to be reliable in elderly critically ill patients [9] and can identify any cardiac dysfunction or tissue hypoperfusion early. Bleeding in the elderly is usually more severe and lasts longer than in young patients because of atherosclerosis and anticoagulation or antiplatelet therapy. Interventional angio-embolization or operative intervention should be considered earlier than in young patients with similar injuries. The volume and rate of intravenous fluid administration should be monitored closely, because the physiologic margin between hypovolemia and overloading and pulmonary edema is very narrow. Central venous pressure or noninvasive volume status monitoring should be used liberally.

Prevention of hypothermia, by means of warm fluid administration or warming devices, should be initiated soon after admission to the emergency department. The limited thermoregulatory response which occurs with aging results in early hypothermia that can aggravate acidosis and coagulopathy resulting in increased mortality.

If CT scan or other radiological evaluation is required, the patient should be monitored continuously during the procedure, because of the high risk of sudden cardiorespiratory decompensation, which is potentially lethal. Due to the reduced renal physiological reserves, it is essential to avoid the nephrotoxic effects of intravenous contrast by reducing the amount of administered contrast medium and using nonionic, iso-osmolar medium. Good hydration, as well as bicarbonate and acetylcysteine administration, may play a protective role in reducing contrast-induced nephropathy.

Specific Injuries

Penetrating Injuries to the Head

Gunshot wounds to the head are the most common injuries in suicide attempts in the elderly. They are found in approximately 55 % of suicide attempts in the patients 65 years or older [2]. The mortality in this group of patients exceeds 90 %, and only tangential temporoparietal injuries have a possibility of survival [10]. In patients surviving for more than a few hours, there is a high incidence of coagulopathy and diabetes insipidus. These conditions should be monitored closely and treated aggressively [11, 12].

Penetrating Injuries to the Neck

These injuries should be evaluated and managed according to the usual principles applicable to all patients with this type of trauma. Victims with "hard" signs of vascular trauma (active bleeding, unexplained shock, expanding or pulsatile hematoma, absent or severely diminished peripheral pulse) or hard signs of aerodigestive injuries (respiratory distress, air bubbling through the wound, hemoptysis) should undergo emergency operative exploration. The remaining patients with "soft" signs of vascular or aerodigestive injuries (small hematomas, slow bleeding, mild shock, subcutaneous emphysema, hoarseness, odynophagia) and patients with proximity injuries to vital structures should be evaluated by CT angiography, endoscopy, and esophagography, as indicated. Overall, fewer than 15–20 % of victims with penetrating neck injuries require surgical intervention [13].

Penetrating Chest Trauma

The evaluation and management of these injuries should be performed along the standard ATLS guidelines. Victims with significant hemodynamic instability, clinical or FAST findings of cardiac tamponade, massive hemothorax, and immediate blood loss from the chest (>1,000–1,200 ml) require emergency thoracotomy or median sternotomy. Hemodynamically stable patients with gunshot wounds should undergo CT scan evaluation, and in cases with a bullet tract near the esophagus or tracheobronchial tree, an endoscopy and/or esophagography should be performed. Diagnostic laparoscopy should be considered in all asymptomatic patients with penetrating trauma to the left thoracoabdominal area, in order to evaluate for diaphragmatic injury. Overall, about 90 % of stab wounds and 80 % of gunshot wounds can be safely managed with tube thoracostomy alone. Transmediastinal gunshot wounds pose special problems because of the high incidence of significant injuries. Hemodynamically stable patients should be evaluated by means of CT angiography and in the appropriate cases by additional investigations such as endoscopy and/or esophagography. About 70 % of hemodynamically stable patients with transmediastinal gunshot wounds can be managed nonoperatively [14, 15].

Penetrating Abdominal Trauma

The abdomen together with the chest is the most common body area injured after penetrating trauma following assault in the elderly. The basic principles in the initial evaluation and management are the same as in the rest of the trauma victims, irrespective of age. However, as described above, early and aggressive monitoring, careful resuscitation, and liberal ICU admission are critical, even in stable-appearing patients. Patients with hemodynamic instability, peritonitis, or an unevaluable abdomen because of associated head or spinal cord injuries should undergo an emergency laparotomy [16]. The remaining patients should be evaluated by FAST and CT scan exams. A positive FAST is not an absolute indication for laparotomy, if the victim is hemodynamically stable and has no signs of peritonitis. The CT scan can provide valuable information about peritoneal violation and injuries to the solid or hollow viscera. Some trauma centers practice nonoperative management in penetrating injuries to the liver, kidney, or spleen in carefully selected patients [17]. A laparoscopy should be considered in asymptomatic patients with left thoracoabdominal injuries in order to diagnose any diaphragmatic injuries. Prospective studies have shown that in asymptomatic patients with left thoracoabdominal penetrating injuries, about 26 % of stab wounds and 13 % of gunshot wounds are associated with a diaphragmatic injury [18]. Overall, about 50 % of stab wounds to the anterior abdomen, 85 % of stab wounds to the back, 25 % of gunshot wounds to the anterior abdomen, and 65 % of gunshot wounds to the back can be managed nonoperatively [19–21].

The management of specific intra-abdominal injuries follows standard techniques. However, damage control procedures should be used more liberally in the elderly patients.

Outcomes

Old age is an independent risk factor for death or permanent disability following injury. Reduced physiological reserves, anatomical weakening, and comorbid conditions account for the poor outcomes in the elderly population [1, 7, 10]. Figure 28.2 shows the mortality rate stratified by age groups

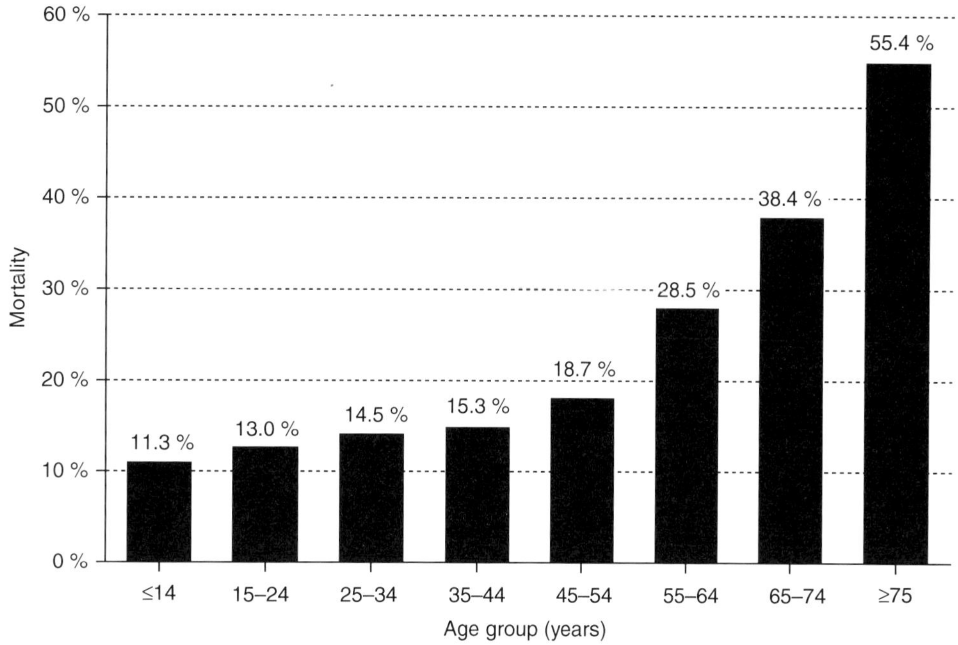

Fig. 28.2 98,242 gunshot injuries: mortality rate stratified by age groups (Reproduced, with permission, from the author)

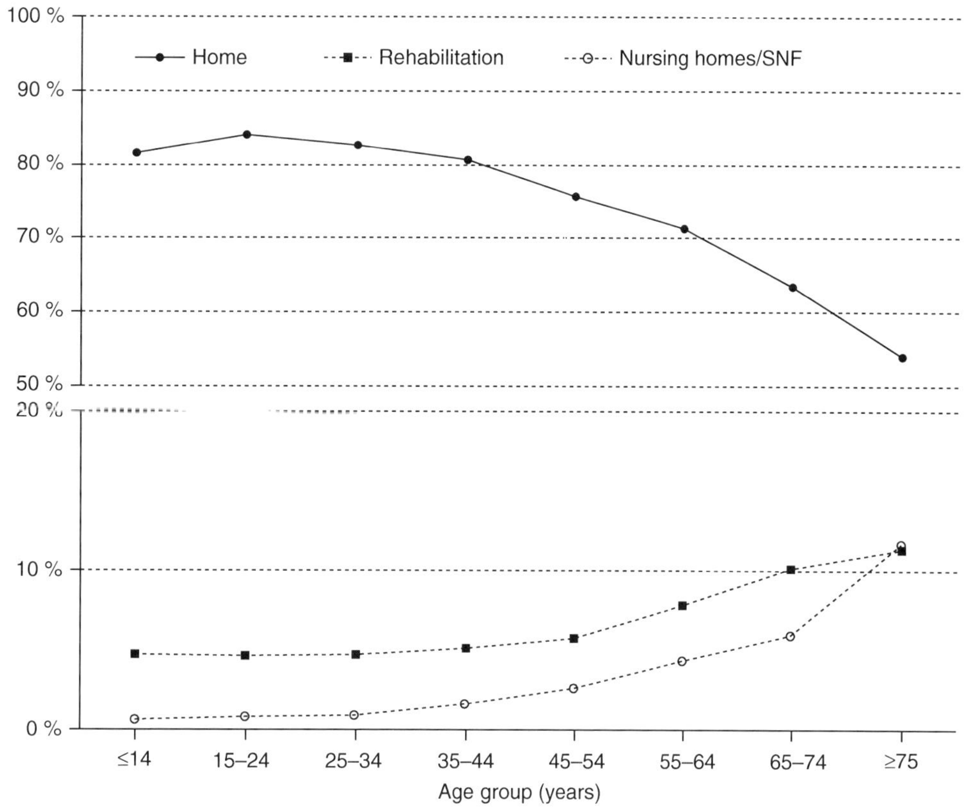

Fig. 28.3 Discharge disposition in patients with gunshot wounds stratified by age groups. There is a significant decrease in the proportion of survivors discharged home beginning at the age of 45 years (Reproduced, with permission, from the author)

in patients with gunshot wounds and shows a stepwise increase in the mortality rate with advancing age, in both assault-related and self-inflicted injuries [2]. Patients suffering self-inflicted injuries have a significantly higher mortality (60 %) than assault-related injuries (25 %) or unintentional penetrating injuries (9 %) [2]. Victims of gunshot injuries surviving to discharge require more intensive utilization of hospital resources, including ICU and hospital length of stay [2].

Finally, survivors in the older age groups are significantly less likely to return to normal and much more likely to require admission to a skilled nursing facility or rehabilitation center (Fig. 28.3). Even for those that do achieve independent living, significant residual disability in quality of life metrics can be expected after injury [22].

Conclusions

Penetrating trauma in the elderly is fairly rare, but it accounts for a significant number of deaths, especially in suicide attempts. Elderly victims have limited physiological reserves, and the mortality is much higher than in young patients. The initial clinical examination may be misleading, and unfortunately small mistakes interpreting physical examination data can be catastrophic. For these reasons, it is important that age alone with a suspicious mechanism of injury should be a criterion for the highest level of trauma activation. Early, advanced cardiorespiratory monitoring, timely execution of all diagnostic tests while constantly monitoring vital signs, and liberal criteria for ICU admissions should be practiced in this population.

References

1. Demetriades D, Kimbrell B, Salim A, Velmahos G, Rhee P, Preston D, et al. Trauma deaths in a mature urban trauma system: is trimodal distribution a valid concept? J Am Coll Surg. 2005; 201:343–8.
2. Lustenberger T, Inaba K, Schnuriger B, Barmparas G, Eberle B, Lam L, Talving P, Demetriades D. Gunshot injuries in the elderly: patterns and outcomes. A National Trauma Databank analysis. World J Surg. 2011;35:528–34.
3. Center for Disease Control and Prevention. National center for injury prevention and control. Suicide. Facts at a glance, Atlanta, 2008.
4. Demetriades D, Murray J, Sinz B, Myles D, Chan L, Sathyaragiswaran L, Noguchi T. Epidemiology of major trauma and trauma deaths in Los Angeles County. J Am Coll Surg. 1998; 187:373–83.
5. Demetriades D, Sava J, Alo K, Newton E, Velmahos G, Murray J. Old age as a criterion for trauma team activation. J Trauma. 2001;51:754–6.
6. Demetriades D, Karaiskakis M, Velmahos G, Alo K, Newton E, Murray J. Effect on outcome of early intensive management of geriatric trauma patients. Br J Surg. 2002;89:1319–22.
7. Heffernan DS, Thakkar RK, Monaghan SF, Ravindran R, Adams CA, Kozloff MS. Normal presenting vital signs are unreliable in geriatric blunt trauma victims. J Trauma. 2010;69:813–20.
8. Pracht EE, Langland OB, Flint L. Survival advantage for elderly trauma patients treated in a designated trauma center. J Trauma. 2011;71:69–77.
9. Brown C, Shoemaker W, Wo C, Chan L, Demetriades D. Is noninvasive hemodynamic monitoring appropriate for the elderly critically injured patient? J Trauma. 2005;58:102–7.
10. Demetriades D, Kuncir E, Murray J, Velmahos G, Rhee P, Chan L. Mortality prediction of head abbreviated injury score and Glasgow Coma Scale: analysis of 7,764 head injuries. J Am Coll Surg. 2004;199:216–22.
11. Talving P, Benfield R, Hadjizacharia P, Inaba K, Chan L, Demetriades D. Coagulopathy in severe traumatic brain injury: a prospective study. J Trauma. 2009;66:55–61.
12. Hatzizacharia P, Beale E, Inaba K, Chan L, Demetriades D. Acute diabetes insipidus in severe injury: a prospective study. J Am Coll Surg. 2008;207:477–84.
13. Demetriades D, Theodorou D, Cornwell E, Berne T, Asencio J, Belzberg H, Velmahos G, Weaver F, Yellin A. Evaluation of penetrating injuries of the neck: prospective study of 223 patients. World J Surg. 1997;21:41–7.
14. Demetriades D, Velmahos GC. Penetrating injuries of the chest: indications for operation. Scand J Surg. 2002;91(1):41–5.
15. Cornwell 3rd EE, Kennedy F, Ayad IA, Berne TV, Velmahos G, Asensio J, Demetriades D. Transmediastinal gunshot wounds. A reconsideration of the role of aortography. Arch Surg. 1996; 131(9):949–52.
16. Inaba K, Demetriades D. The nonoperative management of penetrating abdominal trauma. Adv Surg. 2007;41:51–62.
17. Demetriades D, Hadjizacharia P, Constantinon C, Brown C, Inaba K, Rhee P, Salim A. Selective non-operative management of penetrating solid organ injuries. Ann Surg. 2006;244:620–8.
18. Murray JA, Demetriades D, Asensio JA, Cornwell 3rd EE, Velmahos GC, Belzberg H. Occult injuries to the diaphragm: prospective evaluation of laparoscopy in penetrating injuries to the left lower chest. J Am Coll Surg. 1998;187(6):626–30.
19. Demetriades D, Rabinowitz B. Indications for operation in abdominal stab wounds. A prospective study of 151 patients. Ann Surg. 1987;205:129–32.
20. Demetriades D, Velmahos G, Cornwell E, Berne T, Cohen S, Bhasin P. Selective non-operative management of gunshot wounds of the anterior abdomen. ArchSurg. 1997;132:178–83.
21. Velmahos G, Demetriades D, Foinnini E, Tutevossian R, Cornwell E, Asensio J. A selective approach to the management of gunshot wounds to the back. Am J Surg. 1997;174:342–6.
22. Inaba K, Goecke M, Sharkey P, Brenneman F. Long-term outcomes after injury in the elderly. J Trauma. 2003;54(3):486–91.

Critical Care Epidemiology and Outcomes/Resource Use in the Elderly

29

Samantha L. Tarras and Lena M. Napolitano

Growth of the Elderly Population

Elderly is defined as age ≥65 years by the World Health Organization and the United States Census Bureau [1]. According to the 2010 US Census data, the population with age ≥65 years is 38.6 million (21.8 million females, 16.8 million males) comprising 13.1 % of the total population. The elderly population continues to increase (Fig. 29.1) [2].

The USA has seen a rapid growth in its elderly population during the twentieth century. There has been an 11-fold increase in the number of Americans age ≥65 years, with 35 million in 2000 vs. 3.1 million in 1900. For the same years, the ratio of elderly to the total population jumped from 1/25 to 1/8. The trend is guaranteed to continue in the coming century as the "baby-boom" generation grows older. Between 1990 and 2020, those aged 65–74 is projected to grow 74 %.

The elderly population explosion is a result of an impressive increase in life expectancy. When the nation was founded, the average American could expect to live to the age of 35. Life expectancy at birth had increased to 47.3 by 1900, and the average American born in 2000 can expect to live to the age of 77.

The "oldest old" (those age ≥85) are the most rapidly growing elderly age group (Fig. 29.2). Between 1960 and 1994, they increased 274 % (three million, 10 % of elderly, 1 % of population) compared to 100 % increase in the elderly and a 45 % increase in the entire population. It is expected the oldest old will number 19 million in 2050, comprising 24 % of the elderly and 5 % of all Americans.

S.L. Tarras, MD
Department of Surgery,
Wayne State University/Detroit Medical Center,
4S-13 Detroit Receiving Hospital,
4201 St. Antione, Detroit, MI 48201, USA
e-mail: starras@med.wayne.edu

L.M. Napolitano, MD, FACS, FCCP, FCCM (✉)
Department of Surgery, University of Michigan Health System,
1C340A-UH, University Hospital, SPC 5033,
1500 E. Medical Center Drive, Ann Arbor, MI 48109-5033, USA
e-mail: lenan@med.umich.edu, lenan@umich.edu

Critical Care Resource Use in the Elderly

Elderly patients (age >65 years) currently comprise 42–52 % of ICU admissions and account for almost 60 % of all ICU days in the USA [3]. In addition, 40 % of Medicare patients who die are admitted to the ICU during their terminal illness, with decedents accounting for 25 % of all Medicare expenditures. Thus, a significant amount of critical care resources are used at the end of life caring for elderly patients.

Current estimates predict that by 2050, the percentage of the population older than 80 years will double, which will lead to an increasing demand for healthcare resources, including intensive care [4]. In a large multicenter cohort study of 57 ICUs across New Zealand and Australia, elderly (age ≥80 years) patient ICU admissions increased roughly 6 % per year between 2000 to 2005 and represented approximately 14 % of total admissions in 2005 [5].

Although increasing numbers of very elderly patients are requiring ICU care, few large sample studies have investigated ICU admission of very elderly patients. An observational cohort study from 15 hospitals in France examined interhospital variability of ICU admission rates from the

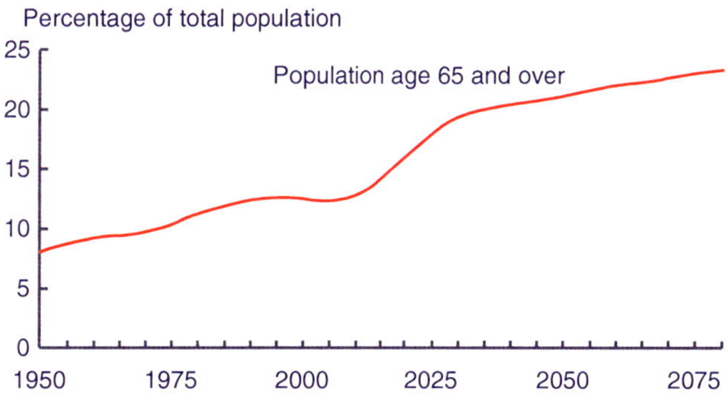

Fig. 29.1 Growth in the elderly population in the USA (*Source*: Social Security Administration, Office of the Chief Actuary. *Note*: Projections based on intermediate assumptions of the *The 2003 Annual Report of the Board of Trustees of the Federal Old-Age and Survivors Insurance and the Federal Disability Insurance Trust Funds*)

J.A. Yelon, F.A. Luchette (eds.), *Geriatric Trauma and Critical Care*,
DOI 10.1007/978-1-4614-8501-8_29,

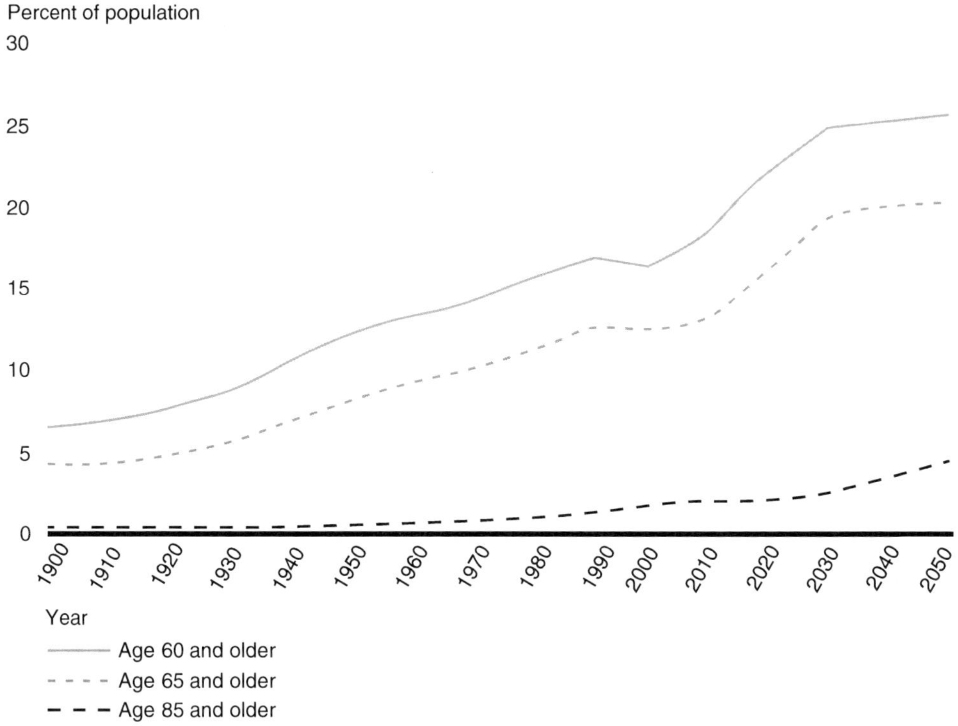

Fig. 29.2 Growth in elderly vs. super-elderly population in the USA (*Source*: GAO analysis of U.S. Census Bureau data by the Administration on Aging)

emergency department and its association with elderly patients' (age >80) outcomes over a 1-year period. Rates of patients deemed eligible for ICU admission ranged from 5.6 to 38.8 % across the participating centers, and this variability persisted after adjustment for patients' characteristics. Despite this variability, no association between level of ICU eligibility and either in-hospital death or 6-month death or functional deterioration was identified. In France, the likelihood that an elderly person will be admitted to an ICU varies widely from one hospital to another, and influence of ICU admission on elderly patients' outcome remains unclear [6].

Critical Care Outcomes in the Elderly

ICU mortality for those older than 65 years (36.8 %) is significantly higher when compared to that for those less than 45 years old (14.8 %). In addition, elderly patients discharged from the ICU to subacute facilities have a higher mortality rate than similar patients discharged home.

In a study of 484 patients admitted to medical, surgical, and coronary ICUs in a large urban teaching hospital, it was determined that one-third (1/3) of adults older than 64 years admitted to the ICU die within 6 months of hospital discharge. Independent predictors of death at 6 months were number of days during the 30 days before hospitalization that the patient felt their "physical health was not good" on the health-related quality of life survey [odds ratio = 1.08; confidence interval 1.04–1.12], a higher Acute Physiology and Chronic Health Evaluation II score [OR 1.09; 95 % CI 1.06–1.12], and chronic pulmonary disease as a comorbidity [OR 2.22; 95 % CI 1.04–4.78]. Among survivors at 6 months, health-related quality of life had significantly worsened over time in the oldest patients, but improved in the youngest survivors [7].

A larger study has confirmed similar findings [8]. A matched, retrospective cohort study was conducted using a 5 % sample of Medicare beneficiaries older than 65 years. There were 35,308 ICU patients who survived to hospital discharge. The ICU survivors had a higher 3-year mortality (39.5 %; $n=13{,}950$) than hospital controls (34.5 %; $n=12{,}173$) (adjusted hazard ratio [AHR], 1.07 [95 % CI, 1.–1.10]; $p<.001$) and general controls (14.9 %; $n=5{,}266$) (AHR, 2.39 [95 % CI, 2.31–2.48]; $p<.001$).

Those receiving mechanical ventilation had substantially increased mortality (57.6 % [1234 ICU survivors] vs. 32.8 % [703 hospital controls]; AHR, 1.56 [95 % CI, 1.40–1.73]), with risk concentrated in the 6 months after the quarter of hospital discharge (6-month mortality, 30.1 % ($n=645$) for those receiving mechanical ventilation vs. 9.6 % ($n=206$) for hospital controls; AHR, 2.26 [95 % CI, 1.90–2.69]). Discharge to a skilled care facility for ICU survivors (33.0 %; $n=11{,}634$) and hospital controls (26.4 %; $n=9{,}328$) also was associated with high 6-month mortality (24.1 % for ICU survivors and hospital controls discharged to a skilled care facility vs. 7.5 % for ICU survivors and hospital controls discharged home; AHR, 2.62 [95 % CI, 2.50–2.74]; $p<.001$ for ICU survivors and hospital controls combined).

This study confirmed that there is a large US population of elderly individuals who survive the ICU stay to hospital discharge but who have a high mortality over the subsequent years in excess of that seen in comparable controls. The risk is concentrated early after hospital discharge among those who require mechanical ventilation.

Planned Surgical vs. Medical and Unplanned Surgical ICU Admissions

Elderly patients requiring ICU admission after planned surgery have better long-term outcomes compared to elderly medical and unplanned surgical ICU admissions. This is likely related to the ability to optimize the elderly patient physiologically for surgical intervention.

Guidelines were recently published for optimal preoperative assessment of the geriatric surgical patient from the American College of Surgeons National Surgical Quality Improvement Program and the American Geriatrics Society. The guidelines recommend and specify 13 key issues of preoperative care for the elderly: cognitive impairment and dementia; decision-making capacity; postoperative delirium; alcohol and substance abuse; cardiac evaluation; pulmonary evaluation; functional status, mobility, and fall risk; frailty; nutritional status; medication management; patient counseling; preoperative testing; and patient-family and social support system [9].

Outcome Measures: Mortality vs. Long-Term Functional Outcomes

ICU survival may not be the most appropriate endpoint when evaluating the role of critical care, particularly in the elderly. The goal of critical care medicine is to restore patients to a level of function similar to that of their preadmission status. A practical goal, therefore, is to define the most accurate criteria for identification of elderly ICU patients most likely to benefit from ICU care regardless of age.

A study of long-term outcome in medical patients aged 80 or over following admission to an ICU documented a hospital mortality rate of 55 % with only 47 % of the ICU patients still alive at 2 years. Interestingly, factors independently associated with mortality were SAPS II score at ICU admission and the McCabe score. Conversely, functional status prior to admission (as assessed by Knaus or Karnofsky scores) was not associated with long-term mortality. In long-term survivors, SF-36 physical function scores were poor, but scores for pain, emotional well-being, and social function were not much affected. In addition, the group that was discharged had increased mortality compared to the general population of the same age not admitted to an ICU [10].

A prospective cohort study from a 10-bed, medical-surgical ICU in a 460-bed, tertiary, university hospital in France examined the outcome, functional autonomy, and quality of life of elderly patients (≥70 years, $n=75$) hospitalized for more than 30 days in an ICU. The survival rate was 67 % in the ICU and 47 % survived to discharge. Independence in activities of daily living was decreased significantly after the ICU stay, except for feeding. However, most patients remained independent (class A of the activities of daily living index) with the possibility of going home. Perceived Quality of Life scores remained good, even if the patients estimated a decrease in their quality of life for health and memory. Return to society appeared promising regarding patient self-respect and happiness with life. The estimated cost per survivor was of 55,272 EUR ($60,246 US). This study suggested that persistent high levels of ICU therapeutic intensity were associated with a reasonable hospital survival in elderly patients experiencing prolonged mechanical ventilatory support. These patients presented a moderate disability that influenced somewhat their perceived quality of life. These results are sufficient to justify prolonged ICU stays for elderly patients [11].

Elderly Critical Care Trauma Outcome and Resource Utilization

Elderly patients are at high risk for mortality after injury. According to 2010 National Vital Statistics Report preliminary data, accidental death was the nineth leading cause of death for those greater than 65 years old, with 15 % of these accidental deaths from motor vehicle collisions. Elderly trauma patients have increased mortality risk compared to younger trauma patients in all injury severity categories (Fig. 29.3).

A review of 26,237 blunt trauma patients admitted to all trauma centers ($n=26$) in one state over 24 months confirmed that elderly (age ≥65 years, $n=7,117$) patients had significantly higher mortality rates than younger (age <65 years) trauma patients after stratification by Injury Severity Score (ISS), revised trauma score, and other preexisting comorbidities. Age greater than 65 years was associated with a two- to threefold increased mortality risk in mild (ISS <15, 3.2 % vs. 0.4 %; <0.001), moderate (ISS 15–29, 19.7 % vs. 5.4 %; <0.001), and severe traumatic injury (ISS ≥30, 47.8 % vs. 21.7 %; <0.001) compared with patients younger than 65 years. Logistic regression analysis confirmed that elderly patients had a nearly twofold increased mortality risk (OR 1.87; confidence interval, 1.60–2.18; <0.001). Elderly patients also had significantly longer hospital LOS after stratifying for severity of injury by ISS

Fig. 29.3 Data from National Trauma Data Bank, Case Fatality Rate by Injury Severity Score and age (American College of Surgeons NTDB)

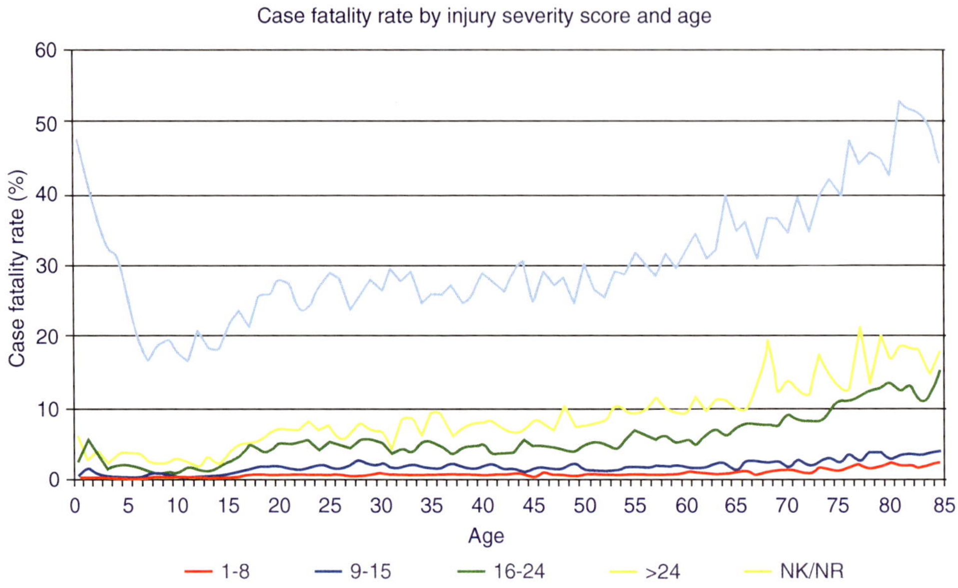

(1.9 fewer days in the age 18–45 group, 0.89 fewer days in the age 46–64 group compared with the age over 64 group). Mortality rates were higher for men than for women only in the ISS <15 (4.4 % vs. 2.6 %, <0.001) and ISS 15–29 (21.7 % vs. 17.6 %, = 0.031) groups. ICU LOS was significantly shorter in elderly patients with ISS ≥30. This study confirmed age as an independent predictor of mortality in trauma after stratification for injury severity in this largest study of elderly trauma patients to date. Interestingly, elderly patients with severe injury (ISS >30) had decreased ICU resource use secondary to associated increased mortality rates [12].

In a single-center Level I trauma center study, it was confirmed that age alone was associated with increased odds of being admitted to the hospital, independent of injury severity and other physiologic parameters. A total of 451 (8.68 %) elderly patients were 65 years or older; 62 % of the total population was admitted. Elderly patients had a significantly higher hospital admission rate (86.7 %; $p<0.001$). Multivariate analysis showed that age over 64 years (OR 3.76), head injury (OR 5.3), ISS (OR 17.5), Glasgow Coma Scale score on arrival (OR 0.753), and initial systolic blood pressure (OR 0.987) were significant independent factors predictive of hospital admission ($p<0.001$). Elderly patients were also admitted to the ICU at a higher rate (60.9 % vs. 38.5 %, $p<0.001$) and were more likely to remain there for a longer period of time. Greater than 75 % of the elderly patients stayed for over 3 days. This has implications for trauma centers that see a significant proportion of geriatric trauma patients and for trauma systems that must prepare for the "aging of America" [13].

Trauma benchmarking efforts benefit from development of a geriatric-specific model for risk-adjusted analyses of trauma center outcomes. A total of 57,973 records of elderly patients (age older than 65 years) with data from the National Trauma Data Bank (NTDB) and the National Sample Project were used to construct a multivariable logistic regression model, which was compared with the American College of Surgeons Committee on Trauma's Trauma Quality Improvement Project's (TQIP) existing model. Additional analyses were performed to further objectively quantify the physiologic differences between geriatric patients and their younger counterparts. The geriatric-specific and TQIP mortality models shared several covariates: age, ISS, motor component of the Glasgow Coma Scale, and systolic blood pressure. This new model additionally used temperature and the presence of mechanical ventilation. This geriatric-specific regression model compared with the TQIP approximation (0.85 vs. 0.77; $p=0.048$). Spline analyses demonstrated that elderly patients appear to be less likely to tolerate relative hypotension with higher observed mortality at initial systolic blood pressures of 90–130 mmHg. Although the TQIP model includes a single-age component, these data suggest that each variable needs to be adjusted for age to more accurately predict mortality in the elderly. Clearly, a separate geriatric model for predicting outcomes is not only warranted, but necessary [14].

Super-Elderly Trauma Patients

The fastest growing segment of the population is the "super-elderly," i.e., those greater than 85 years old. It is projected that those 85 years and older will double from 2000 to 2030. By 2050 this age group will be five times larger than in 2000 and will make up a little over 4 % of the total population.

Despite this growth there is little information of trauma outcomes in this group.

In a retrospective cohort study from a countywide trauma registry, overall mortality of very elderly trauma patients ($n=455$, mean age 85.9 years, range 80–101) was 10 %, with head injury and injury severity as independent risk factors for increased mortality. They also confirmed that very elderly patients admitted to trauma centers (Level I and II) had better outcomes than non-trauma centers, especially in the high injury severity (ISS 21–45) cohort (mortality 56 % vs. 8 % survival; $p<0.01$) [15].

Another study compared the post-injury outcomes of super-elderly patients ($n=422$, age ≥80 years) to elderly patients ($n=898$, age 60–79 years) treated at a Level I Trauma Center after adjustment for gender, mechanism of injury, Glasgow Coma Scale, ISS, and admission vital signs. Super-elderly patients had significantly higher risk-adjusted in-hospital mortality compared with elderly patients [13.4 % vs. 7.7 %, adjusted OR 1.94 (95 % CI 1.14, 3.31), $p=0.015$]. Of patients surviving hospitalization, super-elderly patients experienced shorter ICU and hospital length of stay but were more likely to require discharge to another level of care, defined as nursing facility, acute rehabilitation facility, or long-term acute care facility (AOR 3.78, CI 2.75–5.28, $p<0.0005$). Importantly, super-elderly patients were more likely than elderly patients to die during hospitalization as a result of withdrawal of medical support (9.5 % vs. 5.5 %, $p=0.007$) [16].

Performance Improvement in Elderly Trauma

Given the high mortality rate for elderly trauma patients, attention to modifiable risk factors in establishing a performance improvement program is imperative. Delays in recognizing the special needs of older trauma patients may result in suboptimal care.

We have reported our performance improvement efforts in elderly trauma care. In 2004 (baseline data), the in-hospital mortality rate for the most severely injured trauma patients (ISS >24) at our trauma center was 30 %, consistent with the reported mortality rate from the NTDB for patients with this severity of injury. Over 5 years, our mortality rate decreased significantly for severely injured patients with an ISS > 24–18 %, representing a 12 % absolute reduction in mortality ($p=0.011$). During the same 5-year time period, the proportion of elderly patients cared for at our trauma center increased from 23.5 % in 2004 to 30.6 % in 2008 ($p=0.0002$), while there was a significant reduction in mortality over this time period. Class I trauma activations increased significantly from 5.5 % in 2004 to 15.5 % in 2008. A greater percentage of patients were admitted to the ICU (25.8 % vs. 30.4 %) with no difference in the mechanism of injury throughout the 5 years. Trauma Quality Improvement Program (TQIP) data for our institution confirmed improved trauma outcomes with observed-to-expected ratio and 95 % confidence intervals of 0.64 (0.42–0.86) for all patients, 0.54 (0.15–0.91) for blunt single-system patients, and 0.78 (0.51–1.06) for multisystem patients [17].

One method to improve trauma geriatric outcome is to establish *geriatric trauma patient care protocols*. These protocols are created from evidence-based guidelines that serve to reduce variation in care. Patient care protocols have been found to positively impact patient care with reduced duration of mechanical ventilation, shorter LOS in the ICU and shorter overall hospitalization time, reduced mortality, and reduced health care costs.

A single-institution study documented that use of new protocols helped guide practical changes in geriatric trauma care that resulted in a 32 % decrease in LOS for elderly trauma patients. The four protocols implemented were a VAP bundle, massive transfusion protocol, reversal of coagulopathy protocol, and rib fracture protocol [18].

Some trauma centers have created a dedicated *geriatric trauma service*. This concept was studied in a Level II Trauma Center and documented a significant decrease in the ED LOS, ICU LOS, decreased time from ED to OR, decreased hospital stay, and decreased mortality (3.8 % vs. 5.7 %). There was also a significant decrease in pneumonia, respiratory failure, and UTI rates [19]. Other institutions have been able to show similar results once standard protocols are initiated in the care of geriatric patients [20].

A number of trauma centers have developed an inpatient geriatric trauma consultation service (GTCS), a proactive geriatric consultation model aimed at preventing and managing age-specific complications, and discharge planning for elderly patients admitted to the trauma service. A report by Fallon and colleagues in 2006 documented that geriatricians identified 14 % of patients who presented with alcohol issues; 36 % of patients exhibited signs of delirium; and 46 % of patients presented with a new medical condition(s). Geriatricians assisted with advanced care planning in 15 % of cases; disposition decisions to promote function in 49 %; made medication changes in 65 %; decreased inappropriate medications in 20 %; and assisted with pain management in 42 %. Trauma surgeons followed 91 % of one or more recommendations. They concluded that outcomes of older patients can be improved through geriatricians' expertise by addressing new and existing medical issues and reducing hospital-acquired complications such as functional decline, falls, delirium, and death [21].

A recent single-center before ($n=238$)/after ($n=248$) case series documented that the rate of adherence to recommendations made by the GTCS team was 93.2 %. There were fewer consultation requests made to Internal Medicine and Psychiatry in the post-GTCS group. Interestingly, there were no differences in any of the prespecified complications except delirium (50.5 % pre-GTCS vs. 40.9 % post-GTCS, $p=0.05$). Among patients admitted from home, fewer were discharged to long-term care facilities among the post-GTCS group (6.5 % pre-GTCS vs. 1.7 % post-GTCS). This study documented that a proactive geriatric consultation model for elderly trauma patients may decrease delirium and discharges to long-term care facilities. Future studies should include a multicenter randomized trial of this model of care [22].

Most recently, the American College of Surgeon published the ACS TQIP Geriatric Trauma Management Guidelines. This document summarizes efforts to improve elderly trauma outcome, including initial evaluation (Table 29.1), standardizing when to obtain a geriatric consultation (Table 29.2), focus on medication management (Table 29.3), and pain control and delirium avoidance (Table 29.4). It serves as an important repository of performance improvement information relevant to the care of the elderly injured patient [23].

Table 29.1 Consideration in initial trauma evaluation of elderly patients

The primary survey for the elderly is the same as for any injured patient, but the secondary survey should emphasize the following: • Determine medications that affect initial evaluation and care Coumadin Clopidogrel Other anticoagulants ASA Beta blockers ACE inhibitors
• Consider common, acute, nontraumatic events that could complicate the patient's presentation, including: Acute coronary syndrome (EKG) Hypovolemia/dehydration Urinary tract infection Pneumonia Acute renal failure Cerebrovascular event Syncope
Lab assessment: • Hypoperfusion is often underappreciated in the elderly. Base deficit should be assessed expediently to identify those patients in occult shock who need resuscitation, abbreviated evaluation, and admission to an intensive care unit. The following panel of laboratory studies is suggested for all elderly patients with injury: Lactic acid or blood gas (arterial or venous) for baseline base deficit PT/PTT/INR Renal function (BUN, Cr, estimated GFR) Blood alcohol level Urine toxicology screen Serum electrolytes

Table 29.2 Criteria for geriatric consultation

Develop criteria for early geriatric consultation and geriatric expertise on the multidisciplinary trauma care team
If the response to two or more of the following questions is "yes," geriatric consultation should be obtained: • Before you were injured, did you need someone to help you on a regular basis? • Since the injury, have you needed more help than usual to take care of yourself? • Have you been hospitalized for one or more nights during the past 6 months? • In general, do you have problems seeing well? • In general, do you have serious problems with your memory? • Do you take more than three different medications every day?

Table 29.3 Geriatric trauma patients are at particular risk for medication-related adverse events

Establish past medication history • Attempt to communicate with the patient's immediate family and physician • Document the patient's complete medication list, including over-the-counter and complementary/alternative medication
Use the following geriatric medication prescribing recommendations: • Follow Beers Criteria. Use Beers Criteria in decision making about pharmacotherapy. • Discontinue nonessential medications • Continue medications with withdrawal potential, including selective serotonin reuptake inhibitors (SSRIs), tricyclic antidepressants, benzodiazepines, antipsychotics, monoamine oxidase inhibitors (MAOIs), beta blockers, clonidine, statins, and corticosteroids • Continue β-blocker or start if indicated • Continue statins when appropriate • Adjust doses of medications for renal function based on glomerular filtration rate

Table 29.4 Pain control and delirium avoidance in elderly trauma patients

Effective pain management can be a central determinant of success in the drive to improve pulmonary and toilet functions, optimize mobility, and mitigate delirium **The following pain medication strategies are recommended**: • Use elderly appropriate medications and dose • Avoid benzodiazepines • Monitor use of narcotics; consider early implementation of patient-controlled analgesia • Consider early use of nonnarcotics, including NSAIDs, adjuncts, and tramadol Epidural algesia may be preferable to other means for patients with multiple rib fractures to avoid respiratory failure

Outcomes in Special Populations

Respiratory Failure Requiring Mechanical Ventilation

The incidence of acute respiratory failure (ARF) in the 65–84 age group is twice that of the 55–64 year old group [24]. Since respiratory failure is a common reason for ICU admission in the elderly, examination of outcomes is important. Underlying etiology of ARF is no different than those for younger patients, but the ICU and hospital courses may be very different.

A large prospective observational study evaluated patients ($n=514$) greater than 65 years old who presented to the ED for acute dyspnea. Only 29 % were admitted to the ICU. The main causes of ARF were cardiogenic pulmonary edema (43 %), community-acquired pneumonia (35 %), acute exacerbation of chronic respiratory disease (32 %), pulmonary embolism (18 %), and acute asthma (3 %); 47 % had more than two diagnoses. In-hospital mortality was 16 %. A missed diagnosis in the ED was noted in 101 (20 %) patients. The accuracy of the diagnosis of the emergency physician ranged from 0.76 for cardiogenic pulmonary edema to 0.96 for asthma. An inappropriate treatment occurred in 162 (32 %) patients and led to a higher mortality (25 % vs. 11 %; $p<0.001$). In a multivariate analysis, inappropriate initial treatment (OR 2.83, $p<0.002$), hypercapnia greater than 45 mmHg (OR 2.79, $p<0.004$), creatinine clearance less than 50 (OR 2.37, $p<0.013$), elevated B-type natriuretic peptide (OR 2.06, $p<0.046$), and clinical signs of ARF (odds ratio 1.98, $p<0.047$) were predictive of death. The rates of ICU admission and mortality (25 % vs. 11 %, $p<0.001$) were significantly higher in patients with an inappropriate initial ED treatment and error in initial diagnosis. Most of the difference in mortality occurred within a few days of admission [25].

Older studies examining outcomes of elderly patients requiring mechanical ventilation reported ICU risk-adjusted mortality as 38 % and all-cause mortality 60, 63, and 67 % at 6, 12, and 18 months, respectively [26]. More recent studies have reported ICU mortality rates between 31 and 52 % for 6 month post-discharge [27].

Prolonged mechanical ventilation (greater than 21 days) is associated with even higher rates of mortality in the elderly. One year out from prolonged mechanical ventilation, 67 % of those older than 65 years had died. The cost of prolonged mechanical ventilation, although this study also included patients less than 65 years old, per 1 year survivor was $423,596 [28].

In a study of functional outcomes after mechanical ventilation, only 11 % of geriatric patients were doing well and achieved a Functional Independence Measure (FIM) scale score greater than or equal to 90 at 1 year [29]. This cohort also had poor survival rates of 33 % at the end of hospitalization and 22 % at 1 year. Are we able to predict which elderly patients will have improved outcome on mechanical ventilation? In a study of critically ill mechanically ventilated medical patients, severity of acute illness and chronic comorbidities, but not age, were independent predictors of ICU and hospital mortality [30]. As intensivists, we should then focus on determining the cause of ARF and implement appropriate management based on the disease etiology.

Respiratory Failure Requiring Noninvasive Ventilation

Noninvasive ventilation (NIV) is frequently used for the management of ARF in very old patients (≥80 years), often in the context of a do-not-intubate order (DNI). A number of studies have examined the efficacy of NIV and its impact on long-term outcome.

A prospective cohort study of all patients admitted to the medical ICU of a tertiary hospital during a 2-year period and managed using NIV. Characteristics of patients, context of NIV, and treatment intensity were compared for very old and younger patients. Six-month survival and functional status were assessed in the very old patients. During the study period, 1,019 patients needed ventilatory support and 376 (37 %) received NIV. Among them, 163 (16 %) very old patients received ventilatory support with 60 % of them successfully managed using NIV compared with 32 % of younger patients ($p<0.0001$). Very old patients received NIV more frequently with a DNI order than in younger patients (40 % vs. 8 %). Such cases were associated with high mortality for both very old and younger patients. Hospital mortality was higher in the very old than in younger patients but did not differ when NIV was used for cardiogenic pulmonary edema, acute-on-chronic respiratory failure (20 % vs. 15 %), and in postextubation (15 % vs. 17 %) out of a context of DNI. Six-month mortality was 51 % in very old patients, 67 % for DNI patients, and 77 % in setting of NIV failure and subsequent endotracheal intubation. Of the 30 hospital survivors, 22 lived at home and 13 remained independent for activities of daily living. This study confirmed that very old patients managed using NIV have an overall satisfactory 6-month survival and functional status, except for endotracheal intubation after NIV failure [31].

The effectiveness of NIV in treating patients with ARF is related to the ability to diminish endotracheal intubation, the reduction of ventilator-associated lung infections, as well as related mortality. A specific issue is the outcome of NIV in patients admitted to the ED for ARF who receive a DNI order because of severe acute illness or advanced age. Recent data show that elderly patients (mean age 81 years) with ARF who have a DNI order can be successfully treated by NIV, as demonstrated by a survival rate of 83 %. The positive outcome was confirmed by a subsequent 3-year observation that demonstrated an overall survival rate of 54 %. These findings clearly suggest that NIV treatment in elderly patients may be effective, even in presence of a DNI order [32].

Critical Care Resource Utilization and Physiology of Aging

The most common organ systems that require support in the critically ill are cardiac, pulmonary, and renal, and the physiology of these systems changes significantly in the elderly, resulting in increased need for organ support and critical care resource utilization in these patients.

Cardiac Physiology

There is a lack of cardiac reserve once a person reaches the age of 70. Other structural changes are a progressive decrease in the number of myocytes and an increase in myocardial collagen content. Autonomic tissue is replaced by connective tissue and fat, and fibrosis causes conduction abnormalities through the intranodal tract and the Bundle of His. Clinically this contributes to the increased incidence of sick sinus syndrome, atrial arrhythmias, and bundle branch blocks. The older heart also becomes less responsive to sympathetic stimulation. Therefore to increase cardiac output in the aged heart, the stroke volume has to increase by increasing ventricular filing (preload). Elderly patients are very sensitive to fluid status and even minor hypovolemia can induce cardiac dysfunction. Arteries become stiffer with age which results in a compensatory myocyte enlargement and left ventricular hypertrophy. This leads to diastolic dysfunction which accounts for the majority of heart failure in patients over 80 years. Resting heart rate is the same as seen in younger patients; however, the chronotropic response to exercise decreases with age. Diastolic ventricular filling is dependent on atrial contraction which is why atrial fibrillation is poorly tolerated particularly in the elderly patient population, especially if diastolic dysfunction is present. Furthermore, age is a significant risk factor for coronary artery disease and its associated complications. As a person ages, atypical presentations of cardiac ischemia and dysfunction are more prevalent and may go unrecognized or silent in greater than 40 % of patients older than 75 years old. Chapter 2 reviews in detail the impact of aging on cardiac physiology.

Pulmonary Physiology

Changes both in chest wall mechanics and lung compliance alter pulmonary physiology. Structural changes of kyphosis and vertebral collapse decrease chest wall compliance, and decrease in muscle strength can result in reduction of inspiratory and expiratory force as much as 50 %. Total lung capacity and vital capacity decline in the elderly while the residual volume and functional residual capacity are increased. Within the lung parenchyma, there is a loss of elasticity with collapse of small airways and uneven alveolar airflow with air trapping. The alveolar to arterial difference for oxygen (Aa gradient) increases significantly with aging due to this ventilation-perfusion mismatch. Control of ventilation is also affected by aging. The respiratory centers response to hypoxia and hypercapnia decreases by 50 and 40 %, respectively. With aging, the respiratory reserve declines just as with respect to cardiac reserve. These pulmonary changes result in increased incidence of acute respiratory dysfunction and failure requiring noninvasive or invasive mechanical ventilation. Please see Chap 3 for a detailed discussion of the physiologic changes of the pulmonary system with aging.

Renal Function

Between the ages of 25 and 85 years, approximately 40 % of the nephrons become sclerotic. While the remaining functional units hypertrophy in a compensatory manner, there is a decline in the glomerular filtration rate (GFR). However, the serum creatinine remains unchanged as one ages because of the concomitant decrease in lean body mass and decrease in creatinine production. In the critically ill, the GFR may be affected by other factors such as nephrotoxic medications and muscle breakdown from sepsis, trauma, and immobility. The aging kidney also has diminished capacity to regulate fluid and acid–base status. This is thought to be due to a decline in activity of renin-angiotensin system and decreased responsiveness to antidiuretic hormone. The elderly patient is therefore at high risk for development of hypovolemic shock. Finally, as many ICU medications undergo renal excretion, dose adjustment is required in elderly patients with diminished GFR to avoid toxic levels.

Efforts to Improve Elderly Outcomes

As critical care treatment and organ support continues to improve, we must examine efforts to improve elderly patient-centered outcomes in the ICU, which is not always consistent with ICU survival.

Advance Directives/POLST

It is important to establish goals of care in elderly patients as soon as possible and ideally before admission to an ICU. We must aspire to make certain that all of our patients have advance directives, so that treatment goals are in line with patient's wishes.

Most recently, some states have mandated that all patients should have physician orders for life-sustaining treatment (POLST) [33]. POLST was originally developed in Oregon in 1991 to create a coordinated system for eliciting, documenting, and communicating the life-sustaining treatment wishes of seriously ill patients. There are 12 states that have endorsed POLST programs and 28 states in the development stages. The POLST document is completed by the health care professional with a patient or surrogate decision maker. How this differs from an advance directive is that it gives clear orders to a physician who might not be familiar with the patient and specifies what to do if the patient is confronted by a serious illness. Advance directives can be vague or not specific enough (not to prolong dying through artificial means, feeding tube vs. no feeding tube, for example) and are usually not filled out in the presence of a health care professional to encourage a discussion between the patient's family and physician.

The form includes a section on cardiopulmonary resuscitation, whether to resuscitate or do not resuscitate in the event of a cardiopulmonary arrest. The second section is about medical interventions, whether to perform comfort measures vs. limited additional intervention (usually means no ICU involvement) vs. full treatment. The second section also includes the decision of whether to transfer to a hospital or not. The third section is about medically administered nutrition, such as no tube, no permanent tube, or a defined trial of nutrition. The last section is the signature section that is to include both the patient and the physician. A copy of this form is included in the medical record, and another copy is to remain with the patient as they transfer across settings of care. In California and Oregon, these forms are maintained in a registry that can be access by emergency personnel and any hospital 24 h a day.

Studies have documented that POLST use significantly reduces unwanted hospitalizations, provides treatment consistent with patient's wishes more than 90 % of the time, and decreases the medical errors in their care. Eighty-five percent of transfers to a hospital are because the nursing facility could not control the patient's suffering. In several studies the POLST form is embraced by heath care professionals. In comparison to those that have a power of attorney for health care appointed, those with POLST were more likely to die in a nursing home and die from a terminal or chronic illnesses, saving the cost of a hospital admission. Concerns that some patients and/or their families have voiced is that the form might be misplaced or not be honored outside of the nursing home. This study was from North Carolina where there is not a government-maintained registry as in California and Oregon.

Delirium Prevention, Diagnosis, and Management

An important area for improvement in the care of the critically ill elderly is the prevention, recognition, and treatment of delirium. Delirium is characterized by inattention and acute cognitive dysfunction. It is extremely common in the ICU setting. The incidence can reach as high as 70–87 % of elderly patients admitted to the ICU.

Risk factors for delirium are numerous; however, there are specific ones that have the potential to be modified. These included sensory impairment, such as not providing a patient with their glasses or hearing aid, or not speaking loudly enough, in order for a patient to hear. Immobilization is another risk factor; this not only includes restraints but excess catheters, tubes, and IVs that place the patient a risk for a fall, so they are less likely to get out of bed. Medications, pain, and sustained sleep deprivation are risk factors for delirium in the elderly. After controlling for baseline patient characteristics and etiological factors, patients with delirium have poorer outcomes, and the more severe the episode, the worse the outcome.

Specific risk factors for dementia during a critical illness in elderly have been determined. A cohort study of a random 5 % sample of Medicare beneficiaries who received intensive care in 2005 and survived to hospital discharge, with 3 years of follow-up was conducted. Over the 3 years of follow-up, dementia was newly diagnosed in 4,519 (17.8 %) of 25,368 patients. After accounting for known risk factors, having an infection (adjusted hazard ratio (AHR) = 1.25; 95 % CI, 1.17–1.35), or a diagnosis of severe sepsis (AHR = 1.40; 95 % CI, 1.28–1.53), acute neurologic dysfunction (AHR = 2.06; 95 % CI, 1.72–2.46), and acute hemodialysis (AHR = 1.70; 95 % CI, 1.30–2.23) were all independently associated with a subsequent diagnosis of dementia. No other measured ICU factors, such as need for mechanical ventilation, were independently associated [34].

The most commonly used screening tool for delirium is the Confusion Assessment Method for the ICU (CAM-ICU). This has high sensitivities of 93–100 % and high specificities of 98–100 % when performed by trained critical care nurses. In addition, most ICU patients when they experience delirium are characterized by the hypoactive subtype and so often go unrecognized but are still at risk for prolonged ICU course and increase risk of complications.

It is estimated that 30–40 % of cases of delirium are preventable, and we should strive to prevent the adverse outcomes associated with delirium. One strategy that can be initiated is the Hospital Elder Life Program (HELP). It includes maintaining orientation to surroundings; meetings needs for nutrition, fluids, and sleep; promoting mobility within the limitations of physical condition; and providing visual and hearing adaptations for patients with sensory impairments. This program decreases the development of delirium from 15 % in the control group vs. 9.9 % in the intervention group. This program also decreased the total number of episodes and days of delirium in the hospital and hence decreased overall costs and resource utilization. The complications of delirium include aspiration, pressure ulcers, pulmonary emboli, and decreased oral intake.

Another measure used to decrease the risk of delirium is proactive geriatric consultations. This measure was shown to decrease the risk of delirium by 40 % in acute hip fractures. In addition, hospital staff education about delirium and its management can reduce delirium rates and/or duration.

Once delirium develops, goals should be made to decrease its duration and prevention of any harm to the patient by themselves. First-line delirium treatment is always nonpharmacological strategies, including providing a quiet patient care setting with minimal noise, minimal sleep interruptions, and support from family members or people that the patient is familiar with to reorient them. Other methods to help patients sleep include providing a glass of warm milk or herbal tea, relaxation tapes or relaxing music, and finally a back massage. If these methods do not work, then pharmacological strategies must be added to the treatment regimen, and this is particularly true with those in hyperactive delirium, where the agitation could be harmful.

Several national quality agencies have used delirium as a marker for quality of care and patient safety. Delirium is an important independent determinant of hospital stay, mortality, rates of nursing home placement and functional, and cognitive decline. Delirium results in increased nursing time per patient, higher per day hospital cost, and increased length of hospital stay. In addition, many of these patients will go to nursing facilities or additional home health care which will add to increase costs. Thus, if delirium can be prevented in one patient, cost saving up to $64,000 per year can be appreciated.

Nutrition Support

With the aging process there are physiological changes and social factors that play a role in nutrition in the elderly. Dietary inadequacy is present in 7–21 % of community elderly from poor enteral intake. As a person ages their sense of smell and taste decrease, leading to a decreased desire for food. Loss of appetite in the elderly is referred to as the physiological anorexia of aging and may predispose to protein and energy undernutrition. In addition there is impaired absorption of some micronutrients and mineral, especially vitamins B12 and D, calcium, and iron. The social factors of isolation, poverty, loss of spouse, and alcoholism also may contribute to reduced food intake. Thus, when elderly patients present to the hospital, they are already undernourished and critical illness may worsen their malnourished state. Early and prompt attention to nutrition in the elderly critically ill patient is of utmost importance [35].

Infection Prevention

Infection and sepsis are common complications that occur in critically ill elderly patients, and all efforts to prevent these infectious complications should be implemented [36]. Most ICUs focus on infection prevention directed at catheter-associated urinary tract infection (CA-UTI), ventilator-associated pneumonia (VAP), and central line-associated bacteremia (CLABSI). The compendium of strategies for prevention of healthcare-associated infections in Acute Care Hospitals provides an evidence-based foundation for infection prevention [37].

Conclusion

Elderly patients comprise an increasing percentage of ICU admissions requiring significant critical care resource utilization. Aging is associated with a progressive increase in the risk of ICU death. A significant amount of critical care resources are used at the end of life in elderly patients. It is imperative to determine goals of care in all elderly patients considered for ICU admission. Efforts to decrease resource utilization in elderly patients require prevention of complications (infection, delirium, respiratory failure) and performance improvement strategies, including use of protocols, geriatric consultation, and specialized elderly units. Optimal goals of care in elderly ICU patients should be consistent with patient desires.

References

1. http://www.census.gov/compendia. Accessed 1 June 2012.
2. http://www.census.gov/population/socdemo/statbriefs/agebrief.html. Accessed 1 June 2012.

3. Marik PE. Management of the critically ill geriatric patient. Crit Care Med. 2006;34(Suppl):S176–82.
4. Nguyen YL, Angus DC, Boumendil A, Guidet B. The challenge of admitting the very elderly to intensive care. Ann Intensive Care. 2011;1:29.
5. Bagshaw SM, Webb SA, Delaney A, George C, Pilcher D, Hart GK, Bellomo R. Very old patients admitted to intensive care in Australia and New Zealand: a multi-centre cohort analysis. Crit Care. 2009;13(2):R45.
6. Boumendil A, Angus DC, Guitonneau AL, Menn AM, Ginsburg C, Takun K, Davido A, Masmoudi R, Doumenc B, Pateron D, Garrouste-Orgeas M, Somme D, Simon T, Aegerter P, Guidet B, ICE-CUB study group. Variability of intensive care admission decisions for the very elderly. PLoS One. 2012;7(4):e34387. doi:10.1371/journal.pone.0034387. Epub 2012 Apr 11.
7. Khouli H, Astua A, Dombrowski W, Ahmad F, Homel P, Shapiro J, Singh J, Nallamothu R, Mahbub H, Eden E, Delfiner J. Changes in health-related quality of life and factors predicting long-term outcomes in older adults admitted to intensive care units. Crit Care Med. 2011;39(4):731–7. doi:10.1097/CCM.0b013e318208edf8.
8. Wunsch H, Guerra C, Barnato AE, Angus DC, Li G, Linde-Zwirble WT. Three-year outcomes for Medicare beneficiaries who survive intensive care. JAMA. 2010;303(9):849–56. doi:10.1001/jama.2010.216.
9. Chow WB, Rosenthal RA, Merkow RP, Ko CY, Esnaola NF, American College of Surgeons National Surgical Quality Improvement Program; American Geriatrics Society. Optimal preoperative assessment of the geriatric surgical patient: a best practices guideline from the American College of Surgeons National Surgical Quality Improvement Program and the American Geriatrics Society. J Am Coll Surg. 2012;215(4):453–66. doi:10.1016/j.jamcollsurg.2012.06.017. Epub 2012 Aug 21.
10. Roch A, Wiramus S, Pauly V, Forel JM, Guervilly C, Gainnier M, Papazian L. Long-term outcome in medical patients aged 80 or over following admission to an intensive care unit. Crit Care. 2011;15(1):R36. doi:10.1186/cc9984. Epub 2011 Jan 24.
11. Montuclard L, Garrouste-Orgeas M, Timsit JF, Misset B, De Jonghe B, Carlet J. Outcome, functional autonomy, and quality of life of elderly patients with a long-term intensive care unit stay. Crit Care Med. 2000;28(10):3389–95.
12. Taylor MD, Tracy JK, Meyer W, Pasquale M, Napolitano LM. Trauma in the elderly: intensive care unit resource use and outcome. J Trauma. 2002;53(3):407–14.
13. Peschman J, Neideen T, Brasel K. The impact of discharging minimally injured trauma patient: does age play a role in trauma admission? J Trauma. 2011;70(6):1331–6. doi:10.1097/TA.0b013e31821693e2.
14. Hranjec T, Sawyer RG, Young JS, Swenson BR, Calland JF. Mortality factors in geriatric blunt trauma patients: creation of a highly predictive statistical model for mortality using 50,765 consecutive elderly trauma admissions from the national sample project. Am Surg. 2012;78(12):1369–75.
15. Meldon SW, Reilly M, Drew BL, Mancuso C, Fallon Jr W. Trauma in the very elderly: a community-based study of outcomes at trauma and nontrauma centers. J Trauma. 2002;52(1):79–84.
16. Bennett KM, Scarborough JE, Vaslef S. Outcomes and health care resource utilization in super-elderly trauma patients. J Surg Res. 2010;163(1):127–31. doi:10.1016/j.jss.2010.04.031. Epub 2010 May 21.
17. Sarkar B, Brunsvold ME, Cherry-Bukoweic JR, Hemmila MR, Park PK, Raghavendran K, Wahl WL, Wang SC, Napolitano LM. American College of Surgeons' Committee on Trauma performance improvement and patient safety program: maximal impact in a mature trauma center. J Trauma. 2011;71(5):1447–53. doi:10.1097/TA.0b013e3182325d32; discussion 1453–4.
18. Frederickson TA, Renner CH, Swegle JR, Sahr SM. The cumulative effect of multiple critical care protocols on length of stay in a geriatric trauma population. J Intensive Care Med. 2013;28(1):58–66. doi:10.1177/0885066611432420. Epub 2012 Jan 23.
19. Mangram AJ, Mitchell CD, Shifflette VK, Lorenzo M, Truitt MS, Goel A, Lyons MA, Nichols DJ, Dunn EL. Geriatric trauma service: a one-year experience. J Trauma Acute Care Surg. 2012;72(1):119–22. doi:10.1097/TA.0b013e318241f0ba.
20. Bourg P, Richey M, Salottolo K, Mains CW. Development of a geriatric resuscitation protocol, utilization compliance, and outcomes. J Trauma Nurs. 2012;19(1):50–6. doi:10.1097/JTN.0b013e31822b80f5.
21. Fallon Jr WF, Rader E, Zyzanski S, Mancuso C, Martin B, Breedlove L, DeGolia P, Allen K, Campbell J. Geriatric outcomes are improved by a geriatric trauma consultation service. J Trauma. 2006;61(5):1040–6.
22. Lenartowicz M, Parkovnick M, McFarlan A, Haas B, Straus SE, Nathens AB, Wong CL. An evaluation of a proactive geriatric trauma consultation service. Ann Surg. 2012;256(6):1098–101. doi:10.1097/SLA.0b013e318270f27a.
23. ACS TQIP Geriatric trauma management guidelines. 2013. http://www.facs.org/trauma/ntdb/tqip.html.
24. Fagon JY. Acute respiratory failure in the elderly. Crit Care. 2006;10(4):151.
25. Ray P, Birolleau S, Lefort Y, Becquemin MH, Beigelman C, Isnard R, Teixeira A, Arthaud M, Riou B, Boddaert J. Acute respiratory failure in the elderly: etiology, emergency diagnosis and prognosis. Crit Care. 2006;10(3):R82. Epub 2006 May 24.
26. Dardaine V, Constans T, Lasfargues G, Perrotin D, Giniès G. Outcome of elderly patients requiring ventilatory support in intensive care. Aging (Milano). 1995;7(4):221–7.
27. Dardaine V, Dequin PF, Ripault H, Constans T, Giniès G. Outcome of older patients requiring ventilatory support in intensive care: impact of nutritional status. J Am Geriatr Soc. 2001;49(5):564–70.
28. Cox CE, Carson SS, Lindquist JH, Olsen MK, Govert JA, Chelluri L, Quality of Life After Mechanical Ventilation in the Aged (QOL-MV) Investigators. Differences in one-year health outcomes and resource utilization by definition of prolonged mechanical ventilation: a prospective cohort study. Crit Care. 2007;11(1):R9.
29. Lieberman D, Nachshon L, Miloslavsky O, Dvorkin V, Shimoni A, Lieberman D. How do older ventilated patients fare? A survival/functional analysis of 641 ventilations. J Crit Care. 2009;24(3):340–6. doi:10.1016/j.jcrc.2009.01.015.
30. Tang EY, Hsu LF, Lam KN, Pang WS. Critically ill elderly who require mechanical ventilation: the effects of age on survival outcomes and resource utilisation in the medical intensive care unit of a general hospital. Ann Acad Med Singapore. 2003;32(5):691–6.
31. Schortgen F, Follin A, Piccari L, Roche-Campo F, Carteaux G, Taillandier-Heriche E, Krypciak S, Thille AW, Paillaud E, Brochard L. Results of noninvasive ventilation in very old patients. Ann Intensive Care. 2012;2(1):5. doi:10.1186/2110-5820-2-5.
32. Riario-Sforza GG, Scarpazza P, Incorvaia C, Casali W. Role of noninvasive ventilation in elderly patients with hypercapnic respiratory failure. Clin Ter. 2012;163(1):e47–52.
33. www.polst.org.
34. Guerra C, Linde-Zwirble WT, Wunsch H. Risk factors for dementia after critical illness in elderly medicare beneficiaries. Crit Care. 2012;16(6):R233.
35. Martindale RG, McClave SA, Vanek VW, McCarthy M, Roberts P, Taylor B, Ochoa JB, Napolitano L, Cresci G, American College of Critical Care Medicine; A.S.P.E.N. Board of Directors. Guidelines for the provision and assessment of nutrition support therapy in the adult critically ill patient: Society of Critical Care Medicine and American Society for Parenteral and Enteral Nutrition: Executive Summary. Crit Care Med. 2009;37(5):1757–61.
36. To KB, Napolitano LM. Common complications in the critically ill patient. Surg Clin North Am. 2012;92(6):1519–57. doi:10.1016/j.suc.2012.08.018.
37. http://www.shea-online.org/HAITopics/CompendiumofStrategiestoPreventHAIs.aspx.

Cardiovascular/Invasive Monitoring

30

Jay Menaker and Thomas M. Scalea

Introduction

The older or elderly population, those over the age of 65 years of age [1–4], represent one of the fastest growing segments of the US population. In 2010, more people were older than 65 than at any previous time in US history [5]. It is estimated that by the year 2030, the population of elderly is expected to double as compared to 2000 and account for almost 20 % of the US population [6]. Additionally, it is predicted that by the year 2025, individuals older than 85 years, the oldest-old, will number more than seven million [7]. This increase in the number of elderly is multifactorial and is due in large part to the advances in medicine which have resulted in a longer life expectancy.

Physiologic Changes

As people age their physiologic reserve decreases. This loss of physiologic reserve is a slow process of deterioration often starting in the fourth decade of life and continues with increasing age. Despite this decrease in organ function, most elderly people can compensate physiologically to meet the needs of daily activities under normal condition. However, when stressed by illness, including traumatic injury, the physiologic demand may be excessive with a limited ability to compensate and mount the appropriate cardiovascular response to ensure adequate perfusion. The rate of physiologic change is variable from organ to organ and individual to individual [8].

Age is a major risk factor for the development of cardiovascular disease (CVD), and as such many elderly patients have some degree of CVD. CVD has been shown to be responsible for more than 40 % of deaths in patients over the age of 65 years [9]. Age-related changes in the myocardium affect anatomical as well as physiologic and electrophysiologic activity of the heart [10]. With aging, there is a decrease in myocardial contractility and ventricular compliance for a given preload as a result of loss of myocytes and increased myocardial collagen [11]. Autonomic tissue is replaced with connective tissue and fat, while fibrosis of the myocardium results in conduction abnormalities. The change in the conduction system increases the incidence of dysrhythmias including sick sinus syndrome, bundle branch blocks with resultant atrial arrhythmias which may be a cause for subsequent syncope in the elderly [12–14].

As one ages, systolic blood pressure increases due to augmented afterload from stiffening of the outflow tract. During times of physiologic stress, such as acute illness or injury, these changes result in decreases in peak ejection fraction and cardiac output [11, 15–17]. Compounding the situation is that between the ages of 20 and 85 years of age, it is estimated that maximal heart rate decreases by as much as 30 % [18]. Additionally aged myocardium does not respond as well to increased levels of endogenous and exogenous catecholamines [19]; thus, cardiac output in the elderly must be augmented by increasing ventricular filling and stroke volume rather than an increase in heart rate [11, 20]. This reliance on adequate volume (preload) makes the elderly very sensitive to even minimal hypovolemia which may result in cardiac collapse. However, one must be vigilant during times of volume resuscitation in the elderly and balance the need for adequate cardiac output with the potential for pulmonary edema due to decreased ventricular compliance.

J. Menaker, MD, FACEP (✉) • T.M. Scalea, MD, FACS
Division of Trauma/Surgical Critical Care, Department of Surgery, University of Maryland School of Medicine, R Adams Cowley Shock Trauma Center, 22 South Greene Street, T1R60, Baltimore, MD 21201, USA
e-mail: jmenaker@umm.edu; tscalea@umm.edu

J.A. Yelon, F.A. Luchette (eds.), *Geriatric Trauma and Critical Care*,
DOI 10.1007/978-1-4614-8501-8_30, © Springer Science+Business Media New York 2014

Atrial Fibrillation

Atrial fibrillation (AF) is the most common postoperative arrhythmia occurring in 3.7–6.7 % of patients [21–24]. Advanced age has been shown to be independently associated with a higher incidence of AF. AF is associated with higher daily fluid requirements, prevalence of severe infections, and the need for vasoactive and inotropic support [24]. It has been shown to be associated with significantly longer intensive care unit (ICU) and hospital length of stay (LOS) as well as increased mortality [23, 24].

The etiology for the development of AF can be multifactorial. Underlying myocardial disease in the elderly along with increased systemic inflammation can cause further myocardial dysfunction causing AF [25]. Increased intravascular volume from large volume resuscitation may dilate the left atrium and increase the risk of AF. Alternatively, hypovolemia leading to an increased adrenergic state can increase the likelihood of AF [26]. Regardless of the cause, atrial fibrillation in the geriatric critically ill patient appears to be a marker of severity of illness as demonstrated by higher Simplified Acute Physiologic Scores II, nursing workload in the ICU (OMEGA), and mortality [24].

There is a wide variation in the treatment of elderly patients with AF [27]. Clinicians should investigate for any treatable causes including thyroid dysfunction, electrolyte abnormalities, or acute cardiac ischemia. Therapy goals include rate control, rhythm control, and the prevention of thromboembolism.

Elderly patients in the ICU with AF often become hemodynamically unstable as a result of the loss of the atrial contribution to ventricular filling and stroke volume which leads to a decreased cardiac output [27]. Those with hypotension, angina, or heart failure should be immediately cardioverted. In contrast, the hemodynamically stable patient without symptoms can be treated pharmacologically. Currently, there are a number of treatment options available. Amiodarone has become the initial drug of choice for atrial fibrillation. It is a class III antiarrhythmic agent that depresses atrioventricular conduction and controls the ventricular rate. Side effects include bradycardia, thyroid dysfunction, as well as drug interaction, specifically warfarin. Intravenous (IV) amiodarone has been associated with acute elevation in liver enzymes; however, levels normalize with discontinuation of the IV form. Additionally, long-term amiodarone use has been associated with the development of pulmonary fibrosis. Dronedarone, similar to amiodarone, has been studied for rate and rhythm control in AF. It reduces morbidity and mortality in inpatients at risk for development of AF, however, is contraindicated in patients with acute severe heart failure [28]. Other pharmacological options include β-blockers and calcium channel blockers (CCB). Beta-blockers may be more appropriate for postoperative hyperadrenergic states, while CCB, specifically diltiazem, may be more appropriate for patients with severe asthma or chronic obstructive pulmonary disease. Side effects of CCB include hypotension, heart failure, and heart block.

Digoxin, one of the oldest antiarrhythmic agents for AF, is still used by many clinicians. Digoxin works by slowing down conduction at the atrioventricular node by parasympathetic activation. It may be the ideal pharmacological choice if patients have simultaneous heart failure or left ventricular dysfunction. Digoxin may have a synergistic effect with β-blockers or CCB. Unfortunately, digoxin has many drug-drug interactions which often limit its use in critically ill patients. Additionally, digoxin is renally metabolized, and drug levels need to be closely monitored and adjusted accordingly in patients with abnormal renal function.

If patients do not respond to pharmacological interventions and remain in AF, cardioversion is sometimes required. Patients who remain in AF for more than 48–72 h have an increased risk of atrial clot formation. Prior to cardioversion, it is recommended that a transesophageal echocardiogram be performed to evaluate for an atrial thrombus. Once successfully cardioverted, systemic anticoagulation is required. Clinicians need to take into account the risks of systemic anticoagulation in the critically ill geriatric patient including falls risks and drug interactions. Alternatively, additional medical attempts at rate control alone may be safer in this patient population.

Myocardial Ischemia/Infarction

Age and preexisting cardiovascular disease predispose the elderly to cardiac complications when critically ill. Cardiac complications have been reported to range from 12 to 16.7 % in this patient population especially for those over the age of 80 years [29–31]. Cardiac complications are one of the more common causes of mortality in the elderly surgical patient, and for those over the age of 80 years, myocardial infarction (MI) has been shown to be the leading cause of postoperative death [32]. The prevalence of postoperative MI in the elderly ranges between 0.1 and 4 % [33–35]. The majority of MIs occur within 72 h after conclusion of the operation [33].

Beta-blockers are thought to be the mainstay of treatment to help prevent perioperative cardiac complications in the elderly. By decreasing heart rate and afterload, the shear forces on the atherosclerotic vessels are reduced. These changes to the cardiovascular system also minimize the chances of plague rupture, which is the etiology of up to 50 % of perioperative heart attacks [36]. Additionally β-blockers assist in minimizing ventricular dysrhythmias, improve myocardial oxygen balance, and decrease sympathetic tone, leading to fewer perioperative cardiac complications. In 2002, Auerbach and Goldman reviewed the efficacy of perioperative β-blockade in reducing myocardial ischemia, infarction, and cardiac-related mortality [37]. The authors concluded that there was a benefit with β-blockade in preventing perioperative cardiac morbidity. In 2008 the Perioperative Ischemic Evaluation (POISE) study group evaluated the use perioperative β-blockade and concluded that although the treatment group had significantly lower rates of MI, there was a significantly higher death rate and stroke rate in the patients receiving β-blockers [38].

As a result of the vast literature on the use of β-blockers in the perioperative period, there is little consensus as the appropriate patient population that would benefit from their use. Some authors believe patients having one or two risk factors (high risk surgery, known ischemic heart disease, history of congestive heart failure or cerebrovascular disease, baseline creatinine >2 mg/dL) would benefit, while others believe patients with more than three risk factors are more appropriate [36, 39, 40]. As a result of the existing literature, the American Heart Association/American College of Cardiology Foundation has modified the recommendation for the use of β-blockers in the perioperative period [41, 42].

Hemodynamic Monitoring

During times of acute illness or trauma, many elderly patients cannot appropriately augment their cardiac output, and therefore, systemic vascular resistance is increased to maintain perfusion [43]. As a result, elderly patients may demonstrate a normal blood pressure, while having severely depressed and compromised cardiac function leading to overall poor systemic perfusion. In a study of geriatric trauma patients, Scalea and colleagues demonstrated as many as 50 % geriatric trauma patients who appeared clinically stable with "normal" blood pressure had unrecognized cardiogenic shock and a poor outcome [44]. Using a pulmonary artery catheter, resuscitation was optimized using volume, inotropes, and afterload reduction, and survival increased from 7 to 53 %. The authors determined that identifying occult shock early in the geriatric population with the use of invasive monitoring improves survival.

The question as to the ideal method for hemodynamic monitoring in the elderly, or any critically ill patient, is an ongoing dilemma. Unfortunately, there is scant data specifically looking at invasive monitoring in the elderly, and as such, data must be extrapolated from existing literature based on various patient populations. The pulmonary artery catheter (PAC) has long been considered the gold standard of hemodynamic monitoring. It was first described and used in 1970 by Doctors Swan and Ganz [43]. However, the studies evaluating its utility to improve patient outcomes are variable with some showing no effect [45–47]; some concluding mortality rates are decreased with the use of a PAC [44, 48, 49], and others reporting increased morbidity and mortality [50]. It has been suggested by some experts that the reason for the variable outcomes with the use of the PAC is the incorrect interpretation of the hemodynamic parameters and subsequent clinical decision making [51–53].

Continuous Central Venous Oximetry

Research and development has focused on creating devices that are less invasive but can still provide accurate and useful hemodynamic information. Continuous central venous oximetry ($ScvO2$) has been used as a surrogate for mixed venous oxygen saturation ($SvO2$) provided with a PAC. Using a modified central venous catheter with fiber-optic technology, clinicians are able to continuously monitor venous blood oxygenation in the superior vena cava. Although ScvO2 and SvO2 do not correlate absolutely, they have been shown to correlate with one another [54, 55]. Additionally, the use of ScvO2 can help identify global tissue hypoxia allowing earlier intervention in the clinical course and thus affecting outcome [56, 57]. Additionally, it has potential for time and cost savings as well as less morbidity compared to the PAC.

Pulse Contour Analysis

Another alternative to the PAC is pulse contour analysis. The idea is based on the Windkessel model first described by Otto Frank in 1899 [58]. It is based on the principle that stroke volume can be continuously estimated, on a beat-to-beat basis, using arterial waveform obtained from an arterial line. Calculations using the area under the curve of the systolic arterial pressure waveform allowed development of an algorithm for monitoring stroke volume [59]. Limitations of pulse contour technology include its accuracy in patients with irregular cardiac rhythms, right heart failure, spontaneous breathing, and mechanical ventilation using low tidal volumes (<8 mL/kg body weight) [60].

Examples of devices using pulse contour technology include the FloTrac™ (Edwards Lifesciences, Irvine, CA). It provides continuous cardiac output, stroke volumes, and stroke volume variation. The device does not require a central venous access, only an arterial catheter. The technology concept is based on arterial waveform analysis and the principle that pulse pressure is proportional to stroke volume [61], thus deriving a cardiac output on a beat-to-beat basis. Studies by Cannesson et al. and Button et al. showed clinically acceptable agreement between the PAC and FloTrac™ [62, 63]. Others, however, have had less favorable results [64].

The PiCCO™ (PULSION Medical Systems, Munich, Germany) is another pulse contour analysis device. Unlike the FloTrac™, it requires both an arterial line and a central venous catheter. The arterial line must be placed in either the femoral or axillary artery. The PiCCO™ system can provide clinicians with similar data to that of the FloTrac™; however, it also has the ability to measure a number of volumes including intrathoracic blood volume (ITBV), global end diastolic volume (GEDV), and extravascular lung water (EVLW). These volumes have been shown to better measure cardiac preload than traditional values including central venous pressure (CVP) and pulmonary capillary wedge pressure (PCWP) [65, 66]. Additionally, ITBV and GEDV are not affected by mechanical ventilation. Unfortunately, unlike the FloTrac™ which does not need any calibration, the PiCCO™ system requires calibration on a regular basis depending on the hemodynamics of the patient. A study by Della Rocca and colleagues compared the PAC and the PiCCO™ and found that these two methods yielded similar measurements [67]. A study by Uchino et al. looked at outcomes when using a PiCCO™ versus using a PAC. The authors concluded that the choice of monitoring did not influence major outcomes [68].

Despite much effort, an accurate and reliable marker to guide fluid management has yet to be determined. Traditional measurements of preload including CVP and PCWP have not been shown to reliably predict cardiac preload and the need for volume to optimize cardiac function [69]. A study by Boulain and colleagues demonstrated that passive leg raises (PLR) change pulse pressure and can predict the need for fluid administration in mechanically ventilated patients [61]. As stated previously, pulse pressure is proportional to stroke volume, thus allowing pulse contour technology to calculate a stroke volume variation (SVV). SVV has been used to try to answer the never-ending, possible unanswerable critical care question, "is a patient wet or dry"? Some believe it to be a good marker of fluid responsiveness in patients and may be the simplest way to predict fluid responsiveness [70]. In general, a lower SVV implies adequate fluid balance, while elevated measurements of SVV imply the need for volume resuscitation. Both the FloTrac™ and PiCCO™ systems can calculate SVV. Studies have demonstrated that the PiCCO™ system can predict fluid responsiveness in a variety of clinical situations [71, 72]. In contrast, studies evaluating the ability of FloTrac™ system to predict volume responsiveness are more varied [62, 63, 73]. One study compared the FloTrac™ device to the PiCCO™ system for predicting fluid responsiveness and concluded that both had a similar accuracy [74].

What is the exact threshold of SVV for determining fluid responsiveness? Unfortunately, the literature has yet to answer this question [74]. A report by Berkenstadt and colleagues determined a SVV value of 9.5 % or more will predict an increase in stroke volume [75]. Suehiro and Okutani determined a SVV cutoff value of 10.5 % to predict fluid responsiveness [76]. When comparing values derived from the FloTrac™ to those of the PiCCO™, Hofer and colleagues found that although both equally predicted fluid responsiveness, the FloTrac™ had a lower threshold of 9.6 % versus 12.5 % for the PiCCO™ [74]. In general, normal SVV values are thought to be 10–15 %.

Echocardiography

The role of ultrasound and echocardiography continues to grow and expand in the critical care setting. Information about cardiac function, fluid status, and inferior vena cava diameter and collapsibility can rapidly be attained at the bedside. This information allows for reliable monitoring of intravascular volume in mechanically ventilated patients [77]. The gold standard to evaluate cardiac function is transesophageal echocardiography (TEE); however, it is invasive and requires specialized training to perform. Transthoracic echocardiography (TTE) however is less invasive, requires less specialized training, and can effectively assess cardiac function. Handheld echocardiography (HHE) using a smaller device has been shown to be as accurate and as clinically beneficial as the TTE [78].

The first focused echocardiography ultrasound protocol for non-cardiologists was the "Focused Assessment with Transthoracic Echocardiography" (FATE) [79]. The authors demonstrated the ability to describe the hemodynamics of patients as well as the ability to optimize care. Since then a number of similar protocols have been created. In 2008, Gunst et al. used the "Bedside Echocardiographic Assessment in Trauma" (BEAT) to compare function and volume status in critically ill patients with a PAC [80]. The authors demonstrated a significant correlation of cardiac index and CVP between the two modalities. However, as stated previously, CVP has been suggested to be a poor measurement of volume status. In 2011, the "Focused Rapid Echocardiographic Examination" (FREE) was first described by Ferrada and colleagues [81]. It was designed to be performed by both surgeons and intensivists. It is a "transthoracic examination, which incorporates hemodynamic information from the echo with the patient's clinical scenario to generate broad treatment recommendations about fluid, inotropic agents and vasopressors" [81]. When compared to PAC, the FREE was found to have similar results in the measurement of cardiac index; however, when compared to the FloTrac™, there was less agreement, especially in patients with low (<40 %) ejection fractions [82].

Conclusion

The population of those over the age of 65 years continues to increase. Aging is associated with a decrease in physiologic reserve, and when stressed by acute illness, the cardiovascular system is unable to effectively compensate and meet the physiologic demand to ensure adequate perfusion. Underlying cardiac dysfunction becomes more pronounced, and complications including cardiac dysrhythmia, myocardial ischemia, and infarction occur. Early aggressive hemodynamic monitoring has been shown to improve survival in the elderly patient population; however, the optimal method by which to do this has yet to be definitively determined.

References

1. Osler T, Baker SP, Long W. A modification of the injury severity score that both improves accuracy and simplifies scoring. J Trauma. 1997;43:922–6.
2. Champion HR, Copes WS, Buyer D. Major trauma in geriatric patients. Am J Public Health. 1989;79:1278–82.
3. Grossman MD, Miller D, Scaff DW. When is elder old? Effect of preexisting conditions on mortality in geriatric trauma. J Trauma. 2002;52:242–6.
4. Taylor MD, Tracy JK, Meyer W. Trauma in the elderly: intensive care unit resource use and outcome. J Trauma. 2002;53:407–14.
5. US Census Bureau. 2010. The older population: 2010. 2010 Census Briefs. http://www.census.gov/prod/cen2010/briefs/c2010br-09.pdf. Accessed 19 Apr 2012.
6. US Census Bureau. 65+ in the United States: 2005. http://www.census.gov/prod/2006pubs/p23-209.pdf. Accessed 19 Dec 2012.
7. United States Census Bureau. U.S. population projections. 2008 national population projections. http://www.census.gov/population/www/projections/2009summarytables.html. Accessed 19 Apr 2012.
8. Boss GR, Seegmiller JE. Age related physiologic changes and their clinical significance. West J Med. 1981;135:434–40.
9. Lakatta EG. Age-associated cardiovascular changes in health. Impact on cardiovascular disease in older persons. Heart Fail Rev. 2002;7:29–49.
10. Harris R. Cardiovascular diseases in the elderly. Med Clin North Am. 1983;67:379–94.
11. Morley JE, Reese SS. Clinical implications of the aging heart. Am J Med. 1989;86:77–86.
12. Marik PE. Management of the critically ill geriatric patient. Crit Care Med. 2006;34:S176–82.
13. Rosenthal RA, Kavic SM. Assessment and management of the geriatric patient. Crit Care Med. 2004;4:S92–105.
14. Watters JM, McClaran JC. The elderly surgical patient. In: The American College of Surgeons: care of the surgical patient, vol. 1. New York: Scientific American; 1991.
15. Pisani MA. Consideration in the caring for the critically ill older patient. J Intensive Care Med. 2009;24:83–95.
16. Sollott SJ, Lakatta EG. Normal aging changes in the cardiovascular system. Cardiol Elder. 1993;1:349–58.
17. Stratton JR, Levy WC, Cerqueira MD, et al. Cardiovascular response to exercise. Effects of aging and exercise training in healthy men. Circulation. 1994;59:1648–55.
18. Lakatta EG, Levy D. Arterial and cardiac aging: major shareholders in cardiovascular disease enterprises: part II: the aging heart in health: links to heart disease. Circulation. 2003;107:346–54.
19. Lakatta EG. Age-related alterations in the cardiovascular response to adrenergic mediated stress. Fed Proc. 1980;39:3173–7.
20. Green JS, Crouse SF. Endurance training, cardiovascular function and the aged. Sports Med. 1993;16:331–41.
21. Ryu JK. Postoperative atrial fibrillation after noncardiothoracic surgery: is it different from after cardiothoracic surgery? Korean Circ J. 2009;39:93–4.
22. Brathwaite D, Weissman C. The new onset of atrial arrhythmias following major noncardiothoracic surgery is associated with increased mortality. Chest. 1998;114:462–8.
23. Polanczyk CA, Goldman L, Marcantonio ER. Supraventricular arrhythmia in patients having noncardiac surgery: clinical correlates and effect on length of stay. Ann Intern Med. 1998;129:279–85.
24. Seguin P, Signouret T, Laviolle B. Incidence and risk factors of atrial fibrillation in a surgical intensive care unit. Crit Care Med. 2004;32:722–6.
25. Court O, Kumar A, Parrillo JE. Clinical review: myocardial depression in sepsis and septic shock. Crit Care. 2002;6:500–8.
26. Edwards JD, Wilkins RG. Atrial fibrillation precipitated by acute hypovolemia. BMJ. 1987;294:283–4.
27. Mead GE, Elder AT, Faulkner S. Cardioversion for atrial fibrillation: the views of consultant physicians, geriatricians and cardiologists. Age Ageing. 1999;28:73–5.
28. Patel C, Yan GX, Kowey PR. Dronedarone. Circulation. 2009;120:636–44.
29. Seymour DG, Pringle R. Post-operative complications in the elderly surgical patient. Gerontology. 1983;29:262–70.
30. Pedersen T, Eliasen K, Henriksen E. A prospective study of risk factors and cardiopulmonary complications associated with anaesthesia and surgery: risk indicators of cardiopulmonary morbidity. Acta Anaesthesiol Scand. 1990;34:144–55.
31. Liu LL, Leung JM. Predicting adverse postoperative outcomes in patients aged 80 years or older. J Am Geriatr Soc. 2000;48:405–12.
32. Djokovic JL, Hedley-Whyte J. Prediction of outcome of surgery and anesthesia in patients over 80. JAMA. 1979;242:2301–6.
33. Plumlee JE, Boettner RB. Myocardial infarction during and following anesthesia and operation. South Med J. 1972;65:886–9.
34. Pedersen T, Eliasen K, Henriksen E. A prospective study of mortality associated with anaesthesia and surgery: risk indicators of mortality in hospital. Acta Anaesthesiol Scand. 1990;34:176–82.
35. Seymour DG. Medical assessment of the elderly surgical patient. Rockville: Aspen Systems Co; 1986. p. 80.
36. Kertai MD, Bax JJ, Klein J. Is there any reason to withhold beta blockers from high risk patients with coronary artery disease during surgery? Anesthesiology. 2004;100:4–7.
37. Auerbach AD. Goldman L, β-Blockers and reduction of cardiac events in noncardiac surgery. JAMA. 2002;287:1435–44.
38. Devereaux PJ, Yang H, Yusuf S, Guyatt G, Leslie K, Villar JC, et al. Effects of extended-release metoprolol succinate in patients undergoing non-cardiac surgery: a randomised controlled trial. Lancet. 2008;371:1839–47.
39. Priebe HJ. Perioperative myocardial infarction – aetiology and prevention. Br J Anaesth. 2005;95:3–19.
40. Lindenauer PK, Pekow P, Wang K. Perioperative beta-blocker therapy and mortality after major noncardiac surgery. N Engl J Med. 2005;353:349–61.
41. Fleisher LA, Beckman JA, Brown KA, et al. ACC/AHA 2006 guideline update on perioperative cardiovascular evaluation for noncardiac surgery: focused update on perioperative beta-blocker therapy: a report of the American College of Cardiology/American Heart Association Task Force on Practice Guidelines (Writing Committee to Update the 2002 Guidelines on Perioperative Cardiovascular Evaluation for Noncardiac Surgery): developed in collaboration with the American Society of Echocardiography, American Society of Nuclear Cardiology, Heart Rhythm Society, Society of Cardiovascular Anesthesiologists, Society for Cardiovascular Angiography and Interventions, and Society for Vascular Medicine and Biology. Circulation. 2006;113:2662–74.
42. Fleisher LA, Beckman JA, Brown KA, et al. 2009 ACCF/AHA focused update on perioperative beta blockade incorporated into the ACC/ AHA 2007 guidelines on perioperative cardiovascular

evaluation and care for noncardiac surgery: a report of the American College of Cardiology Foundation/American Heart Association Task Force on Practice Guidelines. Circulation. 2009;120:e169–276.
43. Oleske DM, Wilson RS, Bernard BA. Epidemiology of injury in people with Alzheimer's disease. J Am Geriatr Soc. 1995;43: 741–6.
44. Scalea TM, Simon HM, Duncan AO, et al. Geriatric blunt multiple trauma: improved survival with early invasive monitoring. J Trauma. 1990;30:129–34.
45. Swan HJC, Ganz W, Forrester J. Catheterization of the heart in man with the use of a flow directed balloon-tipped catheter. N Engl J Med. 1970;283:447–51.
46. Wu AW, Rubin HR, Rosen MJ. Are elderly people less responsive to intensive care? J Am Geriatr Soc. 1990;38:621–7. CVP and PCWP – BA.
47. Tuman KJ, McCarthy RJ, Spiess BD, DaValle M, Hompland SJ, Dabir R, et al. Effect of pulmonary artery catheterization on outcome in patients undergoing coronary artery surgery. Anesthesiology. 1989;70:199–206.
48. Sandham JD, Hull RD, Brant RF, Knox L, Pinero GF, Doig CJ, et al. A randomized, controlled trial of the use of pulmonary artery catheters in high risk surgical patients. N Engl J Med. 2003; 348:5–14.
49. Boyd O, Grounds RM, Bennett ED. A randomized clinical trial of the effect of deliberate perioperative increase of oxygen delivery on mortality in high-risk surgical patients. JAMA. 1993;270:2699–707.
50. Savino JA, Del Guercio LR. Preoperative assessment of high-risk surgical patients. Surg Clin North Am. 1985;65:763–91.
51. Polanczyk CA, Rohde LE, Goldman L, Cook EF, Thomas EJ, Marcantonio ER, et al. Right heart catheterization and cardiac complications in patients undergoing noncardiac surgery: an observational study. JAMA. 2001;286:309–14.
52. Shoemaker WC, Appel PL, Kram HB. Prospective trial of supranormal values of survivors as therapeutic goals in high risk surgical patients. Chest. 1988;94:1176–86.
53. Iberti TJ, Fischer EP, Leibowitz AB. A multicenter study of physicians' knowledge of the pulmonary artery catheter. Pulmonary Artery Catheter Study Group. JAMA. 1990;264:2928–32.
54. Reinhart K, Kuhn HJ, Hartog C. Continuous central venous and pulmonary artery oxygen saturation monitoring in the critically ill. Intensive Care Med. 2004;30:1572–8.
55. Goodrich C. Continuous central venous oximetry monitoring. Crit Care Nurs Clin North Am. 2006;18:203–9.
56. Rady MY, Rivers EP, Martin GB. Continuous central venous oximetry and shock index in the emergency department: use in the evaluation of clinical shock. Am J Emerg Med. 1992;10:538–41.
57. Scalea TM, Hartnett RW, Duncan AO, Atweh NA, Phillips TF, Sclafani SJ, et al. Central venous oxygen saturation: a useful clinical tool in trauma patients. J Trauma. 1990;30:1539–43.
58. Otto F. Die Grundform des arteriellen Pulses. Zeitung für Biologie. 1899;37:483–586.
59. Wesseling KH, Smith NT, Nichols WW. Beat-to-beat cardiac output from the arterial pressure pulse contour. In: Feldman SA, Leigh JM, Spierdijk J, editors. Measurement in anaesthesia. Leiden: Leiden University Press; 1974. p. 148–64.
60. Porhomayon J, El-Solh A, Papadakos P. Cardiac output monitoring devices: an analytic review. Intern Emerg Med. 2012;7:163–71.
61. Boulain T, Achard JM, Teboul JL. Changes in BP induced by passive leg raising predict response to fluid loading in critically ill patients. Chest. 2002;121:1245–52.
62. Cannesson M, Attof Y, Rosamel P. Comparison of FloTrac cardiac output monitoring system in patients undergoing coronary artery bypass grafting with pulmonary artery cardiac output measurements. Eur J Anaesthesiol. 2007;24:832–9.
63. Button D, Weibel L, Reuthebuch O. Clinical evaluation of the FloTrac/Vigileo system and two established continuous cardiac output monitoring devices in patients undergoing cardiac surgery. Br J Anaesth. 2007;99:329–36.
64. Saraceni E, Rossi S, Persona P, Dan M, Rizzi S, Meroni M, et al. Comparison of two methods for cardiac output measurement in critically ill patients. Br J Anaesth. 2011;106:690–4.
65. Boussat S, Jacques T, Levy B, Laurent E, Gache A, Capellier G, et al. Intravascular volume monitoring and extravascular lung water in septic patients with pulmonary edema. Intensive Care Med. 2002;28:712–8.
66. Bindels AJ, van der Hoeven JG, Graafland AD. Relationships between volume and pressure measurements and stroke volume in critically ill patients. Crit Care. 2000;4:193–9.
67. Della Rocca G, Costa MG, Coccia C, Pompei L, Di Marco P, Vilardi V, et al. Cardiac output monitoring: aortic transpulmonary thermodilution and pulse contour analysis agree with standard thermodilution methods in patients undergoing lung transplantation. Can J Anaesth. 2003;50:707–11.
68. Uchino S, Bellomo R, Morimatsu H, Sugihara M, French C, Stephens D, et al. PAC/PiCCO Use and Likelihood of Success Evaluation [PULSE] Study Group Pulmonary artery catheter versus pulse contour analysis: a prospective epidemiological study. Crit Care. 2006;10:R174.
69. Kumar A, Anel R, Bunnell E, Habet K, Zanotti S, Marshall S, et al. Pulmonary artery occlusion pressure and central venous pressure fail to predict ventricular filling volume, cardiac performance or the response to volume infusion in normal subjects. Crit Care Med. 2004;3:691–9.
70. Michard F. Changes in arterial pressure during mechanical ventilation. Anesthesiology. 2005;103:419–28.
71. Marx G, Cope T, McCrossan L, Swaraj S, Cowan C, Mostafa SW. Assessing fluid responsiveness by stroke volume variation in mechanically ventilated patients with severe sepsis. Eur J Anaesthesiol. 2004;21:132–8.
72. Hofer CK, Muller SM, Furrer L. Stroke volume and pulse pressure variation for prediction of fluid responsiveness in patients undergoing off-pump coronary artery bypass grafting. Chest. 2005;128:848–54.
73. de Waal EE, Rex S, Kruitwagen CL. Stroke volume variation obtained with FloTrac/Vigileo fails to predict fluid responsiveness in coronary artery bypass graft patients. Br J Anaesth. 2008; 100:725–6.
74. Hofer CK, Senn A, Weibel L. Assessment of stroke volume variation for prediction of fluid responsiveness using the modified FloTrac™ and PiCCO plus™ system. Crit Care. 2008;12:R82.
75. Berkenstadt H, Margalit N, Hadani M, Friedman Z, Segal E, Villa Y, et al. Stroke volume variation as a predictor of fluid responsiveness in patients undergoing brain surgery. Anesth Analg. 2001;92:984–9.
76. Suehiro K, Okutani R. Stroke volume variation as a predictor of fluid responsiveness in patients undergoing one-lung ventilation. J Cardiothorac Vasc Anesth. 2010;24:772–5.
77. Feissel M, Michard F, Faller JP. The respiratory variation in inferior vena cava diameter as a guide to fluid therapy. Intensive Care Med. 2004;30:1834–7.
78. Vignon P, Chastagner C, François B, Martaillé JF, Normand S, Bonnivard M, et al. Diagnostic ability of handheld echocardiography in ventilated critically ill patients. Crit Care. 2003;7:R84–91.
79. Jensen MB, Sloth E, Larsen KM. Transthoracic echocardiography for cardiopulmonary monitoring in intensive care. Eur J Anaesthesiol. 2004;21:700–7.
80. Gunst M, Ghaemmaghami V, Sperry J, Robinson M, O'Keeffe T, Friese R, et al. Accuracy of cardiac function and volume status estimates using bedside echocardiographic assessment in trauma/critical care. J Trauma. 2008;65:509–16.
81. Ferrada P, Murthi S, Anand RJ. Transthoracic focused rapid echocardiographic examination: real-time evaluation of fluid status in critically ill trauma patients. J Trauma. 2011;70:56–62.
82. Murthi SB, Hess JR, Hess A. Focused rapid echocardiographic evaluation versus vascular catheter-based assessment of cardiac output and function in critically ill trauma patients. J Trauma. 2012;72:1158–64.

Part IV

Critical Care Management of the Elderly Patient

31 Pulmonary Critical Care and Mechanical Ventilation

Stephanie R. Goldberg and Ajai K. Malhotra

Aging has a negative impact on all organ systems in the body. Age-related diminution in physiology is felt on the respiratory system the earliest [1], and trauma to the chest has a disproportionate influence on outcomes following injury at all ages [2]. In addition to this direct impact chest trauma has on outcomes, even in the absence of direct chest injury, adequate oxygenation is critical to cellular homeostasis of all injured tissues/organs with the injured brain being at greatest risk of even brief periods of hypoxemia during the immediate post-injury period. For these reasons adequate pulmonary care following injury is critically important not only from the respiratory standpoint but also for overall recovery.

Age-Related Changes to Respiratory Physiology

While this subject is addressed in detail in other chapters, a brief review here is important to fully understand the basis of pulmonary care in the elderly especially following injury. The respiratory system consists of two fundamental elements: (1) a gas exchange mechanism in the lung that leads to inspired oxygen being transferred from the alveolus into the blood and carbon dioxide being transferred in the opposite direction and (2) the rib cage, respiratory muscles, and neural mechanisms that govern the act of breathing including the brain stem that responds to levels of oxygen and carbon dioxide in the blood [3]. Both elements of the respiratory system change with age in a manner that reduces reserve and our ability to increase the delivery of oxygen to the tissues following injury. In the lung while the total lung volume remains relatively constant, there is a decrease in vital capacity primarily caused by an increase in residual volume [4]. This directly limits the degree to which minute ventilation can be increased to facilitate greater oxygen delivery and removal of carbon dioxide. At the same time the closing volume increases, so even minor chest trauma leads to alveolar collapse and increased shunting resulting in a ventilation-perfusion (V/Q) mismatch [5]. In the chest wall, respiratory muscles participate in the overall decline in muscle mass with aging, limiting the ability to take deep breaths and effectively clear the airways of secretions [6]. Also the sensitivity of the brain stem to hypoxemia and hypercarbia is diminished leading to decreased respiratory drive. In addition to these age-related physiological changes, older patients may also have pulmonary comorbidities that further diminish respiratory function. Finally, all narcotic analgesics used for pain control, to a lesser or greater degree, diminish respiratory drive [7]. In summary, there is less drive, diminished strength, and poorer gas exchange setting the stage for respiratory failure.

Principles of Pulmonary Care in the Elderly

Certain principles apply to any elderly patient admitted to the hospital for any reason but are especially pertinent after injury. These are:

1. Optimizing gas exchange
2. Preventing aspiration
3. Prevention of pulmonary infections
4. Early detection of deterioration
5. Early detection and prompt therapy of pulmonary infection
6. Assistance with ventilation if required:
   (a) Noninvasive ventilation
   (b) Endotracheal intubation and assisted ventilation

S.R. Goldberg, MD
Department of Surgery, Virginia Commonwealth University, 980454, Richmond, VA 23298, USA
e-mail: sgoldberg@mcvh-vcu.edu

A.K. Malhotra, MDDNB, FRCS, FACS (✉)
Department of Surgery, VCU Medical Center, 1200 East Broad Street, 15th fl. East, 980454, Richmond, VA 23298, USA
e-mail: akmalhot@mcvh-vcu.edu

J.A. Yelon, F.A. Luchette (eds.), *Geriatric Trauma and Critical Care*,
DOI 10.1007/978-1-4614-8501-8_31, © Springer Science+Business Media New York 2014

7. Liberation from mechanical ventilation and extubation
8. Role of tracheostomy
9. Ethical considerations and end of life care

Optimizing Gas Exchange

Gas exchange in the lung is dependent upon ventilation of the alveolus and perfusion of the ventilated alveolus or V/Q matching. Over time, there is an age-related decrease in the partial pressure of oxygen in arterial blood (PaO_2) at the rate of 4 mmHg per decade without any change in the partial pressure of alveolar oxygen (PAO_2) or partial pressure of arterial carbon dioxide ($PaCO_2$) [8]. This is due to decreased efficiency of gas exchange across the respiratory membrane caused by increased thickness and reduced surface area, decreasing from nearly 75 m^2 at age 20–60 m^2 by age 70 [9].

Simple measures that maintain V/Q matching to ensure adequate V/Q matching include:

1. Preventing atelectasis
   (a) Raising the head of the bed to 30°: Semirecumbent position is the preferred positioning adopted by the Institute for Healthcare Improvement in their ventilator bundle [10, 11]. Since patients in the supine position have lower spontaneous tidal volumes on pressure support ventilation than those in an upright position, it has been assumed that a semirecumbent position may facilitate ventilatory efforts [11, 12].
   (b) Incentive spirometry: A normal alveolar sac measures 0.3 mm in diameter. During normal breathing the alveolar sac inflates and then deflates, but does not completely collapse. The inflation and deflation stimulates surfactant production, a key to maintaining adequate compliance. Complete collapse of the alveolus leads to alveolar damage (see atelectrauma below) and reduces surfactant production thus making re-expansion difficult. Incentive spirometers, or sustained maximal inspiration devices, encourage deep breathing by augmenting pulmonary ventilation through the re-expansion, or recruitment of alveoli [13]. The routine use of incentive spirometers has been shown to be effective in reducing pulmonary complications [14–16].
2. Providing adequate analgesia while minimizing sedation: Poor pain control may result in respiratory splinting and contribute to diminished inspiratory effort, while parenteral administration of narcotics depresses the cough reflex and may be sedating and limit the patient's ability to clear airway secretions. These indirect effects on pulmonary function commonly lead to atelectasis and V/Q mismatch. A multimodal approach to analgesia consisting of epidural pain control, local analgesic delivery (i.e., topical lidocaine patches), and local nerve blocks is effective at minimizing narcotic use [17].
3. Encouraging pulmonary toilet: Pulmonary toilet (or hygiene) refers to a set of therapies that facilitate clearance of secretions from the airways. Nasotracheal or endotracheal suctioning, chest physiotherapy and percussion, and prone positioning are widely accepted adjuncts to facilitate the removal of secretions from the tracheobronchial tree and prevent atelectasis [18, 19].

Preventing Aspiration

Aspiration is a common cause of respiratory failure among the elderly and occurs when oropharyngeal and/or gastric contents that may carry pathogens enter the airway. Chemical aspiration of gastric content results in a sterile chemical pneumonitis that damages type I pneumocytes impeding gas exchange, reduces surfactant production which results in alveolar collapse, and makes the patient prone to the development of microbial pneumonia – usually bacterial but sometimes viral or fungal. Risk factors contributing to aspiration include the positioning of the head of the bed <30°, presence of a nasogastric tube, enteral feeds (especially via a nasogastric tube), mechanical ventilation longer than 7 days, Glasgow Coma Score less than 9, and thermal injury [20–24].

Measures to prevent aspiration include:

1. Raising the head end of the bed 30°: Head of bed elevation has been incorporated in ventilator bundles and has been shown to decrease the rate of ventilator-associated pneumonia from 34 to 8 % in the semirecumbent position. This effect is most likely due to a reduction in aspiration [10]. Unless contraindicated, this is a low-cost approach to preventing aspiration.
2. Encouraging pulmonary toilet: Regular pulmonary toilet consisting of suctioning and chest physiotherapy facilitates removal of secretions.
3. Delivery of enteral nutrition distal to the pylorus: Although the exact mechanism remains unknown, nasogastric tubes have been associated with aspiration explained by reduction in the lower esophageal sphincter pressure. Mechanically ventilated patients who undergo early gastrostomy have been shown to have a lower incidence of ventilator-associated pneumonia compared with nasogastric tube-fed patients with stroke or closed head injury [25]. If nasogastric tubes are to be used, frequent assessments are necessary to confirm that the tubes are in the appropriate position in the stomach; tubes with the tip in the esophagus have been associated with aspiration [26].

4. Closely monitoring enteral feeding: Monitoring residual volumes to detect non-tolerance early and using intestinal tubes (post-ligament of Treitz, if possible) are good measures to reduce the chances of aspiration. Gastric residual volumes in excess of 200–250 cc every 4 h indicate intolerance, and the feedings should be stopped until tolerance returns [27–29]. Other signs and symptoms of intolerance include abdominal pain, bloating, and distention [30].

Prevention of Pulmonary Infections

Respiratory infections are a common complication in the elderly and contribute to significant morbidity and mortality, especially in the presence of underlying comorbidities [31, 32]. The most common pathogen is bacterial, followed by viral, and then atypical pathogens, or fungi. There are numerous mechanisms for clearing infected material from the upper airways – mucociliary escalator, cough reflex, etc. All of these are diminished with age which make the geriatric patient more prone to the development of a pulmonary infection. The problem is more pronounced in the mechanically ventilated patient as the protective mechanisms are completely eliminated. Pooling of oropharyngeal and regurgitated gastric secretions just above the balloon of the endotracheal tube results in micro-aspiration [33]. The gastric secretions very often are colonized as a result of reduced production of gastric acid with aging or the common use of acid-inhibiting drugs (proton pump inhibitors, histamine receptor-2 blockade). Studies have shown that these supraglottic secretions harbor pathogenic organisms and that the upper airway of the intubated patient becomes colonized by such organisms within 3–5 days of intubation.

The following measures should be taken to prevent the development of pulmonary infection in any elderly patient admitted to the hospital:

1. All measures noted above to prevent aspiration.
2. Strict hand washing by healthcare providers. Hand hygiene is an important tool in the prevention of nosocomial infections, especially pneumonia. Strict hand washing should be employed to prevent cross-contamination between patients [34].
3. Minimizing the use of antacid medications. Administration of acid-reducing medications increases the risk of pneumonia by neutralizing gastric acidity. This alteration of an innate host defense mechanism allows for bacterial overgrowth in the stomach [35].
4. Strict oral hygiene. Routine oral decontamination with agents such as chlorhexidine gluconate decreases bacterial proliferation in the oropharynx and may decrease the incidence of ventilator-associated pneumonia [36].
5. Consideration for specialized endotracheal tubes that have mechanisms for aspirating supraglottic secretion and/or tubes impregnated with silver. A specialized endotracheal tube has been developed to address the proposed mechanisms for the development of VAP which suggest micro-aspiration of colonized secretions that collect just above the balloon of the endotracheal tube. To reduce this from occurring, a Hi-Lo endotracheal tube allows for continuous aspiration of the pooled secretions from the supra- and infraglottic areas. The use of these tubes in an ICU setting has been shown to increase the time for development of VAP [37–39]. Another method addresses the role of biofilm which develops on the endotracheal tube. These endotracheal tubes have silver impregnation on the surface of the endotracheal tubes. The silver ion is bacteriostatic and has been shown to reduce the incidence of VAP. The efficacy of both tubes has been demonstrated in a large multicenter randomized study [40].
6. Use of ventilator bundle protocols for all ventilated patients. Prevention of nosocomial infections, including pneumonia, relies on a comprehensive set of interventions "bundled" together to achieve more significant outcomes than possible if each were implemented individually. One of the most widely accepted is the VAP bundle promoted by the IHI. The bundle consists of (i) elevation of the head of bed, (ii) daily "sedation vacation" and assessment of readiness to extubate, (iii) appropriate ulcer and deep venous thrombosis prophylaxis, and (iv) oral hygiene with chlorhexidine swabs. Thorough education of physicians, nursing staff, and respiratory therapists is necessary to ensure proper implementation of these bundles in an effective manner. If consistently used, the VAP bundle has been shown to decrease the rate of VAP [41].

Early Detection of Deterioration

Despite all measures, some patients, especially the elderly trauma patients, will experience deterioration of their pulmonary function. The earlier this deterioration is detected and appropriate therapy provided, outcome will be improved. Therefore, all healthcare providers involved with such patients should be aware of the early subtle signs of impending respiratory failure. These include (i) alteration in mental status – caused by neurologic event or sepsis; (ii) alteration in vital signs – heart rate, blood pressure, respiratory rate, and pulse oximeter saturations; and (iii) all subtle signs of stroke and myocardial infarction – the elderly may not manifest the more obvious signs/symptoms of these conditions. The use of rapid response teams has been shown to improve outcomes when subtle signs and symptoms of respiratory compromise are identified by the bedside nurse [42]. Lastly, specific to the respiratory system, the use of the incentive spirometer is an excellent method for reducing the incidence of respiratory complications. However, if the volume of air moved as shown by the incentive spirometer is not increasing or actually decreasing, it may be an early indicator of a developing problem and should lead to a careful evaluation of the patient [43].

Early Detection and Prompt Therapy of Pulmonary Infection

Infection may present in a vastly different manner in elderly patients compared to the young due to altered pulmonary reserve [44]. Elderly patients with infections may fail to manifest a fever or leukocytosis. Instead, alterations in behavior including agitation and altered mentation may be the only signs and symptoms of an infection. In any elderly patient with subtle or overt signs/symptoms of infection, a systematic search should be instituted to identify the source of the infection and if detected to treat it appropriately. From a respiratory standpoint, infection could occur anywhere from the supraglottic area – sinusitis or pharyngitis – to the infraglottic airways in the form of tracheobronchitis and pneumonia. If a respiratory infection is suspected, then appropriate specimen for culture should be obtained and empiric antimicrobials initiated. Additionally, any unnecessary tubes in the aerodigestive tract should be removed if at all possible. For sinusitis and pharyngitis in a non-intubated patient, a sputum culture is usually an adequate specimen. In contrast, the diagnosis of pneumonia is made with the combination of clinical signs and laboratory studies such as fever, leukocytosis, new or changing infiltrate on chest radiograph, and productive sputum with predominant growth of a single pathogen. If based on clinical and radiographic criteria, pneumonia is suspected, a deep tracheal aspirate should be obtained and empiric antimicrobials initiated. The choice of the empiric therapy is based primarily on whether the patient has or has not had contact with any healthcare facility or use of antimicrobials over the past 90 days. Patients admitted for less than 5 days and who have not had any contact with a healthcare facility or used antimicrobials over the past 90 days can be treated with standard therapy for community-acquired pneumonia. On the other hand, a patient who has been critically ill for 5 days, or who has had contact with a healthcare facility and/or used antimicrobials in the past 90 days, the possibility of hospital-acquired organisms should be strongly considered. In such situations empiric therapy should cover MRSA and hospital-acquired resistant gram-negative organisms like Pseudomonas, Enterobacter, and Acinetobacter.

The diagnosis of pneumonia in an elderly, traumatized, ventilated patient poses additional challenges. Leukocytosis and fever are nonspecific and, as noted above, may be absent in the elderly; infiltrates on chest radiograph too are nonspecific and may be due to other conditions such as cardiac pathology or pulmonary contusion. Sputum culture may be positive due to nonpathogenic colonization of the tracheobronchial tree and may not represent a true pathogenic infection. In such situations, the quantitative evaluation of the lower respiratory tract can offer a way of differentiating between nonpathogenic colonization and true VAP (CDC definition: pneumonia occurring in a patient who is or was on the ventilator in the previous 48 h) [45]. The specimen from the lower airways can be obtained by either bronchoalveolar lavage (BAL) or brush specimen and could be obtained bronchoscopically or blindly by specially designed catheters. At the authors' institution, a patient demonstrating any two of the following, fever, leukocytosis, changing infiltrate on x-ray, or productive sputum, undergoes a bronchoscopic-guided BAL for quantitative analysis. Empiric antimicrobials are initiated immediately after obtaining the specimen. There is ample evidence that delay in initiating appropriate antimicrobials in patients with VAP worsens outcomes [46]. If the quantitative cultures demonstrate $\geq 10^5$ microorganisms/ml of BAL fluid, the diagnosis of VAP is confirmed. However, if the results of the quantitative culture are less than $<10^5$, then VAP is considered unlikely, and further investigations for the source of infection are continued. In either case, the empiric antimicrobials are de-escalated. Once the sensitivities return, the spectrum of the antimicrobials is narrowed to an agent with activity against the specific organism and also has excellent tissue concentration. For patients with a quantitative culture that has $<10^5$ microorganisms/ml, antimicrobials are discontinued unless another indication for their continuation is present.

An alternative technique for obtaining a quantitative culture is the blind BAL technique. The exact quantitative threshold for diagnosing VAP and initiation of therapy is not well defined in the literature. While almost all agree that for the brush specimen, 10^3 microorganisms/ml is the correct threshold, for BAL, different institutions use differing thresholds ranging from 10^3 to 10^5 [47]. The duration of therapy of any diagnosed infection is another area of active investigation. There is a move to treat all infections, including pulmonary, based on the patient's clinical response, i.e., reduction in fever, reduction in leukocytosis, and improvement in other signs of sepsis – rather than arbitrary durations [48].

In addition to upper and lower respiratory infection, pulmonary infection may also reside in the pleural space. A known risk factor for empyema is retained hemothorax after insertion of a tube thoracostomy. The presence of blood, a foreign object, and a pathway to the skin offers the perfect conditions for infection of the pleural cavity. Additionally, any parapneumonic effusion can get secondarily infected and turn into an empyema. Any infected fluid within the pleural cavity requires adequate drainage. The drainage can be achieved by a simple thoracostomy tube for a non-loculated effusion. However, if loculated, the success of evacuation of the effusion with a single tube thoracostomy is low, and the patient will require either thoracoscopic or open surgical drainage. Finally, in rare instances, either from a very virulent organism or after a pulmonary embolism has decreased the blood supply to a part of the lung, a lung abscess may develop and require VATS.

Identification of Failure of Therapy

One of the basic tenets of critical care medicine is to identify failure of any therapy early and investigate the cause(s). Failure to respond to treatment of any infection with appropriate antibiotics after 48–72 h of therapy should prompt the critical team investigate for an explanation. The signs consist of failure to improve in signs of sepsis, reduction in fever, and leukocytosis. The causes of failure when treating a pulmonary infection are:

1. Inappropriate antimicrobial therapy. This maybe in the form of (i) an agent that does not target the causative organism; (ii) an agent that has poor tissue penetration, e.g., vancomycin; and (iii) inadequate dosing.
2. Development of resistance by the causative organism.
3. Infection by an organism that was not identified and hence is not being treated. There is a known false-negative rate for BAL in which a causative organism is not identified in the BAL fluid. In such cases, especially if the organism is multidrug resistant, the antimicrobial therapy may not be targeting the organism [49].
4. Development of a new infection, either within the pulmonary system or elsewhere.
5. A possible extrapulmonary source that has been present from the beginning but not identified.

A systemic search should be performed with a thorough physical examination and appropriate imaging studies when there is a treatment failure. From a pulmonary standpoint consideration should be given to all the above factors and also to the possibility that the patient has developed an empyema. Any pleural effusion should be sampled for gram stain along with culture and sensitivity. If the gram stain is diagnostic for empyema, appropriate therapy should be initiated immediately (see above). Additionally, to account for the possibility of a false BAL, a repeat BAL should be performed, and after obtaining the specimen, strong consideration should be given to broadening the antimicrobial coverage. Once again after the culture and sensitivity results are available, antimicrobial therapy should be adjusted.

Assistance with Ventilation if Required

Assistance with ventilation is required when a patient is unable to maintain adequate oxygenation (primary indication) or remove carbon dioxide (secondary indication) by him/herself despite the use of supplemental oxygen. Ventilatory assistance may be provided by noninvasive or invasive methods as discussed in the following sections.

Noninvasive Ventilation

Noninvasive ventilation usually consists of a tight mask around the nose *and/or* mouth, with assistance provided by the apparatus usually in the form of a continuous positive airway pressure (CPAP). It is possible to also provide some degree of pressure support with each patient-initiated breath. Since the mask can be uncomfortable, and the seal unable to tolerate pressures greater than 10 mmHg, the device has limited use. It should only be considered as a temporizing measure. However despite these limitations, the device can be used for a brief period of time: (i) in preparation for formal intubation; (ii) immediately after extubation to decrease the chance of re-intubation; and (iii) in patients where a therapy or intervention can improve the respiratory status over the next few hours, for example, use of a diuretic for pulmonary edema. Attempts to use the device long term for frank respiratory failure have not met with success. If noninvasive ventilation is utilized for one or more of the above three indications, the lowest CPAP ($\leq$10 mmHg) that provides adequate oxygenation (SaO_2 >90 % with respiratory rate <30/min) and is comfortable for the patient should be utilized. If after a few (usually four) hours there is no improvement in the status, the patient is best intubated and ventilatory support provided though mechanical ventilation.

Endotracheal Intubation and Assisted Ventilation

Respiratory failure after trauma or an acute surgical illness and the need for invasive ventilation is one of the most common reasons for an elderly patient to be admitted to a surgical intensive care unit. However, it is increasingly recognized that the therapy itself – mechanical ventilation – may result in or, if already present, worsen the acute lung injury: ventilator-induced lung injury (VILI). Hence, the aim of mechanical ventilation is to provide ventilatory support to the patient without causing or worsening acute lung injury. To achieve this goal some principles should be kept in mind:

1. Avoidance of atelectrauma or shear stress: In the normal state alveoli inflate during inspiration and partially deflate during expiration, but do not collapse. The complete closure of the alveoli and subsequent reopening with inspiration lead to shear stress on the alveolar wall resulting in damage to type I pneumocytes that are essential for gas exchange and the production of surfactant.

2. Avoidance of volutrauma and barotraumas: In elegant animal experiments, it has been demonstrated that alveoli are damaged both by overstretching even if the airway pressures are low (volutrauma) and by excessive pressure even if the volumes are kept low (barotrauma) [50, 51]. Interestingly as the mean tidal volume has decreased over the past decades, the mortality from acute lung injury and ARDS has also decreased. Since so many other changes in critical care have also taken place, it is difficult to ascribe a cause and effect, but the association is certainly present.
3. Avoidance of toxic levels of oxygen within the alveolus: It is well established that 100 % oxygen is toxic to type II pneumocytes and prolonged periods (>24–48 h) of 100 % oxygen within the alveolus would exacerbate the acute lung injury. What is less clear is the safe upper limit of alveolar oxygen levels which avoids toxicity to the type II pneumocytes is 60 % [52].

While a detailed discussion of ventilation is beyond the scope of this chapter, some basic terms and principles are presented below:

1. Mode – Volume vs. pressure-limited ventilation: There are two modes of ventilation. In the volume limited mode, the ventilator delivers a set volume, irrespective of the pressure required although there is a minimum and maximum level. The pressure-limited mode adjusts the pressure within the circuit, irrespective of the amount required to deliver the set tidal volume.
2. Modality – Assist control (AC) vs. synchronous intermittent mandatory (SIMV) vs. CPAP: The AC mode delivers a set number of breaths/minute to the patient. In addition, each patient-initiated breath also results in delivery of the set tidal volume. In the SIMV mode, the ventilator only delivers the set number of breaths/minute allowing the patient initiated breaths provide a spontaneous tidal volume without any augmentation from the ventilator. The CPAP modality is only used in spontaneously breathing patients with CPAP as the only support provided by the ventilator. All breaths are initiated by the patient. Another parameter utilized in conjunction with CPAP is pressure support (PS). With PS, as the patient initiates a breath, the volume of air entrained will increase due to the additional support provided by the ventilator. PS is also utilized with SIMV to support the patient-imitated breaths that are over and above the ventilator set breaths.
3. Positive end-expiratory pressure (PEEP): PEEP is the lowest pressure in the breathing circuit at the end of expiration. The use of PEEP increases residual volume in the lung thus increasing functional residual capacity. This in turn leads to improvement in oxygenation by not allowing complete alveolar collapse at the end of expiration while at the same time preventing atelectrauma. PEEP is transmitted to the thoracic pressure and can have a negative impact on venous return and thus cardiac output. Hence, the lowest level of PEEP (usually 5–10 mmHg but sometimes higher) necessary to maintain adequate oxygenation should be utilized.
4. Inspiration-expiration (I:E) ratio: In normal breathing the I:E ratio is 1:3. At rest and breathing at15 breaths/min, each respiratory cycle is 4 s of which 1 s is required for inspiration allowing 3 s for expiration. One of the methods of improving oxygenation is to increase the proportion of time spent in the inspiratory phase by altering prolonging the inspiratory time on the ventilator. This will increase the amount of time available for the hemoglobin molecule to be fully oxygenated. Like PEEP, equalizing or reversing the I:E ratio does have a negative impact on venous return and cardiac output.

Weaning from Mechanical Ventilation and Extubation

Ventilator weaning begins almost as soon as the patient is intubated. Studies have shown that the process of daily interruption of sedation leading to improved alertness and mentation is a critical practice towards an efficient weaning process. In this setting, spontaneous breathing trials are utilized to assist the clinicians with predicting which patients can be successfully extubatable. One of the most widely accepted tools used for this is the Rapid Shallow Breathing Index (RSBI), described by Yang and Tobin. The RSBI is calculated by dividing the respiratory rate (*f* as breaths/minute) by the tidal volume (tv in liters) – RSBI = *f*/tv. Most ICUs utilize a RSBI ≤ 105 as predictive of successful extubation and proceed to a spontaneous breathing trial [53]. However, in the elderly some have suggested that an RSBI ≤ 130 maybe more appropriate [54, 55].

Role of Tracheostomy

Patients requiring long-term ventilation often undergo tracheostomy. It is felt by many surgeons that tracheotomy is safer for patients requiring prolonged mechanical ventilation. It may also hasten weaning from the ventilator by reducing the amount of dead space ventilation in the circuitry [56, 57]. However, data supporting this view is limited. There are several small studies that demonstrate that early tracheostomy was associated with improved outcomes in the form of ICU and hospital lengths of stay and possibly reduced incidence of pneumonia. However, a meta-analysis failed to demonstrate any benefit [58, 59]. In contrast, tracheostomies are known to be associated with serious short- and long-term complications [60]. Despite these complications, most surgeons consider converting an endotracheal tube to a tracheostomy in patients requiring mechanical ventilation longer than 10 days. As critical care practice has advanced and more elderly patients are surviving the initial phase of ICU care, the number of tracheostomies performed on elderly patients is steadily increasing. The decision to perform a tracheostomy should also take into consideration the long-term goals of therapy – cure or palliation.

Ethical Considerations and End of Life Care

Mechanical ventilation is associated with significant hospital and medical costs. The outcomes for prolonged mechanical ventilation in elderly patients have been shown to be dependent on primary diagnosis at the time of admission and the acute physiologic derangements rather than age [61]. Our ability to provide prolonged ventilatory support may not constitute a reasonable quality of life. Many geriatric patients have their specific medical wishes reflected in a living will. When not available or if the patient is unable to personally articulate their wishes for medical care, it is important to have a multidisciplinary approach to define the goals of care and determine if these are consistent with the patient's beliefs and values. Family members and healthcare providers alike must account for long-term outcomes, quality of life, and baseline functional status. If appropriate, palliative care providers may provide insight into alternative therapies.

References

1. Sharma G, Goodwin J. Effect of aging on respiratory system physiology and immunology. Clin Interv Aging. 2006;1:253–60.
2. Peterson RJ, Tepas 3rd JJ, Edwards FH, et al. Pediatric and adult thoracic trauma: age-related impact on presentation and outcome. Ann Thorac Surg. 1994;58:14–8.
3. Richter T, Ragaller M. Ventilation in chest trauma. J Emerg Trauma Shock. 2011;4:251–9.
4. Crapo RO. The aging lung. In: Mahler DA, editor. Pulmonary disease in the elderly patient. New York: Marcel Dekker; 1993. p. 1–21.
5. Ware JH, Dockery DW, Louis TA, et al. Longitudinal and cross-sectional estimates of pulmonary function decline in never-smoking adults. Am J Epidemiol. 1990;132:685–700.
6. Turner JM, Mead J, Wohl ME. Elasticity of human lungs in relation to age. J Appl Physiol. 1968;25:664–71.
7. Freye E, Levy JV. Use of opioids in the elderly – pharmacokinetic and pharmacodynamics considerations. Anasthesiol Intensivmed Notfallmed Schmerzther. 2004;39:527–37.
8. Francis Jr J. Surgery in the elderly. In: Goldman DR, Brown FH, Guarneri DM, editors. Peri-operative medicine. 2nd ed. New York, USA: McGraw-Hill, Inc.; 1994. p. 385–94.
9. Hall WJ, Ahmed B. Pulmonary disorders. In: Duthie Jr EH, Katz PR, Malone ML, editors. Duthie: practice of geriatrics. 4th ed. Philadelphia: Saunders; 2007. p. 536–76.
10. Drakulovic MB, Torres A, Bauer TT, et al. Supine body position as a risk factor for nosocomial pneumonia in mechanically ventilated patients: a randomised trial. Lancet. 1999;354:1851–8.
11. Institute for Healthcare Improvement. How-to guide: prevent ventilator-associated pneumonia. Cambridge: Institute for Healthcare Improvement; 2012.
12. Niel-Weise BS, Gastmeier P, Kola A, et al. An evidence-based recommendation on bed head elevation for mechanically ventilated patients. Crit Care. 2011;15:R111. doi:10.1186/cc10135.
13. Berman A, et al. Kozier & Erb's fundamentals of nursing: concepts, process, and practice. Boston: Pearson Education, Inc.; 2012.
14. Lawrence VA, et al. Strategies to reduce postoperative pulmonary complications after non cardiothoracic surgery: systematic review for the American College of Physicians. Ann Intern Med. 2006;144:596–608.
15. Pelus S, Kaplan D. What the new guidelines offer for pre-operative risk reduction. Patient Care. 2006;40(10):18–25.
16. Westwood K, et al. Incentive spirometry decreases respiratory complications following major abdominal surgery. Surgeon. 2007;5:339–42.
17. Ullman DA, Fortune JB, Greenhouse BB, et al. The treatment of patients with multiple rib fractures using continuous thoracic epidural narcotic infusion. Reg Anesth. 1989;14:43–7.
18. Allen GS, Coates NE. Pulmonary contusion: a collective review. Am Surg. 1996;62(11):895–900. PMID 8895709.
19. Michaels AJ. Management of post traumatic respiratory failure. Crit Care Clin. 2004;20(1):83–99, vi–vii.
20. Torres A, Serra-Batlles J, Ros E, et al. Pulmonary aspiration of gastric contents in patients receiving mechanical ventilation: the effect of body position. Ann Intern Med. 1992;116:540–3.
21. Orozco-Levi M, Torres A, Ferrer M, et al. Semirecumbent position protects from pulmonary aspiration but not completely from gastroesophageal reflux in mechanically ventilated patients. Am J Respir Crit Care Med. 1995;152:1387–90.
22. Rodriguez JL, Steinberg SM, Luchetti FA, Gibbons KJ, Taheri PA, Flint LM. Early tracheostomy for primary airway management in the surgical critical care setting. Surgery. 1990;108:655–9.
23. Hansen TS, Larsen K, Engberg AW. The association of functional oral intake and pneumonia in patients with severe traumatic brain injury. Arch Phys Med Rehabil. 2008;89:2114–20.
24. Hollingsed TC, Saffle JR, Barton RG, Craft WB, Morris SE. Etiology and consequences of respiratory failure in thermally injured patients. Am J Surg. 1993;166(6):592–6; discussion 596–7.
25. Kostadima E, Kaditis AG, Alexopoulos EI, Zakynthinos E, Sfyras D. Early gastrostomy reduces the rate of ventilator-associated pneumonia in stroke or head injury patients. Eur Respir J. 2005;26:106–11.
26. Metheny NA, Clouse RE, Clark JM, Reed L, Wehrle MA, Wiersema L. pH testing of feeding-tube aspirates to determine placement. Nutr Clin Pract. 1994;9(5):185–90.
27. Bankhead R, Boullata J, Brantley S, et al. Enteral nutrition practice recommendations. JPEN J Parenter Enteral Nutr. 2009;33(2): 122–67.
28. Metheny NA, Schallom L, Oliver DA, Clouse RE. Gastric residual volume and aspiration in critically ill patients receiving gastric feedings. Am J Crit Care. 2008;17(5):512–9.
29. Pinilla JC, Samphire J, Arnold C, Liu L, Thiessen B. Comparison of gastrointestinal tolerance to two feeding protocols in critically ill patients: a prospective, randomized controlled trial. JPEN J Parenter Enteral Nutr. 2001;25(2):81–6.
30. McClave SA, Martindale RG, Vanek VW, et al. Guidelines for the provision and assessment of nutrition support therapy in the adult critically ill patient: Society of Critical Care Medicine (SCCM) and American Society for Parenteral and Enteral Nutrition (A.S.P.E.N.). JPEN J Parenter Enteral Nutr. 2009;33:277–316.
31. Torres A, El-Ebiary M, Riquelme R, et al. Community-acquired pneumonia in the elderly. Semin Respir Infect. 1999;14:173–83.
32. Centers for Disease Control and Prevention (CDC), USA. Pneumonia and influenza death rates, United States 1979–1994. MMWR. 1995;44:535–7.

33. Hamilton VA, Grap MJ. The role of the endotracheal tube cuff in microaspiration. Heart Lung. 2012;41(2):167–72.
34. Doebbeling BN, Stanley GL, Sheetz CT, et al. Comparative efficacy of alternative hand-washing agents in reducing nosocomial infections in intensive care units. N Engl J Med. 1992;327: 88–93.
35. Herzig S, Howell MD, Ngo LH, Marcantonio ER. Acid-suppressive medication use and the risk for hospital-acquired pneumonia. JAMA. 2009;301(20):2120–8.
36. Scannapieco FA, Yu J, Raghavendran K, Vacanti A, Owens SI, Wood K, Mylotte JM. A randomized trial of chlorhexidine gluconate on oral bacterial pathogens in mechanically ventilated patients. Crit Care. 2009;13(4):R117. Epub 2009 Jul 15.
37. Mahul P, Auboyer C, Jospe R, Ros A, Guerin C, el Khouri Z, et al. Prevention of nosocomial pneumonia in intubated patients: respective role of mechanical subglottic secretions drainage and stress ulcer prophylaxis. Intensive Care Med. 1992;18:20–5.
38. Valles J, Artigas A, Rello J, Bonsoms N, Fontanals D, Blanch L, et al. Continuous aspiration of subglottic secretions in preventing ventilator-associated pneumonia. Ann Intern Med. 1995;122: 179–86.
39. Kollef MH, Skubas NJ, Sundt TM. A randomized clinical trial of continuous aspiration of subglottic secretions in cardiac surgery patients. Chest. 1999;116:1339–46.
40. Kollef MH, Afessa B, Anzueto A, Veremakis C, Kerr KM, Margolis BD, et al. Silver-coated endotracheal tubes and the incidence of ventilator-associated pneumonia: the NASCENT randomized trial. JAMA. 2008;300:805–13.
41. Million Lives Campaign. Getting started kit: prevent ventilator-associated pneumonia how-to guide. Cambridge: Institute for Healthcare Improvement; 2008.
42. Ranji SR, Auerbach AD, Hurd CJ, O'Rourke K, Shojania KG. Effects of rapid response systems on clinical outcomes: systematic review and meta-analysis. J Hosp Med. 2007;2(6):422–32.
43. Brown SD, Walters MR. Patients with rib fractures: use of incentive spirometry volumes to guide care. J Trauma Nurs. 2012;19(2): 89–91.
44. Meyer KC. Lung infections and aging. Ageing Res Rev. 2004;3(1):55–67.
45. Guidelines for the management of adults with hospital-acquired, ventilator-associated, and healthcare-associated pneumonia. American Thoracic Society and the Infectious Diseases Society of America. Am J Respir Crit Care Med. 2005; 171:388–416.
46. Iregui M, Ward S, Sherman G, Fraser VJ, Kollef MH. Clinical importance of delays in the initiation of appropriate antibiotic treatment for ventilator-associated pneumonia. Chest. 2002;122(1): 262–8.
47. Riaz OJ, et al. Bronchoalveolar lavage in the diagnosis of ventilator-associated pneumonia: to quantitate or not, that is the question. Am Surg. 2011;77(3):297–303.
48. Chastre J, Wolff M, Fagon JY, Chevret S, Thomas F, WWermert D, et al. Comparison of 8 vs 15 days of antibiotic therapy for ventilator-associated pneumonia in adults: a randomized trial. JAMA. 2003; 290:2588–98.
49. Malhotra AK, Riaz OJ, Duane TM, Aboutanos MB, Goldberg AE, Smalara KM, et al. Subthreshold quantitative bronchoalveolar lavage: clinical and therapeutic implications. J Trauma. 2008;65: 580–8.
50. Webb HH, Tierney DF. Experimental pulmonary edema due to intermittent positive pressure ventilation with high inflation pressures. Protection by positive end-expiratory pressure. Am Rev Respir Dis. 1974;110:556–65.
51. Dreyfuss D, Soler P, Basset G, Saumon G. High inflation pressure pulmonary edema. Respective effects of high airway pressure, high tidal volume, and positive end-expiratory pressure. Am Rev Respir Dis. 1988;137:1159–64.
52. Bitterman H. Bench-to-bedside review: oxygen as a drug. Crit Care. 2009;13(1):205.
53. Yang KL, Tobin MJ. A prospective study of indexes predicting the outcome of trials of weaning from mechanical ventilation. N Engl J Med. 1991;324:1445–50.
54. Breitenbucher A, Ershowsky P, Krieger B. Rapid, shallow breathing is a predictor of weaning outcome in elderly [abstract]. Am Rev Respir Dis. 1992;145(Pt 2):A520.
55. Krieger BP, Isber J, Breitenbucher A, Throop G, Ershowsky P. Serial measurements of the rapid-shallow-breathing index as a predictor of weaning outcome in elderly medical patients. Chest. 1997;112:1029–34.
56. Ranes JL, Gordon SM, Chen P, Fatica C, Hammel J, Gonzales JP, et al. Predictors of long-term mortality in patients with ventilator-associated pneumonia. Am J Med. 2006;119(10):819.
57. Holzapfel L, Chevret S, Madinier G, Ohen F, Demingeon G, Coupry A, et al. Influence of long-term oro- or nasotracheal intubation on nosocomial maxillary sinusitis and pneumonia: results of a prospective, randomized, clinical trial. Crit Care Med. 1993;21(8):1132–8.
58. Devarajan J, Vydyanathan A, Xu M, Murthy SM, McCurry KR, Sessler DI, Sabik J, Bashour CA. Early tracheostomy is associated with improved outcomes in patients who require prolonged mechanical ventilation after cardiac surgery. J Am Coll Surg. 2012;214(6):1008–16.e4.
59. Gomes Silva BN, Andriolo RB, Saconato H, Atallah AN, Valente O. Early versus late tracheostomy for critically ill patients. Cochrane Database Syst Rev. 2012;(3):CD007271.
60. Cavaliere S, Bezzi M, Toninelli C, Foccoli P. Management of post-intubation tracheal stenoses using the endoscopic approach. Monaldi Arch Chest Dis. 2007;67(2):73–80.
61. Meinders AJ, Van Der Hoeven JG, Meinders AE. The outcome of prolonged mechanical ventilation in elderly patients: are the efforts worthwhile? Age Ageing. 1996;25:353–6.

Renal Replacement Therapy (RRT) 32

Sudha P. Jayaraman and Zara R. Cooper

Introduction and Epidemiology

Elderly trauma patients often require intensive care admission for management of acute surgical illnesses and injuries, their comorbidities, or for clinical decompensation. However, the data on rates of renal failure and subsequent renal recovery for geriatric trauma patients is sorely lacking. Several population-based studies have established the increase in prevalence of acute kidney injury (AKI) with age [1–3], and there is growing literature that outlines the risks, causes, and prognosis of acute kidney injury in elderly patients who are hospitalized or critically ill. Elderly trauma patients are at particularly high risk for AKI because of injury-related hypotension and hypovolemia superimposed on decreased physiologic reserve.

People over the age of 65 occupy 55 % of all ICU bed-days in the United States. The BEST Kidney investigators in a recent prospective observational study of over 29,000 ICU patients found that 5.7 % developed AKI in the ICU [4]. Mortality in critically ill patients with AKI is quite high – patients who developed AKI or required renal replacement therapy (RRT) had an overall hospital mortality of 60.3 % [4]. In AKI, delayed nephrology consultation is associated with increased mortality and morbidity, whether or not dialysis is ultimately required [5]. Chertow et al. reported in 2007 that patients who had any increase in serum creatinine by 0.3 mg/dL had at least four times the odds of death and an increase in hospital costs of $4,886 [6]. Therefore, the cost of renal failure, in terms of lives and dollars, is a major problem in the United States and especially in the growing population over the age of 65 (Table 32.1) [7].

S.P. Jayaraman, MD, MSc
Department of Surgery, Brigham and Women's Hospital, 75 Francis Street, Boston, MA 02115, USA
e-mail: sjayaraman@partners.org

Z.R. Cooper, MD, FACS, MSc (✉)
Department of Surgery, Brigham and Women's Hospital, 75 Francis Street, Boston, MA 02115, USA

Trauma Burn and Surgical Critical Care, Brigham and Women's Hospital, 75 Francis Street, Boston, MA 02115, USA
e-mail: zcooper@partners.org; zaracooper1@gmail.com

Definitions

Historically, the definition of AKI has included 35 different terms in the literature [7, 8]. This lack of standardization has greatly impeded the understanding of the epidemiology of kidney dysfunction. Most recently, nephrologists have proposed using the term "acute kidney injury" as a simple and direct description of the process, one that patients can readily understand and one that includes mild and moderate kidney dysfunction along with outright kidney failure. Additionally, the term injury is thought to better represent the pathologic changes occurring in the kidney parenchyma [7]. In 2004, the Acute Dialysis Quality Initiative (ADQI) workgroup published the RIFLE criteria as a method of staging acute kidney injury. They created an acronym for 3 levels of renal dysfunction (*R*isk of renal dysfunction, *I*njury to the kidney, *F*ailure of kidney function) and 2 levels of outcome (*L*oss of kidney function and *E*nd-stage kidney disease). The dysfunction criteria are based on a relative rise in creatinine, the absolute level of urine output, or both. The failure category uses serum creatinine ≥4 mg/dL, to account for the severity of acute renal disease in patients with chronic renal disease whose relative increase in creatinine may not otherwise reflect AKI [9] (Table 32.2).

Table 32.1 Hospital acquired AKI

Increase in serum creatinine level (mg/dL)	Multivariable OR (95 % CI)	Area under ROC curve	Increase in total cost
0.3	4.1 (3.1–5.5)	0.84	$4,886
0.5	6.5 (5.0–8.5)	0.86	$7,499
1.0	9.7 (7.1–13.2)	0.84	$13,200
2.0	16.4 (10.3–26)	0.83	$22,023

Himmelfarb [7]. Reprinted, with permission, from Elsevier Limited
OR odds ratio, *CI* confidence interval, *ROC* receiving operating characteristic

J.A. Yelon, F.A. Luchette (eds.), *Geriatric Trauma and Critical Care*,
DOI 10.1007/978-1-4614-8501-8_32, © Springer Science+Business Media New York 2014

Table 32.2 Staging for AKI-RIFLE and AKIN criteria

	RIFLE	SCr criteria	UOP criteria	AKIN stage	SCr criteria	UOP criteria
Increasing suverity of AKI ↓	R	↑ SCr × 1.5	<0.5 mL/kg/h × 6 h	1	↑ in SCr ≥0.3 mg/dL or ↑ ≥150–200 % from baseline (1.5- to 2-fold)	<0.5 mL/kg/h for >8 h
	I	↑ SCr × 2	<0.5 mL/kg/h × 12 h	2	↑ in SCr to >200–300 % from baseline (>2- to 3-fold)	<0.5 mL/kg/h for >12 h
	F	↑ SCr × 3, or SCr ≥4 mg/dL with an acute rise of at least 0.5 mg/dL	<0.5 mL/kg/h × 24 h or anuria × 12 h	3	↑ in SCr to >300 % (3-fold) from baseline or SCr ≥4 mg/dL with an acute rise of at least 0.5 mg/dL	<0.5 mL/kg/h × 24 h or anuria × 12 h
	L	Persistent loss of kidney function for >4 weeks				
	E	Persistent loss of kidney function for >3 months				

Dennen et al. [10]. Reprinted, with permission, from Wolters Kluwer Health
RIFLE risk, injury, failure, loss, end-stage kidney disease, *AKIN* acute kidney injury network, *SCr* serum creatinine, *UOP* urine output

The predictive value of RIFLE criteria for mortality is a near-linear relationship between the renal dysfunction by RIFLE criteria and hospital mortality. In a retrospective, single-center trial of 20,126 patients, Uchino et al. found that 9.1 % of all patients fell into the risk category, 5.2 % into the injury category, and 3.7 % into the failure category with hospital mortality of 4.4 % for normal patients, 15.1 % for patients falling in the "risk" group, 29.2 % for patients falling in the "injury" group, and 41.1 % for patients falling in the "failure" group. Multivariate logistic regression analysis indicated that RIFLE criteria were predictive for hospital mortality [11]. The RIFLE criteria have been validated in the elderly and in the critically ill [12, 13].

Risk Factors

The etiology of AKI is often multifactorial in geriatric patients. Age-related changes in renal function make the elderly more susceptible to AKI at baseline [14, 15]. In the trauma setting, hypovolemia from under-resuscitation and shock from hemorrhage play important roles in increasing the risk of AKI. Comorbidities such as diabetes, hypertension, cardiovascular disease, congestive heart failure, and especially preexisting chronic kidney disease are additional independent risk factors for developing, and not recovering from, an episode of AKI. Furthermore, the treatment of these conditions often requires the use of nephrotoxic drugs which further enhance the risk of AKI [12]. Intravascular volume depletion from preexisting congestive heart failure or liver disease increases susceptibility to AKI in the setting of trauma and hospitalization [15]. Contrast-induced nephropathy is thought to be a major cause of kidney injury in elderly patients, although the incidence is unknown. Data from the cardiac literature suggests that age greater than 75 years is an independent risk factor for AKI after percutaneous coronary intervention [16]. The risk is further increased in the setting of chronic kidney disease [10, 15]. Medication-induced nephrotoxicity is another major cause of AKI in the elderly who tend to be on multiple medications and have decreased renal clearance due to age-related changes [15, 17]. Rhabdomyolysis which can be seen in severe trauma may put elderly patients at risk for AKI from deposition of myoglobin, hemoglobin, or light chains [15]. Geriatric trauma patients are also at risk for infection from numerous sources, which is another key risk factor for AKI in this population. Lastly, obstructive nephropathy can also contribute to AKI. Older male patients are at particular risk for obstruction from prostatic disease [15] (Fig. 32.1).

Age-Related Changes of the Kidney and Risk of AKI in the Elderly

Many age-dependent changes occur in the kidney. The glomerular filtration rate (GFR) falls by 10 % per decade after age 40 [14, 18, 19]. This is due to age-related functional reductions in the glomerular capillary plasma flow rate, reduction in afferent arteriolar resistance, and increase in glomerular capillary hydraulic pressure. However, serum creatinine levels in elderly patients can remain within the normal range despite gross reductions in GFR [14, 20]. Serum creatinine is reflective of muscle mass and consumption of protein load both of which are decreased in elderly patients thus making it an unreliable measure of renal functional reserve in this patient population. Structural changes within the kidney also occur with aging and result in the loss of renal mass, hyalinization of afferent arterioles, glomerular arterioles, and an increase in the percentage of sclerotic glomeruli and tubulointerstitial fibrosis. By age 70, the loss in renal mass measured by functioning cortical glomeruli due to ischemia ranges

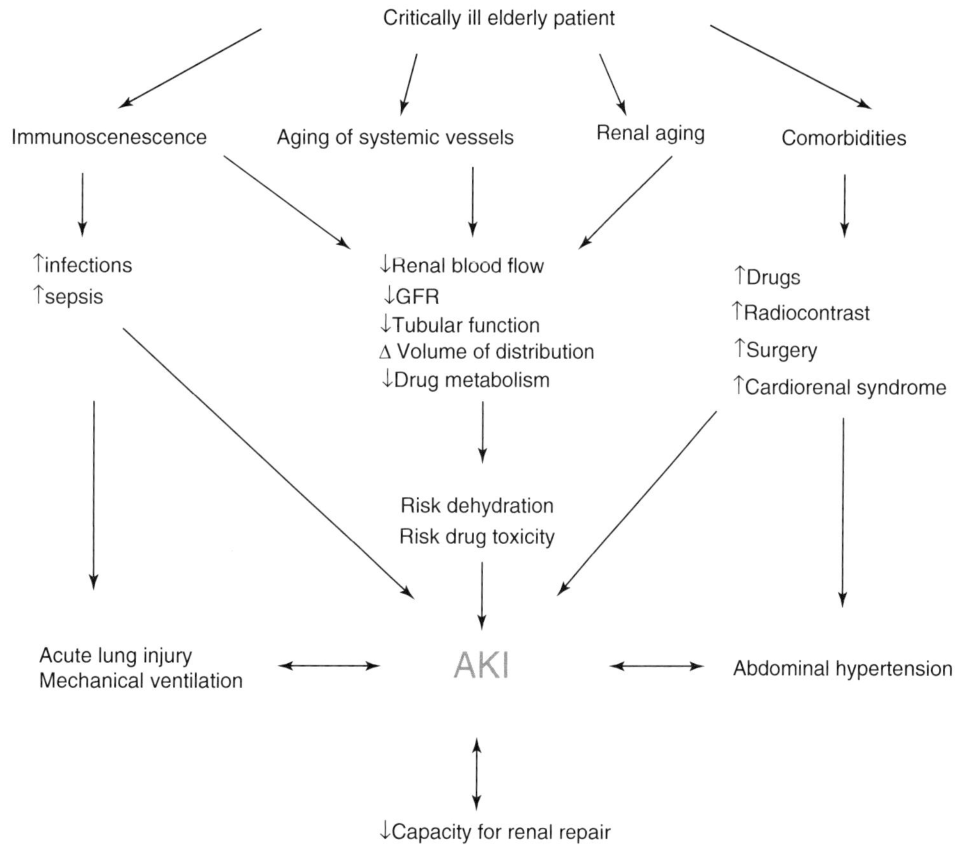

Fig. 32.1 Factors contributing to AKI (Adapted from [12]. Reproduced, with permission, from Springer Science+Business Media)

between 30 and 50 % [15, 19, 21]. Changes in the activity of the renin-angiotensin and nitric oxide systems further lead to loss of urinary concentration and diluting ability, inability to conserve sodium, and decreased plasma renin and aldosterone levels. These changes lead to volume depletion and dehydration, thus making elderly patients more susceptible to AKI when exposed to other risk factors such as trauma, sepsis, or nephrotoxins [19, 21]. With aging, there is also altered activity and responsiveness to vasoactive stimuli. Responses to vasoconstrictor stimuli are enhanced, while vasodilatory responses are impaired which further increases sensitivity to risk factors for AKI. Renal function becomes more dependent on prostaglandin-mediated afferent arteriolar vasodilation with advancing age [19–21]. In the elderly, the traditional features of prerenal AKI such as low urine sodium, low fractional excretion of sodium, low fractional excretion of urea, high urine osmolality, and an elevated blood urea nitrogen/serum creatinine ration are less reliable due to age-related changes in fluid and electrolyte homeostasis. Urine sodium may be over 20 meq/l and urine osmolality less than 500 mOsmol/kg despite intravascular hypovolemia. The inability to concentrate urine may cause inappropriately high urine output. With aging, total body water as a fraction of body weight is also decreased further adding to the risk of AKI [15] (Fig. 32.2).

Chronic Kidney Disease (CKD) and Risk of AKI in the Elderly

Elderly patients with CKD are most susceptible to develop AKI with poor renal recovery because of their decreased renal reserve. Age older than 65 is a risk factor for nonrecovery from AKI and even progression to advanced-stage CKD [17, 22]. Elderly patients with estimated glomerular filtration rate (eGFR) of 45–59 mL/min/1.73 m^2 are at higher risk for AKI compared with their counterparts with eGFR >60 mL/min/1.73 m^2 [1]. Recent data from the Atherosclerosis Risk in Communities Study demonstrated that the adjusted risk of AKI approximately doubles as eGFR declines from 60 to 45 mL/min/1.73 m^2 [9, 23].

Among patients with AKI and baseline GFR <45 mL/min/1.73 m^2, almost half develop ESRD within 30 days, and even those who do not are more likely to develop ESRD within the subsequent 4 years. The annualized risk of ESRD increases to 7–9 % if the AKI occurs in an individual with a preexisting history of CKD [24–26] (Fig. 32.3).

Hypovolemia and Risk of AKI in the Elderly

Intravascular hypovolemia results in AKI due to renal hypoperfusion from decreased effective arterial blood volume.

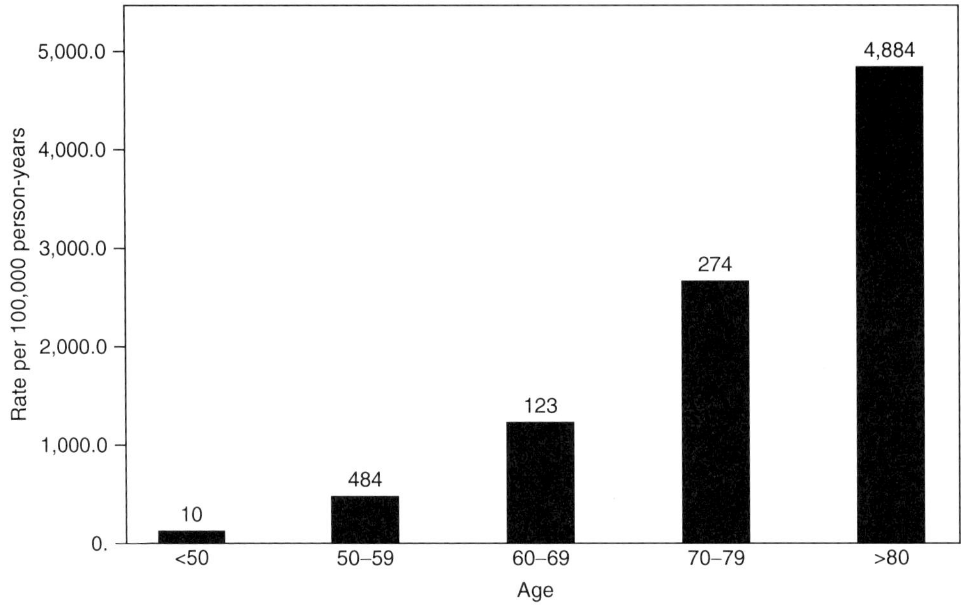

Fig. 32.2 Age and incidence of community-acquired AKI [1] (Reprinted, with permission, from Nature Publishing)

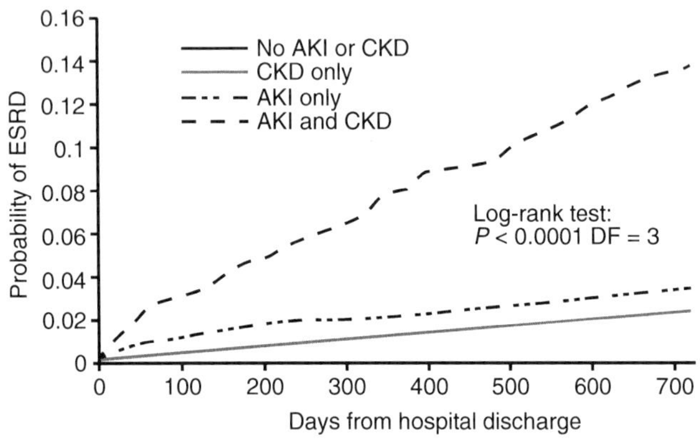

Fig. 32.3 Relationship of AKI and CKD [25] (Reprinted, with permission, from the American Society of Nephrology)

Baseline intravascular hypovolemia from congestive heart disease or liver disease increases the risk of ischemic and nephrotoxic insults in elderly patients who already have physiologic age-related changes as outlined above [14]. Traumatic hemorrhage, third spacing of fluids after operative interventions, and sepsis may result in intravascular volume depletion which increases the risk of AKI [15, 27].

Infection

Elderly are at increased risk for healthcare-associated infections [28, 29], and they also have an increased risk of developing AKI from sepsis [12]. The BEST Kidney investigators reported in their prospective observational study of over 29,000 ICU patients that nearly half of the 5.7 % who developed AKI had septic shock as a likely etiology [4, 30]. Septic AKI is emerging as a separate entity with distinct pathophysiology and outcomes [27].

Drugs and Dye and the Risk of AKI in the Elderly

Medication use may play a significant role in AKI in the elderly. Diuretics and angiotensin-converting enzyme inhibitors used to treat hypertension and congestive heart failure deplete volume which can cause acute kidney injury. NSAIDs are associated with acute tubular necrosis or acute interstitial nephritis. NSAIDs have a longer half-life in the elderly and alter renal hemodynamics by inhibiting the production of vasodilatory prostaglandins and thus increase risk of acute kidney injury [17]. In a nursing home population, NSAIDs were found to increase the risk of AKI by 13 % [31]. Elderly patients also tend to have decreased body mass which increases the risk of AKI associated with NSAID use. Hypersensitivity to medications causes acute interstitial nephritis, a less common cause of AKI. Antibiotics especially penicillins, cephalosporins, and sulfonamides are often implicated.

Contrast-induced nephropathy is a major cause of AKI in hospitalized elderly patients [10, 32, 33]. Older patients with history of CKD particularly have an increased risk of developing CIN. However, recent studies suggest that this may not be the case in trauma patients. McGillicuddy et al. conducted a retrospective review of 1,371 trauma patients and found that intravenous contrast for CT did not result in higher rates of AKI [34]. In another retrospective review of 571 trauma patients admitted to the ICU at a level I trauma center for 48 h, Kim et al. found that nearly 30 % developed AKI. Age over 65years and Injury Severity Score greater than 25 were independent predictors of AKI on multivariate analysis. However, IV contrast did not predict AKI in these patients nor in subgroup analysis of patients >65 years, those who were hypotensive on admission or those who were severely injured (ISS >25) [35].

Obstruction

Postrenal obstruction occurs between the renal pelvis and the urethra. AKI from postrenal obstruction typically occurs in men from benign prostatic hypertrophy or prostate cancer. In women, retroperitoneal and pelvic malignancies are the most important cause of AKI due to obstruction. Space-occupying retroperitoneal lesions such as hematomas or abscesses can also cause ureteral or bladder obstruction in trauma patients. Imaging is essential for diagnosis – ultrasound, CT, or rarely intravenous pyelogram [15].

Workup

A detailed history and physical exam focusing on comorbidities, especially diabetes, hypertension and vasculitides, baseline renal function, and current medications, are essential to assessing the risk for AKI in any given patient. Physical exam should focus on the assessment of volume status and signs of uremia. Laboratory studies should include standard serum complete blood counts, chemistry panels, urine electrolytes, and examination for sediment. Typically a renal ultrasound is used to evaluate for obstructive causes. Rarely, a renal biopsy is necessary to truly establish the diagnosis especially when the cause of AKI is multifactorial [15].

Treatment

Aggressive fluid resuscitation may be needed to correct prerenal causes of AKI. This should be balanced with other conditions such as pulmonary edema, congestive heart failure, and elevated abdominal compartment pressures, which may limit how much volume an individual patient can tolerate. A critical step in treating AKI is to avoid exposure to nephrotoxins and minimize repeated episodes of AKI, which increase the risk of developing oliguric chronic renal failure especially in the elderly.

Diuretics in ARF

The physiologic argument to use diuretics in critically ill patients with AKI is that diuretics increase flow of urine and renal perfusion which reduces continual glomerular injury. Loop diuretics are also thought to decrease metabolic demand of renal tubular cells and reduce oxygen consumption [36]. Furthermore, some papers have shown that oliguric AKI is associated with higher mortality than nonoliguric AKI [36]. However, Karajala et al. conducted a systematic review in 2009 evaluating the role of diuretics in treating AKI and found that diuretics, while useful in managing volume status, do not improve mortality, decrease the need for renal replacement therapy (RRT), or reduce the time for recovery from AKI. Diuretics have a role, in the setting of oliguric AKI, if systemic complications of volume overload such as pulmonary edema are manifested [10, 37].

Indication for RRT

There are several indications for RRT in critically ill patients. RRT can correct electrolyte imbalances, acid/base disturbances, drug toxicity, fluid overload, and uremia [38]. Examples of conditions that may improve with renal support include congestive heart failure, respiratory acidosis from adult respiratory distress syndrome, liver failure, pancreatitis, fluid management in multi-organ failure, lactic acidosis, crush injury, tumor lysis syndrome, and possibly cytokine removal in sepsis [39, 40].

Initiation of RRT in an oliguric patient generally requires evidence of severe hyperkalemia (K >6.5 or rapidly rising levels), severe pulmonary edema, severe acidemia (pH <7.1), uremia, hyponatremia, hypernatremia, hyperthermia, and overdose although specific guidelines for thresholds are lacking [41]. Continuous renal replacement therapy (CRRT), rather than intermittent hemodialysis (IHD), is preferred for critically ill patients with hemodynamic instability. Non renal indications for CRRT are being investigated. Several studies suggest that high-volume hemofiltration may affect levels of inflammatory mediators in sepsis and ARDS although the mechanisms are as yet unclear [39, 40, 42].

Principles of Renal Replacement Therapy

RRT modalities are categorized by mechanisms of fluid and solute removal and by the intermittent versus continuous nature of treatment. Given the lack of definitive outcome data for RRT modality in AKI, current practice is largely dictated by local resources and physician experience.

Fluid Removal – Ultrafiltration

Fluid removal is accomplished through ultrafiltration (UF) in all RRT methods with the exception of peritoneal dialysis (PD). UF uses a pressure gradient to drive fluid across a semipermeable membrane. Factors affecting the UF rate are the transmembrane pressure gradient, membrane water permeability, and membrane surface area.

Solute Removal

The two primary mechanisms of solute removal are diffusion and convection. In hemodialysis, solutes are cleared by diffusion. Diffusion is the movement of a solute from a higher to a lower concentration across a semipermeable membrane. Diffusion is most effective with low molecular weight molecules (<500 Da). The dialysate fluid, which generally contains sodium, bicarbonate, chloride, magnesium, and calcium, runs countercurrent to blood flow, thus maximizing the concentration gradient. The factors affecting the rate of solute clearance are solute molecular weight, flow rates of blood and dialysate, dialysis duration, concentration gradient across the membrane, membrane surface area, and membrane permeability.

Convection, the primary mechanism of solute clearance in hemofiltration, occurs when solutes are "dragged" with water during ultrafiltration. Solutes eliminated by convection include both low molecular weight molecules, such as potassium, phosphates, creatinine, and blood urea nitrogen (BUN), as well as medium molecular weight molecules up to 40,000 Da. Solute clearance is primarily dependent on the ultrafiltration rate, the ultrafiltration coefficient of the membrane, and the sieving coefficient of the solute that is inversely proportional to the molecular weight.

RRT Modalities

Intermittent renal replacement modalities are IHD and sustained low-efficiency dialysis (SLED), also referred to as extended daily dialysis (EDD). The continuous modalities are peritoneal dialysis (PD) and CRRT, which exists in various forms using ultrafiltration, hemodialysis, hemofiltration, hemodiafiltration, and combinations of these. The three primary modalities of RRT used to treat AKI are IHD, CRRT, and SLED. PD, a common modality in chronic kidney disease, is generally not used in the acute setting as it carries an increased risk of peritonitis, cannot be used in patients with recent abdominal surgery or abdominal sepsis, gives insufficient solute clearance in catabolic patients, and reduces respiratory function through impedance of diaphragmatic excursion.

Intermittent Hemodialysis

IHD uses diffusion for solute removal and ultrafiltration for volume removal. In AKI, it is generally performed 3–4 times/week, around 4 h per session, with blood flow rates of 200–300 mL/min and dialysate flow rates of 500–800 mL/min [43]. The advantages include swift solute and volume removal, relatively low cost and complexity, and relatively small anticoagulation requirements due to rapid flow rates. Its primary disadvantage is the risk of hypotension which may be seen in as many as 10 % of patients receiving IHD [43]. The rapid movement of solutes from the extravascular space can also cause cerebral edema, thus IHD is contraindicated in patients with head trauma or hepatic encephalopathy.

Continuous Renal Replacement Therapies

CRRT includes a variety of modalities that use ultrafiltration and may use convection, diffusion, or both. Treatment is 24 h/day with a blood flow of 100–200 mL/min and a dialysate flow of 17–34 mL/min in the case of diffusive technologies [43]. The advantage is a slow shift in both fluid and solutes allowing for better hemodynamic stability and more precise solute concentration control. The gradual nature of solute removal in CRRT makes it less likely to cause cerebral edema [44]. CRRT also has greater cumulative solute removal than IHD due to the longer treatment time.

Replacement solution supplants the ultrafiltrate continuously removed by hemofiltration and hemodiafiltration. Buffers used in the replacement solution are lactate, bicarbonate, or citrate. Lactate and citrate are metabolized by the liver and muscles to produce bicarbonate, which is easily tolerated, but can be unstable in solution. Commercially available bicarbonate solutions are manufactured with a 2-compartment bag to prevent carbonate precipitation during storage. Lactate is stable in replacement solution; however, it may contribute to an existing lactic acidosis in patients with sepsis or liver failure [45]. Citrate provides regional anticoagulation of the hemofilter. The choice of parameters within CVVH offers some flexibility for patients with differing underlying processes [39]. Citrate is successfully used in patients at risk of bleeding, while bicarbonate-based replacement solution is preferred in those with lactic acidosis or liver failure [46].

Slow Low-Efficiency Dialysis/Extended Daily Dialysis

SLED can use the same hemodialysis machines as IHD, but runs for longer periods at slower rates. A usual treatment runs for 6–12 h, with blood flow rate of 200 mL/min, and dialysate flow rate of 300 mL/min. It combines many of the advantages of IHD and CRRT. It is relatively low cost and low complexity since it uses the same technology as IHD; however, it also has the advantages of gradual fluid and solute removal and high total solute removal. In addition, because it is not continuous, other diagnostic and therapeutic procedures can occur between treatments.

RRT Modalities and Outcomes

Data comparing the outcomes of different modalities in AKI continues to be inconclusive, although available data suggest similar survival rates for IHD and CRRT. A meta-analysis by

Kellum et al. in 2002 which examined 14 studies and included 1,400 patients revealed no differences in mortality for CRRT versus IHD. However, on secondary analysis, when controlling for disease severity and study quality, there was a survival advantage with CRRT (RR 0.72; CI, 0.60–0.87, $p<0.01$). The authors concluded that the data were insufficient to make strong recommendations for CRRT in AKI, and a large, randomized clinical trial would be needed to further study outcomes [47]. Another meta-analysis in 2002 found no differences in mortality between IHD and CRRT (IHD vs. CRRT, RR 0.96; CI, 0.85–1.08; $p=0.50$) [48]. Small retrospective studies and recent small randomized prospective trials have all failed to show any survival advantage with the use of CRRT [49–51]. Overall, these studies suggest a lack of survival benefit with CRRT versus IHD, with a possibility of improvement with CRRT in the most severely ill AKI patients.

RRT Dose

While standard dosing targets in ESRD have been developed, dosing targets in AKI are not clear. Studies on dose and schedule of RRT have shown variable results [52–54]. Most recently, the VA/NIH Acute Renal Failure Trial Network (ATN) Study, a multicenter, prospective, randomized, parallel-group trial across 27 institutions, attempted to definitely answer whether high-intensity or low-intensity RRT in critically ill patients resulted in better outcomes as measured by 60-day all-cause mortality. In this study, 1,124 patients were randomized to receive either intensive versus conventional therapy. In the intensive-therapy group, intermittent hemodialysis and sustained low-efficiency dialysis were provided 6 times/week, and continuous venovenous hemodiafiltration was prescribed to provide a flow rate of the total effluent of 35 mL/kg/h, based on the ideal body weight before the onset of acute illness. In the less-intensive strategy, intermittent hemodialysis and SLED were provided 3 times/week (on alternate days except Sunday), and continuous venovenous hemodiafiltration was prescribed to provide a total effluent flow rate of 20 mL/kg/h. The primary end point was death from any cause by day 60. There was no difference between the two groups [55].

Anticoagulation in CRRT

The primary disadvantage of CRRT is the need for continuous heparin anticoagulation to avoid clotting of the hemofilter which increases the risk of bleeding complications. This is a particular issue in geriatric trauma patients who may already be at increased risk for developing bleeding complications. Regional citrate anticoagulation prolongs filter life and has higher efficacy and safety than the alternative method, systemic heparin. It entails a pre-filter infusion of citrate and works by extracorporeal chelation of calcium ions to decrease their availability for calcium-dependent steps in the clotting cascade. Systemic anticoagulation does not occur as the ionized calcium level is restored when blood returning from the extracorporeal system is mixed with venous blood. Rapid metabolism of citrate by the kidney, liver, and muscle restores bicarbonate levels and releases calcium [56]. However, patients with severe liver failure and lactic acidosis may develop citrate toxicity which is characterized as low ionized calcium, elevated total serum calcium, exacerbation of serum acidosis, and an elevation of the anion gap.

A systematic review of studies through June 2005 concluded that, although the quality of available data was poor, it appears that, compared with heparin, anticoagulation with citrate provides better circuit survival time, less bleeding, and some evidence for improved biocompatibility by decreasing activation of coagulation and leukocytes [56]. Two prospective observational trials confirm the trend toward decreased bleeding, although a study in pediatric patients did not demonstrate a benefit in filter clotting time [57, 58]. Citrate anticoagulation can add complexity to CRRT because it can require customized dialysate solutions or replacement fluids and frequent laboratory monitoring, including electrolytes, ionized Ca, and acid/base status [43, 56]. Nonetheless, it is a powerful method for increasing the safety and efficacy of CRRT in AKI. Citrate can cause particular metabolic complications, especially in patients with liver dysfunction and decreased citrate metabolism; however, these are generally not life-threatening and are easily corrected. In addition, available citrate solutions may increase the feasibility of citrate for widespread use and techniques for simpler CRRT protocols. New solutions are continually being developed and tested [59]. A variety of other methods have been studied to address the bleeding risk associated with CRRT and heparin, but are yet to be established as alternatives to heparin and citrate [56].

New Developments in the Treatment of AKI

High-Volume Hemofiltration (HVHF) for Sepsis/SIRS/MODS

Severe sepsis and septic shock are associated with multiple organ dysfunction syndrome (MODS) and mortality in the ICU. Removal of MMW molecules, including pro-inflammatory molecules, via CRRT could be advantageous. However, the benefit of removing inflammatory molecules via CRRT has not been demonstrated [60].

HVHF is an emerging technique that uses specialized CRRT equipment to treat MODS. MODS is associated with a loss of autoregulation of pro- and anti-inflammatory mediators that leads to both "hyperinflammation" and "immunodepression" [61]. Increased clearance of MMW and high molecular weight solutes that make up the inflammatory mediators can be achieved with a high-volume approach [62]. While drug treatments that block a specific mediator have not proven effective, it is postulated that the generalized and nonspecific removal of solutes through HVHF may disrupt the escalation of inflammatory mediators. This theory is described by the "peak concentration hypothesis," the concept that reducing the peaks of soluble mediators by using continuous hemofiltration may interrupt the damage from the pro- and anti-inflammatory processes [63]. Thus far, small and mostly non-randomized studies have pointed to a possible benefit of HVHF in MODS. Machines with a capacity for increased blood flow and increased filter surface area are required. Machines that can safely perform HVHF are now available [63]. A large randomized controlled trial is needed to study the potential benefits of HVHF.

Preventing AKI

The Critical Care Nephrology Working Group of the European Society of Intensive Care Medicine published recommendations in 2010 for the prevention of AKI in adults based on a systematic review of renal-protective strategies in the literature [64]. Some of their key recommendations include:

Volume Expansion: They recommend controlled fluid resuscitation with crystalloids in volume depletion (grade 1C), in patients at risk of contrast nephropathy (grade 1B), and to prevent AKI by certain drugs and avoiding hydroxyethyl starches and albumin. They also suggest the use of bicarbonate solutions in patients at risk of contrast nephropathy when undergoing emergency procedures. They recommend against the use of loop diuretics to prevent or ameliorate AKI (grade 1B evidence).

Vasopressors: The group recommends targeting mean arterial pressures of greater than or equal to 60–65 mmHg or premorbid baseline pressures if available and the use of norepinephrine or dopamine in vasoplegic hypotension (grade 1C). They suggest against using low-dose dopamine to reduce the risk for AKI based on the literature (grade 1A).

Vasodilators: When patients are adequately resuscitated, they suggest using fenoldopam in cardiovascular surgery patients at risk for AKI. They suggest using theophylline instead of fenoldopam or natriuretic peptides for prophylaxis against contrast nephropathy.

Metabolic/Endocrine: They recommend against tight glycemic control in the general ICU population (grade 1A) but suggest using "normal-for-age" glycemic control to prevent AKI (grade 2C). It is recommended that nutritional support for all patients at risk for AKI be provided via the enteral route (grade 2C) and against the use of selenium (grade 1B) or *N*-acetylcysteine (grade 2B) to prevent contrast nephropathy.

Prognosis and Ethical Issues of Treating AKI in the Elderly

The relationship between age and recovery of renal function after AKI is well studied. In a systematic review and meta-analysis in 2008, Schmitt et al. reviewed 17 studies of patients with AKI and used age >65 to predict recovery of kidney function. In the 17 studies, 31.3 % of surviving elderly did not recover renal function as compared to 26 % of patients below the age of 65 (pooled RR 1.28, CI 1.06–1.55, $p<0.05$). The risk of non-recovery was higher in the elderly in studies on intermittent RRT (RR 1.52, CI 1.06–2.17) although looking at continuous RRT, the difference in risk was not statistically significant (RR 1.19, CI 0.85–1.66). When the data was pooled to evaluate recovery at hospital discharge, the elderly had higher risk of non-recovery compared to the young (RR 1.25, CI 1.01–1.54). When follow-up beyond hospital discharge was evaluated, this difference increased (RR 1.57, CI 1.16–2.13). When independence from RRT was used as the end point instead of return to baseline creatinine level, the results persisted in showing that the elderly had a higher risk of non-recovery (RR 1.56, CI 1.18–2.06) [65].

Patients requiring RRT during a critical illness have a reduced survival, particularly in the elderly. The United States Renal Data System reports that patients over the age of 80 who start dialysis for renal failure have a 1-year mortality of 46 % with a median survival time of 15 months for those over 80 years and 8 months for those over 90 years of age. European data is slightly better survival with 1- and 2-year survival for patients over 65 being 69 and 51 %, respectively. In addition to age and underlying disease, comorbidities have a major impact on mortality in the elderly. The survival rate for elderly patients on RRT, who also have cardiovascular disease or diabetes, is lower [66].

Given the high mortality rates associated with RRT in the elderly, the use of RRT in geriatric trauma patients can present ethical challenges. The initiation of RRT and the withdrawal of RRT in this population are controversial. In patients who have a poor prognosis, i.e., a poor quality of life and need for palliative care, including hospice, withholding may be a better alternative to initiating RRT. In patients where renal recovery remains uncertain, clinicians should consider offering a time-limited trial of therapy [67].

Making the transition to permanent dialysis is not straightforward in elderly patients. The Renal Physicians Association and the American Society of Nephrology have published a clinical practice guideline: *Shared Decision-Making in the*

Table 32.3 Recommendations in the clinical practice guideline on "shared decision-making in the appropriate initiation of and withdrawal from dialysis"[a]

Recommendation No. 1: Shared Decision-Making
A patient–physician relationship that promotes shared decision-making is recommended for all patients with either ARF or ESRD. Participants in shared decision-making should involve at a minimum the patent and the physician. If a patient lacks decision-making capacity, decisions should involve the legal agent. With the patient's consent, shared decision-making may include family members or friends and other members of the renal care team.
Recommendation No. 2: Informed Consent or Refusal
Physicians should fully inform patients about their diagnosis, prognosis, and all treatment options, including: (1) available dialysis modalities, (2) not starting dialysis and continuing conservative management that should include end-of-life care, (3) a time-limited trial of dialysis, and (4) stopping dialysis and receiving end-of-life care. Choices among options should be made by patients or, if patients lack decision-making capacity, their designated legal agents. Their decisions should be informed and voluntary. The renal care team, in conjunction with the primary care physician, should insure that the patient or legal agent understands the consequences of the decision.
Recommendation No. 3: Estimating Prognosis
To facilitate informed decisions about starting dialysis for either ARF or ESRD, discussions should occur with the patient or legal agent about life expectancy and quality of life. Depending upon the circumstances (e.g., availability of nephrologists), a primary care physician or nephrologist who is familiar with prognostic data should conduct these discussions. These discussions should be documented and dated. All patients requiring dialysis should have their chances for survival estimated, with the realization that the ability to predict survival in the individual patient is difficult and imprecise. The estimates should be discussed with the patient or legal agent, patient's family, and among the medical team. For patients with ESRD, these discussions should occur as early as possible in the course of the patient's renal disease and continue as the renal disease progresses. For patients who experience major complications that may substantially reduce survival or quality of life, it is appropriate to discuss and/or reassess treatment goals, including consideration of withdrawing dialysis.
Recommendation No. 4: Conflict Resolution
A systematic approach for conflict resolution is recommended if there is disagreement regarding the benefits of dialysis between the patient or legal agent (and those supporting the patient's position) and a member(s) of the renal care team. Conflicts may also occur within the renal care team or between the renal care team and other health care providers. This approach should review the shared decision-making process for the following potential sources of conflict (1) miscommunication or misunderstanding about prognosis, (2) intrapersonal or interpersonal issues, or (3) values. If dialysis is indicated emergently, it should be provided while pursuing conflict resolution, provided the patient or legal agent requests it.
Recommendation No. 5: Advance Directives
The renal care team should attempt to obtain written advance directives from all dialysis patients. These advance directives should be honored.
Recommendation No. 6: Withholding or Withdrawing Dialysis
It is appropriate to withhold or withdraw dialysis for patients with either ARF or ESRD in the following situations:
Patients with decision-making capacity, who being fully informed and making voluntary choices, refuse dialysis or request dialysis be discontinued
Patients who no longer possess decision-making capacity who have previously indicated refusal of dialysis in an oral or written advance directive
Patients who no longer possess decision-making capacity and whose properly appointed legal agents refuse dialysis or request that it be discontinued
Patients with irreversible, profound neurological impairment such that they lack signs of thought, sensation, purposeful behavior, and awareness of self and environment
Recommendation No. 7: Special Patient Groups
It is reasonable to consider not initiating or withdrawing dialysis for patients with ARF or ESRD who have a terminal illness from a nonrenal cause or whose medical condition precludes the technical process of dialysis.
Recommendation No. 8: Time-Limited Trials
For patients requiring dialysis, but who have an uncertain prognosis, or form whom a consensus cannot be reached about providing dialysis, nephrologists should consider offering a time-limited trial of dialysis.
Recommendation No. 9: Palliative Care
All patients who decide to forgo dialysis or for whom such a decision is made should be treated with continued palliative care. With the patient's consent, persons with expertise in such care, such as hospice health care professionals, should be involved in managing the medical, psychosocial, and spiritual aspects of end-of-life care for these patients. Patients should be offered the option of dying where they prefer including at home with hospice care. Bereavement support should be offered to patient's families.

Cohen et al. [67]

[a]Reprinted with permission from the Renal Physicians Association *ARF* acute renal failure, *ESRD* end-stage renal disease

Appropriate Initiation of and Withdrawal from Dialysis in 2000 that provides nine recommendations for the dialysis of patients with AKI and ESRD (Table 32.3). This guideline provides a systematic approach to aiding decision making and resolving ethical conflicts related to renal support and palliative care [67, 68].

References

1. Hsu CY, et al. Community-based incidence of acute renal failure. Kidney Int. 2007;72(2):208–12.
2. Feest TG, Round A, Hamad S. Incidence of severe acute renal failure in adults: results of a community based study. BMJ. 1993;306(6876):481–3.
3. Pascual J, Liano F. Causes and prognosis of acute renal failure in the very old. Madrid Acute Renal Failure Study Group. J Am Geriatr Soc. 1998;46(6):721–5.
4. Uchino S, et al. Acute renal failure in critically ill patients: a multinational, multicenter study. JAMA. 2005;294(7):813–8.
5. Mehta RL, Chertow GM. Acute renal failure definitions and classification: time for change? J Am Soc Nephrol. 2003;14(8): 2178–87.
6. Chertow GM, et al. Acute kidney injury, mortality, length of stay, and costs in hospitalized patients. J Am Soc Nephrol. 2005;16(11): 3365–70.
7. Himmelfarb J. Acute kidney injury in the elderly: problems and prospects. Semin Nephrol. 2009;29(6):658–64.
8. Riviello ED, Christopher K. Critical care nephrology: acute renal failure in the intensive care unit. Nephrol Rounds. 2006;4(10).
9. Bellomo R, et al. Acute renal failure – definition, outcome measures, animal models, fluid therapy and information technology needs: the Second International Consensus Conference of the Acute Dialysis Quality Initiative (ADQI) Group. Crit Care. 2004;8(4):R204–12.
10. Dennen P, Douglas IS, Anderson R. Acute kidney injury in the intensive care unit: an update and primer for the intensivist. Crit Care Med. 2010;38(1):261–75.
11. Uchino S, et al. An assessment of the RIFLE criteria for acute renal failure in hospitalized patients. Crit Care Med. 2006;34(7): 1913–7.
12. Chronopoulos A, et al. Acute kidney injury in elderly intensive care patients: a review. Intensive Care Med. 2010;36(9):1454–64.
13. Joannidis M, et al. Acute kidney injury in critically ill patients classified by AKIN versus RIFLE using the SAPS 3 database. Intensive Care Med. 2009;35(10):1692–702.
14. Rosner MH. The pathogenesis of susceptibility to acute kidney injury in the elderly. Curr Aging Sci. 2009;2(2):158–64.
15. Abdel-Kader K, Palevsky PM. Acute kidney injury in the elderly. Clin Geriatr Med. 2009;25(3):331–58.
16. Mehran R, et al. A simple risk score for prediction of contrast-induced nephropathy after percutaneous coronary intervention: development and initial validation. J Am Coll Cardiol. 2004;44(7):1393–9.
17. Anderson S, et al. Acute kidney injury in older adults. J Am Soc Nephrol. 2011;22(1):28–38.
18. Musso CG, Oreopoulos DG. Aging and physiological changes of the kidneys including changes in glomerular filtration rate. Nephron Physiol. 2011;119 Suppl 1:1–5.
19. Lerma EV. Anatomic and physiologic changes of the aging kidney. Clin Geriatr Med. 2009;25(3):325–9.
20. Weinstein JR, Anderson S. The aging kidney: physiological changes. Adv Chronic Kidney Dis. 2010;17(4):302–7.
21. Long DA, et al. Blood vessels and the aging kidney. Nephron Exp Nephrol. 2005;101(3):e95–9.
22. Coca SG. Acute kidney injury in elderly persons. Am J Kidney Dis. 2010;56(1):122–31.
23. Grams ME, et al. Albuminuria and estimated glomerular filtration rate independently associate with acute kidney injury. J Am Soc Nephrol. 2010;21(10):1757–64.
24. James MT, et al. Glomerular filtration rate, proteinuria, and the incidence and consequences of acute kidney injury: a cohort study. Lancet. 2010;376(9758):2096–103.
25. Ishani A, et al. Acute kidney injury increases risk of ESRD among elderly. J Am Soc Nephrol. 2009;20(1):223–8.
26. Wald R, et al. Chronic dialysis and death among survivors of acute kidney injury requiring dialysis. JAMA. 2009;302(11):1179–85.
27. Bellomo R, et al. Septic acute kidney injury: new concepts. Nephron Exp Nephrol. 2008;109(4):e95–100.
28. Bloomfield MG, Sherwin JC, Gkrania-Klotsas E. Risk factors for mortality in Clostridium difficile infection in the general hospital population: a systematic review. J Hosp Infect. 2012;82:1–12.
29. Ashraf M, Ostrosky-Zeichner L. Ventilator-associated pneumonia: a review. Hosp Pract (Minneap). 2012;40(1):93–105.
30. Bagshaw SM, et al. Septic acute kidney injury in critically ill patients: clinical characteristics and outcomes. Clin J Am Soc Nephrol. 2007;2(3):431–9.
31. Gurwitz JH, et al. Nonsteroidal anti-inflammatory drug-associated azotemia in the very old. JAMA. 1990;264(4):471–5.
32. Kohli HS, et al. Treatment-related acute renal failure in the elderly: a hospital-based prospective study. Nephrol Dial Transplant. 2000;15(2):212–7.
33. Rich MW, Crecelius CA. Incidence, risk factors, and clinical course of acute renal insufficiency after cardiac catheterization in patients 70 years of age or older. A prospective study. Arch Intern Med. 1990;150(6):1237–42.
34. McGillicuddy EA, et al. Contrast-induced nephropathy in elderly trauma patients. J Trauma. 2009;68(2):294–7.
35. Kim DY, et al. Is contrast exposure safe among the highest risk trauma patients? J Trauma. 2011;72(1):61–7.
36. Bagshaw SM, Bellomo R, Kellum JA. Oliguria, volume overload, and loop diuretics. Crit Care Med. 2008;36(4 Suppl):S172–8.
37. Karajala V, Mansour W, Kellum JA. Diuretics in acute kidney injury. Minerva Anestesiol. 2009;75(5):251–7.
38. Mehta RL. Indications for dialysis in the ICU: renal replacement vs. renal support. Blood Purif. 2001;19(2):227–32.
39. Mehta RL. Continuous renal replacement therapy in the critically ill patient. Kidney Int. 2005;67(2):781–95.
40. Ricci Z, et al. Practice patterns in the management of acute renal failure in the critically ill patient: an international survey. Nephrol Dial Transplant. 2006;21(3):690–6.
41. Palevsky PM, Berns JS, Sheridan AM. Renal replacement therapy (dialysis) in acute kidney injury (acute renal failure) in adults: indications, timing, and dialysis dose. In: Basow D, editor. UpToDate. Waltham; 2012.
42. Schetz M. Non-renal indications for continuous renal replacement therapy. Kidney Int Suppl. 1999;72:S88–94.
43. O'Reilly P, Tolwani A. Renal replacement therapy III: IHD, CRRT, SLED. Crit Care Clin. 2005;21(2):367–78.
44. Ronco C, et al. Brain density changes during renal replacement in critically ill patients with acute renal failure. Continuous hemofiltration versus intermittent hemodialysis. J Nephrol. 1999;12(3): 173–8.
45. Heering P, et al. The use of different buffers during continuous hemofiltration in critically ill patients with acute renal failure. Intensive Care Med. 1999;25(11):1244–51.
46. Palsson R, Laliberte KA, Niles JL. Choice of replacement solution and anticoagulant in continuous venovenous hemofiltration. Clin Nephrol. 2006;65(1):34–42.
47. Kellum JA, et al. Continuous versus intermittent renal replacement therapy: a meta-analysis. Intensive Care Med. 2002;28(1):29–37.
48. Tonelli M, Manns B, Feller-Kopman D. Acute renal failure in the intensive care unit: a systematic review of the impact of dialytic modality on mortality and renal recovery. Am J Kidney Dis. 2002;40(5):875–85.
49. Waldrop J, et al. A comparison of continuous renal replacement therapy to intermittent dialysis in the management of renal insufficiency in the acutely III surgical patient. Am Surg. 2005;71(1):36–9.

50. Uehlinger DE, et al. Comparison of continuous and intermittent renal replacement therapy for acute renal failure. Nephrol Dial Transplant. 2005;20(8):1630–7.
51. Gasparovic V, et al. Continuous renal replacement therapy (CRRT) or intermittent hemodialysis (IHD) – what is the procedure of choice in critically ill patients? Ren Fail. 2003;25(5):855–62.
52. Schiffl H. Daily haemodialysis for acute renal failure. Curr Opin Nephrol Hypertens. 2002;11(6):589–92.
53. Ronco C, et al. Effects of different doses in continuous veno-venous haemofiltration on outcomes of acute renal failure: a prospective randomised trial. Lancet. 2000;356(9223):26–30.
54. Bouman CS, et al. Effects of early high-volume continuous venovenous hemofiltration on survival and recovery of renal function in intensive care patients with acute renal failure: a prospective, randomized trial. Crit Care Med. 2002;30(10):2205–11.
55. Palevsky PM, et al. Intensity of renal support in critically ill patients with acute kidney injury. N Engl J Med. 2008;359(1):7–20.
56. Oudemans-van Straaten HM, et al. Anticoagulation strategies in continuous renal replacement therapy: can the choice be evidence based? Intensive Care Med. 2006;32(2):188–202.
57. Bagshaw SM, et al. Is regional citrate superior to systemic heparin anticoagulation for continuous renal replacement therapy? A prospective observational study in an adult regional critical care system. J Crit Care. 2005;20(2):155–61.
58. Brophy PD, et al. Multi-centre evaluation of anticoagulation in patients receiving continuous renal replacement therapy (CRRT). Nephrol Dial Transplant. 2005;20(7):1416–21.
59. Tolwani AJ, et al. Simplified citrate anticoagulation for continuous renal replacement therapy. Kidney Int. 2001;60(1):370–4.
60. Kellum JA, et al. The first international consensus conference on continuous renal replacement therapy. Kidney Int. 2002;62(5):1855–63.
61. Kellum JA, et al. Consensus development in acute renal failure: the acute dialysis quality initiative. Curr Opin Crit Care. 2005;11(6): 527–32.
62. Ronco C. Recent evolution of renal replacement therapy in the critically ill patient. Crit Care. 2006;10(1):123.
63. Ronco C, et al. Interpreting the mechanisms of continuous renal replacement therapy in sepsis: the peak concentration hypothesis. Artif Organs. 2003;27(9):792–801.
64. Joannidis M, et al. Prevention of acute kidney injury and protection of renal function in the intensive care unit. Expert opinion of the Working Group for Nephrology, ESICM. Intensive Care Med. 2010;36(3):392–411.
65. Schmitt R, et al. Recovery of kidney function after acute kidney injury in the elderly: a systematic review and meta-analysis. Am J Kidney Dis. 2008;52(2):262–71.
66. Del Vecchio L, Locatelli F. Ethical issues in the elderly with renal disease. Clin Geriatr Med. 2009;25(3):543–53.
67. Cohen LM, et al. Renal palliative care. J Palliat Med. 2006;9(4):977–92.
68. Claure-Del Granado R, Mehta RL. Withholding and withdrawing renal support in acute kidney injury. Semin Dial. 2011;24(2): 208–14.

Nutrition Support

33

Robert D. Barraco, Michael D. Pasquale,
and Ryan A. Lawless

Introduction

The Current State

The American population continues to age as confirmed by the Federal Interagency Forum on Aging-related Statistics [1]. They noted that in 2008, 39 million people in the USA were over the age of 65, comprising approximately 13 % of the population. Additionally, 5.7 million Americans were over the age of 85. Advances in medicine have increased the average life expectancy, and current information suggests that if a person lives to the age of 65, they can be expected to live another 18.5 years. However, one of the "side effects" of this aging process is the increased prevalence of chronic health conditions and the decline in function of our elderly (>65 years). Twenty-five percent of the elderly population has difficulty with at least one activity of daily living (bathing, dressing, getting in/out of a chair, walking, using a toilet), and 42 % report at least one functional limitation, which includes the ability to feed oneself. In nursing care facilities, 15 % of the elderly patients require assistance with feeding [3]. In general, elderly Americans met or exceeded federal dietary quality standards for only 3 of 12 nutritional components (whole fruit, total grain, and meat and beans) as determined by the Healthy Eating Index – 2005 [1]. Protein-energy malnutrition occurs in up to 10 % of elderly living at home and up to 70 % of hospitalized elderly [2]. Based on the aging of our population and the limitations associated with this aging, efforts must be focused on improving nutritional support.

Nutritional Assessment

Nutritional Scales

Over 200 equations predictive of resting energy expenditure currently exist in the literature. The original equations for resting energy expenditure in humans were derived from healthy human subjects at rest and were subsequently adjusted for illness. Due to a number of confounding factors which include but are not limited to obesity, cachexia, edema, and surgery, calculated values are inaccurate by as much as 55 % when predicting daily needs [4].

Indirect calorimetry is the most accurate method to determine resting energy expenditure and caloric needs in the ICU patient [5]. In 1919, the Harris-Benedict equation, which utilizes the variables of height, weight, age, and sex, was derived using data from indirect calorimetry that had been performed in healthy subjects. Once the resting energy expenditure is determined, an illness-based variable multiplier is used to approximate the patient's caloric needs. This equation has been shown to be unreliable when applied to malnourished and critically ill patients and frequently underestimates the caloric requirements when compared to indirect calorimetry [5]. The available evidence suggests that the Harris-Benedict equation should not be used for patients in an ICU setting.

The Ireton-Jones equation, published in 1992, was derived from a multivariate regression analysis including the variables age, weight, sex, and the presence/absence of trauma or burns. The original equation appeared to overestimate needs and was revised in 1997 in an attempt to increase its accuracy compared to indirect calorimetry. The 1997 revision performed poorly in younger and obese patients and in

R.D. Barraco, MD, MPH, FACS, FCCP (✉)
Department of Surgery, Lehigh Valley Health Network, 1240 S Cedar Crest Blvd, Suite 308, Allentown, PA 18103, USA
e-mail: robert_d.barraco@lvhn.org

M.D. Pasquale, MD
Department of Surgery, Lehigh Valley Health Network, 1240 S Cedar Crest Blvd, Suite 308, Allentown, PA 18103, USA
e-mail: michael.pasquale@lvh.com

R.A. Lawless, MD
Department of General Surgery, Lehigh Valley Health Network, 1240 S Cedar Crest Blvd, Suite 308, Allentown, PA 18103, USA
e-mail: ryan_a.lawless@lvhn.org, ryanlawless@gmail.com

J.A. Yelon, F.A. Luchette (eds.), *Geriatric Trauma and Critical Care*,
DOI 10.1007/978-1-4614-8501-8_33,

general was felt to underestimate caloric needs. While the original equation is generally the preferred of the two, neither has been shown to be very accurate when compared to indirect calorimetry [6].

Swinamer et al. derived an equation using variables that contribute >3 % of energy expenditure: total body surface area, age, respiratory rate, tidal volume, and temperature. While the accuracy of this equation is better than others (45–55 %), it is not utilized frequently because it is cumbersome and not user friendly [4].

A group at Penn State University developed an equation using data from mechanically ventilated, medical/surgical critical care patients in 1998 [7]. The original equation utilized the patient's adjusted body weight in the setting of obesity; however, a modified version was derived in 2003 specifically for obese patients, which led to improved accuracy in that population. The accuracy of the PSU [m] equation is 93 % in the nonobese elderly and 67 % in the obese elderly mechanically ventilated medical/surgical/trauma patient. No stress factor adjustment is necessary for either of these equations, and they are more user friendly than the Ireton-Jones equations [7].

Modified equation:

$$\text{RMR}\ (\text{kcal/day}) = \text{Mifflin} - \text{St Jeor}\ (0.71) + \text{Tmax}(85) + \text{Ve}(64) - 3{,}085$$

Original equation:

$$\text{RMR}\ (\text{kcal/day}) = \text{MSJ}(0.96) + \text{Tmax}(167) + \text{Ve}(31) - 6{,}212$$

Mifflin-St Jeor [6]

$$\text{Male}: 10(\text{wt}) + 6.25(\text{ht}) - 5(\text{age}) + 5$$

$$\text{Female}: 10(\text{wt}) + 6.25(\text{ht}) - 5(\text{age}) - 161$$

(RMR = resting metabolic rate, Tmax = maximum body temperature, Ve = minute ventilation, wt = weight in kilograms, ht = height in meters) [6]

The American College of Chest Physicians (ACCP) consensus statement in 1997 recommends 25 kcal/kg of usual body weight for calculating resting energy expenditure to avoid overfeeding. The calculation for obese individuals (BMI >25 using ACCP definitions) should utilize ideal body weight (Male IBW = 50 kg + 2.3 kg for each inch >60 in., Female IBW = 45.5 kg + 2.3 kg for each inch >60 in.). Underweight patients (BMI <16) are at increased risk for refeeding syndrome. The calculation for REE in this setting should utilize the actual body weight for the first 7–10 days and then the ideal weight thereafter. For example, a 70 kg male with a BMI of 25 has a resting energy expenditure of 70 kg × 25 kcal/kg or 1,750 kcal [8].

Metabolic Requirements

Physiologic Changes

While aging decreases the basal metabolic rate (BMR), physiologic aging does not progress at the same rate in all individuals. It is agreed that between the ages of 30 and 70 years, the BMR decreases by approximately 16 % and body composition changes such that there is increased fat and decreased protein content [9, 10]. Lean body mass for the average 30-year-old is approximately 45 % of total body weight (TBW) and for a 70-year-old is approximately 27 % TBW, while the total body fat is 14 % of TBW for age 30 and 30 % of TBW for age 70 [11].

A number of factors impact on appetite as patients' age. The incidence of dysgeusia and dysosmia increases secondary to the decreasing number of taste buds, peripheral olfactory atrophy, and less saliva production. The first taste buds to be lost detect sweet and salt quality with bitter and sour diminishing later. Due to these changes food begins to taste bitter and not smell appetizing [3, 9, 12]. Additionally, the physiologic regulation of appetite is a complex neural and hormonal network involving the autonomic nervous system, enteric nervous system, and hypothalamic-pituitary-adrenal axis in homeostatic balance. This balance is disrupted with chronic diseases, cancers, inflammatory processes, and polypharmacy, resulting in an overall decrease in appetite [12].

Renal function declines with age and 40 % of nephrons are sclerotic by the age of 85. This process is accelerated in patients with diabetes, hypertension, dyslipidemia, and/or atherosclerosis. As renal function declines, the ability to regulate fluid balance and acid/base status deteriorates, and dehydration can occur as the kidney is unable to respond to renal sodium and water losses. This is likely secondary to a decreased responsiveness to ADH and decreased renin-angiotensin system activity, as well as diminished thirst [3, 13].

The gastrointestinal tract also undergoes age-related changes that include esophageal dysmotility from a change in peristalsis, chronic atrophic gastritis, intestinal bacterial overgrowth, and chronic constipation. All of the above-mentioned factors, as well as laxative abuse, impact the intake and absorption of nutrients [9, 10]. Dyspepsia frequently occurs in the elderly and is most commonly related to peptic ulcer disease, gastroesophageal reflux, or gastric cancer [13]. Lactase, an essential enzyme in the digestion of dairy products, is produced in lesser amounts in the elderly, which leads to lactose intolerance resulting in stomach cramps and diarrhea. These factors contribute to malnutrition and vitamin/mineral deficiencies in the geriatric population [3]. Malnutrition, in turn, increases the incidence of complications such as wound failure/infection and nosocomial infections when combined with age-related reductions in skin integrity and immunocompetence. In an ICU setting these complications are associated with negative outcomes and potentially death [9, 10].

Common Deficiencies

The aging population is at risk for deficiencies in many vitamins and nutrients. Decreased appetite, the inability to chew certain foods (e.g., fresh fruits and vegetables), and the increased incidence of lactose intolerance are contributing factors to these deficiencies (Table 33.1).

Vitamin D deficiency in the elderly is multifactorial with decreased consumption of vitamin D-fortified dairy products occurring secondary to an increased incidence of lactose intolerance. Further, less exposure to sunlight disrupts the conversion of vitamin D to the active form. This can be more pronounced in institutionalized patients who have limited exposure to direct sunlight. Finally, as the kidney ages, its ability to convert vitamin D to the active form also decreases. In order to prevent vitamin D deficiency, it should be supplemented (600 IU daily) in the diet, and efforts should be directed at providing the elderly with more exposure to sunlight [11, 13].

Red meat is the primary source of vitamin B12, and deficiencies may be related to food cost, dietary caloric restrictions, and difficulty with mastication due to poor dentition. Twenty percent of the geriatric population are deficient in vitamin B12 [13]. Decreased gastric acid secretion related to aging and/or the use of acid-reducing medications diminishes intrinsic factor production which can lead to atrophy of the gastric mucosa. Intrinsic factor is essential for the release of vitamin B12 from its carrier protein as well as absorption. Signs and symptoms of vitamin B12 deficiency include anemia, neuropathy, and dementia [11, 13].

Vitamin K deficiency is not prevalent in the geriatric population; however, certain medications may lead to an inadequate absorption such as anticoagulants, antibiotics, and sulfa drugs. This vitamin should be kept in mind when starting these medications in the intensive care setting [11].

Nutritional Monitoring

There is no standard way to measure malnutrition in the hospitalized elderly patient. There are screening tools to help identify those individuals at risk. Screening is important due to the adverse effects of malnutrition on outcomes. Patients presenting malnourished have increased hospital stays, more complications, and higher mortality rates. In this section, we will discuss risk factors, screening tools, and biochemical markers of malnutrition.

Risk Factors

Risk factors for malnutrition in the elderly include those unrelated to age and those related to age [2]. Factors unrelated to age include cancer, chronic and severe organ failure, gastrointestinal diseases, alcoholism, chronic infectious and/or inflammatory diseases, as well as all factors likely to cause one or more of the following: a reduction in food intake, an increase in energy requirements, and malabsorption.

Risk factors related to age include psychological, social and environmental factors such as depression, grieving, financial hardship, and admission to a long-term care facility. Oral, dental, and swallowing disorders can contribute to

Table 33.1 Common deficiencies [39]

Deficiency	Etiology	Symptoms/signs	Recommendation
Vitamin D	1. Increased incidence of lactose intolerance 2. Decreased intake 3. Decreased sunlight exposure 4. Decreased renal conversion of vitamin D to the active form	Bone pain, muscle weakness	600 IU
Vitamin B12	1. Decreased intake of red meat due to cost, difficulty with mastication, caloric restriction 2. Atrophic gastritis	Anemia, neuropathy, dementia	Adequate dietary intake with supplementation if necessary
Vitamin K	1. Anticoagulant use 2. Antibiotic use 3. Sulfa medications	Easy bruising/bleeding, hematuria, hematochezia	Adequate dietary intake with supplementation if necessary
Calcium	1. Hormonal changes in women (postmenopausal) 2. Inadequate intake	Osteoporosis	800–1,200 mg/day
Water	1. Diminished thirst sensitivity 2. Fluid loss through diarrhea/vomiting not replaced	Altered mental status, hypotension	30 cc/kg/day

malnutrition. Dementia and other neurological disorders put the elderly at increased risk. Acute problems that result from trauma such as pain, fractures, and surgery increase the risk for malnutrition the elderly.

Screening Tools

Screening for malnutrition includes evaluating risk factors, appetite and food intake, comparing weights as possible, and calculating body mass index. These may contribute to the diagnosis of malnutrition, but will not be obtainable in the obtunded trauma patient.

The Mini Nutritional Assessment (MNA) has been used as a standard for screening the elderly for malnutrition risk and is recommended in the 2007 evidence-based guideline from France. Questions address various areas and include appetite, meals, and weight loss. It also contains objective measurements of calf and midarm circumference. There is also a short form, the MNA-SF, which contains only 6 items [38]. An even shorter subset focusing on dietary habits, called the MNA-3, is suggested as the most important component of screening [14].

Albumin

Visceral protein stores can be assessed by serum albumin concentration. Albumin is a plasma protein that maintains plasma oncotic pressure and a carrier protein for multiple elements and drugs. Testing serum levels is routinely available and the normal range is between 3.5 and 5 g/dL. The half-life of serum albumin is approximately 20–21 days; therefore, loss of protein stores will be reflected in the serum level at that time. Serum albumin is a reliable marker in the absence of liver disease, renal disease, prolonged bed rest, infection/sepsis, and cancer. However, these ailments are frequently comorbidities for many of the geriatric patients that enter critical care units [11, 15].

The assay of C-reactive protein may assist in interpreting the albumin result when an inflammatory process is involved. Serum albumin may distinguish between two forms of malnutrition: that due to a deficiency in food intake (albumin may be normal) and that due to inflammation and a catabolic state, with a rapid fall in serum albumin [2].

Transferrin

Transferrin is a protein that binds iron for transport to the bone. Its levels are affected by total body iron storage [15]. With aging, body tissue iron stores increase leading to a decrease in transferrin levels in healthy individuals. However, malnourished elderly patients with decreased protein and low iron stores may express a normal transferrin level. The 8–10-day half-life makes transferrin a good choice to assess the nutritional status of younger individuals, but should not be used in the geriatric population [10]. Normal serum values are between 200 and 400 mg/dL [15].

Prealbumin

Prealbumin is a visceral protein synthesized by the liver that binds thyroxine. The half-life of prealbumin is approximately two days making it a promising biochemical marker of protein storage and ideal for short-term nutritional assessment. Normal serum levels are between 18 and 40 mg/dL [11, 15].

Total Lymphocyte Count

Depressed total lymphocyte count can be a marker of malnutrition as it is used as a measure of immunocompetence. However, the total lymphocyte count can be altered by a wide variety of factors including hypoalbuminemia, infection, chronic comorbid conditions, and malignancy. The normal range is greater than 1,500 cells/mm^3 [11]. Total lymphocyte count is not an adequate indicator of nutritional status in the geriatric populations as it is affected by the factors mentioned above [16].

Diagnosis of Malnutrition

Per the French Guideline on Protein-Energy Malnutrition, the diagnosis of malnutrition is based on one or more of the following criteria: [2] weight loss ≥5% in 1 month or ≥10% in 6 months, body mass index <21 (a BMI ≥21 does not exclude the diagnosis of malnutrition), serum albumin concentrations <35 g/L, and MNA score <17.

Severe malnutrition may be diagnosed by one or more of the following criteria:

weight loss of ≥10% in 1 month or ≥15% in 6 months, BMI <18 , and serum albumin <30 g/L. Severe malnutrition requires rapid nutritional management.

Nutritional Requirements (See Table 33.2)

Carbohydrates

Half of the average Western diet consists of calories derived from carbohydrates. The body is able to store approximately 1,200 cal in the liver and muscle in the form of glycogen. These stores are immediately available and depleted within three days of starvation. This process begins between 8 and

Table 33.2 Nutritional requirements [39]

Variable	Requirement	70 kg nonstressed patient	70 kg ICU patient
Calories	25 kcal/kg/day	1,750 kcal	1,750 kcal
Protein	1.0–1.5 g/kg/day	70 g = 280 kcal	105 g = 420 kcal
Fat	20–30 % daily caloric intake (20 %)	38 g = 350 kcal	38 g = 350 kcal
Carbohydrates	Makes up the rest of daily caloric intake	1,750 – (280 + 350) = 1,120 kcal [kcal/4 = 280 g]	1,750 – (420 + 350) = 980 kcal [kcal/4 = 245 g]
Intravenous fluid	25–30 cc/kg/day	2,100 cc/day	2,100 cc/day
Vitamin E	10 IU/day		
Vitamin C	200 mg/day		
Zinc	2.5–5 mg/day		
Copper	0.3–0.5 mg/day		
Selenium	20–60 mcg/day		

16 h postprandially. Glycogenolysis occurs as insulin levels decrease, mobilizing glucose from hepatic stores. Alanine is also essential for this process in muscle and is used for gluconeogenesis as muscle cannot mobilize glucose from glycogen for lack of glucose-6-phosphatase [12]. The ability to metabolize glucose diminishes with age, leading to chronically elevated blood glucose levels and the development of advanced glycosylation end products (AGEs). AGEs promote fibrosis, decrease connective tissue flexibility, and change the extracellular matrices of the heart, kidney, skin, and central nervous system. These changes result in many of the common comorbid conditions in the geriatric population: neuropathy, nephropathy, cardiomyopathy, atherosclerosis, etc [12]. Therefore, it is recommended that elderly individuals consume complex carbohydrates rather than simple sugars [11].

Proteins

The average adult requires 0.8 g of protein per kilogram body weight daily. The body is able to store protein in large amounts. However, only 50 % of the proteins can be utilized without serious consequences. Over 50 % depletion of protein stores is incompatible with life [12]. In the stress state, the body may require up to 1.5 g/kg/day to support wound healing, immune function, etc. Furthermore, patients whom are bedbound, or institutionalized, require more than average protein to maintain nitrogen balance. This is not intuitive as one may believe that since lean muscle mass decreases in the elderly population, protein requirements would follow suit. However, the amount of nitrogen retained by the body decreases with decreased caloric intake, and in order to maintain positive nitrogen balance, additional protein must be provided. The average elderly person requires 1.0 g/kg/day of protein in order to maintain skeletal muscle protein metabolism which requires a larger amount of essential amino acids [11, 17]. Finally, only 25 % of undernourished patients achieve protein and energy requirements by day 4 of their hospitalization [18]. Protein intake is essential and should not be overlooked.

Lipids

Up to 40 % of the calories that make up the average Western diet are from fat. This is 10 % in excess of the daily requirement and is approximately 600 unnecessary kilocalories daily. The greatest amount of energy storage in the body is in the form of fat. During starvation, free fatty acids are released in the normal state; however, in the elderly patient, the mobilization of fat does not occur as readily leading to excess protein breakdown and sarcopenia [11, 17]. Fat is a requirement in every diet, but should not exceed 30 % of total caloric intake. If being administered parenterally, triglyceride levels should be monitored and elevated levels should prompt a reduction of infusion.

Vitamins and Minerals

Vitamin E, vitamin C, zinc, copper, and selenium are vitamins and minerals that have been shown to improve outcomes in critically ill surgical patients receiving nutritional support. A variety of combinations of the antioxidant vitamins and minerals administered have shown a decrease in mortality. Studies have also shown that adding selenium to the nutritional source reduces mortality in sepsis and septic shock [19, 20].

Calcium

Calcium is used to maintain bone health and structure and to minimize the risk of fractures in the elderly. Osteoporosis is aggravated by age-related hormonal changes, particularly in women. Total bone mass decreases with age and inadequate intake leading to lower vertebral, hip, femoral, and cervical spine fractures. This affects women more so than men secondary to gender-specific hormonal changes, dieting, childbearing, breastfeeding, and life longevity. Calcium requirements increase with age. The recommendation for calcium intake is 800–1,200 mg/day with supplementation if levels cannot be maintained with diet [9, 13].

Fluids

Dehydration is a major concern in the geriatric population. Cellular dehydration and hypovolemia are the two main factors involved in thirst regulation. Thirst sensitivity decreases with age leading to high risk for dehydration. The recommended fluid intake is 30 mL of fluid per kilogram of body weight. This amount increases substantially in patients with vomiting or diarrhea and should be based on clinical findings [11].

Glutamine

Glutamine is the essential nutrient used by intestinal epithelium for maintenance of function. Enterocytes, lymphocytes, and macrophages utilize glutamine to maintain intracellular levels of ATP. In critical illness, the gut is susceptible to loss of mucosal integrity, increasing the risk of bacterial translocation, sepsis, and death. Adding glutamine (0.3–0.5 g/kg/day) to enteral formulas has been shown to decrease hospital mortality in burn and mixed ICU patients [20, 22].

Indications for Nutritional Support

All patient admitted to the hospital should be screened for the risk of malnutrition. The rationale for screening all patients stems from studies showing increased complication rate, mortality rate, and length of stay in malnourished patients (ASPEN-1). The goal of aggressive early nutritional support is the maintenance of immunological integrity, preservation of lean body mass, and aversion of metabolic complications [19, 21].

Patients with oral/esophageal obstructions, dysphagia, psychomotor diseases (Parkinson's disease, Huntington's disease, multiple sclerosis, dementia), polytrauma, poor dentition, and xerostomia have difficulty consuming nutrients orally. Patients with loss of appetite, depression, decreased metabolism with aging, and decreased colonic motility lose the desire to eat. Even though patients may eat, the caloric intake may be inadequate. Contributing factors include infections (e.g., urinary tract), polypharmacy, and electrolyte imbalances [11, 19, 22].

"At risk" patients, as determined by initial screening, should then have their nutritional status assessed. Traditional nutritional assessments include anthropometry and laboratory values such as albumin, prealbumin, transferrin, and total lymphocyte count. The assessed values are valid in "normal" patients outside and can be useful within the critical care arena.

Anthropometric data obtained should include height (cm), weight (kg), body mass index (kg/cm^2), and skinfold measurements to determine fat and protein stores. There is a great deal of variability in these measurements between physicians and even when repeated by the same physician. A trained technician or physician should obtain these measurements with validity testing performed often. The measurements obtained are more useful in the outpatient setting [11].

Laboratory values are discussed within the nutritional monitoring section of this chapter. The values are more for nutritional monitoring rather than determination of nutritional status as most are acute phase reactants affected by a patients' metabolic state.

Other important nutritional assessment parameters include the patients' normal weight and any recent weight loss, pre-illness caloric intake, the severity of their disease state, comorbid conditions, and gastrointestinal function. Once a patient is identified as being malnourished, interventions should be made in the form of enteral nutrition, parenteral nutrition, or supplementation (Table 33.3) [19].

Table 33.3 Methods of nutritional support [39]

	Indications	Route of administration	Pros	Cons
Enteral	"If the gut works, use it"	Oral (preferred), nasogastric, nasoenteric, gastrostomy, jejunostomy	Decreases rate of infectious comorbidities, decreases length of stay, preservation of mucosal integrity	Aspiration, vomiting, electrolyte imbalance, hyperglycemia, hyperosmolar diarrhea, clogging of delivery system, mechanical bowel obstruction, bowel perforation/tube dislodgement
Parenteral	Well nourished – after 7 days without enteral nutrition Malnourished – preoperatively and continue into postoperative period	Central venous access (peripheral insertion vs. central venous catheter)	Restoration of nitrogen balance and anabolic state	Access complications (pneumothorax, hemothorax, infection, venous thrombosis), electrolyte imbalance, hepatic dysfunction

Enteral Nutrition

Surgical dogma has dictated, "if the gut works, use it." This simple statement has been backed by many studies throughout the literature. The enteral route of nutrition administration is preferred for multiple reasons. Studies have shown a decreased rate of infectious comorbidities including pneumonia, central venous catheter infection, and abdominal abscess in trauma. Decreased length of stay and cost has also been shown. Other benefits include the preservation of intestinal mucosal integrity [19]. Feeding enterocytes promotes the release of endogenous hormones, blood flow, and secretory IgA immunocytes. Without these factors gut permeability increases leading to a breakdown in the mucosal defense system and the theoretical risk of bacterial translocation, systemic infection, and multiorgan system failure [19]. Enteral nutrition can be delivered via nasogastric and nasojejunal tubes or gastrostomy and jejunostomy tubes.

When should enteral nutrition be initiated? The general answer to this has to do with the patient's nutritional status, timing of presentation to the hospital, and the procedure to be performed. In the case of elective surgery, if the patient is determined to be protein malnourished, nutritional support should be initiated 10 days preoperatively [23]. However, emergent/unplanned admissions do not have the luxury of extensive preoperative planning, and the answer becomes when the patient is hemodynamically stable and fully resuscitated with a time frame between 24 and 48 h from admission. Feedings should not be started nor initiated if the patient is hemodynamically unstable or under resuscitated secondary to the risk of ischemic bowel. Patients requiring vasopressors to maintain adequate perfusion should not be started on enteral nutrition unless the vasopressor requirement has been stable. Initiating enteral feedings for patients on a stable vasopressor dose warrants close monitoring for intolerance [19].

Old surgical dogma included the presence of bowel sounds as criteria for the initiation of enteral nutrition. The absence of bowels sounds has not been shown to be associated with enteral nutrition intolerance and should not be used as criteria for initiation. Gastric residuals are often checked during the infusion of tube feedings as an indicator of tolerance. The literature has shown that a range of aspirate between 200 and 500 cc is elevated [3, 19]. However, tube feedings should not be held, and interventions to promote gastric emptying and decrease aspiration risk should be initiated unless the patient is showing signs of intolerance (pain, distention, absent flatus). These interventions include administration of a prokinetic agent, elevating the head of the bed, and possibly inserting a small bowel feeding tube. Gastric residuals >500 cc should prompt cessation of enteric feeding with the intent of attempting again in the near future after the initiation of the interventions mentioned above [19].

There are many formulations of enteral nutrition from predigested amino acid-based formulations to immune-modulating formulations. With so many different options and new products coming to the market, what should be used and when? Immune-modulating enteral formulations contain arginine, glutamine, nucleic acids, omega-3 fatty acids, and antioxidants. These formulations are beneficial in major elective general surgery, trauma (ISS >20), burn, obese patients (BMI >30), and head and neck cancer patients in the intensive care setting on mechanical ventilation. Benefits include decreased time on mechanical ventilation, infectious morbidities, and hospital length of stay. There was no significant impact on mortality. These benefits were more profound in patients that were determined to be malnourished preoperatively and started on supplemental nutrition 7 days prior to surgery [19].

Another subset of patients are those with adult respiratory distress syndrome (ARDS) or acute lung injury (ALI). Enteral formulations with an anti-inflammatory lipid profile are beneficial to this subset. The formulation includes omega-3 fatty acids (eicosapentaenoic acid), fish oil, borage oil, and gamma-linolenic acid. Benefits include decreased ICU length of stay, time on mechanical ventilation, and organ failure. However, no significant impact on mortality was found [19].

Protein is important for wound healing, maintenance of immune function, and maintenance of lean body mass. Supplementation for patients with a BMI <30 should occur to increase the protein consumption to 1.2–2.0 g/kg/day. This is especially beneficial in patients with negative nitrogen balance, which is the preferred method to determine need for protein supplementation rather than albumin, prealbumin, transferrin, and total lymphocyte count [19].

Complications of enteral nutrition arise from the formulation, infection, or route of delivery. Formulation complications include diarrhea, vomiting, constipation, aspiration, hyperglycemia, and electrolyte imbalance. At times, patients may have diarrhea secondary to an infectious etiology while on tube feedings; therefore, if a patient develops loose stools, it should be immediately investigated. Possible etiologies include hyperosmolar substances/formulation, recent broad-spectrum antibiotics, and Clostridium difficile colitis. Physical exam, fecal white blood cell count, stool quantification, and basic metabolic profile should be obtained [19]. Aspiration is a serious complication and is the most common cause of death after percutaneous gastrostomy tube insertion [3]. Subclinical aspiration can be seen in patients who develop chronic cough with enteral access. In this population changing the nasogastric tube to a nasoenteric tube may decrease the incidence of aspiration.

The mechanics of the route of delivery can also lead to complications. Clogging of the tube with inspissated tube feedings occurs in 18–45 % of tubes placed. This complication prompts attempts at flushing the tube or dissolving the tube feeds with warm water, cola, pancreatic enzyme, and meat tenderizer [24]. In the case of percutaneous endoscopically or surgically placed tubes, mechanical obstructions can occur as the bowel may volvulize around the tube or the balloon may cause a lead point of obstruction at the pylorus or within the small bowel lumen by migration [24, 28]. Also, patients may inadvertently pull the tube out. If the tube has been present long enough for a tract to form between the lumen of the bowel and the exit site (approximately 2 weeks), then reinsertion can be performed. Reinsertion should occur in a timely fashion as the gastrocutaneous tract may obliterate if enough time passes. However, if dislodgement occurs shortly after placement, the tract has not had enough time to form and is likely result in a small bowel or gastric perforation, which is a surgical emergency.

Parenteral Nutrition

The parenteral delivery of nutrition dates to the late 1960s with the work of Dudrick and Rhoads. Infusion of a hypertonic solution with nitrogen and nutrients was shown to sustain nitrogen balance and stimulate growth and development [25, 26]. In patients who are unable to tolerate nutrients orally or enterally, parenteral nutrition should be considered. Throughout the literature, there is a debate regarding when to initiate parenteral nutrition in those who meet criteria. Evidence has shown that initiation of parenteral nutrition preoperatively in a patient with protein malnutrition and continuation postoperatively is beneficial in elective general surgery. In patients who are well nourished preoperatively or prior to admission to the intensive care unit who cannot receive enteral nutrition, parenteral nutrition should be reserved and initiated after 7 days without enteral nutrition [19, 23]. Furthermore, a patient with a nonfunctional gastrointestinal tract should be started on parenteral nutrition [11].

The goal of parenteral nutrition is to restore nitrogen balance and create an anabolic state. Energy requirements are calculated by the equations discussed in the Nutritional Scales section of this chapter. It is recommended that a goal of 80 % of calculated energy expenditure be used as permissive underfeeding, or hypocaloric alimentation, which is beneficial in the critical care setting. Stated benefits include avoidance of the potential for insulin resistance, decreased infectious morbidity, less time requiring mechanical ventilation, and decreased length of stay. Strict glucose control has also been a popular topic in the literature. Current recommendations to maintain blood glucose between 110 and 150 mg/dL have shown decreased rates of sepsis, ICU length of stay, and in-hospital mortality [19].

Parenteral nutrition with hypertonic infusions must be given through a central venous catheter. Insertion of the catheter is not without risk with a complication rate between 5 and 19 % in the literature. Pneumothorax is one of the more frequent complications with a range of 1–1.5 %. The incidence increases with multiple passes of the access needle, insertion of larger catheters, and emergent placement. Malpositioning of the catheter can lead to venous thrombosis or perforation of the vein. Possible vascular injuries include arterial puncture and hematoma, hemothorax, cannulation of the artery leading to stroke or neurologic deficits with infusion, pseudoaneurysms, and arteriovenous fistulas. During insertion, the guidewire can produce cardiac arrhythmias. A small number of the arrhythmias may become symptomatic, but most subside with removal of the guidewire. However, complete heart block and sudden death have been described. Infection of an indwelling catheter is a major complication that can lead to sepsis with a mortality rate of 18 %. Thrombosis increases the rate of infectious complications as well. Great efforts have been made to prevent catheter-related bloodstream infections including strict hand hygiene, surgical preparation with chlorhexidine, sterile precautions during insertion, and catheter removal when no longer required. Indwelling catheters can lead to central venous thrombosis with rates ranging between 33 and 59 %; however, only a small percentage of cases are symptomatic. Over time, mechanical forces on the catheter can lead to fracture and embolization of the catheter. This can also occur during removal of the catheter. Other catheter removal complications include air embolism and hemorrhage [27].

Nutrition in Palliative Care and the Terminally Ill

The goals of nutrition in palliative care must be consistent with those of palliative care in general (See Palliative Care Section at the end of this chapter). To that end, the use of nutrition must improve the quality of life and palliate symptoms. It may be indicated for those patients who are malnourished or may become malnourished during the remaining course of their disease.

Psychosocial Aspects

Patients and loved ones can become distressed over loss of appetite. Meals are often social events. There are many fears and misconceptions surrounding anorexia and cachexia near the end of life. Education and reassurance can help refocus care. Eating will not reverse the terminal illness. In these cases, the body will only take what it needs. The body's needs and ability to metabolize food are altered by the illness and this manifests as decreased intake. This does not shorten life but is a part of the natural process of terminal illness.

Anorexia

In cases of reduced intake, reversible causes should be looked for. These include xerostomia, nausea, constipation, electrolyte disturbances, and psychological barriers such as depression. Altered taste sensation can be addressed by a variety of means. These include altering the temperature or presentation of the food. Using different types of food that are low in urea and spicing or marinating foods may help. Commercial supplements may actually contribute to suppressing appetite. Where possible, the best appetite stimulant is the patient's preferred foods themselves. Pharmacologic appetite stimulants do not affect prognosis but may improve quality of life [29]. Such stimulants include megestrol acetate and dexamethasone.

The most important intervention the care team can offer is to give permission to the patient to eat less. Reducing the stigma of loss of appetite and altering the way in which food is available and meals are offered can help improve intake. Interventions include having smaller, more frequent meals, having food available at all times whenever the patient is hungry, and having patients take part in meal planning.

Cachexia

Cachexia is an effect of disease which causes wasting of protein and energy stores. It is not responsive to hypercaloric feedings. Starvation, on the other hand, is protein and energy deficiency that is not part of a disease process [30]. In cachexia related to terminal illness, of which cancer is the best studied, the process is mediated by cytokines, such as tumor necrosis factor, IL-1 and IL-6 [31–33]. Appetite is suppressed early and hunger pains generally do not occur. Refeeding does not improve functionality or survival. This may not be true of certain subsets of AIDS patients (see Table 33.4) [34].

Table 33.4 Differences between starvation and cachexia of terminal illness [30]

	Starvation	Cachexia of terminal illness
Appetite	Suppressed late	Suppressed early
BMI	Not predictive of mortality	Predictive of mortality
Albumin	Low late	Low early
Cholesterol	May be normal	Low
Total lymphocytecount	Low, responds to refeeding	Low, no response to refeeding
Cytokines	N/A	Elevated
Response to refeeding	Reversible	Resistant

Ethical Decision Making Regarding Artificial Nutrition

The use of artificial nutrition in palliative care is controversial at best. Very few of the terminal illnesses most commonly encountered in the geriatric population show a favorable response to artificial feeding. Patients with dementia and most patients with advanced cancer do not show improvement in outcomes [30]. One subset of patients that may show improvement are those with a head and neck or esophageal cancer [35]. Regarding dementia, the National Institute for Health and Clinical Excellence in Britain recommended the following in their clinical guidelines [36]:

- Encourage people with dementia to eat and drink by mouth for as long as possible.
- Do not generally use tube feeding in severe dementia if dysphagia or disinclination to eat is a manifestation of disease severity.
- Consider nutritional support, including tube feeding, if dysphagia is thought to be transient.
- Apply ethical and legal principles to decisions to withhold or withdraw nutritional support.

Feeding may actually worsen quality of life and the dying process. The by-products, namely, ketones, of the malnourished state can produce a euphoric feeling and reduce hunger pains. Aspiration can lead to pneumonia. Feeding tubes can lead to use of restraints and the complications related to their use [35].

A Cochrane review in 2008 did not find sufficient evidence to make any recommendations for practice with regard to the use of medically assisted nutrition in palliative care patients [37]. Therefore, decisions regarding artificial nutrition must be approached with careful consideration of the clinical situation, the underlying disease, the patient's wishes, and artificial nutrition's possible benefits or burdens.

Summary

The risk of malnutrition rises dramatically in the hospitalized elderly. There are many risk factors related to age and are listed in the table in this chapter. Nutritional deficiencies need to be addressed and requirements maintained. Assessment must be a routine part of the care of the hospitalized elderly. The tables in this chapter will function as a quick reference for practitioners taking key points from the chapter and placing them at your fingertips.

References

1. The Federal Interagency Forum on Aging-Related Statistics. Older Americans 2010: key indicators of well-being. www.agingstats.gov/agingstatsdotnet/main_site/default.aspx. Accessed 1 May 2012.
2. Haute Autorité de Santé, Clinical Practice Guideline, Nutritional support strategy for protein-energy malnutrition in the elderly,

April 2007. http://www.has-sante.fr/portail/upload/docs/application/pdf/malnutrition_elderly_guidelines.pdf.
3. Dorner B, Posthauer ME, Friedrich EK, Robinson GE. Enteral nutrition for older adults in nursing facilities. Nutr Clin Pract. 2011;26(3):261–72.
4. Walker RN, Heuberger RA. Predictive equations for energy needs for the critically ill. Respir Care. 2009;54(4):509–21.
5. Cooney RN, Frankenfield DC. Determining energy needs in critically ill patients: equations or indirect calorimeters. Curr Opin Crit Care. 2012;18:174–7.
6. Frankenfield DC, Coleman A, Alam S, Cooney RN. Analysis of estimation methods for resting metabolic rate in critically ill adults. J Parenter Enteral Nutr. 2009;33(1):27–36.
7. Frankenfield D. Validation of an equation for resting metabolic rate in older obese critically ill patients. J Parenter Enteral Nutr. 2011;35(2):264–9.
8. Cerra FB, Benitez MR, Blackburn GL, Irwin RS, Jeejeebhoy K, Katz DP, Pingleton SK, Pomposelli J, Rombeau JL, Shronts E, Wolfe RR, Zaloga GP. Applied nutrition in ICU patients: a consensus statement of the American college of chest physicians. Chest. 1997;11(3):769–78.
9. Thompson M. Briefs: geriatric nutrition. J Natl Med Assoc. 1980;72(8):795–803.
10. Cutungo CL. The "graying" of trauma care: addressing traumatic injury in older adults. Am J Nurs. 2011;111(11):40–8.
11. Johnston RE, Chernoff R. Geriatrics. In: Matarese LE, Gottschlich MM, editors. Contemporary nutrition support practice. 2nd ed. Philadelphia: Saunders; 2003. p. 377–83.
12. D'Olimpio JT. Chapter 104. Physiology of nutrition and aging. In: Walsh DT, Caraceni AT, Fainsinger R, Foley KM, Glare P, Goh C, Lloyd-Williams M, Nunez Olarte J, Radbruch L, editors. Palliative medicine. 1st ed. Philadelphia: Saunders; 2009.
13. King M, Emery E. Nutrition management of the geriatric patient. Support Line. 2007;29(5):21–8.
14. Kagansky N, Berner Y, Koren-Morag N, Perelman L, Knobler H, Levy S. Poor nutritional habits are predictors of poor outcomes in very old hospitalized patients. Am J Clin Nutr. 2005;82:784–91.
15. Martindale RG, Zhou M, Nutrition and metabolism. In: O'Leary JP, Capote LR, editors. Physiologic basis of surgery. 3rd ed. Philadelphia: Lippincott, Williams & Wilkins; 2002. p. 133–68.
16. Kuzuya M, Kanda S, Koike T, Suzuki Y, Iguchi A. Lack of correlation between total lymphocyte count and nutritional status in the elderly. Clin Nutr. 2005;24(3):427–32.
17. Paddon-Jones D, Rasmussen BB. Dietary protein recommendations and the prevention of sarcopenia: protein, amino acid metabolism and therapy. Curr Opin Clin Nutr Metab Care. 2009;12(1):86–90.
18. Leistra E, Willeboordse F, van Bokhorst MAE, Visser M, Haans-van der Oord A, Weijs PJM, Oostenbrink A, Evers AM, Kruizenga HM. Predictors for achieving protein requirements in undernourished hospital patients. Clin Nutr. 2011;30(4):484–9.
19. McClave SA, Martindale RG, Vanek VW, McCarthy M, Roberts P, Taylor B, Ochoa JB, Napolitano L, Crescit G, ASPEN Board of Directors, American College of Critical Care Medicine. Guidelines for the provision and assessment of nutrition support therapy in the adult critically ill patient. J Parenter Enteral Nutr. 2009;33(3):277–316.
20. Read J, Clarke S. Chapter 107. Clinical nutrition. In: Walsh DT, Caraceni AT, Fainsinger R, Foley KM, Glare P, Goh C, Lloyd-Williams M, Nunez Olarte J, Radbruch L, editors. Palliative medicine. 1st ed. Philadelphia: Sauders; 2009.
21. Jacobs DG, Jacobs DO, Kudsk KA, Moore FA, Oswanski MF, Poole GV, Sacks GS, Scherer LR, Sinclair KE. Practice management guidelines for nutritional support of the trauma patient. J Trauma. 2004;57:660–79.
22. Mueller C, Cimpher C, Ellen DM, ASPEN Board of Directors. A.S.P.E.N. Clinical guidelines: nutrition screening, assessment, and intervention in adults. J Parenter Enteral Nutr. 2011;35(1):16–24.
23. Silk D, Green CJ. Perioperative nutrition: parenteral versus enteral. Curr Opin Clin Nutr Metab Care. 1998;1(1):21–7.
24. Grant MJ, Martin S. Delivery of enteral nutrition. AACN clinical issues: advanced practice in acute & critical care, vol. 11(4). 2000. p. 507–16.
25. Dudrick SJ, Wilmore DW, Vars HM, Rhoads JE. Can intravenous feeding as the sole nutrition support growth in the child and restore weight loss in an adult? An affirmative answer. Ann Surg. 1969;169(6):974–84.
26. Dudrick SJ, Wilmire DW, Vars HM, Rhoads JE. Long-term total parenteral nutrition with growth, development, and positive nitrogen balance. Surgery. 1968;64(1):134–42.
27. Kusminsky RE. Complications of central venous catheterization. J Am Coll Surg. 2007;204(4):681–96.
28. Pancorbo-Hidalgo PL, Garcia-Fernandez FP, Ramierez-Perez C. Complications associated with enteral nutrition by nasogastric tube in an internal medicine unit. J Clin Nurs. 2001;10:482–90.
29. Dy M. Enteral and parenteral nutrition in terminally ill cancer patients: a review of the literature. Am J Hosp Palliat Med. 2006;23(5):369–77.
30. Thomas D. Distinguishing starvation from cachexia. Clin Geriatr Med. 2002;18:883–91.
31. Alexander H. Prevalence and pathophysiology of cancer cachexia. In: Portenoy RK, Bruera E, editors. Topics in palliative care. Oxford University Press: New York; 1998. p. 91–129.
32. Inui A. Cancer anorexia-cachexia syndrome: are neuropeptides the key? Cancer Res. 1999;59(18):4493–501.
33. Dunlop RJ, Campbell CW. Cytokines and advanced cancer. J Pain Symptom Manage. 2000;20(3):214–32.
34. Nemechek PM, Polsky B, et al. Treatment guidelines for HIV-associated wasting. Mayo Clin Proc. 2000;75(4):386–94.
35. Ganzini L. Artificial nutrition and hydration at the end of life: ethics and evidence. Palliat Support Care. 2006;4:135–43.
36. National Institute for Health and Care Excellence Clinical Guideline 42 Dementia. www.nice.org.uk/guidance.nice.org.uk/CG42.
37. Good P, Cavenagh J, Mather M, Ravenscroft P. Medically assisted nutrition for palliative care in adult patients. Cochrane Database Syst Rev. 2008;(4):CD006274.
38. http://www.mna-elderly.com/forms/mna_guide_english_sf.pdf.
39. Braga M, Ljungqvist O, Soeters P, Fearon K, Weimann A, Bozzetti F. ESPEN guidelines on parenteral nutrition: surgery. Clin Nutr. 2009;28:378–86.

Pharmacology

34

Wendy L. Wahl and James T. Miller

Introduction

Trauma in the elderly is an ever-increasing event in American society as the population ages and life expectancy continues to increase. With advancing age, acute and chronic medical illnesses increase in frequency with the need for medical therapy. According to the Medicare database, the average patient over 65 years utilizes more than 28 prescriptions annually. The typical resident in a nursing home uses seven prescription medications. Elderly patients living independently consume between two and four drugs prescribed by their physician(s) daily. Many pharmaceutical drugs have short-term and commonly long-term implications for caring for injured patients. Medications used in critical care practice or emergency settings may have altered pharmacokinetics in geriatric patients or interact with medications already used by the patient. This chapter will outline the effect of aging on drug metabolism, commonly used drugs that effect trauma management (antiplatelet and anticoagulants, drugs which affect heart rate), and the effect of medications on delirium and pain control in the elderly patient (Table 34.1).

Pharmacokinetic and Pharmacodynamic Alterations in the Elderly

Significant alterations in pharmacokinetics accompany aging and must be considered when selecting and optimizing medication therapy in the elderly patient. Enteral absorption is minimally affected by the process of aging alone, but subcutaneous and intramuscular absorption may be affected by decreases in total body water and muscle mass in the aged. Decreases in total body water and alterations in plasma protein concentrations change the volume of distribution for many commonly used medications. Elderly patients may require lower doses of hydrophilic agents such as heparin, insulin, and warfarin to account for this change in drug disposition. Hepatic drug metabolism by the cytochrome P450 system is variably affected due to age-related decreases in some isozymes' activity. Drug elimination is the pharmacokinetic process most affected by aging, as glomerular filtration and renal drug elimination are inversely correlated with age. Many commonly prescribed medications require dosage adjustment in patients with renal dysfunction, including most antibiotics, antihypertensives, cardiac glycosides, histamine receptor antagonists, hypoglycemic agents, and analgesics.

Anticoagulation Agents

Early studies on the effects of pre-injury warfarin were derived retrospectively from large databases and were unable to detect differences in outcomes between patients receiving warfarin and control groups. However, when elderly patients with head trauma are considered, most subsequent studies have shown that pre-injury warfarin treatment is associated with injury severity, risk for an intracranial hemorrhage (ICH) after a fall, mortality after ICH, and overall mortality. However, warfarin therapy alone is not necessarily a predictor of adverse outcome. Patients who are more intensively anticoagulated are more likely to present with a Glasgow Coma Scale score (GCS) of less than 13 and have an increased risk of both overall mortality and mortality after ICH. Warfarin does not seem to impose a higher risk of morbidity or mortality on patients without head injury.

Pre-injury anticoagulant therapy often complicates the management of the elderly trauma patient. Warfarin is an inhibitor of the vitamin K epoxide reductase complex

W.L. Wahl, MD (✉)
Department of Surgery, Saint Joseph Mercy Ann Arbor, 5301 E. Huron River Drive, Suite 2482, Ann Arbor, MI 48106-0995, USA
e-mail: wahlwl@trinity-health.org

J.T. Miller, PharmD
Department of Pharmacy Science, University of Michigan Health System, Victor Vaughan Bldg., Rm. 301, 111 E. Catherine Street, Ann Arbor, MI 48109, USA
e-mail: millerjt@med.umich.edu

J.A. Yelon, F.A. Luchette (eds.), *Geriatric Trauma and Critical Care*,
DOI 10.1007/978-1-4614-8501-8_34, © Springer Science+Business Media New York 2014

Table 34.1 Oral agents

	Mechanism of action	Elimination half-life (h)	Clotting factors affected	Laboratory alterations	Potential treatment
Oral agents					
Warfarin	Vitamin K antagonist	20–60	II, VII, IX, X, proteins C and S	PT/INR	Phytonadione, FFP, rFVIIa, PCC, PCC + rFVIIa
Dabigatran	Direct thrombin inhibitor	12–17, prolonged in renal failure	IIa	aPTT, ECT, TT	Hemodialysis, PCC, rFVIIa
Rivaroxaban	Factor Xa inhibitor	5–9, 11–13 in the elderly	Xa	PT/INR	PCC
Apixaban	Factor Xa inhibitor	8–15	Xa	Anti-Xa (apixaban specific)	No data
Aspirin	Platelet aggregation and activation inhibitor via cyclooxygenase-1 and thromboxane A_2 inhibition	15–20 min (duration of activity is the life of the platelet)	None	Platelet response tests[a]	Desmopressin, rFVIIa
Clopidogrel	Platelet aggregation inhibitor via ADP inhibition and subsequent decrease in GPIIb/IIIa activation	6 (active metabolite, 30 min, duration of activity is the life of the platelet)	None	Platelet response tests[a]	Desmopressin, rFVIIa
Prasugrel	Platelet aggregation inhibitor via ADP inhibition and subsequent decrease in GPIIb/IIIa activation	7	None	Platelet response tests[a]	No data
Ticagrelor	Platelet aggregation inhibitor via ADP inhibition and subsequent decrease in GPIIb/IIIa activation	7	None	Platelet response tests[a]	No data
Parenteral agents					
Enoxaparin	Inhibition of IIa and Xa with antithrombin III	4.5–7 (prolonged with renal impairment)	Xa, IIa	Anti-Xa	Protamine, rFVIIa
Fondaparinux	Inhibition of Xa with antithrombin III	17–21 (prolonged with renal impairment)	Xa	Anti-Xa (fondaparinux specific)	rFVIIa

PT/INR prothrombin time/international normalized ratio, *FFP* fresh frozen plasma, *rFVIIa* recombinant activated factor VIIa, *PCC* prothrombin complex concentrate, *aPTT* activated partial thromboplastin time, *ECT* ecarin clotting time, *TT* thrombin time
[a]No current evidence supports the use of platelet response tests to guide therapy

(VKORC) which results in decreased activation of clotting factors II, VII, IX, and X, in addition to proteins C and S. Warfarin, used commonly for the treatment and prevention of thromboembolic diseases, was the only oral anticoagulant available in the United States for many years. Dabigatran is an orally administered direct thrombin inhibitor approved for the reduction of stroke risk and systemic embolism in patients with non-valvular atrial fibrillation. In clinical trials, bleeding complications with dabigatran therapy were similar to rates for warfarin. Potential advantages of dabigatran therapy compared to warfarin include the lack of required therapeutic drug monitoring and fewer drug-drug and dietary interactions. However, dose adjustments are necessary for dabigatran when prescribed for patients with renal failure (creatinine clearance (CrCl) less than 30 mL/min).

Rivaroxaban is an oral factor Xa inhibitor approved for reduction of risk of stroke and systemic embolism in non-valvular atrial fibrillation and prevention of venous thromboembolism (VTE) after knee or hip replacement surgery. Like dabigatran, it requires dose adjustments for renal insufficiency (CrCl less than 50 mL/min). One small pharmacokinetic study showed only a moderate effect of severe renal impairment on elimination half-life. This finding may be due in part to alternate clearance pathways, including hepatic metabolism. Apixaban is another oral factor Xa inhibitor currently marketed in the European Union. There are currently no data that describe the outcomes of injured patients who are receiving either of these anticoagulants.

Aspirin, clopidogrel, and prasugrel are all drugs which decrease platelet activation and aggregation via glycoprotein IIb/IIIa but by different mechanisms. Pre-injury antiplatelet therapy does not seem to impact outcomes of the non-head-injured trauma patient. However, the impact of pre-injury therapy on outcomes in head injury remains controversial and optimal management is unclear. Much of the data describing these patients is retrospective, and few studies have analyzed the offending agents separately.

Several studies have attempted to address the impact of pre-injury antiplatelet therapy on the elderly patient with a head injury. The majority of patients in these studies were only on antiplatelet therapy, but some patients were also using warfarin. This confounder makes it difficult to interpret the data and conclusions. Pre-injury therapy was associated with 18.5–38 % mortality compared to a rate of 8–9.5 % in matched controls. A study from 2002 was the first to report that ASA and warfarin therapy prior to injury were equivalent risk factors for increased morbidity and mortality. Other studies have shown pre-injury clopidogrel, but not ASA, to increase the risk of both being discharged to a long-term care facility and mortality compared to matched controls. In studies that excluded patients using warfarin, pre-injury clopidogrel was associated with an increased necessity for transfusion of blood and also repeat intracranial surgery. Antiplatelet therapy was associated with a higher-grade hemorrhage.

It is logical to conclude that pre-injury anticoagulation or antiplatelet therapy would be risk factors for increased morbidity and mortality. However, coagulopathy is also a known complication of injury, and some authors have suggested that the pre-injury use of anticoagulants or antiplatelet therapy may have a paradoxically protective effect in patients older than 70 years. Data from the only prospective study addressing the effects of pre-injury anticoagulation implies that low-dose ASA (100 mg/day) does not increase the risk of ICH in elderly patients with mild to moderate head injury. There are no data describing outcomes in injured patients treated with the newer agents prasugrel or ticagrelor.

Reversal of Pre-injury Anticoagulation

Vitamin K is the antidote for warfarin toxicity, and when administered intravenously, its effects can be seen within 12–24 h. However, rapid reversal of the anticoagulant effects of warfarin has been shown to decrease progression of ICH and mortality. Administration of fresh frozen plasma (FFP) can begin to normalize coagulation by supplying clotting factors II, VII, IX, and X while awaiting the full effects of reversal with vitamin K. While a targeted therapy, FFP use is fraught with limitations: optimal dosing is unknown, clotting factor concentrations are variable in each unit, the required volumes of FFP to be infused may be problematic for patients with known cardiovascular comorbidities, additional time is required for thawing prior to administration, and time to correction of INR is highly variable.

Prothrombin complex concentrates (PCCs) and recombinant activated factor VIIa (rFVIIa) may be beneficial for emergent reversal. "Three-factor" PCCs available in the United States contain little to no factor VII. "Four-factor" PCCs available in the European Union contain high concentrations of factors II, VII, IX, and X. Although there is little data on the use of PCC, it represents a potentially valuable therapy for patients who require rapid warfarin reversal. Multiple small, nonrandomized studies have shown that four-factor PCC is associated with more rapid reversal of anticoagulation and decreased hematoma expansion compared to FFP in patients with an ICH on warfarin. However, optimal dosing is unknown. Fixed doses of 500–1,040 international units (IU) of factor IX activity are sufficient for reversal, while an open-label study showed that a weight- and INR-adjusted dose was associated with 89 % of patients reaching a target INR within 15 min of administration compared to 43 % ($p < 0.001$) in the group that received the fixed 500 IU dose. Three-factor PCC has been described as insufficient for reversal. Retrospective data suggests that the combination of three-factor PCC with low-dose rFVIIa may be effective. It should be noted though that the half-lives of PCC and rFVIIa are much shorter than that of warfarin, so phytonadione should also be administered for optimal reversal. Because PCC is a pooled plasma product, there remains a remote risk of infection.

There are even fewer studies evaluating the efficacy of rFVIIa in warfarin-associated ICH compared to the data for PCC. In a retrospective study, rFVIIa was effective at reversing anticoagulation in neurosurgical patients who failed phytonadione and FFP, although less than half of the patients had warfarin as the cause of the abnormal coagulation. In another retrospective study of mostly elderly patients with a traumatic ICH who were also therapeutically anticoagulated, rFVIIa was effective at restoring coagulation and was associated with decreased use of FFP. However, there was no difference in mortality rates. There was a trend towards an increased risk of VTE in the group receiving rFVIIa. One small retrospective study concluded that rFVIIa was superior to three-factor PCC for correcting the INR in warfarin-related ICH. Recent guidelines for anticoagulant reversal from the American College of Chest Physicians recommend use of four-factor PCC for restoring coagulation with warfarin-associated bleeding rather than plasma infusion. Prospective studies are needed to describe the optimal dosing, therapeutic agent, and the impact of these therapies on clinical outcomes.

The introduction of dabigatran, rivaroxaban, and likely apixaban presents the trauma surgeon and acute care surgeon with new challenges. Data from prospective trials has suggested that there may be a lower risk of bleeding with these newer agents compared to warfarin. There are no known or recommended reversal agents, however. Data suggests that four-factor PCC reduces hematoma expansion and mortality in mice injected with dabigatran; however, a small study of 12 healthy human volunteers showed that four-factor PCC was unable to reverse the effects of dabigatran. Emergent hemodialysis can remove up to 62 % of circulating dabigatran in 2 h due to its large unbound fraction and should be considered in life-threatening situations. The same study concluded that the effects of rivaroxaban were completely reversed by administration of PCC. However, in a rabbit model of bleeding, both rFVIIa and PCC were able to improve bleeding times, but did not have an impact on the amount of hemorrhage itself. In a small *ex vivo* study of ten healthy patients, rFVIIa, PCC, and factor eight inhibitor bypassing activity (FEIBA) were variably effective at reversing dabigatran and rivaroxaban. An in vitro study showed that clotting assays altered by apixaban were inconsistently reversed by rFVIIa and PCC.

The antithrombin effects of low-molecular-weight heparins may be reversed by protamine, but it has little to no effect on their anti-Xa activity. Protamine doses have been used up to 100 mg (1 mg protamine for each mg enoxaparin given in the preceding 8 h). However, protamine administration is associated with serious complications, including life-threatening hypersensitivity reactions and counterintuitively hemorrhage. Recombinant FVIIa has been used in a number of case reports and laboratory investigations and has been at least partially effective at doses of 20–120 mcg/kg. Several case reports have described clinical success in reversing the anticoagulant effects of fondaparinux with rFVIIa, but results were inconsistent in the largest case series currently published.

Reversal of Pre-Injury Antiplatelet Effects

Platelet transfusion is commonly employed in the management of traumatic intracranial hemorrhage in all injured patients, but particularly the elderly, receiving antiplatelet therapy, despite a lack of data to support its efficacy. Both aspirin and clopidogrel bind irreversibly to platelets causing dysfunction for the life of the platelet. Transfusion is only beneficial by providing functional platelets. Two retrospective studies have shown no benefit with transfusion of platelets on either morbidity or mortality. Platelet transfusion can lead to a number of complications including transfusion-related acute lung injury (TRALI) and infection. In one study, patients receiving platelet transfusion had a subsequent medical decline when compared to the group not transfused. Given the available evidence, platelet transfusion cannot be currently recommended in this setting.

Extrapolating data from other patient populations, several studies have suggested using intravenous desmopressin (DDAVP) to reverse platelet dysfunction although it has not been studied in trauma patients. Desmopressin is known to increase concentrations of von Willebrand factor and factor VIII. It has been used in doses of 0.3–0.4 mcg/kg.

There are numerous assays currently marketed that assess the therapeutic response to antiplatelet agents. Current cardiology literature does not support antiplatelet testing to individualize therapy given the variability between assays and lack of established reference ranges. One study in trauma patients examined point-of-care testing for patients with a reported history of taking clopidogrel. The results confirmed the findings from studies conducted in uninjured patients in that many patients are either noncompliant or nonresponders to antiplatelet therapy. To date, antiplatelet testing cannot be used to guide therapy in the management of traumatic hemorrhage but may have a role for assessing the therapeutic effect of clopidogrel on platelet function at the time of admission and thus select specific patients who may need platelet transfusion.

Beta-Blocker Therapy

Beta-blockers are commonly prescribed in elderly patients as antihypertensives and antiarrhythmics. Studies have concluded there is a survival benefit for patients receiving beta-blocker therapy for cardiac and high-risk vascular procedures. For nonvascular operations, the data for beta-blocker use is less conclusive, where the cardiac events are less, but the mortality rates are not improved compared to those treated perioperatively for cardiac or vascular procedures.

Nonrandomized, cohort-controlled studies in both adult burn and trauma patients have suggested reduced morbidity and mortality. The effects of beta-receptor blockade include decreased cardiac oxygen consumption and hypermetabolism. Additional benefit from antisympathomimetics includes a decrease in systemic and cerebral perfusion pressure. Theorized mechanisms for these effects include suppression of IL-6 production which has been associated with increased mortality for trauma and sepsis patients. A small, randomized trial of patients treated with beta-blockers found lower IL-6 levels. In a study comparing older patients who were case matched for age, Injury Severity Score, Glasgow Coma Scale score, and mechanism of injury concluded that beta-blocker use decreased mortality. A similar study in adult burn patients showed faster rates of healing and reduced hospital length of stay in the group receiving beta-blockers. Patients in these studies who arrived to the hospital on beta-blockers were older and more severely injured.

A subsequent retrospective study that did not use a cohort group or case matching in the study design found that patients admitted on beta-blockers without head injury had higher mortality than those admitted without beta-blocker therapy. There was no difference in the mortality rate for the group admitted on a beta-blocker; however, this group was also more frequently treated with Coumadin and had a higher incidence of vascular diseases. However, in a subset analysis of head injuries, the data suggest a benefit with beta-blocker therapy.

The last study posed the question that beta-blockers may have caused injured patients to appear less ill due to less tachycardia at presentation and that this may have affected their subsequent resuscitation. Alternatively, beta-blocker use in the elderly may have been a surrogate for pre-injury comorbidities.

Potential side effects of beta-blocker therapy may be vasoconstriction and bradycardia due to antagonism of beta-mediated vasodilation and increased risk of vasovagal reaction. The effects of beta-blockers may mask normal tachycardia in response to hemorrhage, an early clinical sign of hypovolemia, so the clinician should seek other signs of hypoperfusion such as acidosis, decreased urine output, and altered mentation since hypotension is a later manifestation of shock.

Delirium and Management in the Elderly

Unlike dementia, which is a chronic confusional state, delirium is an acute confusional state which occurs most commonly in older, hospitalized patients. Acute brain dysfunction, or delirium, occurs in up to 70 % of mechanically ventilated patients in the surgical ICU and recently has been reported in a similar proportion of trauma ICU patients. Delirium has been identified in 15–53 % of older patients undergoing elective surgical procedures and is associated with mortality rates of 22–76 %, equivalent to mortality rates for sepsis and acute myocardial infarction.

Evidence suggests that delirium may be secondary to altered neurotransmission, inflammation, and even chronic stress. Administration of anticholinergic drugs has been shown to cause delirium in both animals and humans. Excess dopaminergic activity may also contribute to delirium as a regulator of acetylcholine, which supports the use of antipsychotic agents for treatment of delirium symptoms.

Multiple studies have concluded that the use of sedatives and analgesics is associated with delirium in the ICU population. In addition, continuous sedative infusions are also associated with increased mechanical ventilator days and intensive care unit lengths of stay. In a study of elderly (mean age 81 years) patients with hip fractures, the group managed with spinal anesthesia and light sedation had 50 % less postoperative delirium than the group managed with a general anesthetic.

Continuous sedation is known to increase the incidence of adverse outcomes. Recent studies evaluate the interplay of analgesic and sedatives in postoperative patients requiring mechanical ventilation. Patients who remain agitated once therapeutic with analgesics were more likely to be experiencing delirium rather than agitation. Sedative medications were only employed if a patient was unable to be maintained safely on the ventilator or was at risk of removing other vital tubes or drains without sedation. This approach is now gaining attention from critical care organizations and requires objective evaluation of patients with standardized tools which assess for pain and delirium screens such as the Confusion Assessment Method for the Intensive Care Unit score. If patients screen positive for delirium, non-pharmacologic treatment should be attempted. Review of medications that have sedative properties or cognitive side effects should be eliminated or the dose reduced, if possible. Metabolic causes for delirium should be corrected such as hypoxia, electrolyte disturbances, hypothyroidism, and sepsis. In patients using a hearing aid or corrective lenses, they should be in place to improve the ability to communicate and orient the patient. Non-pharmacologic methods such as relaxation, music, and restoration of the normal sleep-wake cycle with avoidance of loud noise and bright lights during sleep should be employed as much as possible.

If delirium symptoms persist or progress with the potential for self-harm, pharmacologic therapy should be given. Generally, antipsychotic and atypical antipsychotic agents are the first-line agents for acute delirium not responsive to alternative treatment. Low doses, administered for 2–3 days for maximal effect, should be initiated. The possibility of alcohol or benzodiazepine withdrawal should also be considered. Haloperidol can be given enterally or intramuscularly starting at doses of 0.5–1 mg, repeating enteral doses every 4 h as needed or every 30–60 min for IM dosing, until the desired effect (see Table 34.2) is observed. Monitoring for extrapyramidal symptoms and prolonged QT intervals should be done with a baseline EKG. Haloperidol should not be used for those with a history of neuroleptic malignant syndrome, QT prolongation, or significant liver dysfunction.

Atypical antipsychotic agents such as risperidone and quetiapine are now commonly used in many intensive care settings for agitation. Unlike haloperidol, these agents have only been tested in smaller, uncontrolled studies. The attraction for use is the potentially safer profile related to extrapyramidal motor side effects. The same cautions apply for QT prolongation, and there have been reported increases in mortality for the generalized use of these agents in elderly patients with dementia (Table 34.2).

Pain Medications and Management

It is common for older patients to suffer from sight and hearing loss and cognitive and memory loss either from pathology or medication side effects. These functional alterations may lead to the under- or overtreatment of pain which in turn may cascade into other adverse events such as pneumonia and falls. Some studies support that there are age-related differences in how pain is perceived. Older patients may have reduced responses to mild pain, while the response to severe

Table 34.2 Delirium

Drug	Dose	Adverse effects	Comments
Haloperidol	Initial episode	QT prolongation, torsades de pointes	Not FDA labeled for intravenous use
	2 mg IV (may double dose and repeat every 15–30 min until delirium controlled)	Extrapyramidal symptoms (EPS)	PO, IV, and IM administration available
	Maintenance	Hypotension	
	25 % of last bolus dose given every 6–8 h after initial episode controlled	Sedation	
		Neuroleptic malignant syndrome (NMS)	
Quetiapine	25–200 mg PO twice daily	QT prolongation	Along with olanzapine, most sedating atypical antipsychotic due to antihistaminic effects
		Sedation	No parenteral product available
		NMS[a]	
Olanzapine	2.5–5 mg PO daily	QT prolongation	Along with quetiapine, most sedating atypical antipsychotic due to antihistaminic effects
		Sedation	PO, SL, IM administration available
		NMS[a]	
Ziprasidone	20–40 mg PO/IM every 6–12 h	QT prolongation	Atypical antipsychotic most likely to increase QT interval
		NMS[a]	PO, IM administration available

FDA Food and Drug Administration, *SL* sublingual
[a]Atypical antipsychotics have lower risk of NMS than haloperidol due to less preferential dopamine receptor inhibition

pain may be exaggerated. These alterations in pain perception make pain management in the elderly more challenging than in younger patients. Higher pain thresholds for less severe pain may lead to delays in diagnosis or missed diagnoses. In addition, heightened responses to severe pain may lead to overtreatment.

Adverse reactions with opioids are common in the elderly and may have much more dire consequences than in the younger population. Drowsiness, motor instability, and dizziness often are poorly tolerated in the geriatric patient population. Common side effects of opioids in the elderly include constipation, nausea, and vomiting; impaired judgment; sedation; reduced psychomotor function; and respiratory depression. For all opioids, these factors can be reduced by using agents with a short half-life, lower starting doses, longer intervals between doses, and cautious incremental increase in dose while titrating for adequate analgesia.

There are no well-controlled studies that address which opioids treat pain most effectively in the elderly population and more specifically for elderly trauma patients. The route and dose of narcotic should be selected based on the patient's renal and hepatic function, severity of pain, hospital setting, and response to treatment. The only guidelines which address pain management in the elderly were published by the American Geriatric Society in 2002 which were for chronic pain, but many of the recommendations are still valid for acute pain management. Pain medication should be administered through the least invasive route which controls the pain. Introduce only one agent at a time at a low dose before titrating to a higher dose. Allow sufficient time between doses given changes in drug availability and metabolism. Provide appropriate monitoring to ensure adequate pain control without overtreatment with adverse effects. Alternatives to opiate administration should be considered when possible. An example would be placement of an epidural catheter for management of rib fracture pain rather than treatment only with parenteral narcotics.

Summary

There are very few pharmacologic studies that specifically address treatment considerations for elderly trauma patients. For any medication administered in the elderly population, knowledge of potential drug-drug interactions, reduced metabolism, and the potential for accentuated side effects should be monitored. Consideration for consultation from a gerontologist, particularly for those with delirium and dementia, and participation of clinical pharmacists may aid the trauma surgeon and surgical intensivist in the complex pharmacologic management of these patients.

Bibliography

Abood GJ, Luchette FA. The management of the trauma patient with medically-altered coagulation. Am Surg. 2008;74:784–92.

Ageno W, Gallus AS, Wittkowsky A, Crowther M, Hylek EM, Palareti G. Oral anticoagulant therapy: antithrombotic and prevention of thrombosis, 9th ed: American College of Chest Physicians

Evidence-Based Clinical Practice Guidelines. Chest. 2012;141: e44S–88.
Altman R, Scazziota A, Lourdes DE, Herrera M, Gonzalez C. Recombinant factor VIIa reverses the inhibitory effect of aspirin or clopidogrel on in vitro thrombin generation. J Thromb Haemost. 2006;4:2022–7.
American Geriatric Society. The management of persistent pain in older persons. J Am Geriatr Soc. 2002;50:S205–24.
Arbabi S, Ahrns KS, Wahl WL, et al. Beta-blocker use is associated with improved outcomes in adult burn patient. J Trauma. 2004;56: 265–9.
Arbabi S, Campion EM, Barker M, Dimo M, Hemmila MR, Ahrns KS, Niederbichler AD, Wahl WL. Beta blocker use is associated with improved outcomes in adult trauma patients. J Trauma. 2006;62: 56–62.
Bonville DJ, Ata A, Jahraus CB, Arnold-Lloyd T, et al. Impact of preinjury warfarin and antiplatelet agents on outcomes of trauma patients. Surgery. 2011;150:861–8.
Breitbart W, Marotta R, Platt MM, et al. A double—blind trial of haloperidol, chlorpromazine and lorazepam in the treatment of delirium in hospitalized AIDS patients. Am J Psychiatry. 1996;153:231–7.
Brewer ES, Reznikov B, Liberman RF, et al. Incidence and predictors of intracranial hemorrhage after minor head trauma in patients taking anticoagulant and antiplatelet medication. J Trauma. 2011; 70:E1–5.
Broadhurst C, Wilson K. Immunology of delirium: new opportunities for treatment and research. Br J Psychiatry. 2001;179:288–9.
Campbell PG, Sen A, Yadla S, Jabbour P, Jallo J. Emergency reversal of antiplatelet agents in patients presenting with an intracranial hemorrhage: a clinical review. World Neurosurg. 2010;74:279–85.
Delafuente JC. Pharmacokinetic and pharmacodynamic alterations in the geriatric patient. Consult Pharm. 2008;23(4):324–34.
Downey DM, Monson B, Butler KL, Fortuna Jr GR, Saxe JM, Markert RJ, McCarthy MC. Does platelet administration affect mortality in elderly dead-injured patients taking antiplatelet medications? Am Surg. 2009;75:1100–3.
Dwyer LL, Han B, Woodwell DA, Rechsteiner EA. Polypharmacy in nursing home residents in the United States: results of the 2004 National Nursing Home Survey. Am J Geriatr Pharmacother. 2010;8:63–72.
Eagle KA, Froehlic JB. Reducing cardiovascular risk in patients undergoing noncardiac surgery. N Engl J Med. 1996;335:1761–3.
Eerenberg ES, Kamphuisen PW, Sijpkens MK, Meijers JC, Buller HR, Levi M. Reversal of rivaroxaban and dabigatran by prothrombin complex concentrate: a randomized, placebo-controlled crossover study in healthy subjects. Circulation. 2011;124:1573–9.
Eikelboom JW, Hirsh J, Spencer FA, Baglin TP, Weitz JI. Antiplatelet drugs: antithrombotic therapy and prevention of thrombosis, 9th ed: American College of Chest Physicians Evidence-Based Clinical Practice Guidelines. Chest. 2012;141:e89S–119.
Ely EW, Shintani A, Truman B, et al. Delirium as a predictor of mortality in mechanically ventilated patients in the intensive care unit. JAMA. 2004;291:1753–62.
Ely EW, Inouye SK, Bernard DR, et al. Delirium in mechanically ventilated patients: validity and reliability of the confusion assessment method for the intensive care unit (CAM-ICU). JAMA. 2001;286:2703–10.
Escolar G, Arellano-Rodrigo E, Reverter JC, et al. Reversal of apixaban induced alterations of hemostasis by different coagulation factor concentrates: studies in vitro with circulating human blood. 2012. http://circ.ahajournals.org/content/early/2012/06/20/CIR.0b013e3182611cc2.citation.
Fortuna GR, Mueller EW, James LE, Shutter LA, Butler KL. The impact of preinjury antiplatelet and anticoagulant pharmacotherapy on outcomes in elderly patients with hemorrhagic brain injury. Surgery. 2008;144:598–605.
Friese RS, Barber R, McBride D, Bender J, Gentilello LM. Could beta-blockade improve outcome after injury by modulating inflammatory profiles? J Trauma. 2008;64:1061–8.
Garcia DA, Baglin TP, Weitz JI, Samama MM. Parenteral anticoagulants: antithrombotic therapy and prevention of thrombosis, 9th ed: American College of Chest Physicians Evidence-Based Clinical Practice Guidelines. Chest. 2012;141:e24S–43.
Gibson SJ, Helme RD. Age-related differences in pain perception and report. Clin Geriatr Med. 2001;17:433–56, v–vi.
Gibson SJ, Farrell M. A review of age differences in the neurophysiology of nociception and the perceptual experience of pain. Clin J Pain. 2004;20:227–39.
Godier A, Miclot A, Le Bonniec B, et al. Evaluation of prothrombin complex concentrate and recombinant activated Factor VII to reverse rivaroxaban in a rabbit Model. Anesthesiology. 2012;116(1): 94–102.
Herndon DN, Hart DW, Wolf SE, et al. Reversal of catabolism by beta-blockade after severe burns. N Engl J Med. 2001;345:1223–9.
Holbrook A, Schulman S, Witt DM, et al. Evidence-based management of anticoagulant therapy: antithrombotic therapy and prevention of thrombosis, 9th ed: American College of Chest Physicians Evidence-Based Clinical Practice Guidelines. Chest. 2012;141: e152S–84.
Holland L, Warkentin TE, Refaai M, Crowther MA, Johnston MA, Sarode R. Suboptimal effect of a three-factor prothrombin complex concentrate (Profilnine-SD) in correcting supratherapeutic international normalized ratio due to warfarin overdose. Transfusion. 2009;49:1171–7.
Inouye SK. Delirium in older persons. N Engl J Med. 2006;354: 1157–65.
Inouye SK, Bogardus Jr ST, Charpentier PA, et al. A multi-component intervention to prevent delirium in hospitalized older patients. N Engl J Med. 1999;340:669–76.
Ivascu FA, Howells GA, Junn FS, Bair HA, Bendick PJ, Janczyk RJ. Rapid warfarin reversal in anticoagulated patients with traumatic intracranial hemorrhage reduces hemorrhage progression and mortality. J Trauma. 2005;59:1131–9.
Ivascu FA, Howells GA, Junn FS, Bair HA, Bendick PJ, Janczyk RJ. Predictors of mortality in trauma patients with intracranial hemorrhage on preinjury aspirin or clopidogrel. J Trauma. 2008;65: 785–8.
Jones K, Sharp C, Mangram AJ, Dunn EL. The effects of preinjury clopidogrel use on older trauma patients with head injuries. Am J Surg. 2006;192:743–5.
Juliebø V, Bjøro K, Krogseth M, et al. Risk factors for preoperative and postoperative delirium in elderly patients with hip fracture. J Am Geriatr Soc. 2009;57:1354–61.
Kennedy DM, Cipolle MD, Pasquale MD, Wasser T. Impact of preinjury warfarin use in elderly trauma patients. J Trauma. 2000;48(3): 451–3.
Khorsand N, Veeger NJ, Muller M, et al. Fixed versus variable dose of prothrombin complex concentrate for counteracting vitamin K antagonist therapy. Transfus Med. 2011;21:116–23.
Kollef MH, Levy NT, Ahrens TS, Schaiff R, Prentice D, Sherman G. The use of continuous IV sedation is associated with prolongation of mechanical ventilation. Chest. 1998;114:541–8.
Kubitza D, Becka M, Mueck W, et al. Effects of renal impairment on the pharmacokinetics, pharmacodynamics, and safety of rivaroxaban, an oral, direct Factor Xa inhibitor. Br J Clin Pharmacol. 2010;70(5):703–12.
Lat I, McMillian W, Taylor S, et al. The impact of delirium on clinical outcomes in mechanically ventilated surgical and trauma patients. Crit Care Med. 2009;37:1898–905.
Lavoie A, Ratte S, Clas D, Demers J, Moore L, Martin M, Berferon E. Preinjury warfarin use among elderly patients with closed head injuries in a trauma center. J Trauma. 2004;56:802–7.

Liu MY. Protective effects of propranolol on experimentally head-injured mouse brains. J Formos Med Assoc. 1995;94:386–90.
Lombard SA, Robbertze R. Perioperative use of β-blockers in the elderly patient. Anesthesiol Clin. 2009;27:581–97.
Lundström M, Olofsson B, Stenvall M, et al. Postoperative delirium in old patients with femoral neck fracture: a randomized intervention study. Aging Clin Exp Res. 2007;19:178–86.
Mangano DT, Layug EL, Wallace A, et al. Effect of atenolol on mortality and cardiovascular morbidity after noncardiac surgery. Multicenter Study of Perioperative Ischemia Research Group. N Engl J Med. 1996;335:1713–20.
Mathieson T, Benediktsdottir K, Johnsson H, Lindqvist M, von Holst H. Intracranial traumatic and non-traumatic haemorrhagic complications of warfarin treatment. Acta Neurol Scand. 1995;91: 208–14.
Mina AA, Bair HA, Howells GA, Bendick PJ. Intracranial complications of preinjury anticoagulation in trauma patients with head injury. J Trauma. 2002;53:668–72.
Mohammadi AA, Bakhshaeekia A, Alibeigi P, et al. Efficacy of propranolol in wound healing for hospitalized burn patients. J Burn Care Res. 2009;30:1013–7.
Mountain D, Sistenich V, Jacobs IG. Characteristics, management and outcome of adults with major trauma taking pre-injury warfarin in a Western Australian population from 2000 to 2005: a population-based cohort study. Med J Aust. 2010;193:202–6.
Neideen T, Lam M, Brasel KJ. Preinjury beta blockers are associated with increased mortality in geriatric trauma patients. J Trauma. 2008;65:1016–20.
Ohm C, et al. Effects of antiplatelet agents on outcomes for elderly patients with traumatic intracranial hemorrhage. J Trauma. 2005;58:518–22.
Ott MM, Eriksson E, Vanderkolk W, Christianson D, Davis A, Scholten D. Antiplatelet and anticoagulation therapies do not increase mortality in the absence of traumatic brain injury. J Trauma. 2010;68:560–3.
Pandharipande P, Cotton BA, Sintani A, et al. Motoric subtypes of delirium in mechanically ventilated surgical and trauma intensive care unit patients. Intensive Care Med. 2007;33:1726–31.
Pergolizzi J, Böger RH, Budd K, et al. Opioids and the management of chronic severe pain the elderly: consensus statement of an international expert panel with focus on the six clinically most often used World Health Organization step III opioids (buprenorphine, fentanyl, hydromorphone, methadone, morphine, oxycodone). Pain Pract. 2008;4:287–313.
Pieracci FM, Eachampati SR, Shou J, Hydo LJ, Barie PS. Use of long-term anticoagulation is associated with traumatic intracranial hemorrhage and subsequent mortality in elderly patients hospitalized after falls: analysis of the New York State Administrative Database. J Trauma. 2007a;63:519–24.
Pieracci FM, Eachampati SR, Shou J, Hydo LJ, Barie PS. Degree of anticoagulation, but not warfarin use itself, predicts adverse outcomes after traumatic brain injury in elderly trauma patients. J Trauma. 2007b;63:525–30.
Pisani MA, McNicoll L, Inouye SK. Cognitive impairment in the intensive care unit. Clin Chest Med. 2003;24:727–37.
Poldermans D, Boersma E. Beta-blocker therapy in noncardiac surgery. N Engl J Med. 2005;353:412–4.
Roache V. Etiology and management of delirium. Am J Med Sci. 2003;325:20–30.
Robinson BRH, Mueller EW, Henson K, Branson RD, Barsoum S, Tsuei BJ. An analgesia-delirium-sedation protocol for critically ill trauma patients reduces ventilator days and hospital length of stay. J Trauma. 2008;65:517–36.
Sarode R, Matevosyan K, Bhagat R, Rutherford C, Madden C, Beshay JE. Rapid warfarin reversal: a 3-factor prothrombin complex concentrate and recombinant factor VIIa cocktail for intracerebral hemorrhage. J Neurosurg. 2012;116(3):491–7.
Sivamini RK, Pullar CE, Manabat-Hidalgo CG, et al. Stress-mediated increases in systemic and local epinephrine impair skin wound healing: potential new indication for beta blockers. PLoS Med. 2009;6:e12.
Smith SC, Blair SN, Bonow RO, et al. AHA/ACC Scientific Statement: AHA/ACC guidelines for prevention heart attack and death in patients with atherosclerotic cardiovascular disease: 2001 update. A statement for healthcare professional from the American Heart Association and the American College of Cardiology. Circulation. 2001;104:1577–9.
Spektor S, Agus S, Merkin V, Constantini S. Low-dose aspirin prophylaxis and risk of intracranial hemorrhage in patients older than 60 years of age with mild or moderate head injury: a prospective study. J Neurosurg. 2003;99:661–5.
van Aart L, Eijkhout HW, Kamphuis JS, et al. Individualized dosing regimen for prothrombin complex concentrate more effective than standard treatment in the reversal of oral anticoagulant therapy: an open, prospective randomized controlled trial. Thromb Res. 2006;118:313–20.
Watanabe M, Siddiqui FM, Qureshi AI. Incidence and management of ischemic stroke and intracerebral hemorrhage in patients on dabigatran etexilate treatment. Neurocrit Care. 2012;16:203–9.
Zhou W, Schwarting S, Illanes S, et al. Hemostatic therapy in experimental intracerebral hemorrhage associated with the direct thrombin inhibitor dabigatran. Stroke. 2011;42:3594–9.

Rehabilitation Concerns in Geriatric Trauma

35

Nancey Trevanian Tsai and Samir M. Fakhry

Introduction

The aging population faces a number of challenges due to changes in anatomy, physiology, and cognition as well as varying availability of social and financial support. Events that would have limited effects on younger patients are magnified in older patients. A common example is a ground level fall, which is a relatively minor event for a young person but, in an older individual is more likely to result in serious pathologies with high mortality rates, such as hip fracture [1]. A number of factors are contributory. Muscle tone and coordination decrease with age. Memory and judgment are affected negatively as is cognitive functioning. Decreased visual and hearing acuity, balance, and response time affect the ability to operate vehicles increasing the risk of a motor vehicle crash (MVC) [2]. The older patient is also more prone to depression, delirium, and dementia. These conditions are not only more common in the geriatric population but are increasingly diagnosed when they are hospitalized [3].

Rehabilitation and Functional Restoration

Many patients in the aging population require rehabilitation as a result of injuries incurred during routine activities that they had performed for many years, but which have become more difficult as they develop more intrinsic barriers. As society has become less "nuclear," fewer intergenerational families cohabitate and the elderly have less support and supervision making them more prone to injury. Furthermore, as a result of this deterioration of multigenerational households, once injury has been sustained, there are fewer family members readily available to assist in functional activities and/or supervision. Seniors generally desire to maintain as much independence as possible, sometimes to their detriment and that of the immediate caregiver groups. With longer and active lifestyles becoming more common, it is likely that the incidence of injury in the elderly will increase resulting in more demand for rehabilitation services for this special population.

It is safe to assume that one of the most important goals of any hospital admission is to discharge the patient safely to a functional environment. For many patients, being able to return to their homes represents the final destination when recovered. Furthermore, length of stay is a quality indicator at many facilities. For the elderly patient, returning to their home, while psychologically fulfilling, may not address the needs for therapies and more intensive rehabilitation after injury.

Discharge planning should optimally begin at the time of admission. Frequently a social worker or case manager evaluates the patient's pre-injury state of wellness at an early stage to consider all of the options available to the patient and to assist the team with discharge plans. Early on, the team uses assessment and prognostic tools in order to establish the likely level of independence at the time of discharge for each patient. All members of the team are responsible for assessing the need for assistance based upon their expertise and experience with the disease and injuries and for communicating it to the admitting service. A viable discharge from the acute inpatient setting is typically contingent upon meeting certain medical criteria and on ensuring that the patient will not require readmission to the hospital due to discharge to an unsafe environment and/or inability to follow through with the treatments prescribed. In the future, it is anticipated that the Centers for

N.T. Tsai, MD
Department of Neurosurgery, Medical University of South Carolina, 96 Jonathan Lucas Street, CSB 301, Charleston, SC 29425-6130, USA
e-mail: tsain@musc.edu

S.M. Fakhry, MD, FACS (✉)
Department of Surgery, Medical University of South Carolina, 96 Jonathan Lucas Street, CSB 426 MSC 613, Charleston, SC 29425-6130, USA
e-mail: fakhry@musc.edu

J.A. Yelon, F.A. Luchette (eds.), *Geriatric Trauma and Critical Care*,
DOI 10.1007/978-1-4614-8501-8_35, © Springer Science+Business Media New York 2014

Medicare and Medicaid Services (CMS) will track these results and adjust (i.e., decrease) reimbursement to treating facilities based upon readmissions of any type within 1 month of discharge.

The aging patient frequently has multiple challenges specific to the injury and comorbidities that prevent successful independent living. For example, hypertension and diabetes tend to have higher prevalence in this population, and both are linked to microvascular disease that, when manifest in the brain, contributes to dementia. Patients may seem relatively functional in known environments where many tasks are automatic, but demonstrate severe cognitive deficits when removed from their usual environment. Additionally, the cortical atrophy of the brain reduces the volume of the brain relative to the calvarium and can lead to indolent subdural hemorrhages, which, coupled with the increased incidence of falls, lead to devastating injuries from a minor injury. Not infrequently, financial burdens limit the extent to which the patient is able to obtain assistance for activities of daily living. Family or other designated caregivers may be unwilling or unable to provide 24-h supervision. Available evidence and common sense would suggest that well-developed, actively involved family networks are linked to decreased rates of institutionalization [4]. This is true for those family members and/or caregivers willing and able to offer ongoing, reliable, hands-on assistance to their love ones. In many cases, however, the patient's primary support system is not readily available or is not located close to the patients preferred residence, thereby creating a dilemma for the patient and their family potentially delaying discharge. These challenges should be identified early and options presented to the patient or designated decision maker(s), such as the healthcare power of attorney.

Rehabilitation Assessment

There are a number of discharge environments available for the patient to transition to prior to returning to their home. Criteria for admission are largely based upon expected functional outcomes as well as funding availability. The Centers for Medicare and Medicaid Services (CMS) designates the diagnoses that they accept as appropriate for rehabilitation. This changes as CMS reviews the claims made on an annual basis, which is to say that admission criteria incur potentially significant changes annually for acute inpatient rehabilitation facilities (IRF), subacute and skilled nursing facilities (SNF), and long-term acute care (LTAC) facilities. Although helpful, it is not expected that non-rehabilitation physicians understand the subtleties of this system. This necessitates a strong working relationship with rehabilitation specialists to assure timely discharge of the injured patient. To further complicate the matter, not all insurance policies cover the gamut of rehabilitation services, such as inpatient, subacute or skilled nursing facility, or even outpatient therapies. For example, patients on Medicaid in South Carolina are often surprised to learn that their policy does not provide outpatient physical therapy (PT). Clearly, the patient with good resources will have the most options available. Later in this chapter, we will provide an overview of the different rehabilitation settings.

As the patient's condition progresses during the hospitalization, there is increased involvement of the interdisciplinary functional restoration team. Early involvement of the physiatrist facilitates care and communication with the patient and the caregivers regarding the options for discharge. Physical medicine and rehabilitation (PM&R) specialists can suggest the best setting for continued care and facilitate the transition to those destinations. However, if the goal is for eventual discharge to home or another permanent living arrangement, it is the responsibility of every member of the entire medical team to be part of that plan to discuss potential barriers with the patient and/or caregivers.

Patients can be assessed for function in the following manner [5]:

1. Identify the diseases and injuries and their sequelae that are affecting activities of daily living (ADLs) to include eating, grooming, dressing, voiding/evacuating, mobility, and cognition. Are there range of motion or weight-bearing restrictions that will impact the patient's ability to do those activities? Do they have appropriate mentation to attend to tasks safely? (Functional Independence Measure (FIM™))
2. Identify barriers to performing ADLs and their completion, such as meal preparation, safety awareness, and entering/exiting the home or rooms in the home. What assistive devices may improve adaptive function and is it financially feasible to obtain them?
3. Identify need for caregivers, especially if relative independence is not expected at the time of discharge. At what level of care will the patient's caregivers be willing to take them home?
4. Identify additional education and training needs. Is additional training or therapy indicated prior to discharge to their previous living situation?

For the patient with significant impairments or disabilities, a consultation from PM&R services may be indicated to delineate the subtleties of progress and recovery. Brain injuries, strokes, and spinal cord injuries involve complex functional issues for the patient, significant educational and physical assistance commitments for the caregivers, and community resource requirements that the interdisciplinary team will need to navigate.

Function is measured in a number of ways. Most inpatient therapists and physiatrists will use elements of the FIM™ or Functional Independence Measure. The full FIM consists of

Table 35.1 Functional Independence Measure Instrument™: developed by the University of Buffalo, a proprietary, subscription-based instrument to measure and document function

Contains 18 items composed of: 13 motor tasks 5 cognitive tasks (considered basic activities of daily living)
Dimensions assessed include: Eating Grooming Bathing Upper body dressing Lower body dressing Toileting Bladder management Bowel management Bed to chair transfer Toilet transfer Shower transfer Locomotion (ambulatory or wheelchair level) Stairs Cognitive comprehension Expression Social interaction Problem solving Memory
Tasks are rated on a 7-point ordinal scale: 7 – Independent: able to perform task independently 6 – Modified independent: able to perform task independently, but requires extra time 5 – Supervised: able to perform task with setup, may need verbal cues for safety and sequencing 4 – Minimal assistance: Requires assistance for up to 25 % of the task 3 – Moderate assistance: Requires assistance for 26–50 % of the task 2 – Maximal assistance: Requires assistance for 51–75 % of the task 1 – Total assistance: Requires assistance for greater than 76 % of the task
Scores range from 18 (lowest) to 126 (highest) indicating level of function
Scores are generally rated at admission and discharge

18 items measured on a 7-point scale (see Table 35.1 and Fig. 35.1). Other measurement systems exist, but CMS has adopted FIM as the primary tool determining the patient's functional level in the rehabilitation setting.

The Interdisciplinary Functional Restoration Team

There are a number of allied health members who are active in the functional restoration process. Each has their own scope of practice and may make suggestions to the primary team based upon their specialty.

Occupational Therapist (OT)

Occupational therapists work with therapeutic use of everyday life activities to participate in the home, school, work, and community settings, addressing physical, cognitive, psychosocial, and other aspects of performance that affect health, well-being, and quality of life. These professionals include:

- Occupational therapy aide/assistant (OTA): Aides are frequently trained on the job, while assistants have an associate-level degree; in some states, the latter clinician is required to have licensure in order to practice.
- Occupational therapist (OT): A baccalaureate- or masters-level degree in an occupational therapy course of study.
- Doctor of Occupational Therapy (Dr. OT): Possess a doctorate-level degree with a dissertation defense in occupational therapy.

Physical Therapist (PT)

Physical therapists examine functional limitation, disability, or other health-related conditions to determine a diagnosis, prognosis, and intervention in order to alleviate impairment through use of exercise, manual therapies, adaptive measures, and modalities. These professionals include:

- Physical therapy aide/assistant (PTA): Aides are frequently trained on the job, while assistants have an associate-level degree; in some states, the latter is required to have licensure in order to practice.
- Physical therapist (PT): This individual has obtained a baccalaureate- or masters-level degree in physical therapy.
- Doctor of Physical Therapy (DPT): The doctorate level degree is awarded after defending a dissertation in physical therapy.

Physiatrist

A physician (M.D., D.O.) with graduate medical education in Physical Medicine and Rehabilitation. Their educational focus is on function and independence in treating nerve, bone, and muscle injuries and illness. They are interdisciplinary team leaders, considering a broad range of medical, socioeconomic, neuropsychological, and cultural factors and barriers that affect a patient's ability to recover and function independently. There are subspecialty designations in Traumatic Brain Injury (TBI), Spinal Cord Injury (SCI), Electrodiagnostics (EMG) and Neuromuscular Medicine, Pain Medicine, Palliative Care, and Sports Medicine. Not all physiatrists participate in acute/subacute inpatient rehabilitation, as many maintain pure outpatient, procedural-based

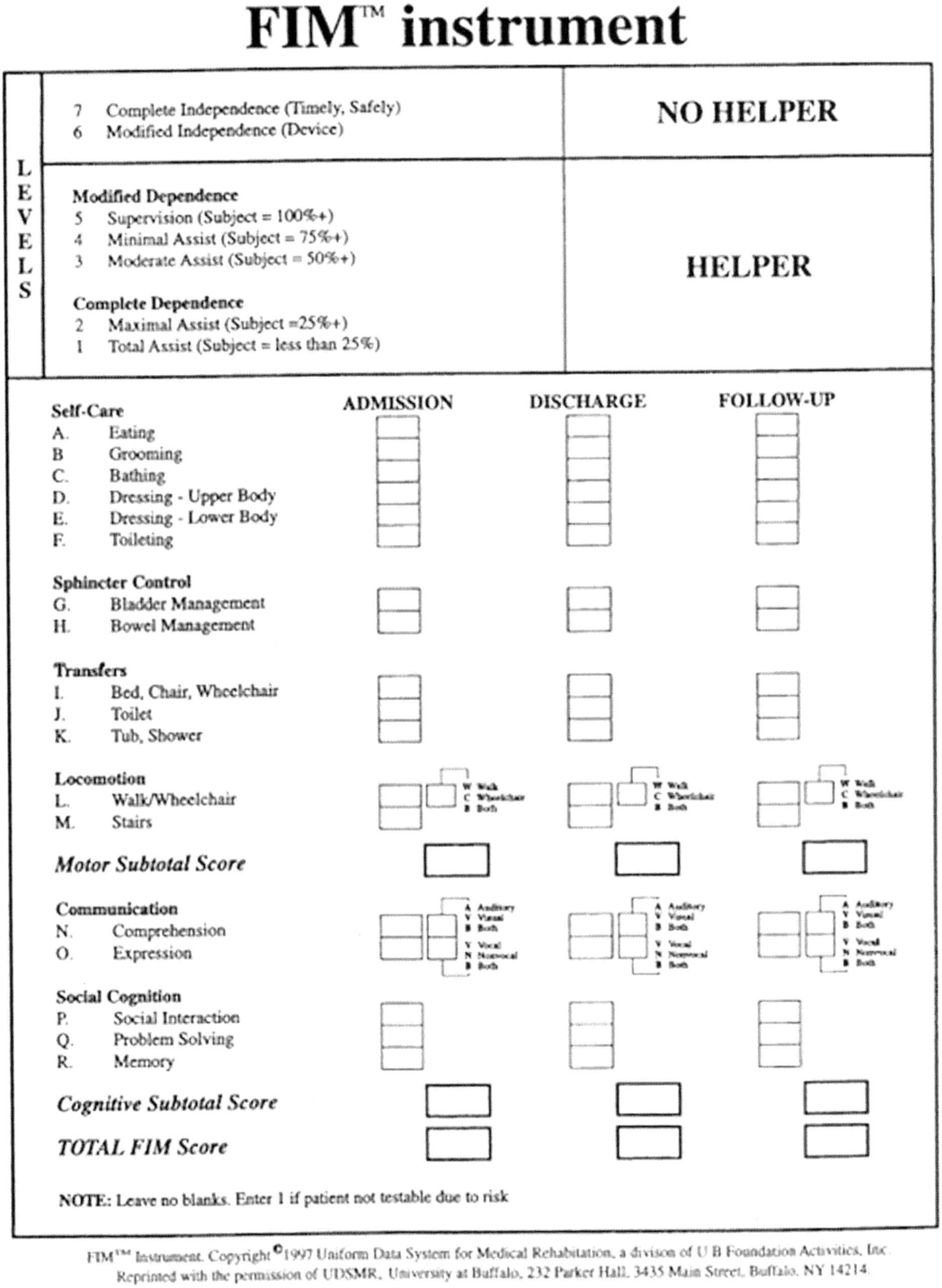

FIM™ instrument

LEVELS		
	7 Complete Independence (Timely, Safely) 6 Modified Independence (Device)	NO HELPER
	Modified Dependence 5 Supervision (Subject = 100%+) 4 Minimal Assist (Subject = 75%+) 3 Moderate Assist (Subject = 50%+) **Complete Dependence** 2 Maximal Assist (Subject = 25%+) 1 Total Assist (Subject = less than 25%)	HELPER

	ADMISSION	DISCHARGE	FOLLOW-UP
Self-Care			
A. Eating			
B. Grooming			
C. Bathing			
D. Dressing - Upper Body			
E. Dressing - Lower Body			
F. Toileting			
Sphincter Control			
G. Bladder Management			
H. Bowel Management			
Transfers			
I. Bed, Chair, Wheelchair			
J. Toilet			
K. Tub, Shower			
Locomotion			
L. Walk/Wheelchair	W Walk C Wheelchair B Both	W Walk C Wheelchair B Both	W Walk C Wheelchair B Both
M. Stairs			
Motor Subtotal Score			
Communication			
N. Comprehension	A Auditory V Visual B Both	A Auditory V Visual B Both	A Auditory V Visual B Both
O. Expression	V Vocal N Nonvocal B Both	V Vocal N Nonvocal B Both	V Vocal N Nonvocal B Both
Social Cognition			
P. Social Interaction			
Q. Problem Solving			
R. Memory			
Cognitive Subtotal Score			
TOTAL FIM Score			

NOTE: Leave no blanks. Enter 1 if patient not testable due to risk

Fig. 35.1 FIM instrument

practices. Practitioners who typically interface with hospital-based teams are in general rehabilitation and are available on a consultative basis.

Medical Social Worker (MSW)

Medical social workers have an in-depth understanding of the resources available to the patient based upon available funding, area (e.g., county) of residence, and related factors. They communicate those options to the patient and the team. They are frequently expert communicators who gather environmental and contextual information, explain the barriers and challenges to patients and their caregivers, and confirm the final discharge plan.

Speech-Language Pathologist (SLP)

These individuals have a graduate-level degree with clinical certification to treat patients with speech, swallowing, and cognitive deficits through use of therapeutic exercises, adaptive strategies, and devices.

Special Considerations in the Geriatric Population

The aging population is typically injured by lower energy force [5–9]. For example, falls are usually from standing or sitting, and compression fractures may occur after sneezing, coughing, or other normal physiologic activities. This occurs because of the effect of aging on bone metabolism resulting in osteoporosis. Furthermore, aging may be responsible for degenerative changes in various organs that will limit the patient's potential for rehabilitation. Changes to the central nervous system that occur in the geriatric patient include a decline in cognition, gait instability, and incontinence/urgency with poor skin integrity. These preexisting conditions amplify the challenges that lead to successful community reentry once the patient recovers from an injury.

Cognitive Decline

Cognitive deficits in the aging population typically involve memory, orientation, and/or judgment [10, 11]. Memory deficits can result from primary progressive diseases, such as Alzheimer disease, or cumulative processes, such as small vessel brain disease or multiple traumatic or anoxic events. Cognitive declines are magnified with each additional injury to the head. A communication challenge to families and caregivers is to convey the idea that while the patient may seem to be independent performing routine daily activities, they may have had a decline in cognition for many years. It is important to note that short-term memory is primarily affected, while long-term memory is maintained, even with dementia.

Unfortunately, with impairment of short-term memory, new tasks taught to enforce safety in mobility may only be learned through repetition and supervision. The rehabilitation team frequently engages in scheduled tasks that are in keeping with the patient's baseline activities and teaches safe strategies to avoid future injuries. It is not uncommon that patients perform better upon discharge home, as familiar environments can provide reminders for activities and precautions.

Gait Instability and Balance

One of the hallmarks of aging is the phenomenon of falling [13–16]. The rising incidence of idiopathic falls in the elderly is still a medical enigma and is likely multifactorial. Not uncommonly, older people fall while performing routine activities, such as getting to the bathroom or transferring while bathing. Prevention of falls includes assessing the home for loose rugs, items close to the ground (e.g., grandchildren toys, pets) that may not be seen easily in dim lighting or with a decline in vision, and smooth flooring that can lead to slippery surfaces when wet, such as tile or wood floors.

Trauma in the aging population typically occurs at lower speeds and heights. Falls from standing due to decreased balance can cause multiple fractures due to loss of bone density. Hip fractures are associated mortality rates of 50 % over 1 year. Degenerative spondylosis increases with age and contributes to a number of conditions associated with increased risk for falling. Cervical myelopathy due to stenosis or vertebral fractures can contribute to falling and result in spinal cord injury. Central cord syndrome is common and can occur with minimal injury. Atrophy of brain mass potentiates tears of bridging veins in the subdural space, which leads to further decline in mentation that can then contribute to falling. Prevention of falls and known contributing factors can help to prevent related injuries.

Prior to discharge, it behooves the clinical team to discuss with patients some of the abovementioned barriers. As quality benchmarks are predicated on decreasing readmissions to the hospital, it becomes essential to limit the ways that patients might incur further injuries in their home through prevention and preemptive preparation. Currently, the literature is equivocal on Tai Chi and other exercises for fall prevention, although it is largely accepted that the patient who stays the most active and mindful is typically less prone to fall. For patients with frequent falls, balance and proprioceptive therapies might be suggested [17, 18]. There are PTs who specialize in this complex process and can be of tremendous benefit to the patient and their families.

Continence and Urgency

Another phenomenon that is more prevalent with advancing age is that of urinary urgency. For men, prostatic hypertrophy and/or malignancy can lead to incomplete bladder emptying with the subjective sensation of urgency and frequency. For women, especially those who have had children and/or gynecological surgery, the integrity of the perineum and external sphincters may have been disrupted, leading to stress and urge incontinence [19, 20]. Additionally, many aging patients are on diuretics and other medications that alter ability to hold or excrete urine. Careful consideration to the time of day when those medications are taken will also improve duration of uninterrupted sleep at night. For example, it is not uncommon for furosemide to be prescribed as multiple doses each day. Knowing that its pharmacokinetics occurs within 6 h, the last dose each day should be taken at least 6 h before bedtime to promote good sleep hygiene. It should not be surprising that with declining dexterity in clothing management and nocturnal frequency are factors that make the bathroom one of the more dangerous rooms in the home for the elderly.

When approaching a patient with continence issues, it is important to identify whether the patient has a spastic bladder, detrusor atony, sphincter incompetency/dysynergia, or outlet obstruction. This can be identified during the inpatient setting by performing bladder scans to determine the bladder volume index and/or post-void residuals. If bladder volumes are consistently low with frequency, then the patient may benefit from an anticholinergic medication. If the bladder volumes are high post-void, it may be that the patient needs to decompress the bladder for a time and use medications that either promotes detrusor tone (e.g., bethanechol) or maintains an open sphincter to allow complete emptying (e.g., tamsulosin). A urology consult should be obtained for the patient with an enlarged prostate or intrapelvic organ prolapse. For most patients, performing bladder scans is a noninvasive way to identify and potentially treat continence problems for the aging patient.

Timed voiding is an easy way for many patients and their caregivers to manage continence. One simple way to avoid incontinence is to offer the aging patient regular times for elimination such as upon awakening, after each meal, and at bedtime. This allows for the opportunity to void and evacuate at least four times a day and is concurrent with activities already requiring supervision, set up, or assistance.

Skin Integrity

Aging is associated with a loss of subcutaneous adipose tissue. This in combination with certain medications that are commonly prescribed for the geriatric patient with concomitant cardiopulmonary disease such as anticoagulants and inhaled steroids increases the risk for skin breakdown, particularly in the sedentary patient [21]. Additionally, incontinence and widespread use of impermeable briefs trap moisture against the skin over bony prominences such as the sacrum and ischial tuberosities leading to an increased incidence of decubitus ulcers. Timed voiding, as described above, is one way to limit the use of briefs by allowing regular micturition and evacuation. For those patients with limited cognition and mobility, a condom or indwelling catheter may be considered, although these are associated with higher risks of urinary tract infections, which can also exacerbate preexisting cognitive dysfunction. It is important to counsel the patient and caregivers on the importance of checking the skin and minimizing the use of impermeable briefs when possible.

Social Structure and Support

As mentioned earlier, more and more children are opting to move away from their parents in the course of seeking educational and employment opportunities. Thus, it is not uncommon that the aging patient lives without siblings and/or children in the same community. Even when children do reside in the same neighborhood, they are not available for constant supervision or assistance of their parents. Americans are living longer because of improved medical care, but it does not necessarily mean that their quality of life or independence is preserved. Independent and assisted living communities have become more commonplace to address this sense of isolation. These facilities are not without substantial cost, however. It is not uncommon for independent living apartments to cost thousands of dollars in monthly rent. The cost escalates with additional services. To avoid leaving their home, friends and neighbors or even extended families that have remained in the area assist the elderly with ADL. However, varying levels of commitment from these individuals over the long term should be expected and clarified by a team representative.

A word should be mentioned about bereavement as a chronic condition. It is not uncommon for the aging patient to experience a slow erosion of their social support, including that from their spouse. Depression can adversely affect one's motivation and willingness to participate. There may be a profound desire to not continue living, and efforts should be made to address the psychological barriers to successful rehabilitation. These conditions are commonly magnified by decreased metabolic and endocrine function. If psychiatry or neuropsychology services are available, consultation can be beneficial both to address the psychological issues and identify potential endocrine and/or neurophysiological contributors to the depression and dysthymia.

Consulting Rehabilitation

An appropriate rehabilitation consultation request should have the following elements:

1. Primary and secondary diagnoses
2. Weight-bearing restrictions and/or other restriction with their duration (e.g., sternal precautions for 6 weeks (post CABG) or NWB for 8 weeks (lower extremity fractures))
3. Comorbidities and contraindications to relatively physically demanding activities
4. At least one discharge plan and setting with caregivers identified as indicated

Any rehabilitation request should be accompanied with at least one viable discharge plan. Rehabilitation is what patients do when temporarily discharge to a therapy providing facility prior to transitioning to the final destination of home. Even amongst the most experienced physicians, rehabilitation can represent a "black box" where a patient is admitted and after improvement are discharged to home. Additionally, while patients can make significant functional improvements, they may not reach complete independence, especially if they have not been independent for quite some time. Consistent conveyance and communication of realistic goals and expectations is the responsibility of the physiatrist and the multidisciplinary team.

Rehabilitation Settings and Criteria for Services

There are different levels of care for rehabilitation services, just as there are different levels of care in hospitals. After admission to a rehabilitation facility, patients may require intensive therapies on a daily basis or may only tolerate a few sessions a week. The patient's insurance carrier will frequently dictate the setting of the post-acute rehabilitation based upon the coverage provided in the insured's policy (see Fig. 35.2). Additionally, it may be helpful to think of the different levels of rehabilitation as a continuum of care; in reality, it is common for a patient to start at an acute inpatient rehabilitation center, transition to a skilled nursing facility, then be discharged to home with home-based therapy, and transitioned to outpatient therapies. This treatment course may require several months after the index acute illness (see Table 35.2).

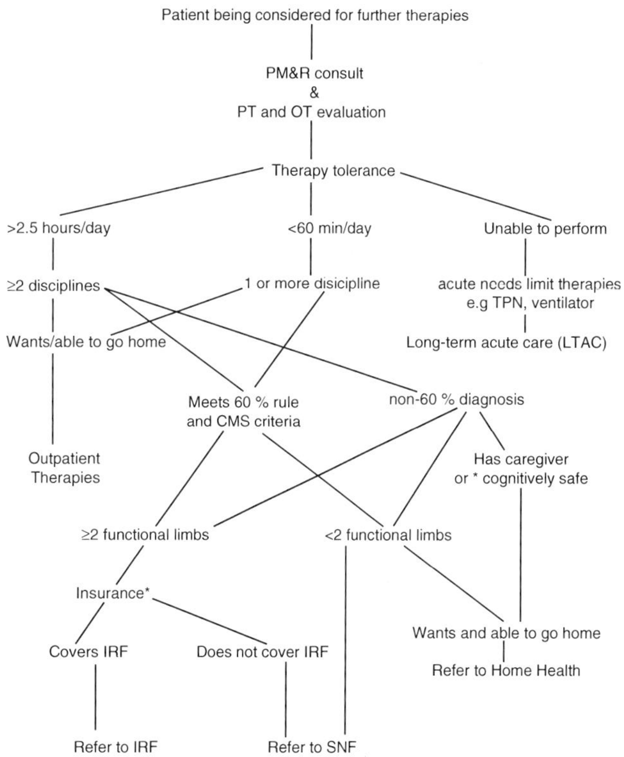

Fig. 35.2 Patient being considered for further therapies

Acute Inpatient Rehabilitation Facility (IRF)

Those who are able to tolerate intensity therapies and demonstrate a high likelihood of significant functional improvements are referred to an IRF. The requirements for admissions to rehabilitation hospitals are strict, and the costs are high (see below). Cost per day varies geographically. For the uninsured, the average cost is approximately $3,500 per day but may be negotiable.

Skilled Nursing Facilities (SNF)

Those who have limited tolerance for therapy, such as those with poor endurance, pain management difficulties, and/or limited ability to learn skills compatible with safe, independent living, are referred to nursing homes. An example of a typical situation where this is appropriate would be for a patient who's weight-bearing status will not change for at least 6–12 weeks after a fracture. Once there is adequate healing, the patient would then begin either inpatient or outpatient therapy. Some SNFs have *subacute therapies services* available, so that the patient will be able to get *at least 180 min of therapies a week*. Many subacute facilities strive

Table 35.2 Overview of typical settings for continued rehabilitation efforts

Rehabilitation option	Typical length of stay	Services/requirements	Insurance coverage
Inpatient rehabilitation facility (IRF)	~10–14 days on average; model systems* (see below) can provide longer stays	Require and are able to tolerate high-intensity therapies at the rate of at least 3 h/day or 15 h/week	Medicare: covers 14 CMS diagnoses
		Must require at least two therapy modalities: PT, OT, and/or SLP	Commercial: varies by plan; requires pre-authorization
		Must require rehab nursing	Medicaid: no
		Must have completed all medical and surgical procedures, are medically stable, and require continued medical supervision	
		Demonstrate high likelihood of significant functional improvements	
		Must have viable discharge plan upon completion of IRF stay	
Model systems IRF	Individually assessed during stay	National Institute on Disability and Rehabilitation Research (NIDRR) funded facilities that receive funding for establishing models for treatment of certain diagnoses (i.e., TBI, SCI)	Medicare: covers typical diagnoses
		Maintain databases on patient treatments and outcomes for the purposes of research and innovative outcomes	Commercial: varies Medicaid: no
Skilled nursing (SNF)/	~20 days, but can be up to 100 days	Require and are able to tolerate some therapies up to 180 min/week	Medicare: covers most diagnoses
Subacute rehabilitation		Many SNFs will work more with patients who are preparing for IRF stay	Commercial: varies by plan; requires pre-authorization
		PT, OT, +/– SLP usually available at most facilities	Medicaid: varies by state
Long-term acute care (LTAC)	Depends on pathology; most take ventilated patients	No therapy requirements, although many offer it in preparation for IRF/SNF	Medicare: covers most diagnoses
		Requires continued physician supervision with 24 h nursing	Commercial: varies by plan; requires pre-authorization
			Medicaid: typically no
Home health	Depends on progress and prognosis	Patients must be home bound and willing to receive care and/or therapies in their home	Medicare: covers most diagnoses
			Commercial: varies
			Medicaid: typically covers
Outpatient therapies	Depends on progress	Goal is to restore function to baseline including requirements for employment	Medicare: covers
			Commercial: varies
			Medicaid: no

Coverage for each option vary by state and by specific insurance plan

to offer patients who are making progress more therapies in order to prepare them for acute IRF admissions, but they are not obligated to do so. Others are able to do less intense therapies over longer periods of time for those patients who are otherwise sedentary at home or live with assistance. Again, the cost varies geographically by location. For those individuals without coverage, the average cost is approximately $500 per day.

Long-Term Acute Care (LTAC)

Certain patients require specific acute needs, but less intensity of care than provided at an acute care hospital. The typical patient who requires the services of a LTAC facility is medically "stable" but ventilator dependent or requires long-term antibiotic therapy or protracted nutrition supplementation. There is no requirement to offer rehabilitative therapies, although many LTAC facilities will have limited therapy services to prepare patients for discharge to an IRF. The cost for these services varies by facility.

Home Health Services

These are skilled services provided in the patient's home. Requirements for these services are that the patient is homebound and must be willing to receive the services in their home. Skilled services include PT, OT, SLP (not available in all areas), nursing care, wound care (not available in all areas), social worker, and/or aide services. Typically, services are provided up to 3 days a week. There is geographical variation in the cost for these services.

Outpatient Therapies

For patients who are mobile and not restricted to their residency, many services are available as an outpatient. They are typically more intense than home health services and offer a greater variety of therapeutic modalities. Patients will frequently incur a co-payment even with insurance coverage.

Hospice

Occasionally, a patient will be assessed to be within 6 months of his/her expected life span. In this case, it is appropriate to consult palliative care services to see if the patient qualifies for hospice services either in their own home, a caregiver's home, or at a hospice facility. A patient can enter and exit a hospice arrangement as their disease process declares itself, and it would be important to communicate this to the patient and their family members. Palliative care service specialists are now versed in such diverse topics as chronic pain management and end-of-life care.

Therapy Prescription and Insurance Coverage

For patients fortunate enough to be discharged home successfully with good support systems while requiring continued therapy, a well-written therapy prescription can be very beneficial to bringing the patient back to their functional status or better. While it is not uncommon for therapists to see prescriptions that say nothing more than "Evaluate and treat," a proper therapy prescription should have the following elements:

1. Specific diagnosis and ICD-9 code to assist with authorization.
2. Frequency and duration of each treatment; most Medicare prescriptions need to be updated monthly.
3. Limitations (e.g., ROM, weight-bearing), precautions, and contraindications to exercise and activity.
4. Specific protocols or treatments desired (if known).
5. Physician signature and date.

The aging patient who has sustained an injury frequently will need to "qualify" for inpatient rehabilitation. There are many rules and regulations that govern IRFs, not to mention misconceptions about their capabilities and logistics on the part of the referring physician as well as the patient and their family. The aging patient will typically have Medicare coverage and qualify for most options including admission to an inpatient rehabilitation facility. However, a patient who requests an IRF referral must still meet the criteria and be able to tolerate the rigorous treatment plan. CMS has identified policies regarding intensive, inpatient rehabilitation services [22]. The services must be reasonable and necessary for the treatment of the patient's condition. In addition, it must be reasonable and necessary to provide these services on an inpatient basis, rather than in a less intensive setting. There are eight specific criteria that the patient must satisfy:

1. *Medically stable, having completed all interventions and workups, and requiring close medical supervision by a physician with experience in PM&R*: The process of inpatient rehabilitation is rigorous and is very different from the acute hospital stay. Patients are asked to have energy expenditures of 3–7 metabolic equivalents (METs) in their evaluation. For reference, each metabolic equivalent is defined as the amount of oxygen consumed for a particular activity, where 1 MET = 3.5 mL O_2 per kg body weight. Three METs is equivalent to walking at a slow pace, and 7 METs would correlate with hiking. As such, it is highly advisable that older patients have adequate hemoglobin and hematocrit levels to support exercise at this level to avoid any risk for cardiac ischemia. They should be able to consume enough nutrition to account for the activity. Additionally, they should have the fewest number of impediments to therapy, such as intravenous lines, catheters, drains, and or continuous feeding tubes so that they will be able to manage their clothing and equipment with minimal risk of injury.
2. *24 hours a day need for rehabilitation nursing*: These patients are typically medically stable, but require careful monitoring of vital signs, oxygen saturation, intake and output, etc., as they adapt to daily activities from a state of relative recumbence. Rehabilitation nurses are also the first line of defense for safety awareness and the patient's pain management needs.
3. *Be able to tolerate an intense level of rehabilitation service (3 h a day, at least 5 days a week, or 15 h per week)*: Many patients who have had a long inpatient stay would appear to be ideal candidates for intense inpatient rehabilitation. In fact, such patients are frequently unable to tolerate the intense level of activity delivered at these centers because of muscle deconditioning, residual injuries that are still incompletely healed, residual cognitive dysfunction from brain injury, exacerbation of preexisting physical or cognitive impairments, and other commonly encountered residua of multiple trauma. This is especially relevant in the geriatric population. It is a common misconception that patients undergoing outpatient procedures are immediately ready for rehabilitation in all cases. Many of the patients who are discharged home the same day of a surgical procedure will be at relative bed

rest for several days, and performing a relatively high level of activity may interrupt their healing process. Furthermore, many elderly patients led very sedentary lifestyles at pre-injury baseline and may not tolerate an intense activity regardless of their medical condition.

4. *A multidisciplinary team approach to delivery of the program*: The patient requires at least two therapeutic modalities, to include PT, OT, and/or SLP. Although there are other members of the rehabilitation team, such as recreational therapists and neuropsychologists who are not infrequently involved, the services they provide do not count toward the "3 h a day" rule.
5. *A coordinated program of care*: A daily schedule that outlines their activities and weekly goals must be documented.
6. *A significant practical improvement must be likely* (e.g., an increase in FIM score): Inpatient rehabilitation is a costly but effective way to restore function, teach adaptive strategies, and patient/caregiver safety. Patients referred to IRFs should have significantly declined from baseline functional status and demonstrate potential for improvement. Physiatrists have training and experience assessing these prognostic indicators and can be a very helpful resource to determining long-term outcome. If a patient is not expected to make any improvements, they should not be referred for this expensive resource.
7. *The rehabilitation goals must be realistic*: Most intensive rehabilitation occurs in a very short amount of time. Patients should have enough physical and cognitive ability, endurance, social support, and desire to participate actively to make the most out of this experience. The end goals have to be achievable and commensurate with all of the supporting factors.
8. *A reasonable length of stay* (LOS): Average LOS for most rehabilitation centers is around 2 weeks. For some injuries and diseases, this can be longer. However, it may be helpful to know that Medicare usually has to make exceptions for stays longer than 20 days.

The CMS also specified diagnoses that qualify a patient for admission to an IRF. Currently, there is a mandate that at least 60 % of the patients admitted for care into an IRF will have one of the following diagnoses:

1. Stroke
2. Congenital deformity
3. Spinal cord injury
4. Amputation
5. Brain injury
6. Major multiple trauma (with internal organ damage)
7. Hip fracture
8. Burns
9. Neurological disorders
10. Active polyarticular arthritis with multiple joint involvement which limits functional activities that cannot be addressed adequately on an outpatient basis
11. Systemic vasculidities refractory to aggressive, sustained treatment with declining function
12. Severe advanced osteoarthritis involving two or more joints (excluding replaced joints) that significantly impairs function in mobility and/or self-care, which has failed conservative therapies and the patient is not a candidate for other treatments
13. Knee and/or hip replacement if one or more of the following are met:
    (a) Bilateral joint replacement
    (b) Morbid obesity (BMI >50)
    (c) Age ≥85 years old

Since the 60 % rule is for all of the admissions over 1 year, it is not uncommon for an IRF to limit admissions that do not fall into the above categories at times of the year, usually just prior to the end of the fiscal year, in order to maintain compliance with CMS rules. Should CMS decide to increase that percentage to 75 % as has been proposed recently [22], there may be even more restrictions on trauma patient admission into IRFs.

Challenges and Future Directions

Many of the challenges in assessing the aging patient for rehabilitative care are related to the ever-changing guidelines, rules, and regulations. The CMS has specific rules regarding the various settings for rehabilitation which may be changed annually as they continue to assess the efficiency and efficacy of services. Additionally, insurance companies frequently change their coverage as laws and negotiations with providers change. In addition to dealing with the challenges in providing the standard of care, the rehabilitation team is limited by reimbursement rules and regulations. The functional restoration resources available to the patients are largely dictated by nonphysician entities with which the patient has to interface unless they have access to large cash reserves. While there are some facilities that have funding provided by the National Institute on Disability and Rehabilitation Research (NIDRR) who provide models for optimal care, only the most financially viable pieces trickle through to the vast majority of general IRFs, SNFs, and other settings. These layers of barriers are seldom encountered by acute clinicians, making the process of selecting the ideal environment for rehabilitation even more frustrating for the admitting physicians. It may help to keep in mind that the rehabilitation process is largely optional, even though the functional benefits are potentially immense.

The members of the rehabilitation team have experience with the most devastating impairments and disabilities and are able to establish realistic functional goals based upon established prognostic indicators. This can be complicated in the elderly patient as they may have baseline deficits due to the effects of aging on various organs function. For example, posttraumatic amnesia is a common indicator for potential recovery after brain injury. For the patient with preexisting symptoms of memory loss or dementia, this becomes even more difficult to assess. It is safe to assume that the patient will, at best, return to their baseline and should not be expected to exceed it. However, family member expectations are frequently unrealistic, such as their loved one will improve dramatically with prolonged therapy. It is important to communicate realistic and manageable goals with the patient and their caregivers. Rehabilitation team goals are typically conservative, as it is easier to have less assistance than to require more resources.

Using 2012 prices, 1 week of inpatient rehabilitation care is approximately $25,000 depending upon facility and geographic location; 1 week at a subacute is approximately $5,000; each hour of home health and/or outpatient skilled care is between $100 and 150; privately hired aides are between $15 and 20/h. The insurance coverage varies by state and by carrier, and acceptance is largely dictated by authorization of the payer. These are relative costs and may vary by region and payer source.

Generally, the most common cause of frustration is due to the referring physician and case manager not understanding the meaning of "Medical Necessity." PM&R is a specialty that is based upon evidence and research, with predictable outcomes, despite working within the constraints of rules and regulations that vary from state to state. Part of the training involves understanding the criteria set forth by government agencies for admission into more intensive therapies, in addition to addressing the functional needs of each individual patient. Ideally, the rehabilitation potential of the patient should be assessed by a physiatrist through formal consultation, just as any patient needing treatment should be evaluated by the appropriate specialist. The intensity, duration, and final program specifics are determined after the patient is admitted to the rehabilitation center. It is generally inappropriate for a non-physiatrist to promise functional outcomes or determine the length of stay at a rehabilitation facility as that would set up unrealistic expectations by the patient and potential caregivers who may make firm plans based upon faulty information.

Another area of dissonance between the trauma team and the PM&R consultants is the tendency for the former to treat the latter as administrative adjuncts rather than colleagues. Appropriate reasons to consult physiatry include assessing rehabilitation potential and/or the setting in which to perform functional restoration. Physiatrists can assess a patient's expected level of function within a specified length of time and training as a function of the injuries and disease processes at work, limited by the patient's motivation and social support. For example, the American Spinal Injury Association (ASIA) guidelines state that a patient with spinal cord injury (SCI) at the C5 level will be dependent on care unless motor function recovery to at least the C6 level is seen in the first days and weeks after the initial injury. No amount of rehabilitation will change that prognosis with current technology. Furthermore, although C6 is the highest level at which a person with SCI can expect to be somewhat independent [23], it takes someone of tremendous motivation and intelligence to become independent with that level of impairment. As such, part of the rehabilitation consultation is to assess the potential for successful discharge from a coordinated program given the patient's baseline capabilities. The case manager usually has to clarify the specific benefits and settings that are available to the patient, and is indispensible to discharge planning.

Not infrequently, information gathered during the consultation is either incomplete or changes as the discharge approaches. For example, a patient with bilateral lower limb fractures limited to touchdown weight-bearing on both legs and is also non-weight-bearing on one upper extremity cannot perform enough activities with the remaining limb for meaningful rehabilitation 3 h a day (as required for admission to an IRF), but may be able to do some activity for up to 3 h a week (at a subacute facility). When healing allows for weight-bearing, the patient would then become a better candidate for an IRF.

In conclusion, for the aging patient, discharge often requires information and resources outside those typically encountered by the medical professional. Having a knowledgeable social worker and a working relationship with a physiatrist improves the odds of a successful discharge that anticipates barriers and prevents potential readmissions.

Case Scenarios

1. The patient is a 77-year-old male with a history of hypertension and heart disease on aspirin and Plavix who slipped and fell in the kitchen. Initially, he could move his arms and legs, but after crawling to the sofa, he experienced profound weakness of all limbs and loss of sensation. He was found to have a vertebral body fracture at C5 and a small subdural hematoma. A rigid collar was used to keep his cervical spine stable, which he was to wear for at least 6 weeks. His lower limbs regained some activity, much greater than his upper limbs, which were limited to biceps movement only, although not enough for meaningful mobility. His wife is in reasonably good health and very motivated to assist her husband in any way possible.

What are his coexisting diagnoses? He has a central cord syndrome presentation with better function in his lower limbs than in the upper limbs. This would suggest a diagnosis of C5 ASIA C SCI with associated neurogenic bladder. His past medical history includes hypertension and heart disease.

What changes in his medications may be needed? As indicated, the treating team appropriately held anticoagulation. He may now have a significantly reduced need for antihypertensive medication as most patients sustaining a spinal cord injury become relatively hypotensive. There are arguments to be made for using either heparin for VTE prophylaxis in this patient as it is reversible and/or placing an inferior vena cava filter.

What rehabilitation options may be appropriate and why? This patient would receive the greatest intensity of rehabilitation at a model systems SCI unit. Many general rehabilitation facilities may consider a course for caregiver training, to include transfers, bladder/bowel/skin management, and general SCI care education. Another option would be to initially be admitted to a subacute rehabilitation facility until the cervical collar is no longer needed and there is clearance for general rehabilitation on a more productive basis. Home health does not provide the intensity of training or education, but can assist with home safety evaluations and limited caregiver training due to time constraints. It can focus on the essentials to prevent further complications from bladder infections due to the need for catheterization and decubitus formation and aspiration due to limited neck mobility in the rigid collar, as well as provide ongoing assessment for spasticity and other entities that limit future functional training.

2. An 82-year-old female was a loosely restrained passenger in an older model car that drove off the side of the interstate when her husband fell asleep at the wheel. She sustained a right proximal humeral fracture, multiple fractured ribs, right comminuted tibial plateau fracture, left tib-fib fracture, and a splenic laceration. There were no neurovascular injuries. She was assessed and stabilized by the trauma and orthopedic teams. The lower extremity fractures were surgically stabilized and the proximal humeral fracture will be managed conservatively. Her husband sustained minor injuries and was discharged home after observation. He wants to know when she will be discharged and "look after the home" again.

What are her medical and functional issues? She is likely to be limited weight-bearing, if any, on the bilateral lower limbs for several weeks, depending upon her bone health. The right upper limb will also be limited to progressive range of motion exercises after the fracture is healed. Voiding and evacuating will be performed either on a bedpan or on a commode via assisted (e.g., Hoyer Lift) transfers. She is at risk for VTE formation due to the lower limb injuries and operations. She is also at risk for limb contractures unless non-weight-bearing range of motion exercises are commenced.

What rehabilitation settings might be appropriate for her? Given that she has one unrestricted limb, referral to a skilled nursing facility with subacute rehabilitation services would be appropriate. She will benefit from some active, non-weight-bearing exercises, has need for nursing and assistance, but clearly does not have enough therapy requirements initially to fill up 3 h on a daily basis. Although home health is technically available, several considerations make it impractical. She had been the primary caretaker of her home, and being unable to perform tasks that were part of her domestic culture could add to either frustration or lead to adverse outcomes were she to attempt them before completing her healing process. Some long-term acute care facility may consider her as a candidate, but therapy services may not be offered which may limit her functional recovery after fracture healing.

3. A 69-year-old female slipped in her bathroom and had exquisite pain in the left hip. She was found to have a left femoral neck fracture which was stabilize with pins and allowed to weight-bear as tolerated. She has military medical benefits with limited income and lives with her daughter who is available at all times.

What would be the most cost-effective rehabilitation course? Home health can provide a safety evaluation, education in the home to prevent future injuries, and the skilled therapies this patient needs. She has a caregiver available at all times and will be in an environment that is familiar to her. She may consider transitioning to an outpatient program as her mobility and pain management improves.

References

1. Zuckerman JD. Hip fracture. N Engl J Med. 1996;334(23):1519–25.
2. Sims RV, McGwin G, Pulley L, Roseman JM. Mobility impairments in crash-involved older drivers. J Aging Health. 1999;13(3):430–8.
3. Phillips EM, Bodenheimer CF, Roig RL, Cifu DX. Geriatric rehabilitation. 4. Physical medicine and rehabilitation interventions for common age-related disorders and geriatric syndromes. Arch Phys Med Rehabil. 2004;85 Suppl 3:S18–22.
4. Green VL, Ondrich JI. Risk factors for nursing home admissions and exits. J Gerontol. 1990;45(6):S250–8.
5. Tinetti ME. Performance-oriented assessment of mobility problems in elderly patients. J Am Geriatr Soc. 1986;34(2):119–26.
6. Schwab CW, Kauder DR. Trauma in the geriatric patient. Arch Surg. 1992;127:701–6.
7. Kauder DR, Schwab CW, Shapiro MB. Geriatric trauma: patterns, care, and outcomes. In: Moore EE, Feliciano DV, Mattox KL, editors. Trauma. 5th ed. New York: McGraw-Hill; 2004. p. 1041–58.
8. National Center for Injury Prevention and Control. Centers for Disease Control and Prevention. http://www.cdc.gov. Accessed 3 Mar 2013.
9. Blumenthal J, Plummer E, Gambert SR. Trauma in the elderly: causes and prevention. Clin Geriatr. 2010;19(3):21–4.
10. Barker A, Jones R, Jennison C. A prevalence study of age-associated memory impairment. Br J Psychiatry. 1995;167:642–8.
11. Levy R. Age-related cognitive decline. Int Psychogeriatr. 1994;6(1):63–8.

12. Coria F, de Caso JAG, Minguez L, et al. Prevalence of age-associated memory impairment and dementia in a rural community. J Neurol Neurosurg Psychiatry. 1993;56:973–6.
13. Stevens JA. Fatalities and injuries from falls among older adults – United States, 1993–2003 and 2001–2005. MMWR 2006;55(45):1221–24.
14. Vellas BJ, Wayne SJ, Romero LJ, Baumgartner RN, Garry PJ. Fear of falling and restriction of mobility in elderly fallers. Age Ageing. 1997;26:189–93.
15. Stevens JA. Falls among older adults–risk factors and prevention strategies. NCOA Falls Free: promoting a National Falls Prevention Action Plan. Research Review Papers. The National Council on the Aging. J Safety Res. 2005;36(4):409–11.
16. Sterling DA, O'Connor JA, Bonadies J. Geriatric falls: injury severity is high and disproportionate to mechanism. J Trauma. 2001;50(1):116–9.
17. Kannus P, Sievanen H, Palvanen M, et al. Prevention of falls and consequent injuries in elderly people. Lancet. 2005;366(9500):1885–93.
18. Lord SR, Sherrington C, Menz HB, Close JCT. Falls in older people: risk factors and strategies for prevention. Cambridge: Cambridge University Press; 2007.
19. Griffiths DJ, McCraken PN, Harrison GM, et al. Urge incontinence and impaired detrusor contractility in the elderly. Neurourol Urodyn. 2002;21(2):126–31.
20. Grimby A, Milsom I, Molander U, Wiklund I, Ekelund P. The influence of urinary incontinence on the quality of life of elderly women. Age Ageing. 1993;22(2):82–9.
21. Cervo FA, Cruz AC, Poscillico JA. Pressure ulcers: analysis of guideline for treatment and management. Geriatrics. 2000;55:55–60.
22. http://www.cms.gov/Medicare/Medicare-Fee-for-Service-Payment/InpatientRehabFacPPS/Downloads/IRFPAI-manual-2012.pdf. Accessed Oct 24 2013.
23. Kirshblum S, Gonzalez P, Cuccurullo S, et al. Spinal cord injuries. In: Cuccurullo S, editor. Physical medicine and rehabilitation board review. New York: Demos Medical Publishing; 2004. Chapter 7.

End-of-Life Care

36

Karen J. Brasel and Travis P. Webb

Epidemiology

The intensive care unit (ICU) is a site of significant illness and complex patient problems. Many patients are admitted following acute injury or after unforeseen complications associated with surgical treatments. Given the severity of illness of patients arriving to the ICU, it is not surprising that mortality of patients admitted to the ICU is high. Approximately 20 % of all deaths in the United States occur each year in the ICU or within days after transfer from the ICU [1, 2]. Furthermore, most of these deaths are a result of discussions leading to withdrawal or withholding life-sustaining therapies [3–7].

When considering geriatric trauma patients, trauma is the fifth leading cause of death in patients over the age of 65 [8]. Furthermore, though geriatric patients represent only 12 % of the overall trauma population, they account for 28 % of the deaths due to trauma [9]. The effects of age begin to impact mortality at age 45, but for each year increase over age 65, mortality increases by 6 % [10, 11]. Emergency general surgery is also associated with a high risk of death in geriatric patients, with an increase in mortality of two to three times that of nonemergent surgery [12]. Similarly, when compared to younger cohorts undergoing emergency general surgery, mortality of geriatric patients is two to three times greater [13].

Given the challenges in management of elderly surgical patients, it is clear that during a surgeon's career he/she will encounter many patients with end-of-life needs. However, there is much evidence that quality of care at the end of life as perceived by patients and their families suffers [1, 14–17]. Table 36.1 lists common barriers to institution of palliative care measures. Some of these barriers to satisfaction and high-quality end-of-life care include inflated expectations of outcomes held by clinicians and families, uncertainty regarding prognosis, delay in attention to palliative needs, and the lack of an integrated approach to end-of-life care [19]. When considering end-of-life situations, an understanding of issues involving palliative care and the ethical management of patients and their families is necessary to improve the care of the dying patient.

Surgical Buy-In

Several barriers have been identified that hinder a timely and adequate approach to end-of-life care, and one of the greatest barriers is that of surgical culture. The historical surgical culture and approach has been one of a warrior against disease carrying the absolute responsibility to save the patient's life [20]. This culture can act as a barrier to open discussions and decision making. Admitting defeat by allowing a patient to die by withdrawing or withholding life-sustaining interventions is an emotional difficulty that many surgeons are unwilling to face. As a result, surgeons frequently delay end-of-life discussions and palliative care treatment for their patients despite patient or family member requests for these measures. Moreover, many patients and families find that continuation of therapies often proceed beyond a time when they feel it is wanted or even acceptable [21].

The relationship between the surgeon and patient has been described as both a covenant and an implicit contract made preoperatively between a patient and their physician [20, 22]. In an analysis of physicians' opinions regarding the contract between patient and physician, Schwarze et al. found that several important steps occurred during the preoperative surgical planning and discussion. It is during this

K.J. Brasel, MD, MPH (✉)
Department of Surgery, Medical College of Wisconsin,
9200 West Wisconsin Avenue, Milwaukee,
WI 53226, USA
e-mail: kbrasel@mcw.edu

T.P. Webb, MD, MHPE
Trauma & Critical Care Surgery, Froedtert Memorial Lutheran Hospital, Medical College of Wisconsin,
9200 W. Wisconsin Avenue, Milwaukee,
WI 53226, USA
e-mail: trwebb@mcw.edu

J.A. Yelon, F.A. Luchette (eds.), *Geriatric Trauma and Critical Care*,
DOI 10.1007/978-1-4614-8501-8_36, © Springer Science+Business Media New York 2014

Table 36.1 Surgical ICU culture and barriers to palliative care [18]

Surgical ICU characteristics	Barrier to palliative care
Structure and process	
"Open" ICU	No leadership to drive change
Multiple consultants	No standard processes in place
No interdisciplinary team rounds or processes of care	No one person has responsibility for end-of-life decisions or communication
Surgical hierarchy prevails	Interdisciplinary team undermined or devalued
Surgeon has primary relationship with family, not ICU team	Communication in silos leads to conflict and delays in decision making
	Delay in palliative care consult
Surgical patients and disease	
Different disease trajectories: trauma, transplant, surgical oncology, neurosurgery	One palliative care approach does not fit all ICU patients
Lack of clear prognosis for mortality	Triggers for palliative care evaluation need to be disease specific
Lack of quality of life or functional outcome data	Cannot tell who is dying, then cannot do palliative care until very late in course
	Difficult to predict if patient's quality of life will be acceptable to patient's wishes
Families	
Sudden or catastrophic illness	Lack of readiness for end-of-life decisions
High expectation for lifesaving surgery (transplant, cardiovascular)	Unwillingness to accept poor outcome
No knowledge of patient's wishes	Family burdened by decision making
	Intensive need for family support
Surgeons' attitudes	
Palliative care = end-of-life care, only for dying	Palliative care delayed until death imminent
Death is a failure	Avoidance and delay of family meetings and end -of-life decisions
Fear of abandonment	Refuse palliative care consultation
Fear of destroying hope	Avoidance of discussion of bad prognosis
Lack of skill or expertise in communication, pain management	

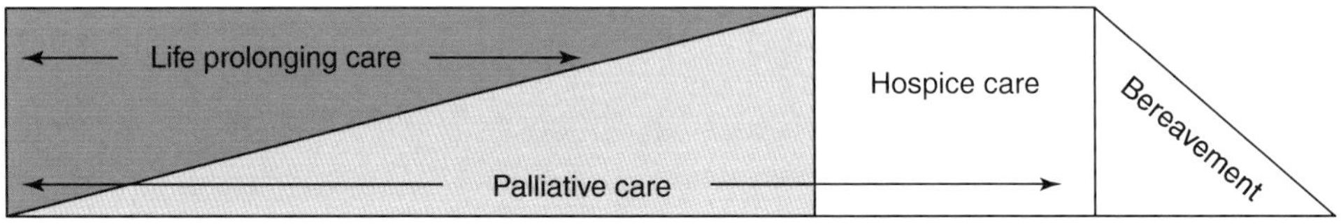

Fig. 36.1 Transition of care from curative to palliative [23]

time when a commitment is made and a contract is created that frequently has important consequences in the postoperative time period [20].

Establishing Goals of Care

The transition of care from curative to palliative does not need to be a dramatic shift in strategy (Fig. 36.1). A patient-centered approach to care should include early discussions with the patient and family regarding goals of care and treatment limitations. These discussions should occur prior to the acute situation when decisions are difficult to make and most frequently the patient is no longer able to voice his or her opinions. In situations where the admission to the hospital or ICU is the initial acute situation, the discussion should occur as soon as possible—ideally, during the initial conversation with the patient and/or family [24]. Communicating clearly and establishing an open dialogue are critical to setting expectations and allowing those with the most at stake to be active participants in healthcare decisions.

One of the first steps is clearly delineating goals of care. Goals of care include the expectations of the patient and surgeon if everything goes as planned as well as if there are significant complications encountered. These goals should include discussions regarding optimal treatment outcomes and what the patient would consider outcomes that they would see as unacceptable. Many patients have opinions regarding quality of life limitations that they have considered privately but never spoken about to family or healthcare providers.

Treatment limitations include setting limits on the aggressiveness with which to sustain life. These limitations may be made considering both the potential for survival and/or the subsequent quality of life. Treatment limitations might include any number of treatment modalities. These limitations are best set while the patient is lucid and able to rationally consider all treatment options.

Do Not Resuscitate

The Do Not Resuscitate (DNR) order is the most commonly recognized treatment limitation. On the surface DNR seems simple to understand and implement; however, there are many nuances to the DNR order that complicate execution of the wishes of the patient. Frequently, DNR orders are not discussed during the preoperative stages of care. Furthermore, most hospitals have rules regarding DNR order holding while the patient is in the operating room. DNR orders may also be complicated to understand as many individuals do not want a portion of resuscitation but would allow other treatment modalities if necessary. For example, a patient may not want chest compressions but would allow intubation or performance of electrical defibrillation. There are stigmata surrounding various resuscitation treatments held by healthcare providers as well as patients. Most patients do not understand the risks and benefits of undergoing CPR in the hospital setting. Similarly, many healthcare providers are uncomfortable "allowing" a patient to die without intervention through heroic measures despite data showing poor outcomes in patients who suffer a cardiorespiratory arrest during hospitalization.

The use of "partial DNR" orders should be discouraged [25]. These orders are intended to provide a tailored approach to an anticipated patient needs and desires; however, because it is impossible to predict all potential patient scenarios, these types of orders frequently lead to nonbeneficial or harmful interventions [25]. For example, a patient may not want chest compressions, but the use of medications without chest compressions during an arrest is extremely unlikely to be of any benefit to that patient. Patient education and physician response to patient emotions and questions are critical [26]. It is up to the physician to provide a recommendation based on medical evidence and patient priorities when establishing code status [26].

Palliative Care Models

Consultative

There are several models of palliative care that have been successful within various institutions and settings. The optimal model depends upon institutional resources and culture. A consultative model describes the use of a consultant palliative care service to provide all or a majority of palliative care needs within an institution [18, 19]. This model works well in settings where few physicians are familiar, adequately trained, or appropriately engaged in palliative management. A consultative service can provide needed resources for patients, families, and their physicians. There are limitations to the ability of a consultative service to provide appropriate coverage for an institution depending upon the size of the organization and the number of healthcare providers on the consultative service.

Triggers

Another model of palliative care similar to and building upon a consultative model is the use of triggers to prompt consultation of a palliative care team. The use of triggers such as number of days spent in the ICU, presence of dementia, and poor prognostic indicators can be used to triage and prompt appropriate resource utilization of the palliative care service [18]. Triggers have, in general, worked better in medical ICUs rather than surgical ICUs [19, 27].

Team Based

Lastly, the most inclusive approach to palliative medicine is to create a culture of team-based palliative management whereby multidisciplinary and interprofessional healthcare teams interact to incorporate palliative care ideals into daily patient care services [18]. Similar to the approach taken by the specialty of geriatrics, palliative care leaders recognize the limitations of a palliative care service and strive to introduce palliative care approaches within all appropriate specialties [18, 19]. Utilizing set orders and care plans or so-called palliative care bundles standing orders aids in the delivery of care without the delay often seen when consulting a new service. Many of these bundles emphasize addressing basic needs important in both palliative care and ICU care on a daily basis—have goals of care been addressed, is pain management optimal, is the patient having respiratory or GI symptoms, and have the patient's and family's spiritual needs been addressed? Incorporating these bundles on a daily basis for all patients in the ICU, regardless of whether they are at the end of life or not, helps establish a culture where optimal palliative care can be delivered [28].

Symptom Management

One of the main concerns of patients and families is that patient treatment ends with palliative care implementation. This misconception must be addressed early and often

Table 36.2 Basic recommendations for pharmacologic treatment based on quality of pain

Pain severity	Drug	Initial dosing (adult, >60 kg)
Mild (VAS 1–3)	Acetaminophen	Maximum = 3,200 mg/24 h
	Aspirin	600–1,500 mg PO qid
	Ibuprofen	Maximum = 3,200 mg/24 h
	Naproxen	250 mg PO bid, Maximum = 1,300 mg/24 h
Moderate (VAS 4–6)	Codeine	30–60 mg PO q 4 h
	Oxycodone	5 mg PO q 4 h
	Tramadol	50–100 mg PO q 4 h
Severe (VAS 7–10)	*Short acting*	
	Morphine	10 mg PO q 2 h, 2–4 mg IV q 2 h
	Hydromorphone	1–3 mg PO, PR q 4 h, 1 mg IV, SC q 4
	Oxycodone	5 mg PO q 4 h
	Oxymorphone	10–20 mg PO q 4 h
	Long acting	
	Morphine SR	15–30 mg PO q 8–12 h
	Oxycodone SR	10 mg PO q 12 h
	Oxymorphone SR	5–10 mg PO q 12 h
	Transdermal fentanyl	12 mcg/h

VAS visual analog scale, *SR* sustained release

during discussions regarding care plans. The hallmark of palliative care is the management of symptoms in order to provide greater patient comfort and quality of life during final days of being. There are a host of options for management of the common symptoms encountered during the stages of death.

The most common symptoms encountered and managed by palliative measures include pain, respiratory distress, gastrointestinal symptoms, and cognitive failure. Pain is a common concern for patients and their families; therefore, assurance that pain will be minimalized is an important step. Basic principles of symptom management include anticipating needs prior to their development, minimizing interventions, and planning alternative routes for administration of medications when oral routes are not feasible.

Pain

Patients and families commonly worry about whether the patient will suffer from pain during the dying process; therefore, allaying fears may be as important as the actual pharmacologic intervention when treating pain. The pharmacologic treatment of pain should follow a "step ladder" approach with escalation of therapies until pain is controlled.

The first step in pain control requires an assessment of the pain and discomfort experienced by the patient. The assessment should include the location, duration, temporal pattern, and modifiers of pain as well as the quality (somatic, visceral, neuropathic), intensity (0–10 scale, 0 = no pain; 10 = worst possible pain), and patient's goal for pain management (0–10 scale, functional, sleep).

Basic recommendations for pharmacologic treatment based on quality of pain are shown in Table 36.2. Non-pharmacologic treatment of pain may include physical modalities, such as massage, heat, cold, stretching and physical therapy, and acupuncture, or behavioral treatments such as relaxation, meditation, music therapy, psychotherapy, reframing, and biofeedback education.

Respiratory Distress

Air hunger or dyspnea in the last stages of dying is common and may be psychologically troubling for family members to witness. The primary treatment of dyspnea in this situation is titration of opioids to increase the patient's comfort of breathing. The opioid dose should be titrated to achieve a respiratory rate between 15 and 20 breaths/min. Supplemental oxygen may provide some relief and should be humidified if used. Oxygen should not be titrated to achieve a pulse oximetry cutoff. Anxiolytics such as diazepam or lorazepam may be of benefit to patients who are also experiencing anxiety or panic as a result of dyspnea. Many dying patients exhibit the "death rattle" due to large amounts of thin, watery respiratory secretions. These secretions should be treated with anticholinergic agents such as centrally acting scopolamine or peripherally acting glycopyrrolate.

Gastrointestinal Symptoms

Nausea and vomiting may occur during the end of life due to a variety of causes. Many surgical patients have bowel obstructions due to functional or anatomic obstructions;

therefore, control of nausea and vomiting becomes a challenge for the treating physician. Intervention may include pharmacologic treatment and non-pharmacologic therapies. Pharmacologic treatment may include a trial and error approach using any number of available antiemetics from various drug classes such as ondansetron, metoclopramide, prochlorperazine, or dronabinol. Nondrug treatment should take into account the acuity and severity of the symptoms. Refractory or severe long-term gastric stasis symptoms may benefit from percutaneous gastrostomy tube placement. Nasogastric tube drainage may suffice for treatment of acute bowel obstruction symptoms but must be weighed against the tube irritation and discomfort.

Cognitive Failure

Cognitive failure during the last stages of dying typically is manifested by worsening delirium or increasing somnolence. Frequently, patients become progressively confused but are typically not mobile or physically active. Therefore, most attention can be directed toward reassurance of both patient and family members. If agitation must be treated, sedatives or anxiolytics may be used to provide sedation and relaxation. Of course, the physician must be aware that escalating doses of opioids or anxiolytics can exacerbate delirium or somnolence.

Withdrawal of Life-Sustaining Treatment

The process of withdrawal of life-sustaining treatment should take into account the above management of symptoms that frequently occur during the final stages of dying. In the ICU, withdrawal of life-sustaining treatment may also include removal of mechanical ventilation as well as withdrawal of artificial hydration and feeding, blood pressure support, antibiotics, blood products, and invasive monitoring and noninvasive monitoring. Often, the decision to withdraw all life-sustaining treatment may be difficult for the family, and an intermediate step of withholding further life-sustaining treatment may be appropriate. Ethically, these two approaches are no different. The goal should be to establish a quiet, peaceful, and supportive environment for both the patient and the family. Once the decision to transition to palliative treatment has been made, the physician should clearly document discussions and plans in the chart.

Removal of mechanical ventilation should be a planned, well-orchestrated event with the presence of physician, respiratory therapist, and nurse in order to assure appropriate symptom control is achieved. Patients should be off of paralytics, but premedication with sedatives and opioids is appropriate to manage dyspnea that may occur upon extubation. In general, family members should also be offered an opportunity to be present during the extubation process.

Communication and Family Meetings

One of the most important aspects of care during the end of life is appropriate communication between caregivers and patients and their families. The emotional toll experienced by all is significant and confusion or unclear messages only worsen this aspect. Families frequently want to know how long the patient has to live, but prognostication is notoriously inaccurate in most patient situations [29]. There are prognostic tools available that will allow for informed discussions with patients, recognizing that no prognostic tool is perfect and that for an individual patient or family the outcome is either 0 or 100 %. Regardless of the prognosis, frequent scheduled meetings with patients and their loved ones has the effect of decreasing the fear of the unknown and the frequently lamented feeling that they are being left in the dark [30]. The transition to end-of-life care is made more easily if frequent meetings have been carried out and a level of familiarity and trust has been developed between the healthcare team and the family. A structured approach to family meetings can ease the delivery of unfavorable news. One approach uses six steps to run a family meeting: (1) select an appropriate setting with introductions and appropriate seating capacity, (2) determine what the family already knows, (3) determine what the family wants to know, (4) deliver information, (5) express empathy, and (6) establish expectations and plan for next steps [31]. A critical aspect of delivery of bad news is for the physician to express and appear empathetic. This requires the healthcare provider to be able to recognize and understand the emotions of the patient and family.

Particularly in the surgical ICU, family meetings directed by intensivists may be perceived as threatening by the primary care team. Although specific diagnoses are often used to determine when family meetings should be held in the medical ICU, a time-based approach works better in the surgical ICU. Patients who remain in the ICU for >72 h are likely to have prolonged ICU stays; often, it is these patients in whom goals of care have not been adequately or appropriately addressed [18]. It is important to emphasize that the reason for family meetings is not to take communication out of the hands of the primary surgeon, but to ensure that all healthcare providers and all family members hear the same thing at the same time. It is also important to ensure that the conversation and outcome of the family meeting is documented in the medical record so it is available to all current and subsequent healthcare providers.

Bereavement and Grief

When death occurs after trauma, emergency general surgery, or an unanticipated ICU stay, it is obviously unexpected. This unexpected nature is a risk factor for complicated grief. Other risk factors include recent loss of another family member, strained relationships or distance between family and the one who died, and separation of the family from their loved one at the time of death [32]. Obviously, much of that is out of the control of the healthcare team.

One factor that is under the control of the healthcare providers is the ability for families to be present at the time of death. This includes facilitating family presence during resuscitative events and ensuring that families have the option to be present throughout the process of withdrawal of life-sustaining therapy if they desire [33].

Another factor that mitigates complicated grief is a formal bereavement program. Services provided through a hospital-based program include physical comforts during the dying process, follow-up from a bereavement coordinator, and cards on major milestones during the first year after death and on the anniversary of the death.

Conclusion

Elderly patients with traumatic injury, emergency general surgery, and unplanned ICU admissions have a much higher mortality than younger patients with the same conditions. Practitioners should have the basic skills to provide optimal end-of-life care to these patients. High-quality care begins with early, open, and honest communication about goals of care and concludes when those goals are met to the best of everyone's ability.

References

1. The SUPPORT Principle Investigators. A controlled trial to improve care for seriously ill hospitalized patients: the Study to Understand Prognoses and Preferences for Outcomes and Risks of Treatments (SUPPORT). JAMA. 1995;274:1591–8.
2. Angus DC, Barnato AE, Linde-Zwirble WT, Weissfeld LA, Watson RS, Rickert T, Rubenfeld GD, Robert Wood Johnson Foundation ICU End-Of-Life Peer Group. Use of intensive care at the end of life in the United States: an epidemiologic study. Crit Care Med. 2004;32:638–43.
3. Cook D, Rocker G, Marshall J, Sjokvist P, Dodek P, Griffith L, Freitag A, Varon J, Bradley C, Levy M, et al. Withdrawal of mechanical ventilation in anticipation of death in the intensive care unit. N Engl J Med. 2003;349:1123–32.
4. Faber-Langendoen K. A multi-institutional study of care given to patients dying in hospitals: ethical practices and implications. Arch Intern Med. 1996;156:2130–6.
5. Keenan SP, Busche KD, Chen LM, McCarthy L, Inman KJ, Sibbald WJ. A retrospective review of a large cohort of patients undergoing the process of withholding or withdrawal of life support. Crit Care Med. 1997;22:1020–5.
6. Sprung CL, Cohen SL, Sjokvist P, Baras M, Bulow HH, Hovilehto S, Ledoux D, Lippert A, Maia P, Phelan D, et al. End-of-life practices in European intensive care units: the Ethicus Study. JAMA. 2003;290:790–7.
7. Prendergast TJ, Claessens MT, Luce JM. A national survey of end-of-life care for critically ill patients. Am J Respir Crit Care Med. 1998;158:1163–7.
8. McMahon DJ, Schwab CW, Kauder D. Comorbidity and the elderly trauma patient. World J Surg. 1996;20:1113–20.
9. Koval KJ, Meek R, Schemitsch E, et al. An AOA critical issue. Geriatric trauma: young ideas. J Bone Joint Surg Am. 2003;85-A:1380–8.
10. Morris Jr JA, MacKenzie EJ, Damiano AM, et al. Mortality in trauma patients: the inter-action between host factors and severity. J Trauma. 1990;30:1476–82.
11. Grossman MD, Miller D, Scaff DW, et al. When is an elder old? Effect of preexisting conditions on mortality in geriatric trauma. J Trauma. 2002;52:242–6.
12. Ansaloni L, Catena F, Chattat R, et al. Risk factors and incidence of postoperative delirium in elderly patients after elective and emergency surgery. Br J Surg. 2010;97(2):273–80.
13. Ingraham AM, Cohen ME, Bilimoria KY, et al. Comparison of 30-day outcomes after emergency general surgery procedures: potential for targeted improvement. Surgery. 2010;148:217–38.
14. Nelson JE, Meier D, Oei EJ, Nierman DM, Senzel RS, Manfredi PL, Davis SM, Morrison RS. Self-reported symptom experience of critically ill cancer patients receiving intensive care. Crit Care Med. 2001;29:277–82.
15. Tilden VP, Tolle SW, Garland MJ, Nelson CA. Decisions about life-sustaining treatment: impact of physicians' behaviors on the family. Arch Intern Med. 1995;155:633–8.
16. Cook DJ, Guyatt GH, Jaeschke R, Reeve J, Spanier A, King D, Molloy DW, Willan A, Streiner DL. Determinants in Canadian health care workers of the decision to withdraw life support from the critically ill. JAMA. 1995;273:703–8.
17. Curtis JR, Treece PD, Nielsen EL, Downey L, Shannon SE, Braungardt T, Owens D, Steinberg KP, Engelberg RA. Integrating palliative and critical care-evaluation of a quality-improvement intervention. Am J Respir Crit Care Med. 2008; 178:269–75.
18. Mosenthal AC, Weissman DE, Curtis JR, et al. Integrating palliative care in the surgical and trauma intensive care unit: a report from the Improving Palliative Care in the Intensive Care Unit (IPAL-ICU) Project Advisory Board and the Center to Advance Palliative Care. Crit Care Med. 2012;40(4):1199–206.
19. Nelson JE. Identifying and overcoming the barriers to high-quality palliative care in the intensive care unit. Crit Care Med. 2006;34(11):S324–31.
20. Schwarze ML, Bradley CT, Brasel KJ. Surgical "buy-in": the contractual relationship between surgeons and patients that influences decisions regarding life-supporting therapy. Crit Care Med. 2010; 38(3):1–6.
21. Katz P. The surgeon as hero: the Scalpel's edge. Boston: Allyn and Bacon; 1999. p. 19–35.
22. Cassell J, Buchman TG, Streat S, et al. Surgeons, intensivists, and the covenant of care: administrative models and values affecting care at the end of life—updated. Crit Care Med. 2003;31:1551–7; discussion 1557–9.
23. Adler EA, Goldfinger JZ, Kalman J, Park ME, Meier DE. Palliative care in the treatment of advanced heart failure. Circulation. 2009;120:2597–606.
24. Mosenthal AC, Murphy PA, Barker LK, Lavery R, Retano A, Livingston DH. Changing the culture around end-of-life care in the trauma intensive care unit. J Trauma. 2008;64:1587–93.

25. Sanders A, Schepp M, Baird M. Partial do-not-resuscitate orders: a hazard to patient safety and clinical outcomes? Crit Care Med. 2011;39:14–8.
26. Loertsher L, Reed DA, Bannonn MP, Mueller PS. Cardiopulmonary resuscitation and do-not-resuscitate orders: a guide for clinicians. Am J Med. 2010;123:4–9.
27. Bradley CT, Brasel KJ. Developing guidelines that identify patients who would benefit from palliative care services in the surgical intensive care unit. Crit Care Med. 2009;37:946–50.
28. Nelson JE, Mulkerin CM, Adams LL, Pronovost PJ. Improving comfort and communication in the ICU: a practical new tool for palliative care performance measurement and feedback. Qual Saf Health Care. 2006;15:264–71.
29. Teno JM, Fisher E, Hamel MB, Wu AW, Murphy DJ, Wenger NS, Lynn J, Harrell Jr FE. Decision-making and outcomes of prolonged ICU stays in seriously ill patients. J Am Geriatr Soc. 2000;48(5): S70–4.
30. Lautrette A, Ciroldi M, Ksibi H, Azoulay E. End-of-life family conferences: rooted in the evidence. Crit Care Med. 2006;34(11):S364–72.
31. Buckman R. How to break bad news. A guide for health care professionals. Baltimore: Johns Hopkins University Press; 1992.
32. Kristensen P, Weisaeth L, Heir T. Bereavement and mental health after sudden and violent losses – a review. Psychiatry. 2012;75(1): 76–97.
33. Tucker TL. Family presence during resuscitation. Crit Care Nurs Clin North Am. 2002;14(2):177–85.

37 Ethics in Geriatric Trauma

Anastasia Kunac and Anne C. Mosenthal

Introduction

Surgical ethics in Western medicine are classically governed by four basic principles: *non-maleficence*, *beneficence*, *autonomy*, *and justice*. As we consider management of the injured geriatric patient, the principle of *double effect* is also of utmost importance. The ethics that underlie contemporary surgical care of the elderly are founded on principles of medicine originating with the Hippocratic Oath. *Beneficence*, *non-maleficence*, and confidentiality, originally described by the earliest records of the oath, continue to be the guiding principles for surgical care into the twenty-first century. These were modified and expanded in 1803 when Thomas Percival created guidelines for physician behavior toward the patient in his treatise, *Medical Ethics*; *or A Code of Institutes and Precepts Adapted to the Professional Conduct of Physicians and Surgeons* [1]. Later in the nineteenth century, the American Medical Association produced its Code of Medical Ethics as a contract that defined the relationship between the physician, the patient, and the public trust, adding the principle of *justice* to beneficence and maleficence [2]. By the mid-twentieth century, the recognition that unprecedented medical advances and research, while potentially beneficial to humanity in general, was not always to the benefit of the individual patient and could be misused or abused. The concept of informed consent became a widespread expectation with the 1972 Patient's Bill of Rights. This heralded a change in medical ethics, as it evolved away from paternalism to embrace *autonomy* as the main guiding principle and value, at least in American health care [3]. Now in the new millennium, as more attention is paid to health-care resource allocation, access, and disparity, the ethical principle of *justice*, or equal distribution of care, is becoming increasingly important to surgical practice as we consider the effects of surgical decision making not just on the individual patient but on the health of the population at large. This is particularly relevant for elderly trauma patients and the surgeons who care for them, as we balance multiple and conflicting ethical priorities in the face of advances in surgery that may not translate into better outcomes for this often frail and compromised group of patients. How this affects surgical decision making for the geriatric trauma patient, and the ethical principles that guide it, is the subject of the ensuing chapter.

Basic Principles of Medical Ethics

Non-maleficence

Primum non nocere; *first, do no harm*. This principle heralds with the Hippocratic Oath in which the physician commits to abstain from doing harm. It gives the physician pause to consider that in some situations, an intervention may cause the patient harm without a net benefit. It is thus important to understand the potential risk of harm of any treatment offered to a patient. In considering the geriatric trauma population, overall mortality is 8 % [4]. For each 1-year increase in age beyond 65, the odds of dying after geriatric trauma increase by 7 % per year [4]. Further, the mortality associated with urgent or emergent operative intervention is two to three times greater in those over age 65 compared to younger patients [5]. This is further increased for the frail elderly; with the availability of frailty scoring systems [6], the surgeon can prognosticate with more accuracy the benefit or harm of emergency surgery in the geriatric trauma patient with significant comorbid conditions. There is most certainly

A. Kunac, MD, FACS
Division of Trauma, Department of Surgery,
Rutgers – New Jersey Medical School,
150 Bergen Street Room M-229,
Newark, NJ 07101, USA
e-mail: anastasia.kunac@rutgers.edu

A.C. Mosenthal, MD, FACS (✉)
Department of Surgery, Rutgers – New Jersey Medical School
185 South Orange Ave, Newark,
NJ 07103, USA
e-mail: mosentac@rutgers.edu

J.A. Yelon, F.A. Luchette (eds.), *Geriatric Trauma and Critical Care*,
DOI 10.1007/978-1-4614-8501-8_37, © Springer Science+Business Media New York 2014

an age-dependent survival decrement [7], and the patients overall outcome should be considered when seeking invasive interventions.

Beneficence

The second ethical principle of *beneficence* goes hand in hand with non-maleficence and also is rooted within the Hippocratic Oath. Beneficence requires that the procedure provided is with the intent of doing good for the patient involved and promotes their overall well-being. One could argue that in the setting of traumatic injury, the intent of the team is always focused toward the good of the patient. In practice, virtually all treatments have some risk of harm, and the practitioner must weigh the potential risks against the intended benefit before proceeding. Frequently, there is conflict between beneficence and non-maleficence, with surgical treatment constituting both, in the same patient. Since beneficence must be weighed against non-maleficence, the effects of the two principles together give rise to the concept of "double effect" which is described in detail later.

Beyond the *intent* to help the patient, beneficence further demands that health-care providers develop and maintain skills and knowledge specific to the patient population that they care for such that they may provide the *best possible care*. One is ethically required to continually update training, maintain appropriate knowledge and skill, consider individual circumstances of all patients, evidence based medicine as it applies to the individual patient, and strive for net benefit. Thus, it is important to understand the challenges specific to the care of the geriatric patient that are discussed elsewhere in this text.

Autonomy

The concept of autonomy is rooted in the right of the individual to make decisions regarding personal matters. It is supported by legal and ethical precedent in the United States, including The Patient's Bill of Rights (American Hospital Association 1972) [8], and The Patient Self-Determination Act of 1990 [9]. Autonomy requires that the patient have autonomy of thought, intention, and action when making decisions regarding health-care procedures. It also justifies the patient's right to refuse any treatment and to be informed of the consequences of the treatment. In order for a patient to make a fully informed decision, he must understand all risks and benefits of the procedure and the likelihood of success. This requires that the patient be well informed during the consent process. Patients may choose among treatment options or refuse care, even if the recommended treatment is lifesaving.

Self-determination in the elderly population may be challenging. Often with advanced age, patients may have diminished decision-making capacity. Patients are however permitted to determine their future health-care decisions by completing a living will or advance directive and identifying a health-care proxy or surrogate. Physicians are legally bound to observe the wishes set forth in a living will in the event that a patient is incapable of making such decisions. Unfortunately, these documents generally do not lay out stipulations for specific clinical scenarios, nor is it easy or straightforward to determine if the actual clinical reality meets the criteria or circumstance intended by the patient in their advance directive. We thus often rely on surrogate decision makers to assist in determining what the wishes of a patient who lacks decision-making capacity might be.

Justice

The fourth ethical principle, *justice*, concerns the distribution of resources that may be scarce and also seeks to protect vulnerable populations. Elderly patients are most certainly a vulnerable population. By virtue of the pathophysiology of aging, geriatric patients have decreased vision and hearing, decreased muscle mass, and decreased balance and proprioception and often have osteoporosis—all of these contribute to an increased risk of traumatic injury and a potentially increased severity of injury. Preexisting medical conditions may contribute to increased morbidity and mortality. Further, cognitive impairment may make it difficult for elderly patients to voice their interests. The ethical principle of justice would mandate that we protect this population as a vulnerable population.

Justice mandates that the burdens and benefits of treatment, even new or experimental treatments must be distributed equally among all groups in society including the aged. Numerous articles suggest a degree of ageism in the treatment of ischemic heart disease and breast cancer [10–12]. We must be careful that treatment decisions are not made in a discriminatory fashion in elderly trauma patients.

Instead of considering age alone when making treatment decisions, the physician may instead utilize measurements of functional status and/or frailty as objective indices of a patient's pre-injury quality of life and potential outcome after injury or surgery [6]. The health-care provider must consider four main areas when evaluating justice: fair distribution of scarce resources, competing needs, rights and obligations, and potential conflicts with established legislation.

Principle of Double Effect

Each clinical situation requires consideration of all four of the above ethical principles (summarized in Table 37.1). Frequently, fulfillment of one principle conflicts with

Table 37.1 Basic principles in medical ethics

Principle	Ethical imperative
Autonomy	Respect the capacity of individuals to make their own choices and act accordingly
Beneficence	Relieve pain and suffering; foster the interests and well-being of other persons and society
Non-maleficence	Do no harm; do not inflict pain or suffering
Justice	Act fairly; distribute benefits and harms equitably

Adapted from Beuchamp and Childress [13]

fulfillment of others. For example, a surgeon may perform an orthopedic procedure with the intent to restore a patient to their previous functional status (beneficence), but may cause further disability or even death from complications related to the procedure (maleficence). Withdrawal of life-sustaining treatment, such as a ventilator, is ethically acceptable if the patient's wishes are to be liberated from burdensome medical treatments. Treatment of pain at the end of life may be beneficial, but is thought to hasten death in some situations. If the *intent* of therapy constitutes beneficence, even if it results in harm, it is ethically justified based on double effect. The principle of double effect allows the surgeon to perform surgery and aggressively treat pain and suffering if the intent is to do good with the understanding that the side effect of the treatment may harm the patient.

Informed Consent

The concept of patient consent for medical procedures evolved over the twentieth century as a reaction to the cruelties committed by Nazi concentration camp "doctors" [14]. Up until the mid-twentieth century, paternalism prevailed, with the physician determining what was best for the patient in most circumstances. The Nuremburg code established the concept of informed consent for research participants to include a requirement that research benefit societal good, patients be informed and volunteer to participate of their own free will without coercion. The consent process as practiced in the developed world is not just a signature on a piece of paper; the process requires a competent doctor, adequate transfer of information, and consent of the patient. In the event that a patient is unable to give consent, a surrogate may consent on the patient's behalf.

The only circumstance under which consent is not required is in the emergent care of a patient who is unable to give consent. While this is perhaps common in the setting of acute traumatic injury, the entitlement to carry out emergency treatment prevails only so long as the treatment is directed toward a life-threatening condition and the patient is unable to participate meaningfully in decision making about his or her condition. Once the immediate threat is addressed, consent for further intervention should be sought. If an individual does not recover consciousness or is cognitively impaired by injury or illness, then physicians may turn to surrogates as with any other impaired patient.

Informed consent is a legal term introduced and defined within FDA regulations in the early 1970s and outlined within the National Research Act in 1974. The basic elements of informed consent include preconditions, information, and consent [14]. Preconditions for informed consent include patient competence to make decisions and the patient's willingness to participate in the consent process. Determination of decision-making capacity is discussed in detail in the next section.

Information is the body of facts provided by the physician or health-care provider to the patient such that the patient has sufficient knowledge to make a decision. The physician is obligated to describe not only the intended treatment or procedure and its benefits, but the associated risks must also be described. In addition, available alternatives to the recommended treatment should be offered, and the patient should be counseled as to the likely course if no treatment or procedure is undertaken at all. The information provided must not only be comprehensive, but must be comprehensible—provided in terms that the patient or their surrogate can easily understand.

The final element of informed consent is the "consent" itself. The patient acknowledges that they understand the procedure or treatment offered and authorizes proceeding with the intended treatment. Consent is usually written but may be given verbally with appropriate documentation of the consent process.

Decision-Making Capacity

A particular challenge with the geriatric population is determining whether the patient has decision-making capacity. While autonomy is valued, and it is certainly preferable to obtain consent from an informed patient directly, the patient must have appropriate insight to make an informed decision. Clinical judgments about decision-making capacity are part of everyday medical practice. A patient who is unconscious is certainly not able to give informed consent, nor is a patient who is delirious or suffers from significant dementia. Other subtle alterations in mental status may lead a clinician to question a patient's decision-making ability. Furthermore, decision-making capacity may fluctuate with a variety of medical conditions or social circumstances.

Formal declarations regarding competence are made by the courts. The following criteria, however, may be useful as a guide to ascertain whether or not an elderly patient has decision-making capacity [16]:

1. *Acknowledgment of Relevant Information*: The patient should understand their diagnosis and the proposed treatment.
2. *Appreciating One's Circumstances*: Patients must be able to acknowledge what disorder or disease process they have and understand how it will impact their life. The patient should be able to answer questions about their illness, the need for treatment, and what the outcome might be with and without treatment. If the patient does not have such insight, they may not be competent to give consent.
3. *Logical Use of Information*: The patient should be able to give evidence that they have recognizable reasons for their views or conclusions. Some views may be the consequence of delirium, dementia, or other disorder. It is not the specific view or belief that is at issue in this determination but the process by which a person has the belief that is important; if the patient came to a decision that is at odds with a physician's recommendation, this is acceptable if the decision was made in a logical fashion. If the decision is based in delusion, one may be concerned about the patient's decision-making ability.
4. *Communication of Choices*: This is a paramount condition of judging competence. The patient must be able to communicate the preference of one choice over another. A patient who says "yes" to every treatment option offered may not be appropriately integrating the information given. The identification of a choice is strengthened by evidence that the choice remains stable over time. That said, a patient may certainly change their mind but should be able to provide a meaningful reason for change.

If the above criteria are not met or if the patient has already been declared incompetent to make decisions by the courts, a surrogate decision maker should become involved in the consent process.

Advance Directives

The Patient Self-Determination Act of 1990 facilitates the right of the patient to make health-care decisions, refuse treatment, and make decisions about their future care by way of an advance directive and/or appointment of a surrogate decision maker. An advance directive is a document, often referred to as a living will, in which a person states his or her wishes regarding medical treatment in the event that they become mentally incompetent or are unable to communicate. Elements of the document frequently include wishes regarding resuscitation, mechanical ventilation, nutrition and hydration assistance, and dialysis and may also include wishes regarding organ or tissue donation. Physicians are obligated to honor the wishes expressed in these written documents so as to honor the patient's autonomy even in a state of diminished capacity.

Surrogate Decision Making

Surgeons are ethically and legally bound to observe the wishes set forth in a living will in the event that a patient becomes incapable of making such decisions. Unfortunately, in practice, specific clinical scenarios are rarely laid out, and paper is a poor substitute for an informed discussion between patient and physician. This has led to a reliance on surrogate decision makers to interpret a patient's living will or advance directive and ensure the patient's wishes are carried out. In the absence of an advance directive, a surrogate may be asked to make a medical decision on behalf of the patient, in consultation with the physician.

Supreme Court decisions in the Karen Anne Quinlan and Nancy Cruzan cases have established that it is consistent with autonomy, beneficence, non-maleficence, and justice if a surrogate decision maker acts based on the patient's best interest or in accordance with the patient's previously expressed wishes [17, 18]. This provides the legal basis not only for treatment decisions, but for decisions to withhold or withdraw life support in patients who are incapacitated.

Do Not Resuscitate

Patients or surrogate decision makers have the right to refuse life-sustaining therapies based on the principle of autonomy. This can include cardiopulmonary resuscitation (CPR). A "DNR" order, or do not resuscitate, is withholding of CPR—this includes management of airway, intubation, and pharmacologic interventions to stimulate the heart, chest compressions, and defibrillation. Based on televised depictions of CPR, the general public, including the elderly, believe that three-quarters of patients survive CPR [19]. The unfortunate reality is that less than 20 % of patients survive CPR and that 10–44 % of those patients that do survive have permanent neurologic impairment.

The Patient Self-Determination Act of 1990 allows patients to refuse medical treatment even if it results in death, and "DNR" may be part of their advance directive. If a patient is unable to direct their own health care, a surrogate may enact a DNR order based on a patient's previously stated wishes. Alternatively, a physician may recommend DNR. The procedure of CPR was never intended for use in patients dying an expected death from a chronic, fatal, medical illness. Physicians are under no obligation to perform the medical procedure of CPR when the procedure is contraindicated.

Futility

Much like the concepts of beneficence and non-maleficence, the concept of futility in medicine also dates back to the time of Hippocrates whereby physicians were advised to "refuse to treat those who are overmastered by their disease, realizing that in such cases medicine is powerless." *Medical futility* has been defined as "a clinical action serving no useful purpose in attaining a specified goal for a given patient" [20]. We can further clarify that medical futility occurs when (1) there is a defined goal, (2) an action is directed at achieving this goal, and (3) there is virtual certainty that the action will fail in achieving this goal [21]. Unfortunately, with modern medical advances physicians in the twenty-first century may be reluctant to claim "certainty" that an action will fail in achieving its goal.

While unlikely, a 70-year-old with a severe traumatic brain injury who underwent craniotomy *might* be restored to an acceptable functional status and an 88-year-old *might* survive postoperative septicemia with multiorgan failure. Modern technologies and advances in medical knowledge have altered our abilities to sustain life. The counter-side is that we also have the ability to prolong death. Thus, in our endeavors where the goals of advanced life support are to prevent premature death by treating reversible illnesses, physicians and families are sometimes caught in a position where the dying process of a patient or loved one is extended and suffering is prolonged.

The American Medical Association states that physicians are not ethically obligated to deliver care that, in their best professional judgment, will not have a reasonable chance of benefiting their patients. These treatments, however, should be discussed with the patient or their surrogate decision maker along with a frank explanation of why the specific treatment is not beneficial. These discussions help to clarify goals of treatment and goals of care. Also, physicians should convey that medical care is NEVER futile, but rather specific therapies may be futile, in that they may not advance the goal or goals of care. In communicating with families, physicians must distinguish between aggressive treatments that may be futile to prolong life and those which are beneficial as they provide comfort. Pain control, respect for patient dignity, and reassurance of the patient and/or surrogate that the medical team will not abandon care even when specific treatments are deemed futile are of utmost importance.

Conclusion

Caring for the geriatric trauma patient is challenging. The elderly are a vulnerable and sometimes frail patient population. While considering treatment plans and seeking procedural consents for these patients, one must adhere to the basic ethical principles of non-maleficence, beneficence, autonomy, and justice. Further, the principle of double effect dictates that if the intent of a planned treatment or procedure is in alignment with basic ethical principles, it may be appropriate to accept that there may be associated secondary effects that are undesirable.

While honoring patient autonomy in the face of severe injury, we must recognize when a geriatric patient is unable to speak for him or herself. The trauma surgeon can navigate difficult medical decisions through shared decision making. This can be accomplished by understanding the patient's wishes via an advance directive or consultation with a surrogate decision maker. While American health care has embraced autonomy, it is incumbent upon health-care practitioners not only to discuss the risks and benefits of specific treatment and procedures with patients and their families but to share with them likely outcomes of disease processes in the injured patient. This may include communication regarding cardiopulmonary resuscitation, DNR orders, or treatments considered futile. As practitioners, we must understand that while a particular procedure might be futile, care of the patient, symptom management, and compassionate communication with surrogate decision makers are never futile.

References

1. Percival T. Medical ethics; or a code of institutes and precepts adapted to the professional conduct of physicians and surgeons. 3rd ed. London: John Churchill 1849. p. 27–66.
2. American Medical Association. Code of medical ethics of the American Medical Association council on ethical and judicial affairs. American Medical Association; Chicago 2006.
3. Doyal L. Surgical ethics. In: Williams NS, Bullstrode CJK, O'Connell PR, editors. Bailey and love's short practice of surgery. London: Hodder Arnold. 2008. p. 119–125.
4. Grossman MD, Miller D, Scaff DW, Arcona S. When is an elder old? Effect of preexisting conditions on mortality in geriatric trauma. J Trauma. 2002;52(2):242–6.
5. Ingraham AM, Cohen ME, Bilmoria KY, Raval MV, Clifford YK, Nathens AB, et al. Comparison of 30-day outcomes after emergency general surgery procedures: potential for targeted improvement. Surgery. 2010;148(2):217–38.
6. Makary MA, Segev DL, Pronovost PJ, Syin D, Bandeen-Roche K, Patel P, et al. Frailty as a predictor of surgical outcomes in older patients. J Am Coll Surg. 2010;210(6):901–8.
7. Jacobs DG, Plaisier BR, Barie PS, Hammond JS, Holevar MR, Sinclair KE, et al. Triage of geriatric trauma. J Trauma. 2003;54(2): 391–416.
8. American Hospital Association. A patient's bill of rights. Chicago: American Hospital Association; 1992.
9. Patient Self-Determination Act of 1990, sections 4206 and 4751 of Omnibus Reconciliation Act of 1990. Public Law 101–508. 5 Nov 1990.
10. Holmes HM. Quality of life and ethical concerns in the elderly thoracic surgery patient. Thorac Surg Clin. 2009;19(3):401–7.
11. Madan AK, Cooper L, Gratzer A, Beech DJ. Ageism in breast cancer surgical options by medical students. Tenn Med. 2006;99(5): 37–8, 41.

12. Madan AK, Aliabadi-Wahale S, Beech DJ. Ageism in medical students' treatment recommendations: the example of breast-conserving procedures. Acad Med. 2001;76(3):282–4.
13. Beuchamp TL, Childress JF. Principles of biomedical ethics. New York: Oxford University Press; 1989.
14. Leclerq WKG, Keulers BJ, Scheltinga MRM, Spauwen PHM, van der Wilt G. A review of surgical informed consent: past, present, and future. A quest to help patients make better decisions. World J Surg. 2010;34:1406–15.
15. National Research Act. Public Law 93–348. 12 July 1974.
16. Murphy T. Ethics in Clerkships; Surrogate Decision Making. University of Illinois at Chicago College of Medicine. [cited 27 Dec 2012]. Available from: http://www.uic.edu/depts/mcam/ethics/surrogate.htm.
17. In re Quinlan, 355 A2d 647 (JN), 429 US 922. 1976.
18. Cruzan v Director, Missouri Department of Health 497 US 261. 1990.
19. Diem SJ, Lantos JD, Tulsky JA. Cardiopulmonary resuscitation on television; miracles and misinformation. N Engl J Med. 1996;334: 1578–82.
20. Kasman DL. When is medical treatment futile? J Gen Intern Med. 2004;19:1053–6.
21. Trotter G. Mediating disputes about medical futility. Camb Q Healthc Ethics. 1999;8:527–37.

Index

J.A. Yelon, F.A. Luchette (eds.), *Geriatric Trauma and Critical Care*,
DOI 10.1007/978-1-4614-8501-8, © Springer Science+Business Media New York 2014

Q

R

Printed by Printforce, the Netherlands